Polysaccharides

Natural Fibers in Food and Nutrition

Edited by
Noureddine Benkeblia

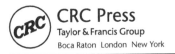
CRC Press
Taylor & Francis Group
Boca Raton London New York

CRC Press is an imprint of the
Taylor & Francis Group, an **informa** business

CRC Press
Taylor & Francis Group
6000 Broken Sound Parkway NW, Suite 300
Boca Raton, FL 33487-2742

First issued in paperback 2017

ISBN-13: 978-1-4665-7181-5 (hbk)
ISBN-13: 978-1-138-03390-0 (pbk)

Library of Congress Cataloging-in-Publication Data

Polysaccharides (CRC Press)
  Polysaccharides : natural fibers in food and nutrition / [edited by] Noureddine Benkeblia.
    pages cm
  Summary: "This book reviews the evidence supporting the influence of plant fibers on our daily life by either having impacts on our nutrition or improving processed foods for human and animal feeding. By bringing new information and updating existing scientific data, this book will also be a consistent source of information for both professional and non-professionals that are involved in food science and technology, nutrition, and even medical sciences related to human health and well-being"-- Provided by publisher.
  Includes bibliographical references and index.
  ISBN 978-1-4665-7181-5 (hardback)
  1. Fiber in human nutrition. 2. Polysaccharides. 3. Plant fibers. I. Benkeblia, Noureddine. II. Title.

QP144.F52P65 2014
572'.566--dc23

2014007203

Visit the Taylor & Francis Web site at
http://www.taylorandfrancis.com

and the CRC Press Web site at
http://www.crcpress.com

A special dedication to my son, Mohamed:
Get well soon and enjoy life with us.

To Zahroucha for your achievements.

Contents

Foreword ix
Preface xi
Editor xiii
Contributors xv

1 Fructan Biosynthesis Regulation and the Production of
Tailor-Made Fructan in Plants 1
JEROEN VAN ARKEL, ROBERT SÉVENIER, JOHANNA C.
HAKKERT, HARRO J. BOUWMEESTER, ANDRIES J. KOOPS,
and INGRID M. VAN DER MEER

2 Dietary Fiber and Its Polyphenol Cotravelers in Healthy Eating:
Seeking the Key Component in Apple Fruit 31
ANTONIO JIMÉNEZ-ESCRIG

3 Agave Fiber Structure Complexity and Its Impact on Health 45
MERCEDES G. LÓPEZ, ALICIA HUAZANO-GARCÍA,
MARÍA CONCEPCIÓN GARCÍA-PÉREZ, and
MARÍA ISABEL GARCÍA-VIEYRA

4 Fructooligosaccharides in *Allium* Species:
Chemistry and Nutrition 75
NOUREDDINE BENKEBLIA

5 Potato Starches: Properties, Modifications, and Nutrition 105
NOUREDDINE BENKEBLIA

6 Potential of the Filamentous Fungi from the Brazilian
 Cerrado as Producers of Soluble Fibers 131
 RITA DE CÁSSIA L. FIGUEIREDO-RIBEIRO, KELLY SIMÕES,
 MAURÍCIO B. FIALHO, ROSEMEIRE A. B. PESSONI,
 MARCIA R. BRAGA, and MARÍLIA GASPAR

7 Polysaccharides from Mushrooms: A Natural Source of
 Bioactive Carbohydrates 149
 ANA VILLARES

8 Polysaccharides from Medicinal Mushrooms for
 Potential Use as Nutraceuticals 171
 IOANNIS GIAVASIS

9 Nonstarch Polysaccharides from Food Grains: Their Structure
 and Health Implications 207
 MURALIKRISHNA GUDIPATI and LYNED D. LASRADO

10 Barley β-Glucan: Natural Polysaccharide for Managing
 Diabetes and Cardiovascular Diseases 233
 PARIYARATH SANGEETHA THONDRE

11 Chicory Fructans in Nutrition and the Formulation of Foods
 Dedicated to Blood Glucose Disorder Management 259
 CATHY SIGNORET and HEIDI JACOBS

12 Dietary Fibers in Gastroenterology: From Prevention to
 Recommendations to Patients 301
 MARTINE CHAMP

13 Soluble Dietary Plant Nonstarch Polysaccharides May Improve
 Health by Inhibiting Adhesion, Invasion, and Translocation
 of Enteric Gut Pathogens 327
 HANNAH L. SIMPSON and BARRY J. CAMPBELL

14 Polysaccharide-Based Structures in Food Plants: Gut and
 Health Effects 347
 JOHN A. MONRO

15 Dietary Polysaccharides for the Modulation of Obesity
 via Beneficial Gut Microbial Manipulation 367
 KANTHI KIRAN KONDEPUDI, MAHENDRA BISHNOI,
 KOTESWARAIAH PODILI, PADMA AMBALAM,
 KOUSHIK MAZUMDER, NIDA MURTAZA, RITESH K. BABOOTA,
 and RAVNEET K. BOPARAI

16 Fructooligosaccharides, Diet, and Cancer Prevention: Myths
 or Realities? 385
 NOUREDDINE BENKEBLIA

17 Polymers of the Plant Cell Wall or "Fiber": Their Analysis in
Animal Feeding and Their Role in Rabbit
Nutrition and Health   399
THIERRY GIDENNE

18 Role of Dietary Polysaccharides in Monogastric Farm
Animal Nutrition   429
VERONIKA HALAS and LÁSZLÓ BABINSZKY

Index   477

Foreword

In a web search for "sugar factory," the site that most closely resembled a factory that makes sugar was a large sugar refinery and its expansion plans in New York City. It is noteworthy that despite our remarkable technological advances, we still cannot duplicate one of the most common activities of the plant kingdom—manufacturing sugar. I do not mean extracting it from plants and purifying it (making it white); that's easy. I mean building sugar molecules with carbon atoms like plants do in photosynthesis. One could argue that there are no man-made sugar factories because it is simply not cost-effective; it would be a losing proposition to compete with plants at this business.

The first time I read about photosynthesis, I thought it seemed impossible that plants could take carbon dioxide and water and, using energy from the sun, produce sugar. These little sugar factories absorb carbon dioxide from the air at a concentration of about 0.04%, amid overwhelming concentrations of nitrogen and oxygen. And, when they are finished, they "discard" oxygen as a waste product!

But they don't stop there, which is what this book is all about. If they don't use the monosaccharide products of photosynthesis directly, they hook them together to form disaccharides, oligosaccharides, and polysaccharides. The types of linkages between monosaccharides make for an incredible diversity of structure and function. Cellulose, starch, fructan, and B-glucan are some of the products of the plant and fungal species described in this book.

This is a unique collection of chapters in that polysaccharides are discussed in the context of potential uses in food and nutrition rather than from a physiological perspective of how they are used by plants. From manipulating plants that produce fructans, to modify the activity of intestinal microbes using nonstarch polysaccharides; a wide array of topics are covered in detail by a number of creative laboratories. As you read about these and other ways to use polysaccharides, I hope you will remember that it is in fact an immeasurable assemblage of small, green, sugar factories all around us that are silently supplying us with these useful molecules.

Professor David Livingston
USDA-ARS – North Carolina State University

Preface

In the plant kingdom, polysaccharides are a complex mixture of materials with very different characteristics, and the mixture varies with plant species. From the simplest sugar or sucrose, which is taken daily and often considered to some extent the first enemy of our health problems despite its crucial role in energy providing, to the most complex polysaccharides, such as fructans, and other oligosugars for which benefits are continuously reported, it is presently admitted that polysaccharides fit well within the current concept of the class of dietary material and could be labelled as "functional foods." The concept of prebiotics, which is topical in food development at this time, is a good example that highlights these benefits. Likely due to their specific properties, polysaccharides affect several functions, contribute to our well-being, and are one of the most important ingredients in food processing. However, and bearing in mind their numerous functional properties, many of their properties and functionalities remain unclear. Moreover, the scientific advances linking diet and health have fostered unprecedented attention to the role of nutrition in health promotion and disease prevention. This is fortunate as considerable evidence indicates that adequate consumption of polysaccharides, mainly fructans and dietary fibers, has a role in preventing many chronic diseases. Although consistent literature exists on different polysaccharides, new analytical techniques and emerging technologies, such as omics, and the progress of medical science are still trying to fill the gap by demonstrating the roles and the effects of these polymers on our life.

Nowadays, polysaccharides are at the forefront of most research because they are vital polymers for human life, and all other living organisms as well, and they are in food processing, health care, and in a large variety of materials, owing to the huge development of bio-based products. Nevertheless, due to the complexity of their synthesis in plants, the highly multidisciplinary character of polysaccharides research, and the very large variety of applications, there is a need for reporting and updating the huge amount of data on these polymers. Therefore, this book aims to contribute one additional "stone to the structure" of polysaccharides science, and the different chapters cover numerous fields from the chemical to the nutritional and medical roles of these polymers.

Professor Noureddine Benkeblia
University of the West Indies, Mona
Editor

Editor

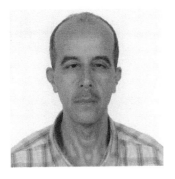

Dr. Noureddine Benkeblia is a professor of crop science; his main research areas are biochemistry and the physiology of fresh crops including preservation technologies. His work is mainly devoted to the metabolism of the carbohydrate, fructooligosaccharides (FOS), during plant development and storage periods. A few years ago, he started using the new concept of system biology—metabolomics—to investigate the mechanisms of biosynthesis, translocation, and accumulation of FOS in Liliaceous plants. Professor Benkeblia earned his BSc, MSc, and doctorate in agricultural sciences (PhD) from the Institut National Agronomique (Algiers, Algeria), and a doctorate in agriculture (PhD) from Kagoshima University, Japan. After a few years of teaching in Algeria, he joined INRA, Avignon (France), as a postdoctoral scientist in 2001. From 2002 to 2007, he worked as a visiting professor at the University of Rakuno Gakuen, Ebetsu (Japan) and a research associate in Hokkaido University from 2005 to 2007. Professor Benkeblia then joined the staff of the Department of Life Sciences, the University of the West Indies, Mona Campus in 2008, continuing his work on the physiology, biochemistry, and metabolomics of fructan-containing plants. He also works on the postharvest physiology and biochemistry of local tropical crops.

Contributors

Padma Ambalam
Department of Biotechnology
Saurashtra University
Gujarat, India

László Babinszky
Department of Feed and Food
    Biotechnology
University of Debrecen
Debrecen, Hungary

Ritesh K. Baboota
National Agri-Food Biotechnology
    Institute (NABI)
Punjab, India

Noureddine Benkeblia
Department of Life Sciences
University of the West
    Indies
Kingston, Jamaica

Mahendra Bishnoi
National Agri-Food Biotechnology
    Institute (NABI)
Punjab, India

Ravneet K. Boparai
Department of Biochemistry
Panjab University
Punjab, India

Harro J. Bouwmeester
Laboratory of Plant Physiology
Wageningen University
Wageningen, the Netherlands

Marcia R. Braga
Instituto de Botânica
Núcleo de Pesquisa em Fisiologia e
    Bioquímica
São Paulo, Brazil

Barry J. Campbell
Department of Gastroenterology
University of Liverpool
Liverpool, United Kingdom

Martine Champ
Western Human Nutrition Research
    Centre (CNRH Ouest)
INRA-Université de Nantes
Nantes, France

Maurício B. Fialho
Instituto de Botânica
Núcleo de Pesquisa em Fisiologia e
  Bioquímica
São Paulo, Brazil

**Rita de Cássia L.
  Figueiredo-Ribeiro**
Instituto de Botânica
Núcleo de Pesquisa em Fisiologia e
  Bioquímica
São Paulo, Brazil

María Concepción García-Pérez
Departamento de Biotecnología y
  Bioquímica
Centro de Investigación y de
  Estudios Avanzados del IPN
Guanajuato, Mexico

María Isabel García-Vieyra
Departamento de Biotecnología y
  Bioquímica
Centro de Investigación y de
  Estudios Avanzados del IPN
Guanajuato, Mexico

Marília Gaspar
Instituto de Botânica
Núcleo de Pesquisa em Fisiologia e
  Bioquímica
São Paulo, Brazil

Ioannis Giavasis
Department of Food Technology
Technological Educational Institute
  (TEI) of Thessaly
Karditsa, Greece

Thierry Gidenne
INRA
Université de Toulouse INPT
  ENSAT and INPT ENVT
Castanet-Tolosan, France

Muralikrishna Gudipati
Department of Biochemistry and
  Nutrition
Council of Scientific and Industrial
  Research
Central Food Technological
  Research Institute (CSIR-CFTRI)
Karnataka, India

Johanna C. Hakkert
Plant Research International
Wageningen UR
Wageningen, the Netherlands

Veronika Halas
Department of Animal Nutrition
Kaposvár University
Kaposvár, Hungary

Alicia Huazano-García
Departamento de Biotecnología y
  Bioquímica
Centro de Investigación y de
  Estudios Avanzados del IPN
Guanajuato, Mexico

Heidi Jacobs
Cosucra Groupe Warcoing SA
Warcoing, Belgium

Antonio Jiménez-Escrig
Department of Metabolism and
  Nutrition
Ciudad Universitaria
Madrid, Spain

Kanthi Kiran Kondepudi
National Agri-Food Biotechnology
  Institute (NABI)
Punjab, India

Andries J. Koops
Plant Research International
Wageningen UR
Wageningen, the Netherlands

Lyned D. Lasrado
Department of Biochemistry and
    Nutrition
Council of Scientific and Industrial
    Research
Central Food Technological
    Research Institute (CSIR-CFTRI)
Karnataka, India

Mercedes G. López
Departamento de Biotecnología y
    Bioquímica
Centro de Investigación y de
    Estudios Avanzados del IPN
Guanajuato, Mexico

Koushik Mazumder
National Agri-Food Biotechnology
    Institute (NABI)
Punjab, India

John A. Monro
Food Industry Science Centre
New Zealand Institute for Plant and
    Food Research Limited
Palmerston North, New Zealand

Nida Murtaza
National Agri-Food Biotechnology
    Institute (NABI)
Punjab, India

Rosemeire A. B. Pessoni
Faculdade da Saúde
Universidade Metodista de São Paulo
São Bernardo do Campo, Brazil

Koteswaraiah Podili
School of BioSciences and
    Technology
VIT University
Tamil Nadu, India

Robert Sévenier
Keygene N.V.
Agro Business Park
Wageningen, the Netherlands

Cathy Signoret
Cosucra Groupe Warcoing SA
Warcoing, Belgium

Kelly Simões
Instituto de Botânica
Núcleo de Pesquisa em Fisiologia e
    Bioquímica
São Paulo, Brazil

Hannah L. Simpson
Department of Gastroenterology
University of Liverpool
United Kingdom

Pariyarath Sangeetha Thondre
Faculty of Health and Life Sciences
Oxford Brookes University
Oxford, United Kingdom

Jeroen van Arkel
Plant Research International
Wageningen UR
Wageningen, the Netherlands

Ingrid M. van der Meer
Plant Research International
Wageningen UR
Wageningen, the Netherlands

Ana Villares
Centro para la Calidad de los
    Alimentos
Instituto Nacional de Investigación y
    Tecnología Agraria y Alimentaria
    (INIA)
Soria, Spain

CHAPTER **1**

Fructan Biosynthesis Regulation and the Production of Tailor-Made Fructan in Plants

JEROEN VAN ARKEL, ROBERT SÉVENIER, JOHANNA C.
HAKKERT, HARRO J. BOUWMEESTER, ANDRIES J. KOOPS,
and INGRID M. VAN DER MEER

Contents

1.1	Introduction	2
1.2	Regulation of Fructan Biosynthesis in Dicot Plants	5
	1.2.1 Localization of Inulin Biosynthesis in the Root	5
	1.2.2 Carbohydrate-Mediated Regulation of Fructan Biosynthesis	6
1.3	Modification of Fructan Synthesis in Fructan-Accumulating Plants	7
	1.3.1 Fructan Biosynthesis in Chicory	7
	1.3.2 Modifying Fructan Biosynthesis in Chicory for a Higher mDP and Yield	9
	1.3.3 Modifying Fructan Biosynthesis in Chicory to Alter the Fructan Type	9
	1.3.4 Modifying Fructan Biosynthesis in Other Plants	10
1.4	Heterologous Production of Fructan in Nonfructan-Accumulating Plant Species	11
	1.4.1 Use of Bacterial Genes in Heterologous Plant Hosts	11
	1.4.2 Use of Plant Genes in Nonfructan-Accumulating Plant Hosts	17
1.5	Tailor-Made Fructan	19
	1.5.1 Sucrose Availability Determines Fructan Yield	19
	1.5.2 Competition of Fructan Accumulation with Starch	20
	1.5.3 Fructan Stability in the New Fructan Storage Organs	20

1.5.4   Fructan Enhances the Drought and Cold Resistance
            of the Platform Crop   21
1.5.5   Platform Crops for Tailor-Made Fructan   22
1.6   Conclusions and Outlook   23
Acknowledgment   24
References   24

1.1 Introduction

Fructan is a polymer that consists of fructose units and a terminal glucose residue. It occurs in a variety of organisms such as bacteria, fungi, and in approximately 15% of flowering plants. Fructan can be divided into three groups based on its linkage type: (1) levan, with β(2-6)-linked fructosyl units—this mainly occurs in bacteria (Dedonder 1966), monocotyledonous plants (where it can also be called phlein) (Bonnett et al. 1997), and also in a member of the order Buxales according to a recent discovery (Van den Ende et al. 2011); (2) inulin, a β(2-1) linear polymer found in dicotyledonous plants (Koops and Jonker 1996); and (3) fructan neo-series, a mixed type of fructan found in Liliaceae (Pollock 1986) where β(2-1) chain elongation occurs at the C1 and C6 positions of the glucose residue. A schematic representation of the fructan biosynthesis reactions occurring in plants and the molecules involved is given in Figure 1.1.

Bacteria use fructan as an energy storage molecule (Burne et al. 1996) and as a protective layer outside the cell. This fructan layer is used by plant pathogenic bacteria to block host–pathogen recognition and protect against bacteriostatic compounds released by collapsed plant cells (Kasapis et al. 1994). *Streptococci*, present in the oral cavity, use the fructan layer as an adhesive leading to the formation of dental plaques, which consist largely of levan-type fructan (Cote and Ahlgren 1993). The biosynthesis of levan in bacteria is brought about by a single enzyme, levansucrase (E.C. 2.4.1.10).

In plants, fructan serves as a reserve carbohydrate and is stored in stems, tubers, or taproots. It has also been suggested that fructan protects plants against stressors such as drought and cold (Pilon-Smits et al. 1995, Pollock 1986). The length of plant fructan varies from 10 to approximately 200 fructosyl units. In Figure 1.2, the inulin pattern of chicory is shown. Variations highly depend on the taxonomic diversity of the fructan-producing plant species. Contrary to bacteria, the biosynthesis of fructan in plants is catalyzed by three different classes of enzymes—sucrose: sucrose 1-fructosyltransferase (EC 2.4.1.99) (1-SST), fructan: fructan 1-fructosyltransferase (EC2.4.1.100) (1-FFT) and fructan exohydrolase (EC.3.2.1.153) (1-FEH) (Edelman and Jefford 1968). 1-SST primarily catalyzes the synthesis of the trisaccharide 1-kestose from two molecules of sucrose. In this reaction, glucose is formed in equimolar amounts to 1-kestose (Figure 1.1). 1-FFT catalyzes the transfer of fructosyl units from 1-kestose, and any other fructan molecule, onto 1-kestose and

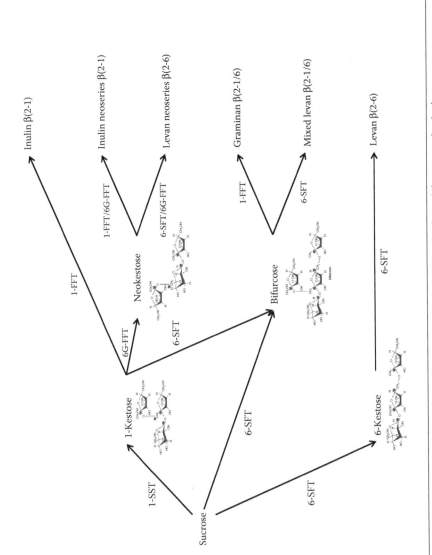

Figure 1.1 Schematic representation of fructan biosynthesis reactions occurring in plants, the molecules and the enzymes involved.

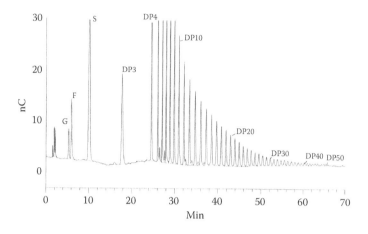

Figure 1.2 High-performance anion exchange chromatography-pulsed amperometric detection (HPAEC-PAD, Dionex) analysis of chicory inulin. The elution positions of glucose (G), fructose (F), sucrose (S), 1-kestose (DP3), DP4, DP10, DP20, DP30, DP40, and DP50 are indicated.

fructan molecules with a higher degree of polymerization (DP) (Figure 1.1). 1-FFT increases the mean degree of polymerization (mDP) when using 1-kestose (the shortest fructan) as a fructosyl donor. This reaction converts 1-kestose into sucrose, which does not constitute a fructan molecule, and a fructosyl unit that is used to elongate a preexisting fructan molecule. Under 1-kestose limiting conditions such as low 1-SST activity, 1-FFT may instead catalyze the transfer of fructosyl units from a fructan molecule onto sucrose (Van den Ende and Roover 1996, Vergauwen et al. 2003). This so-called "back transfer" reaction results in the decrease of the mDP. The third class of enzymes, 1-FEH, catalyzes the degradation of inulin by hydrolyzing terminal fructosyl units resulting in the formation of fructose and a lower DP inulin (Van den Ende et al. 2000). The regulation of fructan biosynthesis is mostly studied in grasses; these studies revealed the central role for sugars in the induction of fructosytransferase genes (Maleux and Van den Ende 2007, Obenland et al. 1991, van Arkel et al. 2012, Winters et al. 1994). In chicory, the induction of fructan biosynthesis has been the subject of several studies. Kusch et al. studied the regulation of 1-SST and 1-FFT in relation to the nitrogen availability (Kusch et al. 2009). Améziane et al. showed the inducibility of 1-SST by light and found a correlation between 1-SST enzyme activity and the concentration of sucrose in the tissue (Améziane et al. 1994). Studies on the regulation of 1-FEH revealed an induction of 1-FEH by cold (Kusch et al. 2009, Michiels et al. 2004) and inhibition of FEH IIa activity by sucrose (Verhaest et al. 2007).

Plant fructan is used for a range of food and nonfood applications (Sévenier et al. 2006) depending on the DP. Short-chain inulin can be used to produce fructose syrup for the sweetening of cold drinks. Long-chain inulin (mDP ≥ 25) is used as a fat replacer, prebiotic and foam stabilizer in food products. Long-chain inulin also provides the starting material for producing carboxymethylinulin, a scavenger of divalent cations in household detergents.

The crop grown for the production of fructan on a commercial scale is chicory. Chicory (*Cichorium intybus* L.) is a biennial taproot-bearing crop; it is sown in spring and the taproots are harvested in autumn of the same year for inulin extraction. At the harvest of the taproots, the mean inulin polymer length is 9–10 and the average yield is about 11,000 kg of carbohydrate per hectare (Wittouck et al. 2002). One of the most important quality parameters of inulin is the polymer length. For certain applications—like fat replacer which requires a minimum DP > 25—the raw inulin extracted from chicory is unsuitable and should be enriched for long polymer molecules, which is a costly process.

Interestingly, it has been observed in chicory that the polymer length in the early growing season is much higher than in autumn when it is harvested. The decrease in polymer length at harvest is caused by catalytic reactions of 1-FFT and 1-FEH; both of these enzymes respond to plant and environmental factors.

Plants that naturally accumulate fructan can also degrade the polymer to remobilize the stored carbon. This catalytic breakdown of fructan is a major drawback in the agricultural production of inulin in chicory. Several solutions to this problem have been proposed, including attempts to genetically modify crops that normally do not metabolize or catabolize fructan. One advantage of using nonfructan accumulating plant species for the commercial production of fructan is that highly productive crop plants, having well-established husbandry and processing chains, can be chosen. Moreover, the introduction of fructan biosynthesis in nonfructan species might render new types and different sizes of fructan not yet present in normal fructan-producing plants—the tailor-made fructan.

This chapter gives an overview on the research of regulation and synthesis of fructan in fructan-accumulating plants and touches upon the introduction of fructan synthesis in nonfructan-accumulating plants. Most of the work on genetic modification of fructan synthesis in fructan-accumulating plants has been performed on chicory. Therefore, an introduction to the inulin metabolism of chicory is given. A wide range of bacterial and plant fructosyltransferase genes have been introduced into many different plants, varying from monocots, such as rice, maize, and sugar cane, to dicots, such as potato, sugar beet, and clover. The effect of the modification or introduction of fructan synthesis will be evaluated on the resulting fructan yield, polymer length, and the linkage type of fructan.

1.2 Regulation of Fructan Biosynthesis in Dicot Plants

1.2.1 *Localization of Inulin Biosynthesis in the Root*

Studies on the localization of inulin biosynthesis in the roots of the dicot plant chicory showed that 1-SST and 1-FFT enzyme activity increased toward the inside of the roots (Kusch 2009). Although in the outer tissues 1-SST and

1-FFT enzyme activity was not absent. This was confirmed by the results of Van Wonterghem, showing that the 1-FFT protein was located in the parenchyma cells surrounding the phloem and more toward the outside of the root (Van Wonterghem et al. 1999). Also inulin crystals were found in radial axis throughout the root (Desmet 1997). In *Taraxacum officinale*, higher fructan enzyme activity and higher inulin accumulation was also found around the phloem tissue, but inulin was also found in the xylem vessels (Van den Ende et al. 2000). Similar results were found for *Helianthus tuberosus* (Ernst 1991) and *Gomphrena macrocephala* (Vieira and Figueiredo-Ribeiro 1993). The transport of inulin throughout the plant is only shown for 1-kestose (Pontis et al. 2002) and not for longer inulin (Turk et al. 1997). This suggests that most inulin biosynthesis and accumulation takes place near the phloem, where sucrose is imported into the root, but is not restricted to this area.

1.2.2 Carbohydrate-Mediated Regulation of Fructan Biosynthesis

From several studies of different plant species, it can be deduced that fructan biosynthesis is regulated by the concentration of monosaccharides (Blacklow et al. 1984, Maleux and Van den Ende 2007, Müller et al. 2000, Ruuska et al. 2008). Other factors like nitrogen status and the developmental phase of the plant have shown to be important factors too (Kusch 2009, Morcuende et al. 2004, van Arkel et al. 2012, Van den Ende et al. 1999). The degradation of fructan has shown to be regulated by temperature and drought. Several studies showed that an increase of FEH expression and activity correlated with these circumstances (delViso et al. 2009, De Roover et al. 2000, Hisano et al. 2004, Kusch et al. 2009, Rao et al. 2011, van Arkel et al. 2012, Wei et al. 2001). The fructan exohydrolase activity of FEH IIa is regulated at the post-transcriptional level and inhibited by sucrose (Verhaest et al. 2007). The inhibition is shown to work via the binding of sucrose to the active site of 1-FEH. The K_i of sucrose is low enough to ensure an effective inhibition of these FEH enzymes under circumstances favorable to fructan accumulation. The major advantage of such regulation, as stated by the authors, is a rapid switch from net fructan synthesis (high sucrose concentrations) to net degradation at low levels of sucrose. This quick response might be especially crucial for the rapid regrowth of grasses after defoliation (Verhaest et al. 2007). Fructosyltransferase gene expression and fructan synthesis was shown to be enhanced in excised leaf blades of grasses upon feeding with sucrose (Cairns et al. 1997, Maleux and Van den Ende 2007, Müller et al. 2000, Wei et al. 2001, Winters et al. 1994) or glucose (Kusch 2009, Suzuki et al. 2012). Recently, it was suggested that high sucrose strength is one of the important factors determining high levels of fructan in wheat (Xue et al. 2012). The authors found a direct correlation between sucrose and the level of fructan. In contrast to grasses, no fructan accumulation is found in leaves of chicory under natural conditions. However, under severe stress conditions, such as drought stress, chicory leaves can accumulate inulin (De Roover et al. 2000). The illumination of excised leaves of chicory was also shown to induce fructan biosynthesis. Améziane et al. showed that the illuminated leaves had higher levels of sucrose and expressed *1-sst*. (Améziane et al. 1994).

To understand how fructosyltransferases are regulated, different studies have analyzed different parts of the regulation process. For example, a central role for small GTPases in sugar signaling has been discovered in a feeding study (Ritsema et al. 2009). Indications that protein kinase, protein phosphatase activities and calcium take part in this regulation process are given by Martinez-Noël et al. and Ritsema et al. (Martínez-Noël et al. 2007, 2009, Ritsema et al. 2009). But also transcription factors and promoter elements involved in sucrose or the developmental regulation of fructan synthesis are important to understand the molecular mechanisms underlying the regulation of fructan biosynthesis. To contribute to the elucidation of this mechanism in chicory, we isolated and studied the sequence of two genomic promoter fragments of *1-fft* and *1-sst* from chicory. The comparison of the promoter sequences with earlier published sequences showed that several well-described regulatory elements involved in sugar regulation are present in *1-sst* and *1-fft* promoter (manuscript in preparation) that are also found in the barley 6-*sft* promoter (Nagaraj et al. 2001). Recent results of an expression correlation study in wheat revealed a positive correlation of *1-sst* and 6-*sft* expression with a group of *myb* genes (Xue et al. 2011). The core DNA-binding sequence in the *1-sst* and 6-*sft* promoters was determined by mutagenesis, and transactivation analysis showed that TaMYB13 is the transcriptional activator of 1-SST and 6-SFT. No TaMYB13 homologues from other fructan accumulating plants are published. The Arabidopsis homologues of TaMYB13, AtMYB59 and to a lesser extent AtMYB48 (Xue et al. 2011), are expressed upon sucrose feeding and under continuous light, as shown in the eFP browser of the Bio-array resource for plant biology (BAR) (Winter et al. 2007). Based on the expression pattern of the TaMYB genes and the finding of Xue et al. that genes involved in fructan and starch synthesis are coregulated in relation to leaf sucrose levels (Xue et al. 2012), it could be hypothesized that the same transcription factors are regulating the expression of the enzymes involved in starch and fructan biosynthesis. The overexpression of TaMYB13-1 in wheat leads to enhanced fructan accumulation suggesting an important role in the upregulation of fructan synthesis genes (Kooiker et al. 2013). This could give clues and tools for further studies on regulation of fructan biosynthesis.

1.3 Modification of Fructan Synthesis in Fructan-Accumulating Plants

1.3.1 Fructan Biosynthesis in Chicory

Chicory is a biannual crop grown for the production of inulin that is stored in the taproot. The taproot starts to thicken seven weeks after sowing, concomitant with the induced activity of the fructan synthesis enzymes, 1-SST and 1-FFT. The activity of 1-SST increases rapidly and reaches its maximum three weeks later (Druart et al. 2001). Ten weeks after sowing, the activity decreases until the end of the growing season (in November) when only 10% of the activity remains (Van den Ende et al. 1996). The activity of 1-FFT follows a different pattern; it increases slowly and stabilizes after four weeks. The activity of 1-FFT remains constant during the rest of the growing season (Van den Ende et al. 2002). In the first few months, mainly short inulin chains are formed as a direct result of the fructosyltransferase activities. Nine weeks after sowing, inulin molecules with a DP of up to 25 are accumulated. At the beginning of September, the mDP reaches a maximum of about 16, and then decreases as reported by Druart et al. (2001). The extent of the decrease depends on the growing conditions (van Arkel et al. 2012) and on the cultivar (Koch et al. 1999). The decrease in mDP is thought to be catalyzed by 1-FFT using, in the absence of 1-SST, incoming sucrose as an acceptor for fructosyl units (Van den Ende et al. 2002). The result is a decrease in mDP but an increase of yield per taproot (van Arkel et al. 2012). Later in the season, the mDP further decreases because of the fructan exohydrolase activity of FEHI that is induced at low temperatures (mid-October) (Michiels et al. 2004, van Arkel et al. 2012). The degradation of inulin is further enhanced by FEHII later in the season, when temperatures of 4°C and below induce this second exohydrolase (Van den Ende et al. 2002). The degradation catalyzed by 1-FFT and 1-FEH that occurs in autumn is highly disadvantageous for industrial inulin production, especially for high DP inulin production.

In summary, from the studies on inulin biosynthesis in chicory it could be concluded that the decline in 1-SST activity combined with the increase in 1-FEH activity negatively influences the mDP.

Several groups focussed on the modification of fructan synthesis in chicory in order to produce high DP inulin with the highest possible yield or fructan with modified linkage types. In our research group, two different approaches to accomplish an increased yield and polymer length have been followed. The first approach to obtain the production of inulin with a higher mDP was by blocking the activity of 1-FEH in the autumn, which might be achieved by down-regulation of FEHI. It was envisioned that the absence of FEHI activity might prevent depolymerization, although a reduction of mDP by 1-FFT and FEHII might still occur. A second approach to enhance the DP was by overexpressing *1-sst* during the growing season. The additional polymerization activity by the extra 1-SST enzyme might maintain a higher concentration of 1-kestose and a lower concentration of sucrose; two factors that might contribute to limiting 1-FFT-mediated depolymerization. Both approaches are discussed in Section 1.3.2.

Other groups focussed on changing the linkage type of fructan in order to modify the fructan produced. Chicory was transformed with genes isolated from species accumulating different types of fructan, such as the *6-sft* from barley (Sprenger et al. 1997) and *6g-fft* from onion (Vijn et al. 1997).

1.3.2 Modifying Fructan Biosynthesis in Chicory for a Higher mDP and Yield

One way of increasing the mDP of chicory inulin was to prevent the reduction of 1-SST activity at the end of the growing season. Earlier results showed that the endogenous 1-SST enzyme is subjected to a regulatory mechanism that mediates a decrease of the enzyme activity during the growing season (van Arkel et al. 2012). Two different *1-sst* genes (*sst-I* and *sst-II*), isolated from *Helianthus tuberosus* (Koops et al. 2003, Van der Meer et al. 1998), were expressed under the control of the CAMV-35S promoter in chicory (unpublished results). Plants harboring an extra *1-sst* gene were grown under field-like conditions to study the effect of the introduced genes. The mDP of inulin and the activity of 1-SST, 1-FFT, and 1-FEH were monitored from September until November, when the reduction of 1-SST activity normally occurs in wild-type chicory, and the fructosyltransferase activity of 1-FFT onto sucrose also takes place. No impairment on growth was observed. Comparison of the control plants with plants harboring the *Helianthus tuberosus* gene *sst-II* showed that the transgene significantly contributed to the total activity of 1-SST. This additional 1-SST activity resulted in a 20% higher mDP in the first 8 weeks of the experiment. Nevertheless, plants harboring the *sst-I* gene did not show elevated levels of 1-SST activity, neither did they show a significant alteration in the mDP. Unfortunately, low temperatures had a comparable effect on the decrease of mDP in both types of transgenics (containing *sst-I* or *sst-II*) and on the wild-type plants. At the end of the growing season the extra *1-sst* gene did not result in longer chains, most probably because of the (early) induction of FEH by low temperatures by the end of the experiment.

Another approach to enhance the mDP of chicory inulin at harvest was to decrease the 1-FEH activity. An *feh-I* antisense fragment driven by the constitutive CaMV 35S promoter was introduced into the chicory. In three independent transgenic lines, cold induction of *feh-I* expression could be inhibited by the antisense *feh-1* expression. However, this decreased 1-FEH induction had only minor effects on the mDP when the transgenics were subjected to a cold treatment, normally inducing specifically *feh-I*. A possible explanation could be that the remaining *feh-I* transcript resulted in enough 1-FEH activity to decrease the mDP.

1.3.3 Modifying Fructan Biosynthesis in Chicory to Alter the Fructan Type

In a study performed by Sprenger et al. (1997), a sucrose, fructan 6-fructosyltransferase (6-SFT), from barley was introduced into the chicory. The aim was to produce the mixed-type fructan. Unfortunately, the composition of inulin in the taproot of the transgenic plants had not been changed. However, excised leaves that were placed in sucrose solutions and illuminated continuously accumulated $\beta(2\text{-}1)$ inulin and $\beta(2\text{-}6)$ fructan (kestose and bifurcose), demonstrating the functionality of barley 6-SFT in chicory. After extended illumination, most of the fructan in the transgenic leaves was of the inulin type and only a small part consisted of the mixed-type fructan. The experiments in leaves showed that most probably 1-FFT out-competes the heterologous 6-SFT for substrate. This competition for substrate could also be the reason for the absence of the mixed-type fructan in the taproots and may result from a lower expression of the *6-sft* (not reported) than the endogenous *1-fft* or from a higher affinity of 1-FFT for the substrate.

In another example of modifying the fructan linkage-type in chicory, the gene encoding onion 6G-FFT was introduced (Vijn et al. 1997). Although the authors did not report on the analysis of fructan accumulation in roots, in excised leaves, in which fructan accumulation was induced, fructan of the neo-series could be detected in addition to the native inulin.

In conclusion, the attempts to modify the inulin metabolism in chicory in order to increase the mDP or to alter the accumulated fructan type comprise the introduction of extra genes and the knockdown of an exohydrolase gene. Although the introduced genes were functional and the knockdown could be detected in the transgenic plants, only slight changes of the expected effect on the mDP or inulin composition were observed. The reasons for this discrepancy could be: (a) the relatively high level of expression of the endogenous inulin biosynthesis genes (unpublished results) as compared to the relatively low expression level of the introduced transgenes; and (b) the mechanism of fructan degradation, which involves three exohydrolase enzymes and 1-FFT, that is highly complex. However, both aspects could be addressed. Strong promoters could be used to drive the expression of the transgenes, for instance, the *1-fft* promoter from chicory. In order to block all exohydrolase activity, three *feh*-genes (*fehIa*, *b*, and *fehII*) may need to be knocked out, preferably by the use of a more effective gene silencing technique like RNAi, or by the use of knock out mutants.

1.3.4 Modifying Fructan Biosynthesis in Other Plants

A few studies on the attempts to modify the fructan composition in other fructan plants than chicory were reported. A study on the expression of a *Bacillus subtilis sacB* in *Lolium multiflorum* revealed that levan could be accumulated in the plant and this consequently disturbed the native fructan pattern. Native high DP fructan was depleted and the profile of lower DP fructan was altered (Ye et al. 2001). The modification of the linkage-type negatively affected the fructan yield. The modification also slowed down plant growth; the flowering plants were stunted and had narrower leaves and poorly developed roots as described by the authors. In contrast, the expression *6g-fft* or *1-sst* from barley in *Lolium perenne* yielded up to 15% more fructan than in wild-type plants; this increased fructan content did not impair the growth of the plant. Differences of the linkage type or changes in the DP profile were not reported. The accumulated fructan was shown to have a positive effect on the freezing tolerance, possibly due to increased amounts of fructan, glucose, and fructose (Hisano et al. 2004). According to Sobolev et al. (2007), transgenic lettuce overexpressing an asparagine synthase from *Escherichia coli* rather unexpectedly accumulated 30 times more fructan than wild-type plants. The aim of this study was to alter the nitrogen status of the plant and eventually enhance growth. It appeared that the whole metabolism of the plant was enhanced, including Krebs's cycle and the fructan biosynthesis, although the nitrogen status was not altered.

The studies described above show that the native fructan composition can significantly be altered in transgenic natively fructan-accumulating plants and that the effect on fructan yield and composition was more pronounced than in the transgenic chicory described earlier, although the different experiments are not fully comparable.

1.4 Heterologous Production of Fructan in Nonfructan-Accumulating Plant Species

There has been an array of alternative industrial crops genetically modified with fructosyltransferase genes for the production of fructan. Table 1.1 summarizes these studies and shows the fructan yield and the characteristics of the transgenic plants. Examples of plants that have been used are tobacco, potato, maize, and sugar beet. Most transgenic plants producing fructan showed a reduced level of sucrose or starch as compared to the wild types. Another characteristic observed in several studies is stunted growth. Fructan production seems to increase at the cost of other carbohydrate synthesis pathways, and in some cases has an impaired effect on the growth.

1.4.1 Use of Bacterial Genes in Heterologous Plant Hosts

Many studies focussed on the introduction of bacterial genes in nonfructan-accumulating plants to produce high DP fructan (Table 1.1). The use of bacterial levansucrases to engineer plants did not prove very successful in terms of fructan yield (Caimi et al. 1997, Ebskamp et al. 1994, Pilon-Smits et al. 1995), although in some studies high amounts of fructan were shown to be accumulated. Van der Meer et al. found 350 mg/g DW levan in transgenic old potato leaves and 50 mg/g DW in growing microtubers when expressing *sacB* from *Bacillus subtilis* (van der Meer et al. 1994). The expression of *lsc* from *Erwinia amylovora* in starch-deficient potato yielded 70–120 mg/g DW of fructan in the tubers (Röber et al. 1996). The DP of the *in planta* produced levan exceeded 25,000 in potato, tobacco, and white clover (Ebskamp et al. 1994, Jenkins et al. 2002, van der Meer et al. 1994). This DP is comparable to what is found in bacteria (van der Meer et al. 1994). Trujillo et al. described the first attempt to express a levansucrase in sugarcane, reporting that PCR-positive plants could be generated but these were not analyzed for fructan accumulation (Trujillo et al. 2000). The expression of levansucrase from *Lactobacillus* resulted in low amounts of levan in sugarcane, as published recently (Bauer

Table 1.1 Fructan Production in Genetically Engineered Crops That Originally Do Not Accumulate Fructan

Crop Transformed	Gene Introduced	Gene's Origin	Enzyme Targeting	Tissue Analyzed	Soluble Sugar Content of the Transformed Tissue			Phenotype Changes	Literature Cited
					Sucrose	Fructan	Glucose		
Maize	sacB	Bacillus amyloliquefaciens	Vacuole	Seeds	NR	10–80 mg/gDW	NR	No effect on the phenotype	Caimi et al. (1996)
Maize	sacB	Bacillus amyloliquefaciens	Cytoplasm	Seeds	NR	16–18 mg/gDW	NR	Severe reduction of seed DW	Caimi et al. (1997)
Maize	1-sst	Helianthus tuberosus	Vacuole	Seeds	2.3 mg/gFW	3.2 mg/gFW	27 mg/gFW	NR	Stoop et al. (2007)
Maize	1-sst + 1-fft	Helianthus tuberosus	Vacuole	Seeds	3.3 mg/gFW	0.6 mg/gFW	10 mg/gFW	NR	Stoop et al. (2007)
Sugar maize (sh2)	1-sst + 1-fft	Helianthus tuberosus	Vacuole	Seeds	24 mg/gFW	20 mg/gFW	4 mg/gFW	NR	Stoop et al. (2007)
Petunia	1-sst	Helianthus tuberosus	Vacuole	Leaf	0.41 mg/gFW	0.47 mg/FW	NR	No effect on the phenotype	Van der Meer et al. (1998)
Petunia	1-fft	Helianthus tuberosus	Vacuole	Leaf	NR	0 mg/FW	NR	No effect on the phenotype	Van der Meer et al. (1998)
Potato	sacB	Bacillus subtilis	Vacuole	Leaves (old)	NR	350 mg/gDW	NR	Reduced starch	Van der Meer et al. (1994)
Potato	sacB	Bacillus subtilis	Vacuole	Microtubers	NR	50 mg/gDW	NR	Reduced starch	Van der Meer et al. (1994)
Potato	sacB	Bacillus subtilis	Vacuole	Leaves	NR	5 mg/gFW	NR	Stunted growth	Pilon-Smits et al. (1996)

Plant	Gene	Source	Localization	Tissue				Phenotype	Reference
Potato	sacB	Bacillus subtilis	Vacuole	Tubers	3–11 mg/gFW	11 mg/gFW	0.5–5 mg/gFW	Reduced starch content and browning	Pilon-Smits et al. (1997)
Potato	sacB	Bacillus amyloliquefaciens	Cytoplasm	Tubers	NR	5–50 mg/gDW	NR	Reduced starch and tuber DW	Caimi et al. (1997)
Potato	1-sst	Cynara scolymus	Vacuole	Tubers	14 μmol/gFW	19 μmol/gFW	NR	NR	Hellwege et al. (1997)
Potato	1-sst + 1-fft	Cynara scolymus	Vacuole	Tubers	15 μmol/gFW	50 mg/gDW	3.9 μmol/gFW	No effect on the phenotype	Hellwege et al. (2000)
Potato	sacB	Bacillus subtilis	Plastid	Leaf	90 μmol/gFW	66 mg/gFW	25 μmol/gFW	NR	Gerrits et al. (2001)
Potato	1-sst	Helianthus tuberosus	Vacuole	Tubers	0.08 mg/gFW	1.4 mg/gFW	2.9 mg/gFW	No effect on the phenotype	Stoop et al. (2007)
Potato	1-sst + 1-fft	Helianthus tuberosus	Vacuole	Tubers	2.0 mg/gFW	2.6 mg/gFW	3.1 mg/gFW	No effect on the phenotype	Stoop et al. (2007)
Starch-deficient potato	lsc	Erwinia amylovora	Vacuole	Tubers	NR	70–120 mg/gDW	82–201 mg/gDW	No effect on the phenotype	Röber et al. (1996)
Starch-deficient potato	lsc	Erwinia amylovora	Apoplasm	Tubers	NR	190 mg/gDW	50 mg/gDW	Reduced tuber FW	Röber et al. 1996
Starch-deficient potato	lsc	Erwinia amylovora	Cytoplasm	Tubers	NR	0 mg/gDW	NR	NR	Röber et al. (1996)

continued

Table 1.1 (Continued) Fructan Production in Genetically Engineered Crops That Originally Do Not Accumulate Fructan

Crop Transformed	Gene Introduced	Gene's Origin	Enzyme Targeting	Tissue Analyzed	Soluble Sugar Content of the Transformed Tissue			Phenotype Changes	Literature Cited
					Sucrose	Fructan	Glucose		
Rice	1-sst	*Triticum* spp.	Vacuole	Leaves	24 mg/gFW	16 mg/gFW	2.2 mg/gFW	No effect on the phenotype, increased total carbohydrate	Kawakami et al. (2009)
Rice	1-sst	*Smallanthus sonchiflius*	Vacuole	Leaves	NR	Visible on TLC	NR	NR	Pan et al. (2009)
Rice	1-sst	*Helianthus tuberosus*	Vacuole	Leaves	NR	Visible on TLC	NR	NR	Pan et al. (2010)
Sugar beet	1-sst	*Helianthus tuberosus*	Vacuole	Leaves	1.8 μmol/gFW	0.9 μmol/gFW	4.8 μmol/gFW	No effect on the phenotype	Sévenier et al. (1998)
Sugar beet	1-sst	*Helianthus tuberosus*	Vacuole	Roots	23 μmol/gFW	110 μmol/gFW	25 μmol/gFW	No effect on the phenotype	Sévenier et al. (1998)
Sugar beet	sacB	*Bacillus subtilis*	Vacuole	Roots/shoot	NR	0.5 mg/gDW	NR	Enhanced drought resistance	Pilon-Smits et al. (1999)
Sugar beet	1-sst + 6-fft	*Allium cepa*	Vacuole	Roots	29 mg/g FW	66.4 mg/gFW	34 mg/gFW	No effect on the phenotype	Weyens et al. (2004)
Sugarcane	lsdA	*Acetabacter diazotrophicus*	Vacuole	NR	NR	NR	NR	No effect on the phenotype	Trujillo et al. (2000)
Sugarcane	1-sst	*Cynara scolymus*	Vacuole	Internodes	470 nmol/gFW	112 nmol/gFW	0.95 nmol/gFW	No change of sucrose pool	Nicholson et al. (2007)
Sugarcane	ftfA	*Lactobacillus sanfranciscensis*	Cytosol/cell wall	Internodes	32–40 mg/gW	0.01 mg/gFW	NR	Reduced total carbohydrate	Bauer et al. (2012)

Sweet potato	lsdA	Acetobacter diazotrophicus	Vacuole	NR	NR	NR	NR	NR	Truijllo et al. (2000)
Tobacco	sacB	Bacillus subtilis	Vacuole	Leaves	0.14 mg/gFW	2.8 mg/gFW	1.5 mg/gFW	No effect on the phenotype	Ebskamp et al. (1994)
Tobacco	sacB	Bacillus subtilis	Vacuole	Leaves	0.3–0.9 mg/gFW	0.05–0.3 mg/gFW	0.5–0.7 mg/gFW	Enhanced drought stress resistance	Pilon-Smits et al. (1995)
Tobacco	6-sft	Hordeum vulgare	Vacuole	Leaves	5–10 mg/gDW	0.05–0.3 mg/gDW	NR	No effect on the phenotype	Sprenger et al. (1997)
Tobacco	6-sft	Hordeum vulgare	Vacuole	Roots	50 mg/gDW	0.5–3 mg/gDW	NR	No effect on the phenotype	Sprenger et al. (1997)
Tobacco	sacB	Bacillus subtilis	Vacuole	Leaves	2–16 mg/gFW	6 mg/gFW	2–12 mg/gFW	Stunted growth and bleached leaves	Turk et al. (1997)
Tobacco	sacB	Bacillus amyloliquefaciens	Cytoplasm (inducible promotor)	Leaves	7 mg/gFW	4 mg/gFW	6 mg/gFW	Necrosis appeared after induction	Caimi et al. (1997)
Tobacco	6-sft	Hordeum vulgare	Vacuole	Leaves	16 mg/gDW	0.17 mg/gDW	25 mg/gDW	NR	Schellenbaum et al. (1999)
Tobacco	6-sft	Hordeum vulgare	Vacuole	Roots	55 mg/gDW	5.5 mg/gDW	10 mg/gDW	NR	Schellenbaum et al. (1999)
Tobacco	levU	Zymomonas mobilis	Cytoplasm	Leaves	NR	Visible on TLC	NR	Enhanced osmotic stress resistance	Park et al. (1999)
Tobacco	sacB	Bacillus subtilis	Plastid	Leaf	NR	20 mg/gFW	NR	NR	Gerrits et al. (2001)

continued

Table 1.1 (Continued) Fructan Production in Genetically Engineered Crops That Originally Do Not Accumulate Fructan

Crop Transformed	Gene Introduced	Gene's Origin	Enzyme Targeting	Tissue Analyzed	Soluble Sugar Content of the Transformed Tissue			Phenotype Changes	Literature Cited
					Sucrose	Fructan	Glucose		
Tobacco	1-sst	Lactuca sativa	Vacuole	Leaves	0.1-3.8 mg/gFW	40–110 ug/gFW	NR	Enhanced freezing tolerance	Hui-Juan et al. (2007)
Tobacco	LsdA	Gluconacetobacter diazotrophicus	Vacuole	Leaves	NR	70 mg/gFW	NR	Older leaves bleached prematurely and became rigid	Banguela et al. (2011)
Tobacco	1-sst, 1-fft or 6-fft	Triticum spp.	Vacuole	Shoots	NR	6.1–10.2 mg/gFW	NR	Tolerance to abiotic stresses	Bie et al. (2012)
Tobacco	1-sst + 1-fft	Triticum spp.	Vacuole	Shoots	NR	36.3 mg/gFW	NR	Tolerance to abiotic stresses	Bie et al. (2012)
Tobacco	1-sst + 6-sft	Triticum spp.	Vacuole	Shoots	NR	610.6 mg/gFW	NR	Tolerance to abiotic stresses	Bie et al. (2012)
Tobacco	1-fft + 6-sft	Triticum spp.	Vacuole	Shoots	NR	29.9 mg/gFW	NR	Tolerance to abiotic stresses	Bie et al. (2012)
Tobacco	1-sst + 1-fft + 6-sft	Triticum spp.	Vacuole	Shoots	NR	75.7 mg/gFW	NR	Tolerance to abiotic stresses	Bie et al. (2012)
White clover	ftf	Streptococcus salivarius	Vacuole	Leaves	1.3 mg/g FW	3.1 mg/g FW	0.6 mg/g FW	Reduced growth	Jenkins et al. (2002)

NR: not reported; eq. hex.: equivalent hexoses.
This table was based on a previously published table (van Arkel, 2013).

et al. 2012). The disadvantage of the accumulation of levan in plants was that in many cases this led to severe alterations of the plants' growth and an aberrant phenotype (Table 1.1) that even occurs in plants that accumulate fructan originally, like *Lolium*, when expressing the *sacB* gene from *Bacillus subtilis* (Ye et al. 2001). Tobacco and potato plants, also expressing the *sacB* gene, had reduced growth (Pilon-Smits et al. 1996, Turk et al. 1997). The potato plants had smaller tubers at harvest and when the fructan concentration was higher than 1% the tubers had a brown phenotype too (Pilon-Smits et al. 1996). Caimi and coworkers reported on tissue necrosis in tobacco and reduced tuber weight in the potatoes upon expression of *sacB* (Caimi et al. 1996). Reduced tuber weight in the potatoes was also reported by Röber et al. (1996). As explanation for the observed phenotype, the authors mentioned that the major part of the fructan was not located in the vacuoles and that the presence of fructan in other cellular compartments may have been detrimental to cell function and the normal development of the transgenic plants. This conclusion was supported by the findings of Caimi (Caimi et al. 1996), who reported a drastic alteration of the kernel phenotype in the *sacB* expressing maize. The dry weight was shown to be 10-fold lower in transgenic seeds as compared to wild-type seeds. However, when the levansucrase was targeted to the vacuole using a sweet potato sporamin vacuole targeting sequence, the accumulation of fructan had no effect on the kernel development (Caimi et al. 1996). When the bacterial *LsdA* was targeted to the plant vacuolar, it also did not alter the phenotype in tobacco, leaves accumulated levan up to 70% of the dry weight. Older leaves, however, bleached prematurely and became rigid (Banguela et al. 2011).

The conclusion from the studies on the expression of bacterial genes in nonfructan-accumulating plants is that the accumulation of levan in plants was shown to be possible, but plant phenotype and fitness was in most cases negatively influenced. The yield remained low in most transgenics, probably because the levansucrase was not targeted to the vacuole.

1.4.2 Use of Plant Genes in Nonfructan-Accumulating Plant Hosts

The expression of fructosyltransferase genes of plant origin in nonfructan-accumulating plants allowed the accumulation of substantial amounts of fructan in the transgenics and did not lead to any alterations in the performance of the host plant; see Table 1.1 for an overview.

1.4.2.1 Introduction of 1-SST into Nonfructan Plants

Various *1-sst* genes originating from different fructan-accumulating plants were introduced into many different nonfructan-accumulating plant species (Table 1.1). Some successful studies will be discussed here in more detail. *Sst-I* from a Jerusalem artichoke was introduced into sugar beet. Carbohydrate analysis of the transgenic plants showed that 90% of the sucrose, normally stored in the taproot of the beet, was converted into fructan. This yielded 110 μmol/g FW fructan, mostly 1-kestose, 1-nystose, and Dp5 (Sévenier et al. 1998). The production of the latter two molecules is normally attributed to 1-FFT activity. However, it had been shown previously that *in vitro* 1-SST alone was able to catalyze the formation of fructan larger than 1-kestose (Koops and Jonker 1996). The 1-SST from globe artichoke was successfully introduced into sugarcane (Nicholson 2007). The yield in sugarcane, however, was only 8–112 nmol/g FW. This small amount of fructan did not negatively influence the sucrose concentration; the sucrose levels in the 1-SST plants were even higher than in wild-type plants. It was stated that carbon partitioning was changed by the accumulation of 1-kestose. The author showed that invertase was not the cause of this low level of 1-kestose, neither was the expression level of the introduced *1-sst*. In rice, three different *1-sst* genes were introduced and shown to be fully functional in the leaves resulting in detectable amounts of fructan (Kawakami et al. 2008, Pan et al. 2009). Kawakami showed that leaves from transgenic rice expressing *1-sst* from *Triticum* spp. accumulated fructan up to 16 mg/g FW. This accumulation of fructan increased the total water-soluble carbohydrate content of the leaves, while the concentration of sucrose was not altered. Effects of the fructan accumulation on the plant performance or grain yield were not reported (Kawakami et al. 2008).

1.4.2.2 Introduction of 6-SFT in Nonfructan Plants   Sucrose:fructan 6-fructosyltransferase (6-SFT) is able to synthesize graminans and phleins. The genes encoding 6-SFT have been isolated from different grasses and introduced into nonfructan plants (Kawakami et al. 2008, Sprenger et al. 1997). Transgenic tobacco and rice plants harboring *6-sft* accumulated kestose and a series of unbranched fructan of the phlein type (Kawakami et al. 2008, Sprenger et al. 1997). This showed that 6-SFT, in the absence of 1-SST, could form fructan in plants. However, the yield, for example in rice, was very low (3.7 mg/g FW) (Kawakami et al. 2008). This low yield could relate to the findings of Duchateau who showed that the enzyme exhibits much higher invertase activity than fructosyltransferase activity when incubated with sucrose as the sole substrate *in vitro* (Duchateau et al. 1995). Since wild-type tobacco and rice plants do not accumulate fructan but do contain sucrose, the 6-SFTs were probably not able to exert sufficient fructosyltransferase activity to accumulate large amounts of fructan in these crops.

1.4.2.3 Introduction of the Complete Fructan Pathway in Nonfructan Plants
Introducing combinations of 1-FFT or 6G-FFT with 1-SST into nonfructan-accumulating plants demonstrated that the pathway is fully transferable. The transgenic plants containing both genes did not only accumulate fructan with a higher DP than the 1-SST-expressing plants but showed inulin chain length distributions comparable to that of the species from which 1-FFT or 6G-FFT originated. Potato, maize, and sugar beet transgenic plants, enriched with the fructan biosynthesis pathway from a Jerusalem artichoke, showed the same

chain length distribution as the Jerusalem artichoke (Koops et al. 2003, Stoop et al. 2007). These results are supported by the findings of Hellwege et al. (2000) showing that the chain length distribution of inulin from a globe artichoke and a Jerusalem artichoke was reflected in a transient plant expression system (tobacco protoplasts) using the respective *1-fft* genes. The introduction of *1-sst* and *6g-fft* from an onion in sugar beet resulted in the accumulation of a branched fructan with a profile closely resembling that from an onion (Weyens et al. 2004), showing that the 6G-FFT-type of FFT also determines the fructan chain length distribution.

A general conclusion of these studies is that the fructan biosynthesis pathway could be transferred into nonfructan-accumulating plants. The genes were fully functional and their expression and accumulation of fructan did not affect the plant phenotype. The chain length distribution of the fructan produced was dependent on the origin of the FFT.

1.5 Tailor-Made Fructan

Tailor-made fructan (the synthesis of fructan with the desired chain length and linkage type) largely relies on the choice of the appropriate genes.

The proof of principal for the tailor-made fructan was delivered with transgenic sugar beet as shown by Koops et al. (2003). Different combinations of *1-sst* genes and *1-fft* genes resulted in sugar beet transgenics with different inulin profiles. The introduction of *1-sst* and *6 g-fft* from an onion in sugar beet showed that tailor-made branched fructan could also be made in sugar beet (Weyens et al. 2004). Beside the origin of the genes used for biosynthesis, the availability of substrate and competition with other carbohydrate biosynthesis pathways are important for the accumulation of fructan.

1.5.1 Sucrose Availability Determines Fructan Yield

The studies described above show that the host crop is crucial in determining the yield. When comparing the potato plants described by Stoop et al. (2007) with the sugar beet described by Sévenier et al. (1998), both harboring the same 1-SST from a Jerusalem artichoke, it became clear that a big difference in yield characterized these two production platforms. The sugar beet accumulated 40 times more inulin than the potato. Similarly, a 55-time higher inulin yield was found in a starch-deficient maize line expressing 1-SST and 1-FFT from Jerusalem artichoke than in the starch-accumulating parent expressing the same genes (Stoop et al. 2007). Both sugar beet and the starch-deficient maize accumulated high levels of sucrose. This positive correlation between the amount of fructan accumulated and the availability of sucrose is also found by Xue et al. in barley-outcrossing populations (Xue et al. 2012). In contrast to maize, it was found that sucrose is the limiting factor; the results on the potato do not show that sucrose is the limiting factor for inulin biosynthesis. This could also mean, as stated by Morandini et al., that the enzymes require a sufficiently high concentration of sucrose to attain a significant enzyme rate (Morandini 2013). In general, it can be concluded that sucrose availability appears to be a determining factor for the fructan yield in these transgenic plants.

1.5.2 Competition of Fructan Accumulation with Starch

Aside from sucrose, many plants used as a platform for the production of fructan also accumulate starch, which might be a competing carbohydrate synthesis pathway using the same substrate as the fructan biosynthesis pathway. The competition between the endogenous starch and fructan biosynthesis appeared clearly when comparing the amounts of fructan accumulated in transgenic starch-deficient maize (storing sucrose) with the amount accumulated in the transgenic maize (starch accumulating) expressing the same fructosyltransferase gene. While the transgenic starch-deficient maize accumulated on average 20 mg/g FW fructan in the kernel, the starch-accumulating transgenic accumulated 60 times less fructan (Stoop et al. 2007). In studies describing potato as the host for the production of fructan, reduced amounts of starch had been reported (Caimi et al. 1997, Pilon-Smits et al. 1996, van der Meer et al. 1994). Moreover, severe reduction of seed weight was reported in maize expressing *sacB* and the reduction in starch content had been explained by the competition between the sucrose synthase and the SacB protein for sucrose (Caimi et al. 1996). Interestingly, Pilon-Smits and coworkers showed that the expression of *sacB* in the potato caused an inverse correlation of starch with the fructan content (Pilon-Smits et al. 1996). It can be concluded from these studies that the production of fructan in starch-accumulating crops is not favorable because the competition for sucrose between the starch production and the fructan biosynthesis will affect the synthesis of both or one of the storage carbohydrates, leading to a reduction in the potential fructan yield.

1.5.3 Fructan Stability in the New Fructan Storage Organs

Next to the availability of substrate and the presence of competing pathways, the absence of degrading enzymes is important for the production of tailor-made inulin in new platform crops. Enzymes capable of degrading fructan are fructan exohydrolases (FEH) present in fructan-accumulating plants that are important for the remobilization of the stored carbohydrates (Van den Ende et al. 2004). In nonfructan plants FEH is not present, although in the sugar beet (leaf) and Arabidopsis FEH homologous are found (Van den Ende et al. 2004) that could play a role in the degradation of the produced fructan. However, invertases may play a more important role in degrading fructan in putative platform crops. Invertases are β-fructofuranosidases that can hydrolyze β-Fru-containing oligosaccharides (Sturm 1999) like inulin. The accumulation of fructan in sugar beet expressing *1-sst* was not hindered by invertase in the taproot due to the complete absence of the enzyme. In leaves however, the fructan yield was only 8% compared to the root, most probably due to fructan degradation by vacuolar invertase (Sévenier et al. 1998). In rice, invertase activity was found in the panicle and the flag leaf. In rice, it is known that several vacuolar invertases have the ability to degrade fructan polymers. However, in peduncle grown under normal circumstances only one invertase gene is expressed (Ji et al. 2007). The possibility to accumulate large amounts of fructan in the peduncle has to be investigated. For transgenic maize expressing fructan biosynthesis genes, it has been proposed that the inulin breakdown at the late stages of kernel development may be related to invertase activity. In maize fructan and starch biosynthesis depletes the sucrose concentration, which upregulates soluble acid invertase *Ivr-1* (Stoop et al. 2007). A study on the stability of fructan in transgenic potato expressing *1-sst* and *1-fft* showed no degradation during tuber development and maturation. Only cold storage of potato tubers resulted in an almost complete breakdown of the accumulated fructan (Stoop et al. 2007). Storage of the potato tubers at low temperatures is known to cause an accumulation of reducing sugars and sucrose, and increase invertase activity (Zrenner et al. 1996). A study on the stability of fructan in maize also showed that the degradation of fructan could also be the result of mechanical damage of the storage cell compartment, as starch granules may destroy the maize vacuolar compartment where the fructan is synthesized and stored. As a possible result, fructan is degraded in the cytoplasm by invertase. This was supported by the observation that inulin production in "high sucrose–low starch" maize lines results in limited or no inulin degradation (Stoop et al. 2007). In conclusion, these data suggest that invertase activity and morphological changes of the storage organ may play a critical role in determining the stability and level of tailor-made inulin polymers produced in both transgenic monocot and dicot crops.

1.5.4 Fructan Enhances the Drought and Cold Resistance of the Platform Crop

Fructan has several food and nonfood applications and, therefore, is harvested from plants. But could it also be beneficial for the crop or for the transgenic plant producing fructan? It has been hypothesized that fructan accumulation could be beneficial to a plant protecting it from drought and cold stress (Pollock 1986). It was shown in the fructan-accumulating perennial ryegrass that the overexpression of *6-sft* or *1-sst* significantly increased the fructan content and, as a consequence, also increased the freezing tolerance (Hisano et al. 2004). Several studies showed that this property is also present in "new" fructan-accumulating plants. Transgenic tobacco and sugar beet, expressing bacterial *sacB*, showed improved drought resistance (Pilon-Smits et al. 1995, 1999). Tobacco also showed enhanced tolerance to osmotic stress when expressing the *sacB* or wheat fructan genes (Bie et al. 2012, Park et al. 1999). The expression of *1-sst* from wheat and *Lactuca sativa*, respectively, in rice and tobacco enhanced chilling and freezing tolerance (Kawakami et al. 2008, Li et al. 2007).

In most cases, the fructan increased the total soluble carbohydrate composition and in this way enhanced the osmotic value and resistance to stress (Hisano et al. 2004, Li et al. 2007, Pilon-Smits et al. 1995). Other studies report on an increase of carbohydrate content only during the stress period, contributing to the stress tolerance (Pilon-Smits et al. 1995, Schellenbaum et al. 1999). Schellenbaum proposed that as a consequence of the alteration of carbon partitioning due to the stress, more sucrose becomes available for fructan synthesis. Based on a study on proline in transgenic fructan-accumulating potato plants, Knipp and Honermeier proposed that the presence of fructan may affect water stress-induced proline accumulation (Knipp and Honermeier 2006).

In conclusion, several examples of transgenic fructan-producing crops show an enhanced tolerance to stress. This aspect can be advantageously exploited in crops such as sugar beet, potato, and rice that are grown in temperate zones where fluctuations in temperature during the growing season can result in drought, freezing, or chilling stress for the plants.

1.5.5 Platform Crops for Tailor-Made Fructan

A well-suited platform crop for fructan production preferably shows a high productivity, possesses a large storage organ, accumulates sucrose and produces little or no starch. Furthermore, a processing chain for extraction of raw material should be available. Sugar beet is able to accumulate high levels of sucrose (200 mg/g FW), resulting in a yield of 10–14 tons/hectare, which almost certainly explains why sugar beet was also shown to be a successful platform for the production of fructan (Koops et al. 2003, Sévenier et al. 1998, Weyens et al. 2004). A pilot study on the processing of the transgenic sugar beet suggests that the fructan extraction process, currently used for chicory inulin, is also applicable for fructan-producing sugar beet (Weyens et al. 2004).

Another potentially powerful platform crop for fructan production is sugarcane (*Saccharum* spp. L.) because it has a high content in sucrose, 500 mg/g DW in mature internodes (Glassop et al. 2010), and a well-established husbandry and processing chain. The sugar production by sugarcane (6–14 tons/ ha) is comparable to sugar beet. Nicholson successfully introduced *1-sst* from globe artichoke into sugarcane and showed 1-kestose production under field-resembling conditions (Nicholson 2007). The yield, however, was at most 112 nmol/g FW, which is 1000 times lower than in transgenic sugar beet expressing *1-sst*. Additional studies will be necessary to address the full potential of sugar cane as a production platform for fructan.

Rice is another interesting platform crop for the production of fructan, since it is grown under different environmental conditions and in other continents than the crops mentioned previously. It has been shown that rice was able to express *1-sst* and *6-sft* genes. Transgenic rice expressing *1-sst* accumulated up to 16 mg/g FW of fructan in leaves (Kawakami et al. 2008). Although fructan concentrations were low in the transgenic rice compared to other fructan-accumulating crops, an interesting approach might be to produce fructan in the leaves of the rice plants, which are normally a waste product, and in this way add extra value to a rest stream. In that case, a new processing chain should be set up to isolate the fructan from the leaves.

In summary, the crops with the highest potential for the production of fructan are sugar beet, sugarcane and, to a lesser extent, rice.

1.6 Conclusions and Outlook

This chapter gives an overview of the research concerning modification of fructan synthesis in fructan-accumulating plants and the introduction of fructan synthesis in nonfructan-accumulating plants. The effects reported on endogenous storage carbohydrates and phenotypes have been described. The different genes and crops used have been evaluated, with a specific focus on the fructan yield. To date, mostly chicory is used for the commercial production of fructan. Chicory, however, shows some disadvantages, such as the breakdown of inulin in autumn and the so far encountered difficulty to modify the native inulin biosynthesis pathway via genetic modification. Both aspects make this crop less suitable for the synthesis of tailor-made fructan.

The limitations seen in chicory for the production of tailor-made fructan are lacking in the described "new platform crops," although those new crops might not yet compete at the production level with chicory (11 tons inulin/ha). On the contrary, the new crops have the advantage of lacking a breakdown mechanism and providing a clean starting point for the tailor-made fructan production. Sugar beet, sugarcane, and rice seem to be the most promising potential production platforms. The production of fructan in these crops could be increased by optimizing the sugar availability in those crops by selecting cultivars with a natural high sugar content as shown by Xue et al. (2012) or by using starch-deficient mutants, as was shown in starch-deficient maize (Stoop et al. 2007). To date a wide spectrum of genes has been isolated from different species allowing the fine tuning of the tailor-made fructan production. Dependent on the desired chain length, genes with a different affinity for a subclass of fructan could be combined in a transgenic plant. A way to produce longer inulin would be to combine 1-SST activity with two different 1-FFTs, one having high affinity for 1-kestose for the synthesis of short polymers, and the second having a relative higher affinity for longer polymers as an acceptor for fructosyl units for further elongation of the polymers. In practice, the genes used could be the *1-sst* and *1-fft* from *Helianthus tuberosus* (Koops and Jonker 1994, 1996) combined with the high DP *1-fft* from *Echinops ritro* (Vergauwen et al. 2003). The overexpression of transcription factors involved in upregulation of fructan biosynthesis would also be a good strategy to increase fructan yield, as shown by Kooiker et al. (2013) and may also result in longer fructan.

A method to accumulate longer inulin in naturally fructan-accumulating plants would be by downregulation of *feh1* expression via antisense or RNAi strategies or by (site-directed) mutagenesis of the *feh1* genes, resulting in lower exohydrolase activity in the plant and thereby less depolymerization of fructan. New mixed types of fructan with putative interesting properties could be synthesized by combining genes from different classes as was anticipated by Sprenger and coworkers when expressing the barley *6-sft* in chicory (Sprenger et al. 1997). Moreover, protein engineering of the fructosyltransferase enzymes by modifications of the active site might allow the production of more and longer fructan in plants. Engineering of the chicory 1-FFT enzyme would lower the affinity for sucrose and fructose as an acceptor substrate and prevent the back transfer of fructosyl units onto these acceptor molecules, thereby leading to a decrease of the mDP. This could be performed by changing critical amino acids near or in the active site of 1-FFT, in a similar way as was performed by Lasseur et al. when changing a 6G-FFT/1-FFT into an 1-SST (Lasseur et al. 2009). Fructosyltransferase enzyme engineering might allow designing tools for tailor-made fructan synthesis with desired properties such as linkage type and polymer length. We showed that many possibilities exist and that some already have been proven for tailor-made fructan synthesis in crops.

Acknowledgment

The authors thank Celine S. Roet for critically reading the manuscript.

References

Améziane, R., A. Limami, and J.-F. Morot Gaudry. 1994. Fructan biosynthesis and SST activity in excised leaves of *Cichorium intybus* L. *Plant Sciences Meeting*, October 12–14, 1994, Saint Malo, France.

Banguela, A., J. G. Arrieta, R. Rodríguez et al. 2011. High levan accumulation in transgenic tobacco plants expressing the *Gluconacetobacter diazotrophicus* levansucrase gene. *J Biotechnol* 154:93–8.

Bauer, R., C. Basson, J. Bekker et al. 2012. Reuteran and levan as carbohydrate sinks in transgenic sugarcane. *Planta* 236:1803–15.

Bie, X., K. Wang, M. She et al. 2012. Combinational transformation of three wheat genes encoding fructan biosynthesis enzymes confers increased fructan content and tolerance to abiotic stresses in tobacco. *Plant Cell Rep* 31:2229–38.

Blacklow, W., B. Darbyshire, and P. Pheloung. 1984. Fructans polymerised and depolymerised in the internodes of winter wheat as grain-filling progressed. *Plant Sci Lett* 36:213–8.

Bonnett, G. D., I. M. Sims, R. J. Simpson, and A. J. Cairns. 1997. Structural diversity of fructan in relation to the taxonomy of the Poaceae. *New Phytol* 136:11–7.

Burne, R. A., Y.-Y. M. Chen, D. L. Wexler, H. Kuramitsu, and W. H. Bowen. 1996. Cariogenicity of *Streptococcus mutans* strains with defects in fructan metabolism assessed in a program-fed specific-pathogen-free rat model. *J Dent Res* 75:1572–7.

Caimi, P. G., L. M. McCole, T. M. Klein, and H. P. Hershey. 1997. Cytosolic expression of the *Bacillus amyloliquefaciens* SacB protein inhibits tissue development in transgenic tobacco and potato. *New Phytol* 136:19–28.

Caimi, P. G., L. M. McCole, T. M. Klein, and P. S. Kerr. 1996. Fructan accumulation and sucrose metabolism in transgenic maize endosperm expressing a *Bacillus amyloliquefaciens* SacB gene. *Plant Physiol* 110:355–63.

Cairns, A. J., G. D. Bonnett, J. A. Gallagher, R. J. Simpson, and C. J. Pollock. 1997. Fructan biosynthesis in excised leaves of *Lolium temulentum* VII. Sucrose and fructan hydrolysis by a fructan-polymerizing enzyme preparation. *New Phytol* 136:61–72.

Cote, G. L. and J. Ahlgren. 1993. Metabolism in microorganisms, Part I. Levan and levansucrase. In *Science and Technology of Fructans*, eds. M. Suzuki and N. Chatterton, 141–168. Boca Raton, FL: CRC Press.

De Roover, J., K. Vandenbranden, A. Van Laere, and W. Van den Ende. 2000. Drought induces fructan synthesis and 1-SST (sucrose: sucrose fructosyltransferase) in roots and leaves of chicory seedlings (*Cichorium intybus* L.). *Planta* 210:808–14.

Dedonder, R. 1966. Levansucrase from *Bacillus subtilis*. In *Methods in Enzymology*, eds. E. F. Neufeld and V. Ginsburg, 500–505. New York: Academic Press.

del Viso, F., A. F. Puebla, C. M. Fusari et al. 2009. Molecular characterization of a putative sucrose: Fructan 6-fructosyltransferase (6-SFT) of the cold-resistant patagonian grass *Bromus pictus* associated with fructan accumulation under low temperatures. *Plant Cell Physiol* 50:489–503.

Desmet, D. 1997. Histologische studie van de witloofwortelstructuur en van *in vitro* geinduceerde meristemen, Toegepaste plantenwetenschappen, Katholieke Universiteit leuven, Leuven, Belgium.

Druart, N., J. De Roover, W. Van den Ende et al. 2001. Sucrose assimilation during early developmental stages of chicory (*Cichorium intybus* L.) plants. *Planta* 212:436–43.

Duchateau, N., K. Bortlik, U. Simmen, A. Wiemken, and P. Bancal. 1995. Sucrose: Fructan 6-fructosyltransferase, a key enzyme for diverting carbon from sucrose to fructan in barley leaves. *Plant Physiol* 107:1249–55.

Ebskamp, M. J. M., I. M. van der Meer, B. A. Spronk, P. J. Weisbeek, and S. C. M. Smeekens. 1994. Accumulation of fructose polymers in transgenic tobacco. *Nature Biotech* 12:272–5.

Edelman, J. and T. Jefford. 1968. The mechanism of fructosan metabolism in higher plants as exemplified in *Helianthus tuberosus*. *New Phytol* 67:517–31.

Ernst, M. 1991. Histochemische Untersuchungen auf Inulin, Stärke und Kallose bei *Helianthus tuberosus* L. (Topinambur). *Angewandte Botanik* 65:319–30.

Glassop, D., L. Ryan, G. Bonnett, and A. Rae. 2010. The complement of soluble sugars in the *Saccharum* complex. *Trop Plant Biol* 3:110–22.

Hellwege, E. M., S. Czapla, A. Jahnke, L. Willmitzer, and A. G. Heyer. 2000. Transgenic potato (*Solanum tuberosum*) tubers synthesize the full spectrum of inulin molecules naturally occurring in globe artichoke (*Cynara scolymus*) roots. *Proc Natl Acad Sci USA* 97:8699–704.

Hisano, H., A. Kanazawa, A. Kawakami et al. 2004. Transgenic perennial ryegrass plants expressing wheat fructosyltransferase genes accumulate increased amounts of fructan and acquire increased tolerance on a cellular level to freezing. *Plant Sci* 167:861–8.

Jenkins, C. L. D., A. J. Snow, R. J. Simpson et al. 2002. Fructan formation in transgenic white clover expressing a fructosyltransferase from *Streptococcus salivarius*. *Func Plant Biol* 29:1287–98.

Ji, X., W. Van den Ende, L. Schroeven et al. 2007. The rice genome encodes two vacuolar invertases with fructan exohydrolase activity but lacks the related fructan biosynthesis genes of the Pooideae. *New Phytol* 173:50–62.

Kasapis, S., E. R. Morris, M. Gross, and K. Rudolph. 1994. Solution properties of levan polysaccharide from *Pseudomonas syringae pv. phaseolicola*, and its possible primary role as a blocker of recognition during pathogenesis. *Carbohydr Polym* 23:55–64.

Kawakami, A., Y. Sato, and M. Yoshida. 2008. Genetic engineering of rice capable of synthesizing fructans and enhancing chilling tolerance. *J Exp Bot* 59:793–802.

Knipp, G. and B. Honermeier. 2006. Effect of water stress on proline accumulation of genetically modified potatoes (*Solanum tuberosum* L.) generating fructans. *J Plant Physiol* 163:392–7.

Koch, K., R. Andersson, I. Rydberg, and P. Åman. 1999. Influence of harvest date on inulin chain length distribution and sugar profile for six chicory (*Cichorium intybus* L.) cultivars. *J Sci Food Agric* 79:1503–6.

Kooiker, M., J. Drenth, D. Glassop, C. L. McIntyre, and G.-P. Xue. 2013. TaMYB13-1, a R2R3 MYB transcription factor, regulates the fructan synthetic pathway and contributes to enhanced fructan accumulation in bread wheat. *J Exp Bot* 64:3681–96.

Koops, A. J. and H. H. Jonker. 1994. Purification and characterization of the enzymes of fructan biosynthesis in tubers of *Helianthus tuberosus* 'Colombia': I. Fructan: Fructan fructosyl transferase. *J Exp Bot* 45(11):1623–31.

Koops, A. J. and H. H. Jonker. 1996. Purification and characterization of the enzymes of fructan biosynthesis in tubers of *Helianthus tuberosus Colombia* (II. Purification of sucrose: Sucrose 1-fructosyltransferase and reconstitution of fructan synthesis *in vitro* with purified sucrose: Sucrose 1-fructosyltransferase and fructan:fructan 1-fructosyltransferase). *Plant Physiol* 110:1167–75.

Koops, A. J., R. E. Sévenier, A. J. Van Tunen, and L. De Leenheer. 2003. Transgenic plants presenting a modified inulin producing profile. Patent WO1999054480 A1, USA.

Kusch, U. 2009. Dissecting the regulation of fructan active enzymes in *Cichorium intybus*. PhD thesis, Heidelberg Institute of Plant Sciences, University of Heidelberg.

Kusch, U., S. Greiner, H. Steininger et al. 2009. Dissecting the regulation of fructan metabolism in chicory (*Cichorium intybus* L.) hairy roots. *New Phytol* 184:127–40.

Lasseur, B., L. Schroeven, W. Lammens et al. 2009. Transforming a fructan: Fructan 6G-fructosyltransferase from perennial ryegrass into a sucrose: Sucrose 1-fructosyltransferase. *Plant Physiol* 149:327–39.

Li, H.-J., A.-F. Yang, X.-C. Zhang, F. Gao, and J.-R. Zhang. 2007. Improving freezing tolerance of transgenic tobacco expressing sucrose: Sucrose 1-fructosyltransferase gene from *Lactuca sativa*. *Plant Cell Tissue Organ Cult* 89:37–48.

Maleux, K. and W. Van den Ende. 2007. Levans in excised leaves of *Dactylis glomerata*: Effects of light, sugars, temperature and senescence. *J Plant Biol* 50:671–80.

Martínez-Noël, G., V. J. Nagaraj, G. Caló, A. Wiemken, and H. G. Pontis. 2007. Sucrose regulated expression of a Ca^{2+}-dependent protein kinase (TaCDPK1) gene in excised leaves of wheat. *Plant Physiol Biochem* 45:410–9.

Martínez-Noël, G. M. A., J. A. Tognetti, G. L. Salerno, A. Wiemken, and H. G. Pontis. 2009. Protein phosphatase activity and sucrose-mediated induction of fructan synthesis in wheat. *Planta* 230:1071–9.

Michiels, A., A. Van Laere, W. Van den Ende, and M. Tucker. 2004. Expression analysis of a chicory fructan 1-exohydrolase gene reveals complex regulation by cold. *J Exp Bot* 55:1325–33.

Morandini, P. 2013. Control limits for accumulation of plant metabolites: Brute force is no substitute for understanding. *Plant Biotechnol J* 11:253–67.

Morcuende, R., S. Kostadinova, P. Pérez et al. 2004. Nitrate is a negative signal for fructan synthesis, and the fructosyltransferase-inducing trehalose inhibits nitrogen and carbon assimilation in excised barley leaves. *New Phytol* 161:749–59.

Müller, J., R. A. Aeschbacher, N. Sprenger, T. Boller, and A. Wiemken. 2000. Disaccharide-mediated regulation of sucrose: Fructan-6-fructosyltransferase, a key enzyme of fructan synthesis in barley leaves. *Plant Physiol* 123:265–74.

Nagaraj, V. J., R. Riedl, T. Boller, A. Wiemken, and A. D. Meyer. 2001. Light and sugar regulation of the barley sucrose: Fructan 6-fructosyltransferase promoter. *J Plant Physiol* 158:1601–7.

Nicholson, T. L. 2007. Carbon turnover and sucrose metabolism in the culm of transgenic sugarcane producing 1-kestose. PhD thesis, University of Stellenbosch, Stellenbosch.

Obenland, D. M., U. Simmen, T. Boller, and A. Wiemken. 1991. Regulation of sucrose-sucrose-fructosyltransferase in barley leaves. *Plant Physiol* 97:811–3.

Pan, W., Y. Sunayama, Y. Nagata et al. 2009. Cloning of a CDNA encoding the sucrose: Sucrose 1-fructosyltransferase (1-SST) from yacon and its expression in transgenic rice. *Biotechnol Biotech Eq* 23:1479–84.

Park, J. M., S.-Y. Kwon, K.-B. Song et al. 1999. Transgenic tobacco plants expressing the bacterial levansucrase gene show enhanced tolerance to osmotic stress. *J Microbiol Biotechnol* 9:213–8.

Pilon-Smits, E., M. Ebskamp, M. J. Paul et al. 1995. Improved performance of transgenic fructan-accumulating tobacco under drought stress. *Plant Physiol* 107:125–30.

Pilon-Smits, E. A. H., M. J. M. Ebskamp, M. J. W. Jeuken et al. 1996. Microbial fructan production in transgenic potato plants and tubers. *Ind Crops Prod* 5:35–46.

Pilon-Smits, E. A. H., N. Terry, T. Sears, and K. van Dun. 1999. Enhanced drought resistance in fructan-producing sugar beet. *Plant Physiol Biochem* 37:313–7.

Pollock, C. J. 1986. Fructans and the metabolism of sucrose in vascular plants. *New Phytol* 104:1–24.

Pontis, H. G., P. González, and E. Etxeberria. 2002. Transport of 1-kestose across the tonoplast of Jerusalem artichoke tubers. *Phytochemistry* 59:241–7.

Rao, R. S. P., J. R. Andersen, G. Dionisio, and B. Boelt. 2011. Fructan accumulation and transcription of candidate genes during cold acclimation in three varieties of *Poa pratensis*. *J Plant Physiol* 168:344–51.

Ritsema, T., D. Brodmann, S. H. Diks et al. 2009. Are small GTPases signal hubs in sugar-mediated induction of fructan biosynthesis? *PLoS ONE* 4:e6605.

Röber, M., K. Geider, B. Müller-Röber, and L. Willmitzer. 1996. Synthesis of fructans in tubers of transgenic starch-deficient potato plants does not result in an increased allocation of carbohydrates. *Planta* 199:528–36.

Ruuska, S. A., D. C. Lewis, G. Kennedy et al. 2008. Large scale transcriptome analysis of the effects of nitrogen nutrition on accumulation of stem carbohydrate reserves in reproductive stage wheat. *Plant Mol Biol* 66:15–32.

Schellenbaum, L., N. Sprenger, H. Schüepp, A. Wiemken, and T. Boller. 1999. Effects of drought, transgenic expression of a fructan synthesizing enzyme and of mycorrhizal symbiosis on growth and soluble carbohydrate pools in tobacco plants. *New Phytol* 142:67–77.

Sévenier, R. E., R. D. Hall, I. M. van der Meer et al. 1998. High level fructan accumulation in a transgenic sugar beet. *Nat Biotech* 16:843–6.

Sévenier, R. E., J. van Arkel, J. C. Hakkert, and A. J. Koops. 2006. Fructan: Nutritional significance, application, biosynthesis, molecular biology and genetic engineering. In *Plant Genetic Engineering, Metabolic Engineering and Molecular Farming*, ed. P. W. Jaiwal, 339–356. Houston: Studium Press.

Sobolev, A. P., A. L. Segre, D. Giannino et al. 2007. Strong increase of foliar inulin occurs in transgenic lettuce plants (*Lactuca sativa* L.) overexpressing the asparagine synthetase a gene from *Escherichia coli*. *J Agric Food Chem* 55:10827–31.

Sprenger, N., L. Schellenbaum, K. van Dun, T. Boller, and A. Wiemken. 1997. Fructan synthesis in transgenic tobacco and chicory plants expressing barley sucrose: Fructan 6-fructosyltransferase. *FEBS Lett* 400:355–8.

Stoop, J. M., J. Van Arkel, J. C. Hakkert et al. 2007. Developmental modulation of inulin accumulation in storage organs of transgenic maize and transgenic potato. *Plant Sci* 173:172–81.

Sturm, A. 1999. Invertases. Primary structures, functions, and roles in plant development and sucrose partitioning. *Plant Physiol* 121:1–8.

Suzuki, T., T. Maeda, S. Grant, G. Grant, and P. Sporns. 2012. Confirmation of fructans biosynthesized *in vitro* from [1–13C]glucose in asparagus tissues using MALDI–TOF MS and ESI–MS. *J Plant Physiol* 170:715–22.

Trujillo, L. E., J. G. Arrieta, G. A. Enríquez et al. 2000. Strategies for fructan production in transgenic sugarcane (*Saccharomyces* spp. L.) and sweet potato (*Ipomoea batata* L.) plants expressing the *Acetobacter diazotrophicus* levansucrase. In *Developments in Plant Genetics and Breeding*, ed. A. D. Arencibia, 194–198. Amsterdam: Elsevier.

Turk, S. C. H. J., K. De Roos, P. A. Scotti et al. 1997. The vacuolar sorting domain of sporamin transports GUS, but not levansucrase, to the plant vacuole. *New Phytol* 136:29–38.

van Arkel, J., R. Vergauwen, R. Sévenier et al. 2012. Sink filling, inulin metabolizing enzymes and carbohydrate status in field grown chicory (*Cichorium intybus* L.). *J Plant Physiol* 169:1520–9.

Van den Ende, W., M. Coopman, S. Clerens et al. 2011. Unexpected presence of graminan- and levan-type fructans in the evergreen frost-hardy eudicot *Pachysandra terminalis* (Buxaceae): Purification, cloning, and functional analysis of a 6-SST/6-SFT enzyme. *Plant Physiol* 155:603–14.

Van den Ende, W., B. De Coninck, and A. Van Laere. 2004. Plant fructan exohydrolases: A role in signaling and defense? *Trends Plant Sci* 9:523–8.

Van den Ende, W., J. De Roover, and A. Van Laere. 1999. Effect of nitrogen concentration on fructan and fructan metabolizing enzymes in young chicory plants (*Cichorium intybus*). *Physiol Plantarum* 105:2–8.

Van den Ende, W., A. Michiels, J. De Roover, and A. Van Laere. 2002. Fructan biosynthetic and breakdown enzymes in dicots evolved from different invertases. Expression of fructan genes throughout chicory development. *Sci World J* 2:1281–95.

Van den Ende, W., A. Michiels, D. Van Wonterghem, R. Vergauwen, and A. Van Laere. 2000. Cloning, developmental, and tissue-specific expression of sucrose: Sucrose 1-fructosyl transferase from *Taraxacum officinale*. Fructan localization in roots. *Plant Physiol* 123:71–80.

Van den Ende, W., A. Mintiens, H. Speleers, A. A. Onuoha, and A. Van Laere. 1996. The metabolism of fructans in roots of *Cichorium intybus* during growth, storage and forcing. *New Phytologist* 132(4):555–63.

Van den Ende, W., J. D. Roover, and A. Van Laere. 1996. *In vitro* synthesis of fructofuranosyl-only oligosaccharides from inulin and fructose by purified chicory root fructan: Fructan fructosyl transferase. *Physiol Plantarum* 97:346–52.

van der Meer, I. M., M. Ebskamp, R. Visser, P. J. Weisbeek, and S. Smeekens. 1994. Fructan as a new carbohydrate sink in transgenic potato plants. *Plant Cell Online* 6:561–70.

Van der Meer, I. M., A. J. Koops, J. C. Hakkert, and A. J. van Tunen. 1998. Cloning of the fructan biosynthesis pathway of Jerusalem artichoke. *Plant J* 15:489–500.

Van Wonterghem, D., W. Van den Ende, and A. Van Laere. 1999. *Proceedings of the 8th Seminar on Inulin*, Lille, France.

Vergauwen, R., A. Van Laere, and W. Van den Ende. 2003. Properties of fructan: Fructan 1-fructosyltransferases from chicory and globe thistle, two Asteracean plants storing greatly different types of inulin. *Plant Physiol* 133:391–401.

Verhaest, M., W. Lammens, K. Le Roy et al. 2007. Insights into the fine architecture of the active site of chicory fructan 1-Exohydrolase: 1-Kestose as substrate vs sucrose as inhibitor. *New Phytol* 174:90–100.

Vieira, C. and R. Figueiredo-Ribeiro. 1993. Fructose-containing carbohydrates in the tuberous root of *Gomphrena macrocephala* St.-Hil. (Amaranthaceae) at different phenological phases. *Plant Cell Environ* 16:919–28.

Vijn, I., A. Van Dijken, N. Sprenger et al. 1997. Fructan of the inulin neoseries is synthesized in transgenic chicory plants (*Cichorium intybus* L.) harbouring onion (*Allium cepa* L.) fructan: Fructan 6G-fructosyltransferase. *Plant J* 11:387–98.

Wei, J.-Z., J. N. Chatterton, and S. R. Larson. 2001. Expression of sucrose: Fructan 6-fructosyltransferase (6-SFT) and myo-inositol 1-phosphate synthase (MIPS) genes in barley (*Hordeum vulgare*) leaves. *J Plant Physiol* 158:635–43.

Weyens, G., T. Ritsema, K. Van Dun et al. 2004. Production of tailor-made fructans in sugar beet by expression of onion fructosyltransferase genes. *Plant Biotechnol J* 2:321–7.

Winter, D., B. Vinegar, H. Nahal et al. 2007. An electronic fluorescent pictograph browser for exploring and analyzing large-scale biological data sets. *PLoS ONE* 2:e718.

Winters, A. L., J. H. H. Williams, D. S. Thomas, and C. J. Pollock. 1994. Changes in gene-expression in response to sucrose accumulation in leaf tissue of *Lolium temulentum* L. *New Phytol* 128:591–600.

Wittouck, D., K. Boone, S. Bulcke et al. 2002. Industriële cichorei. Rumbeke: Onderzoeks- en voorlichtingscentrum voor land- en tuinbouw. *Rumbeke* 1:79–84.

Xue, G.-P., M. Kooiker, J. Drenth, and C. L. McIntyre. 2011. TaMYB13 is a transcriptional activator of fructosyltransferase genes involved in β-2,6-linked fructan synthesis in wheat. *Plant J* 68:857–70.

Xue, G. P., J. Drenth, D. Glassop, M. Kooiker, and C. L. McIntyre. 2012. Dissecting the molecular basis of the contribution of source strength to high fructan accumulation in wheat. *Plant Mol Biol* 81:71–92.

Ye, X. Y., X. W. Wu, H. Z. Zhao et al. 2001. Altered fructan accumulation in transgenic *Lolium multiflorum* plants expressing a *Bacillus subtilis sacB* gene. *Plant Cell Rep* 20:205–12.

Zrenner, R., K. Schüler, and U. Sonnewald. 1996. Soluble acid invertase determines the hexose-to-sucrose ratio in cold-stored potato tubers. *Planta* 198:246–52.

CHAPTER **2**

Dietary Fiber and Its Polyphenol Cotravelers in Healthy Eating

Seeking the Key Component in Apple Fruit

ANTONIO JIMÉNEZ-ESCRIG

Contents

2.1 Dietary Fiber and Its Cotravelers in Fruits   31
    2.1.1 Introduction   31
    2.1.2 Precision on the Undigestible Residue Term   32
    2.1.3 Structural Analysis of Polysaccharides in Cell Walls
           of Dicotyledonous Plants   33
    2.1.4 Phenolic Compounds in Cell Walls of Dicotyledonous Plants   34
2.2 Specific Case of the Apple Fruit (*Malus* × *domestica* Borkh.,
    Rosaceae)   36
    2.2.1 Introduction   36
    2.2.2 *In Vitro* and Animal Models   37
2.3 Conclusions   39
References   40

2.1 Dietary Fiber and Its Cotravelers in Fruits

2.1.1 Introduction

Epidemiological evidences support the concept that diets rich in fruit and vegetables promote health and attenuate or delay the onset of chronic diseases. The range of protective effects ascribed to plant foods is particularly large, especially against consequences of the plurimetabolic syndrome (cardiovascular diseases, diabetes, obesity, renal failure) as well as against some cancers and long-term disabling conditions such as osteoporosis (Aprikian et al. 2003). Earlier epidemiological studies initially associated these health-promoting effects with the presence of dietary fiber, unsaturated fatty acids, certain minerals, and vitamins (Blasa et al. 2010, Cummings et al. 2009). Actually, the health-protective mechanisms of dietary fiber intake are under close examination in the search for a more complete picture taking into account that dietary fiber facilitates the passage of specific material through the digestive tract, which includes other molecules bound to polysaccharides (Jiménez-Escrig et al. 2013, Jones 2010, Kaczmarczyka et al. 2012, Nyström et al. 2007, Saura-Calixto 2011). The association between dietary vegetable intake and chronic diseases is in part attributed to a wide range of plant secondary compounds called phytochemicals, along with dietary fiber. These phytochemicals include lignans, polyphenols, carotenoids, plant sterols, and organosulfur compounds, among other bioactive compounds. As a consequence, an increased consumption of products of vegetable origin has been recommended (Kris-Etherton et al. 2002). Adequate dietary fiber intake in the United States/Canada is set at 31 g/day by the Food and Nutrition Board (FNB), whereas the daily recommended intake for dietary fiber given by the FAO/WHO and the EURODIET project is about 25 g/day (Lunn and Buttriss 2007). In contrast, the per capita intake of dietary fiber in Western countries range is 10–25 g and does not cover the recommendations for the intake of dietary fiber as given by health institutions.

It must be noted that much of the experimental research on the relationship between diet and the health protection exerted by food from vegetable sources has focused on isolated bioactive dietary constituents, such as tocopherols, flavonoids, folates, saponins, or dietary fiber. However, few investigations have simultaneously examined dietary fiber and bioactive compounds in fruits (Eastwood and Kritchevsky 2005). In this sense, there is some disagreement about which entity is the responsible for reduced disease risk: the dietary fiber, the components associated with the fiber residue, or the food matrix with the fiber and the components (Jones 2010).

This chapter will describe health-promoting effects, measured through *in vitro* and rat models, of dietary fiber from peeled and whole fruit, focusing on the concomitant effects of the dietary fiber and its polyphenol cotravelers. The apple fruit was chosen as a temperate fruit model to describe these effects.

2.1.2 Precision on the Undigestible Residue Term

Dietary fiber is not a single compound but a combination of chemical substances with varied composition and structure (Ferguson and Harris 2003, Jiménez-Escrig and Sánchez-Muniz 2000). The definition of dietary fiber has evolved since the publication of Trowell's papers; he defined the new term "dietary fiber" as that portion of food derived from the cell walls of plants and is digested very poorly by human beings (Trowell 1972). Trowell, as a medical doctor, introduces this physiological approach to fiber as a synonym of unavailable carbohydrates to replace the term crude fiber, which is defined as the food residue left after chemical sequential extraction with dilute acid and dilute alkali (Van Soest 1978). However, the debate over developing a comprehensive definition for dietary fiber continues until today (Cummings et al. 2009, Eastwood and Kritchevsky 2005, EU 2008, Jones 2012). A general feature of this debate is whether a wider definition of fiber, including the chemical compounds naturally associated with the structural polysaccharides compounds, should be approved or not. An antioxidant dietary fiber is defined as a product containing a significant amount of natural antioxidants associated with the fiber matrix (Jiménez-Escrig et al. 2001, Saura-Calixto 1998).

2.1.3 Structural Analysis of Polysaccharides in Cell Walls of Dicotyledonous Plants

As Renard et al. (2001) reported, plant cell walls are made up of a complex, porous polysaccharidic material. In fruits and vegetables, they can be described by the type I model of Carpita and Gibeaut (1993) as composed of three interpenetrating but not interconnected networks: a cellulose/xyloglucan framework (50% dry weight (dw)) is embedded in a pectin matrix (25–40% dw), locked into shape by cross-linked glycosylated proteins and lignin (1% dw) (Somerville et al. 2004). Thus, the structural analysis of cell wall polysaccharides in dicotyledons has resulted in the compilation of average structures for the major cell wall polysaccharides: cellulose, hemicellulose, and pectins. Cellulose is present as long unbranched microfibrils composed of hydrogen-bonded chains of 1,4′-β-D-glucose. Hemicelluloses are branched polysaccharides containing backbones of neutral sugars that are capable of hydrogen bonding to the surface of cellulose fibrils. Hemicelluloses, although they share the β-1,4′-diequatorial glycosidic linkage found in cellulose, are more flexible molecules because they have only one of the two interresidue hydrogen bonds that flank the glycosidic linkage in cellulose (Jarvis 2011). The prominent hemicelluloses in fruits are xyloglucans and glucomannans, consisting of 1,4′-linked β-D-glucose units, with 1,2′-linked β-D-xylose side chains or 1,2′-linked β-D-mannose, respectively (Waldron et al. 2003). Pectins from cell walls, far from being just one molecule, are a family of polysaccharides with common features. The most familiar and predominant member is homogalacturonan (HG), composed predominantly of a homopolymer of partially methyl-esterified 1,4-linked α-D-galacturonic acid (GalA), which is known as the "smooth region" of the pectins. A second well-characterized component constitutes the "hairy" region of pectins or rhamnogalacturonan I regions (RGI). Pectins can also contain, with much less frequency, xylogalacturonan and rhamnogalacturonan II (RGII), the latter of which is a highly complex branched that constitutes β-1,4-arabinans, galactans, and arabinogalactans attached to the rhamnose residues. Alkali treatment breaks down the HG backbone and acid treatment cleaves the neutral sugars, preferentially leaving galactans and arabinogalactans. Recent studies on the bioactivity of pectins are beginning to emphasize the potential importance of the galactan containing RGI regions (Maxwell et al. 2012, Ridley 2001, Yapo 2011). The cellulose microfibrils are insoluble because the glucane chains aggregate by means of hydrogen bonding and van der Waals forces to produce crystalline structures of parallel chains. The other polysaccharides are secreted as soluble polymers that diffuse within the aqueous environment of the cell (Somerville et al. 2004).

Plant cell walls are a complex structure surrounding the cytoplasmic membrane of the cells, thus defining their form and their size. They constitute a complex porous material, with specific surface and porosity; in fruits such as apples, they are composed of >90% polysaccharides and are highly hydrophilic (Le Bourvellec and Renard 2005).

Much of the experimental research on the relationship between diet and the health protection exerted by food from vegetable sources has focused on isolated dietary constituents such as tocopherols, flavonoids, folates, saponins, or dietary fiber. The cell wall structure has often been described as a network of cellulosic microfibrils embedded in a matrix of noncellulosic polysaccharides and associated compounds. Some recent studies have pointed out that fiber derived from cereals (Nyström et al. 2007) and fruits (Pinelo et al. 2006) is associated with varying levels of protein, carotenoids, plant sterols, and polyphenols. Few investigations have simultaneously examined dietary fiber and bioactive compounds (Eastwood and Kritchevsky 2005).

2.1.4 Phenolic Compounds in Cell Walls of Dicotyledonous Plants

Polyphenols are natural constituents of plants, some of which are characterized by their high propensity to bind to macromolecules (Watrelot et al. 2013). Two mechanisms of association have been proposed to explain the formation of the complex polysaccharide–phenol entity in the cell walls: (1) Hydrogen bonds between the hydroxyl groups of phenols and the oxygen atoms of the cross-linking ether bonds of sugars present in the cell wall polysaccharides, which enables dextran gels to encapsulate phenols inside their pores; and (2) hydrophobic interactions occurring as a result of the ability of some polysaccharides to develop secondary structures. The formed hydrophobic pockets may be able to encapsulate and complex phenols (Pinelo et al. 2006). Thus, it may be speculated that various phenolic substances, including flavonoids and tannins in dicotyledonous skins, may be deposited and "caught" in the lignin–polysaccharide matrix during the free radical reactions taking place during the lignification process or during the formation of the ether links that interlock the lignin–polysaccharide structures in the cell wall (Pinelo et al. 2008).

However, phenols occurring in plants are not always associated with the plant cell walls, and recent works have demonstrated that phenols can also be found within the cell cytoplasm, inside the cellular vacuoles, or even in (or very near) the cell nucleus. Specifically, it has been reported that polyphenols located within the vacuoles are enclosed by tonoplast and cytoplasmic lipid membranes, which are in turn encapsulated by the plant cell wall. These polyphenols are not only present in free solution inside the vacuoles, but may be linked to the protein matrix forming the vacuolar inclusions (Markham et al. 2001, Pinelo et al. 2008, Rodríguez et al. 2004). Renard and coworkers stated that although some polyphenols can be constitutive of cell walls, such as lignin and ferulic acid in Poaceae or Chenopodiaceae, polyphenols are mainly located in vacuoles (Le Bourvellec et al. 2009). The complexes polysaccharides/polyphenols described in cell walls by Selvendran (1985), at least in the case of the apple cell wall, are artifacts of the isolation procedure related to the adsorption of intracellular polyphenols.

In this sense, fruit processing (such as apple pressing in juices or cider production), environmental stress (such as pathogen attack or injury), and chewing or digestion, involving all of them tissue disruption, leading to, decompartmentalization, and destructuring of tissue cells. As a consequence, compounds contained within the cellular organelles and cytoplasm, such as polyphenols in vacuoles, breach the cellular frontiers and partially bind to extracellular cell walls, forming noncovalently polyphenol–cell wall bonds (Le Bourvellec et al. 2007). This selective mechanism of cell wall-procyanidin adsorption involves weak associations, more precisely a combination of H-bonding and hydrophobic interactions. The binding is fast and spontaneous, and thus will occur whenever tissue degradation happens (Le Bourvellec et al. 2005, 2009, 2012). The structure of the cell walls, a complex porous structure with more or less hydrophilic/hydrophobic domains, played a significant role, as opposed to specific cell wall polysaccharides (Renard et al. 2001).

Among cell wall polysaccharides, pectin displays the strongest affinity to procyanidins. Specifically, the use of dynamic light scattering demonstrates the aggregation of polyphenols in the presence of a fraction of pectin containing a high amount of rhamnogalacturonan II (RGII). When isothermal titration calorimetry is used, strong affinities are recorded between commercial apple pectins (mainly HG) and procyanidins (Watrelot et al. 2013).

In intact plant tissues, cell walls, polyphenols and polyphenoloxidases (PPOs) are present in separated compartments (Renard et al. 2001). Oxidation is one of the consequences of plant tissue destructuration. It allows the enzyme PPO, originally in the plasts, and the substrates (polyphenols and oxygen) to come in contact. In the apple, the main substrates of PPO are caffeoylquinic acid and hydroxycinnamic acid. Procyanidins are not the substrate of PPO, but their primary oxidation entities o-quinones are. The resulting oxidation procyanidins products could have different affinities toward cell walls as compared to the native molecules, and could form covalent bonds with cell walls (Le Bourvellec et al. 2009).

Thus, taking into account that in order for polyphenols in fruits and vegetables to be available for absorption (i.e., become bioavailable) within the human gastrointestinal tract, these compounds must be released from the plant cell (i.e., be bioaccessible). It needs to be stressed that when cells rupture during the processing or oral mastication of fruits and vegetables, the contents, including polyphenols, of the cell will be released. Consequently, interactions between different polyphenols and the food matrix, including the plant cell wall, are likely to affect the bioaccessibility (i.e., the amount released from the food matrix prior to absorption) of polyphenols. This could potentially impact the nutritional content and functional potential of diets (Cheynier 2005, Padayachee et al. 2012a,b, Palafox-Carlos et al. 2011).

Bioactive compounds must be released from the food matrix and modified in the gastrointestinal tract before becoming bioavailable. Bioavailability is defined as the fraction of ingested nutrient that is absorbed and utilized. The overall bioavailability process includes gastrointestinal digestion, absorption, and metabolism (Rodriguez-Roque et al. 2013).

2.2 Specific Case of the Apple Fruit (*Malus × domestica* Borkh., Rosaceae)

2.2.1 Introduction

Apples are one of the most important tree fruit crops grown in the midlatitude climate zones (Cuthbertson et al. 2012). It has been estimated that apples could provide 20–25% of the per capita consumption of fruit polyphenols in the United States as well as 10–30% of the daily intake of fiber and potassium, depending on individual eating habits (Aprikian et al. 2003).

There is a general belief in the health-promoting properties of apples, exemplified in the old saying "an apple a day keeps the doctor away" (Weichselbaum et al. 2010). Apples contain several nutrients and health-promoting constituents, including sugars, sugar-alcohols, organic acids, vitamin C, carotenoids, soluble and insoluble dietary fiber, and polyphenols. Among the polyphenols present in apples are procyanidins (oligo or polymers of flavan-3-ols, (+)-catechin, and mainly (−)-epicatechin linked by interflavan bond), accounting for more than 50% of total polyphenols. The other three main classes of polyphenols are phenolic acids (caffeoylquinic acids), dihydrochalcones (glycosides of phloretins), and monomeric flavan-3-ols (again, mainly (−)-epicatechins) and to a minor extent hydroxycinnamic acids (chlorogenic acids), flavonols (quercetin glycosides), and anthocyanins (Guyot et al. 2003, Lotito and Frei 2004, Neveu et al. 2010, Schieber et al. 2001). The contents of these polyphenols are strongly dependent on their varieties and their maturity. In particular, the total phenolic content, proanthocyanidin, and flavonoid are found in unripe apples in amounts 10 times higher than in ripe apples (Alonso-Salces et al. 2005, Zheng et al. 2009). Interestingly, polyphenols in apples are generally more highly concentrated in the peel than in the pulp. It has been suggested that this high polyphenol concentration of the peel is mainly caused by the defensive role of polyphenols against pathogens, which mainly act on the skin (Lamperi et al. 2008).

Interestingly, the health effects of apples, especially their cholesterol-lowering properties, are ascribed to the combined fiber and polyphenol fractions (Le Bourvellec et al. 2011). In this sense, what has been evidenced is the concept of interaction or synergy between two nutrients in the case of apple pectin and polyphenol fractions; in the case of lowering plasma and liver cholesterol and triglycerides in a rat model, they are more effective in combination than either the apple pectin alone or the apple polyphenol alone (Aprikian et al. 2003).

2.2.2 In Vitro and Animal Models

The relation of hydroxycinnamic acids in the peel and the peeled fruit of Golden delicious varieties have been studied in some detail by *in vitro* assays (Gorinstein et al. 2002). A significantly higher amount of ferulic acid, p-coumaric acid, and caffeic acid is reported in apples with the peel than in peeled apples. Also, the total polyphenols were significantly higher in peels. In addition, Gorinstein and coworkers have measured the content of total dietary fiber [Association of Official Analytical Chemist (AOAC) method] in both fractions (peeled and peels) of the fresh apple fruits, resulting in significantly lower dietary fiber (both soluble an insoluble) in peeled apples than in the peels. In the same study, the *in vitro* antioxidant activities of methanol extracts from the dry powdered peels and pulps of apples are measured by the total radical-trapping antioxidative potential (TRAP) assay, resulting in higher TRAP values in the peel apple fraction than in the pulp apple fraction. A good correlation has been found between TRAP values and total polyphenols, showing TRAP values as providing the best correlation among p-coumaric acid and caffeic acid. In contrast, a poor correlation is observed when the TRAP values are correlated with total dietary fiber content.

In a second stage, Gorinstein and coworkers (Leontowicz et al. 2002, 2003) evaluated the influence of the peel and a peeled apple fruit on the plasma antioxidant capacity in rats. A significant increase in the plasma antioxidant activity is found in the group fed with whole apple in comparison to the control group. In this research, when the antioxidant status is evaluated in the plasma, an increase in the TRAP value and a decrease in the biomarker of lipid oxidation malondialdehyde—measured spectrophotometrically as thiobarbituric reactive substances—are found. It is worth mentioning that these authors state that the correlation between dietary fiber and its antioxidant activity by TRAP assay is very poor. These authors conclude that the *in vivo* and *in vitro* investigations on dietary fiber from the apple do not support the claims that dietary fiber possesses antioxidant properties. Furthermore, they state that the antioxidant potential of dietary fiber in traditional fruits such as apples is questionable, since the antioxidant properties of the whole apple fruit can be attributed to the content of phenolic compounds. This assertion is based on the evidence that the degree of antioxidant potential depends upon the level of total polyphenol.

A recent study describes the effect of three different apple varieties—namely, the Bravo de Esmolfe, the Malápio da Serra, and the Golden that contain different amounts of bioactive compounds—on two biomarkers of cardiovascular diseases in an animal model (Serra et al. 2012). This work correlates these biomarkers with data on apple composition. Good correlations were obtained when comparing the total phenolic contents and antioxidant properties of apples with total cholesterol, low density lipoproteins (LDL)-C, triglycerides, and oxidative-LDL reduction capacity. The highest correlation coefficients were found for catechin, epicatechin, and procyanidin B1, probably due to their capacity to delay lipid absorption. As the authors stated, in contrast to other studies (Aprikian et al. 2003, Leontowicz et al. 2001), the fiber content of apples seems to have no effect on their cholesterol-lowering ability. However, this result could be related to the low levels of fiber present in all fruit diets (<0.6%). Other components in apples such as β-carotene seemed to contribute to the cholesterol-lowering ability of the fruit.

As it is reported (Barth et al. 2005a), a cloudy apple juice showed immunomodulatory activities and further antigenotoxic, antiproliferative properties in colonocytes and significantly reduced preneoplastic lesions in a rat model developed to study colon cancer. The authors have proposed that additive or synergistic effects of apple juice constituents might be responsible for the observed anticancer activities, instead of using single polyphenolic or fiber substances. In order to identify the fractions that contained the bioactive substances of the juice, in a posterior study, the authors have fractionated the cloudy apple juice in a total polyphenol (monomeric and polymeric polyphenols) fraction and a heterogeneous cloud fraction consisting of proteins, fatty acids, polyphenols, and cell wall polysaccharides. The results revealed that the polyphenols alone were not responsible for the observed antiproliferative effect of the cloudy juice as the cloud fraction in a juice-equivalent dosage showed antiproliferative efficacy. These authors state that the cloud particles are heterogeneously composed of lipids, proteins, polysaccharides, and polyphenols with a particle size ranging from 1 to 5 μm. These particles are hydrocolloids with an architectural structure composed of a positively charged nucleus of proteins, which is surrounded and complexed by negatively charged polysaccharides such as pectins. As a whole, these colloids are encapsulated by a hydrate shell. Moreover, they suggest that the polyphenols derived from cloud fraction belong to the group of polymeric procyanidins, on the basis of Le Bourvellec and coworkers' reports showing that the affinity constants of polyphenols with apple pectin were at the highest with high-molecular-weight procyanidins, whereas monomeric apple polyphenols such as hydroxycinnamic acids and (−)-epicatechin do not bind to apple cell wall polysaccharides. Finally, the authors (Barth et al. 2005b, Sembries et al. 2006) conclude first that synergistic effects (interactions) between polyphenols and pectins may be responsible for the high cancer-preventive properties of the cloudy apple juice. And second, the cloud colloids might serve as vectors transferring protection from absorption in the small intestine.

A recent study explores the antiatherogenic effect of different bioactive constituents of apple (polyphenols and dietary fiber) in an animal model of atherosclerosis (Auclair et al. 2008). A crude apple polyphenol extract containing all apple polyphenols in proportions similar to those found in the fruit and an apple fiber extract is administered in the diet of apo E-deficient mice at a level close to the nutritional intake in humans. Although all of the supplemented diets significantly reduced the development of the atherosclerotic plaques in the aortic sinus when compared to the control diet, in the case of apple fibers a higher inhibitory effect than apple polyphenols has been showed. Interestingly, the association of apple fibers and polyphenols does not show a stronger effect than apple fibers alone. These results might be explained by the short-chain fatty acids produced in the colon, which may inhibit smooth muscle cell proliferation and modulate the expression of various genes involved in the oxidative stress and atherosclerosis processes. In the same study, apple fibers and apple polyphenols were found to significantly decrease the concentration of uric acid and reduction power levels in the plasma.

2.3 Conclusions

The contents in dietary fiber and associated compounds polyphenols in the apple fruit are significantly higher in the peels than in the pulp fractions. *In vitro* antioxidant activities in peels of the fruit are significantly higher than in peeled fruit. A whole apple exerts better health-promoting activity than peeled fruit or isolated pectin from the apple in the rat model.

The potential antioxidant activity of dietary fiber in fruits should be clarified. While some authors relate health-promoting properties to certain free and bound bioactive compounds (mainly polyphenols) associated with dietary fiber, no correlation among dietary fiber content and these bioactivities has been clearly described.

Another point of controversy is whether polyphenols are linked to cell walls in the fruit matrix. On the one hand, some authors speculate that various phenolic substances may be "caught" in the lignin–polysaccharide matrix, whereas on the other hand, other authors stress that polyphenols contained within the cellular organelles and cytoplasm, such as procyanidins in apples, breach the cellular frontiers and partially bind to extracellular cell walls during fruit processing, environmental stress, chewing, or digestion.

The clarification of the antioxidant health-promoting role of dietary fiber and its cotraveler bioactive compounds should be focused on the knowledge of the role of food matrix in the retention and the liberation of these molecules through the intestinal lumen.

References

Alonso-Salces, R. M., C. Herrero, A. Barranco, L. A. Berrueta, B. Gallo, and F. Vicente. 2005. Classification of apple fruits according to their maturity state by the pattern recognition analysis of their polyphenolic compositions. *Food Chem* 93:113–23.

Aprikian, O., V. Duclos, S. Guyot et al. 2003. Apple pectin and a polyphenol-rich apple concentrate are more effective together than separately on cecal fermentations and plasma lipids in rats. *J Nutr* 133:1860–5.

Auclair, S., M. Silberberg, E. Gueux et al. 2008. Apple polyphenols and fibers attenuate atherosclerosis in apolipoprotein E-deficient mice. *J Agric Food Chem* 56:5558–62.

Barth, S. W., C. Fahndrich, A. Bub et al. 2005a. Cloudy apple juice decreases DNA damage, hyperproliferation and aberrant crypt foci development in the distal colon of DMH-initiated rats. *Carcinogenesis* 26:1414–21.

Barth, S. W., C. Fahndrich, A. Bub et al. 2005b. Cloudy apple juice is more effective than apple polyphenols and an apple juice derived cloud fraction in a rat model of colon carcinogenesis. *J Agric Food Chem* 55:1181–7.

Blasa, M., L. Gennari, D. Angelino, and P. Ninfali. 2010. Fruit and vegetable antioxidants in health. In *Bioactives Foods in Promoting Health*, ed. R. R. Watson, and V. R. Preedy, pp. 37–58. London: Elsevier.

Carpita, N. C. and D. M. Gibeaut. 1993. Structural models of primary cell walls in flowering plants: Consistency of molecular structure with the physical properties of the walls during growth. *Plant J* 3:1–30.

Cheynier, V. 2005. Polyphenols in food are more complex than often thought. *Am J Clin Nutr* 81:223S–9.

Cummings, J. H., J. I. Mann, C. Nishida, and H. H. Vorster. 2009. Dietary fibre: An agreed definition. *Lancet* 373:365–6.

Cuthbertson, D., P. K. Andrews, J. P. Reganold, N. M. Davies, and B. M. Lange. 2012. Utility of metabolomics toward assessing the metabolic basis of quality traits in apple fruit with an emphasis on antioxidants. *J Agric Food Chem* 60:8552–60.

Eastwood, M. and D. Kritchevsky. 2005. Dietary fiber: How did we get where we are? *Annu Rev Nutr* 25:1–8.

European Union. 2008. Commission Directive 2008/100/EC of 28 October 2008. *Off J Lex* 285:9–12.

Ferguson, L. R. and P. J. Harris. 2003. The dietary fibre debate: More food for thought. *Lancet* 1483:1487–8.

Gorinstein, S., O. Martín-Belloso, A. Lojek et al. 2002. Comparative content of some phytochemicals in Spanish apples, peaches and pears. *J Sci Food Agric* 82:1166–70.

Guyot, S., N. Marnet, P. Sanoner, and J. F. Drilleau. 2003. Variability of the polyphenolic composition of cider apple (*Malus domestica*) fruits and juices. *J Agric Food Chem* 51:6240–7.

Jarvis, M. C. 2011. Plant cell walls: Supramolecular assemblies. *Food Hydrocolloid* 25:257–62.

Jiménez-Escrig, A. and F. J. Sánchez-Muniz. 2000. Dietary fibre from edible seaweeds: Chemical structure, physicochemical properties and effects on cholesterol metabolism. *Nutr Res* 20:585–98.

Jiménez-Escrig, A., E. Gómez-Ordóñez, and P. Rupérez. 2013. Antioxidant and prebiotic effects of dietary fiber co-travelers from sugar Kombu in healthy rats. *J Appl Phycol* 25:503–12.

Jiménez-Escrig, A., A. M. Rincón, R. Pulido, and F. Saura-Calixto. 2001. Guava fruit (*Psidium guajava* L.) as a new source of antioxidant dietary fiber. *J Agric Food Chem* 49:5489–93.

Jones, J. M. 2010. Dietary fibre's co-passengers: Is it the fibre or the copassengers? In *Dietary Fibre: New Frontiers for Food and Health*, ed. J. W. van der Kamp, J. M. Jones, B. V. McCleary, and D. L. Topping, pp. 365–378. Wageningen: Wageningen Academic Publishers.

Kaczmarczyka, M. M., M. J. Miller, and G. G. Freunda. 2012. The health benefits of dietary fiber: Beyond the usual suspects of type 2 diabetes mellitus, cardiovascular disease and colon cancer. *Metab Clin Exp* 61:1058–66.

Kris-Etherton, P. M., K. D. Hecker, A. Bonanome et al. 2002. Bioactive compounds in foods: Their role in the prevention of cardiovascular disease and cancer. *Am J Med* 113:71S–88S.

Lamperi, L., U. Chiuminatto, A. Cincinelli et al. 2008. Polyphenol levels and free radical scavenging activities of four apple cultivars from integrated and organic farmin in different Italian areas. *J Agric Food Chem* 56:6536–46.

Le Bourvellec, C. and C. M. G. C. Renard. 2005. Non-covalent interaction between procyanidins and apple cell wall material. Part II: Quantification and impact of cell wall drying. *Biochim Biophys Acta* 1725:1–9.

Le Bourvellec, C., B. Bouchetb, and C. M. G. C. Renard. 2005. Non-covalent interaction between procyanidins and apple cell wall material. Part III: Study on model polysaccharides. *Biochim Biophys Acta* 1725:10–18.

Le Bourvellec, C., S. Guyot, and C. M. G. C. Renard. 2009. Interactions between apple (*Malus domestica* Borkh.) polyphenols and cell walls modulate the extractability of polysaccharides. *Carbohydr Polym* 75:251–261.

Le Bourvellec, C., J. M. Le Quere, and C. M. G. C. Renard. 2007. Impact of noncovalent interactions between apple condensed tannins and cell walls on their transfer from fruit to juice: Studies in model suspensions and application. *J Agric Food Chem* 55:7896–7904.

Le Bourvellec, C., K. Bouzerzour, Ch. Ginies, S. Regis, Y. Ple, Y., and C. M. G. C. Renard. 2011. Phenolic and polysaccharidic composition of applesauce is close to that of apple flesh. *J Food Compos Anal* 24:537–47.

Le Bourvellec, C., A. A. Watrelot, Ch. Ginies, A. Imberty, and C. M. G. C. Renard. 2012. Impact of processing on the noncovalent interactions between procyanidin and apple cell wall. *J Agric Food Chem* 60:9484–94.

Leontowicz, H., S. Gorinstein, A. Lojek et al. 2002. Comparative content of some bioactive compounds in apples, peaches and pears and their influence on lipids and antioxidant capacity in rats. *J Nutr Biochem* 1:603–10.

Leontowicz, M., S. Gorinstein, E. Bartnikowska, H. Leontowicz, G. Kulasek, and S. Trakhtenberg. 2001. Sugar beet pulp and apple pomace dietary fibers improve lipid metabolism in rats fed cholesterol. *Food Chem* 72:73–8.

Leontowicz, M., S. Gorinstein, H. Leontowitcz et al. 2003. Apple and pear peel and pulp ant their influence on plasma lipids and antioxidant potentials in rats fed cholesterol-containing diets. *J Agric Food Chem* 51:5780–5.

Lotito, S. B. and B. Frei. 2004. Relevance of apple polyphenols as antioxidants in human plasma: Contrasting *in vitro* and *in vivo* effects. *Free Radic Biol Med* 36:201–11.

Lunn, J. and J. L. Buttriss. 2007. Carbohydrates and dietary fibre. *Nutr Bull* 32:21–64.

Markham, K. R., K. S. Gould, and K. G. Ryan. 2001. Cytoplasmic accumulation of flavonoids in flower petals and its relevance to yellow flower colouration. *Phytochemistry* 58:403–13.

Maxwell, E. G., N. J. Belshaw, K. W. Waldron, and V. J. Morris. 2012. Pectine—An emerging new bioactive food polysaccharide. *Trends Food Sci Technol* 24:64–73.

Neveu, V., J. Pérez-Jiménez, F. Vos et al. 2010. Phenol-Explorer: An online comprehensive database on polyphenol contents in foods. *J Biol Databases Curation*, 2010, doi: 10.1093/database/bap024.

Nyström, L., A. M. Lampi, H. Rita, A. M. Aura, K. M. Oksman-Caldentey, and V. Piironen. 2007. Effects of processing on availability of total plant sterols, steryl ferulates and steryl glycosides from wheat and rye bran. *J Agric Food Chem* 55:9059–65.

Padayachee, A., G. Netzel, M. Netzel et al. 2012a. Binding of polyphenols to plant cell wall analogues—Part 1: Anthocyanins. *Food Chem* 134:155–61.

Padayachee, A., G. Netzel, M. Netzel et al. 2012b. Binding of polyphenols to plant cell wall analogues—Part 2: Phenolic acids. *Food Chem* 135:2287–92.

Palafox-Carlos, H., J. F. Ayala-Zavala, and J. A. González-Aguilar. 2011. The role of dietary fiber in the bioaccessibility and bioavailability of fruit and vegetable antioxidants. *J Food Sci* 76:R6–15.

Pinelo, M., A. Arnous, and A. S. Meyer. 2006. Upgrading of grape skins: Significance of plant cell-wall structural components and extraction techniques for phenol release. *Trends Food Sci Technol* 17:579–90.

Pinelo, M., B. Zornoza, and A. S. Meyer. 2008. Selective release of phenols from apple skin: Mass transfer kinetics during solvent and enzyme-assisted extraction. *Sep Purif Technol* 63:620–7.

Renard, C. M. G. C., A. Baron, S. Guyot, and J. F. Drilleau. 2001. Interactions between apple cell walls and native apple polyphenols: Quantification and some consequences. *Int J Biol Macromol* 29:115–25.

Ridley, B. L., M. A. O'Neill, and D. Mohnen. 2001. Pectins: Structure, biosynthesis, and oligogalacturonide-related signaling. *Phytochemistry* 57:929–67.

Rodríguez, R., S. Jaramillo, A. Heredia, R. Guillen, A. Jiménez, and J. Fernández-Bolaños. 2004. Mechanical properties of white and green asparagus: Changes related to modifications of cell wall components. *J Sci Food Agric* 84:1478–86.

Saura-Calixto, F. 1998. Antioxidant dietary fiber product: A new concept and a potential food ingredient. *J Agric Food Chem* 46:4303–06.

Saura-Calixto, F. 2011. Dietary fibre as a carrier of antioxidants: An essential physiological function. *J Agric Food Chem* 59:43–9.

Schieber, A., P. Keller, and R. Carle. 2001. Determination of phenolic acids and flavonoids of apple and pear by high-performance liquid chromatography. *J Chromatogr A* 910:265–73.

Selvendran, R. R. 1985. Developments in the chemistry and biochemistry of pectic and hemicellulosic polymers. *J Cell Sci* 2:51–88.

Sembries, S., G. Dongowski, K. Mehrla, F. Will, and H. Dietrich. 2006. Physiological effects of extraction juices from apple, grape, and red beet pomaces in rats. *J Agric Food Chem* 54:10269–80.

Serra, A. T., J. Rocha, B. Sepodes et al. 2012. Evaluation of cardiovascular protective effect of different apple varieties. Correlation of response with composition. *Food Chem* 135:2378–86.

Somerville, C., S. Bauer, G. Brininstool, M. Facette, T. Hamann, and J. Milne. 2004. Toward a systems approach to understanding plant-cell walls. *Science* 306:2206–11.

Trowell, H. 1972. Isquemic heart disease and dietary fiber. *Am J Clin Nutr* 25:926–32.

Van Soest, P. J. 1978. Dietary fibers: Their definition and nutritional properties. *Am J Clin Nutr* 31:S12–20.

Waldron, K. W., M. L. Parker, and A. C. Smith. 2003. Plant cell walls and food quality. *Comp Rev Food Sci Food Safety* 2:101–9.

Watrelot, A. A., C. Le Bourvellec, A. Imberty, and C. M. G. C. Renardt. 2013. Interactions between pectic compounds and procyanidins are influenced by methylation degree and chain length. *Biomacromolecules* 14:709–18.

Weichselbaum, E, L. Wyness, and S. Stanner. 2010. Apple polyphenols and cardiovascular disease—A review of the evidence. *Nutr Bull* 35:92–101.

Yapo, B. M. 2011. Pectic substances: From simple pectic polysaccharides to complex pectins—A new hypothetical model. *Carbohydr Polym* 86:373–85.

Zheng, H. Z., I. W. Hwang, and S. K. Chung. 2009. Enhancing polyphenol extraction from unripe apples by carbohydrate-hydrolyzing enzymes. *J Zhejiang Univ Sci B* 10:912–9.

CHAPTER 3

Agave Fiber Structure Complexity and Its Impact on Health

MERCEDES G. LÓPEZ, ALICIA HUAZANO-GARCÍA,
MARÍA CONCEPCIÓN GARCÍA-PÉREZ, and
MARÍA ISABEL GARCÍA-VIEYRA

Contents

3.1	Agave	46
3.2	Fructans	47
	3.2.1 Definition	47
	3.2.2 Classification and Degree of Polymerization	48
	3.2.3 Relevance of Fructans	48
3.3	Agave Fructans	49
	3.3.1 Structures	49
	3.3.2 Species	49
3.4	Plant Age	53
3.5	Analytical Tools	55
	3.5.1 Thin Layer Chromatography	55
	3.5.2 High-Performance Anion Exchange Chromatography–Pulsed Amperometric Detection	56
	3.5.3 Derivatization of Fructans to Partially Methylated Alditol Acetates	56
	3.5.4 Matrix-Assisted Laser Desorption/Ionization Time of Flight Mass Spectrometry	56
	3.5.5 Nuclear Magnetic Resonance: ^{13}C-NMR and ^{1}H-NMR	57
	3.5.6 Midinfrared Spectroscopy	58
3.6	Probiotic Studies	58
	3.6.1 Growth of Probiotic Bacteria in Fructans of Different *Agave* Species	58

3.7 Mice Studies 63
    3.7.1 Agave Fructans Impact on the Health of Mice 63
    3.7.2 Modulation of Lipid and Glucose Metabolism by Agave Fructans 64
    3.7.3 Homeostasis of the Hormones Involved in Satiety with Agave Fructans 65
    3.7.4 Agave Fructans on Calcium and Magnesium Absorption 67
3.8 Future Potential 68
References 69

3.1 Agave

The *Agave* genus is a member of the Agavaceae family that consists of nine genera. This family includes ancient plants that have supported the Mesoamerican man since the first inhabitants (around 9000 years ago) until the present time (Colunga-García et al. 1993). Agave is one of the most exploited genera, due to its high integral utilization and the diverse and unique characteristics of many of its species, which have been used as food, fiber, sweeteners, supplement ingredients, and even as house construction material, among many other applications.

Metl is the náhuatl word that prehispanics used for this "sacred" plant, Agave a gift from the goddess. On the other hand, Agave (from the Greek *noble* and Latin *admirable*) was the word used by Charles Linneo to describe this genus (1753), which is in reference to the admirable ability of these plants to grow in extremely dry environments. Agave plants, however, can also be found in many ecosystems, such as productive highlands and areas of high humidity (Gentry 1998). Mexico is considered the origin center of evolution and diversification of the *Agave* genus, since a large number of *Agave* species are found here. The *Agave* genus includes approximately 166 species and is the largest genus in the Agavaceae family that consists of nine genera and approximately 293 species (Roberfroid 2007, Roberfroid et al. 1998). Figure 3.1 shows some Agave fields and some *Agave* species commonly grown in Mexico.

Many *Agave* species are the raw material used in the production of alcoholic beverages. Carbohydrates stored in Agave stems are hydrolyzed by heat and then fermented; this practice dates to around 1300 b.c., when the Aztec civilization fermented the sap that emanated after an Agave stem incision. Curiously, pulque—the product obtained from this practice—is consumed even now as a nutritious beverage, especially by people living one component of the metabolic syndrome, including diabetic, due to the presence of nondigestible carbohydrates (Colunga-García et al. 1993). After the Spaniards arrived to the new continent, the distillation process was introduced, giving rise to well-known Mexican distillated beverages such as tequila and mezcal.

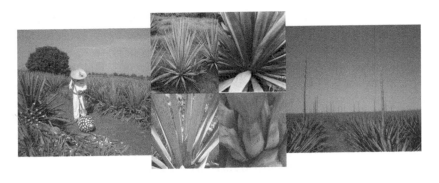

Figure 3.1 Agave fields and *Agave* species commonly found in Mexico.

One of the most appreciated characteristics of Agave plants is their outstanding water-soluble carbohydrate (WSC) content, which represents around 80% of their weight on a dry basis (Mancilla-Margalli and López 2002, Nobel et al. 1998). It is now known that the great majority of these carbohydrates are formed by agavins, branched fructans molecules (López et al. 2003). These carbohydrates are mainly constituted of fructans, which represent more than 60% of the total WSC, while less than 40% are glucose, fructose, and sucrose, which are used commercially for the production of Agave syrup and flour (Mancilla-Margalli and López 2006). More importantly, Agave fructans have been reported as prebiotics *in vitro* and *in vivo* since they have shown many beneficial health-promoting effects (Huazano-García and López 2013, Santiago-García and López 2009, Urías-Silvas and López 2009, Urías-Silvas et al. 2008).

3.2 Fructans

3.2.1 Definition

Fructans are fructose-based oligosaccharides and polysaccharides with a glucose residue derived from sucrose. Fructan synthesis occurs in bacteria, fungi, about 45,000 species of angiosperms, approximately 15% of flowering plants, species belonging to selected families of both monocots and dicots. Fructans of distinct origin can differ based on their degree of polymerization (DP), the type of linkage between adjacent fructose units, the position of the glucose residue, and the presence of branches (Banguela and Hernández 2006, Van den Ende 2011). Fructans are accumulated in the vacuole as reserve carbohydrates (Wiemken 1986). Their functions in plants are not limited to storage energy; they also might protect plants against freezing/drought stresses by stabilizing cell membranes (Hincha et al. 2002, 2003, Valluru and Van den Ende 2008, Vereyken et al. 2001). They have also been implicated in vegetative developmental processes and osmoregulation issues (Spollen and

Nelson 1994). In addition, their cryoprotective role has been demonstrated in cereals such as oat and wheat (Livingston and Henson 1998). Fructans have also been implicated in tolerance to drought, mainly in grasses and in transgenic tobacco and sugar beet plants (Amiard et al. 2003, Pilon-Smits et al. 1995, Pilon-Smits et al. 1999, Thomas and James 1999). Fructans are water-soluble, nondigestible, and fermentable carbohydrates, which have interesting metabolic effects (e.g., decrease in fat mass development, steatosis, and glycemia) (Urías-Silvas et al. 2008). Fructans have several potential applications in the food and non-food industries. Different types of fructan biosynthetic enzymes, termed fructosyltransferases (FTs), can explain the diversity of fructans in plants (Lasseur et al. 2006, Tamura et al. 2009). Depending on the plant species, a more complex cocktail of FTs with distinct substrate specificities is needed as 1-sucrose:sucrose fructosyltransferase (1-SST), 1-fructan:fructan fructosyltransferase (1-FFT), 6-sucrose:fructan fructosyltransferase (6-SFT), and 6G-fructan:fructan fructosyltransferase (6G-FFT) within the monocots (Prud'homme et al. 2007).

3.2.2 Classification and Degree of Polymerization

Five major types of fructans have been identified according to the way β-fructofuranosyl units are linked: (1) linear inulin with β(2-1)-fructofuranosyl linkages, found mainly in chicory; (2) levan (or phlein) with β(2-6) linkages found mainly in grasses; (3) graminans, which are mixed fructans containing linear inulin and levan (generally, they are branched fructans like those found in wheat); (4) inulin neoserie, which contains a glucose moiety between two fructofuranosyl units extended by β(2-1) linkages, present in onion and asparagus; and (5) levan neoserie, formed by β(2-1)- and β(2-6)-linked fructofuranosyl units on either end of a central sucrose molecule, reported in oat (Vijn and Smeekens 1999). A new sixth type, called agavins, are highly branched fructans containing all the β-linked fructofuranosyl units mentioned above. Fructans are generally present as polydisperse mixtures present in the vegetative tissues with different DPs. Several authors have observed that the distribution pattern along the length of fructan polymers depends on environmental and developmental conditions, and also on the species type (Van Loo et al. 1995). Fructans with a short degree of polymerization (SDP) are considered as fibers with high prebiotic potential and with an increasing demand in the functional food market, while fructans with a long degree of polymerization (LDP) also have a good potential with applications in the nonfood industry (Banguela and Hernández 2006).

3.2.3 Relevance of Fructans

The analysis of fructan structures and the study of their physiological roles on development and adaptability in higher plants have led to the speculation that their structures might be tightly related to their functions (Nagaraj et al. 2004). For example, inulin is the only fructan type in dicots that is stored in reserve vegetative organs and is depolymerized and mobilized to cover the energy demand of the whole plant, as sprouting and inflorescence (Bieleski 1993, Machado de Carvalho and Dietrich 1993). In monocots, the high fructan structure variability observed may be related to other physiological roles such adaptability, since a cryoprotective role of graminans has been demonstrated in oat, wheat, and other cereals (Livingston and Henson 1998); a major tolerance to drought conditions has been shown in levans accumulated in transgenic plants (Pilon-Smits et al. 1995). Chatterton and Harrison (2003) suggested that the structural variation found in *Agropyron cristatum* is crucial to the tolerance of this grass to dry conditions. Something similar might occur in the *Agave* species; since a wide fructan structural variation has been documented already, stored fructans in the stems might be a response to an adaptability factor. It can be concluded that in the *Agave* genus, the predominance of highly complex fructan types may reflect the peculiar adaptability processes that these species undergo (Mancilla-Margalli and López 2006).

3.3 Agave Fructans

3.3.1 Structures

Agaves are plants whose carbohydrates have been used in a wide variety of applications but mainly the elaboration of alcoholic beverages such as tequila and mezcal (López and Mancilla-Margalli 2007). The first report on the presence of fructans in *Agave* pines was in 1888, *Agave vera cruz* and *Agave americana* being the most studied species (Bathia and Nandra 1979, Chatterton and Harrison 2003, Mancilla-Margalli and López 2006, Sánchez-Marroquín and Hope 1953). It was reported that *A. vera cruz* fructans were conformed of a mixture of inulins and some branched molecules (Dorland et al. 1977, Srinivasan and Bathia 1953, Srinivasan and Bathia 1954). On the other hand, Bathia and Nandra (1979) reported inulin as the main storage carbohydrate in *A. Americana*; however, Ravenscroft et al. (2009) redefined the fructan structures for this species as a neoseries class with β(2-1) and β(2-6) linkages. In the case of *A. deserti*, the presence of a DP5 fructan in the vascular tissue with neokestose as the principal fructooligosaccharide (FOS), a fructan of DP3 with an internal glucose moiety, was reported for the first time (Wang and Nobel 1998).

3.3.2 Species

3.3.2.1 Agave tequilana Weber Blue Variety
Sánchez-Marroquín and Hope (1953) described the fructans of the *Agave tequilana* Weber blue variety as inulins. Fifty years later, López et al. (2003) published that the *A. tequilana* Weber blue variety in fact contains a complex mixture of fructans, where the less abundant fructan type was the inulin type. These authors using different analytical techniques demonstrated that the fructans present in *A. tequilana* were not inulins but rather were complex and highly branched molecules with

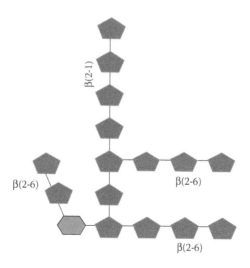

Figure 3.2 Proposed fructan structure of *Agave* species; these branched fructans have been called agavins.

both β(2-1) and β(2-6) linkages in which the presence of both internal (neo-series fructans) and external (graminans fructans) glucose units was reported (Figure 3.2) (López et al. 2003). Mancilla-Margalli and López (2006) evaluated the content of fructans in five different *Agave* species commonly used in Mexico in the production of alcoholic beverages (Figure 3.3). Fructan values found in those *Agave* species were in the range of 360–735 mg/g on a dry weight basis; these amounts are higher than most reported in fructan-storing plants such as dahlia and chicory (350 and 240 mg/g on dry weight, respectively) (Mancilla-Margalli and López 2006, Turner et al. 2006, Van Waes et al. 1998). The same authors reported that abiotic factors such as climate, rainfall, altitude, and soil affect the content of fructans stored in Agave stems (Mancilla-Margalli and López 2006). On the other hand, Agave plants from the same species but grown in distinct environments presented significant differences on the fructan content, this was very evident in the *A. tequilana* from Jalisco and those grown in Guanajuato, which are neighboring states. Plants grown in Jalisco presented almost 72% of fructan while those grown in Guanajuato regions presented only 50%. This difference was explained as a result of changes in altitude, where the uptake of CO_2 and, consequently, carbohydrate accumulation is favored (Mancilla-Margalli and López 2006, Ruiz-Corral et al. 2002).

In general, fructans in Agaves represent 60% and up to 85% of WSC on a dry weight basis (Figure 3.4). Other important carbohydrates in Agaves are glucose, fructose, and sucrose, mono- and disaccharides closely related with the fructan metabolism, which are stored mainly in the stems of Agaves but can also be found in the leaves (Wang and Nobel 1998). Mancilla-Margalli

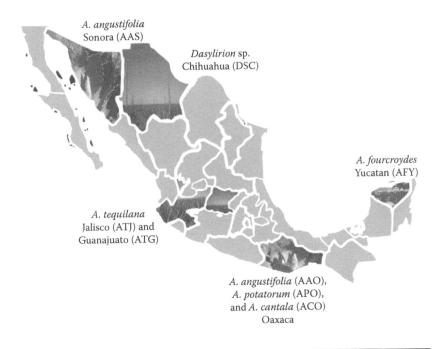

Figure 3.3 Mexican territory and some *Agave* species highly used for the elaboration of alcoholic beverages and nowadays for the production of agavins, soluble fibers.

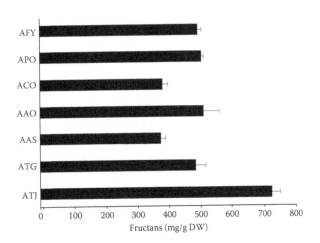

Figure 3.4 Fructan content determined in the stem of different *Agave* species. All plants were collected in different geographic zones of Mexico: ATJ, *Agave tequilana*; ATG, *A. tequilana*; AAS, *A. angustifolia*; AAO, *A. angustifolia*; ACO, *A. cantala*; APO, *A. potatorum*; AFY, *A. fourcroydes*.

Table 3.1 Classification of Agave Fructans by Their Degree of Polymerization and Graminans:Agavins Ratio of Each Group

Classification		Estimated DP	α-ᴅ-Glc*p*	*i*-α-ᴅ-Glc*p*
Group I	At-J	18.12	0.20	0.79
	Aa-S	13.07	0.18	0.82
	Aa-O	31.75	0.21	0.79
	Ap-O	15.34	0.17	0.83
Group II	Ac-O	11.17	0.33	0.67
	Af-Y	6.66	0.31	0.69
	Dsp-C	9.09	0.38	0.62
Group III	At-G	7.13	0.52	0.48
Standards	Dv	37.43	1	nd
	Ac	4.79	0.66	0.34

Note: nd—not determined.

and López (2006) found that fructan structures in Agaves varied as a function of plant species and growing regions, reporting a structural comparison of fructans from several species of *Agave* grown in different regions of Mexico. These species are classified as economically important for the country and include the *Agave tequilana* (Jalisco and Guanajuato), *A. angustifolia* (Oaxaca and Sonora), *A. potatorum* and *A. cantala* from Oaxaca, and *A. fourcroydes* from Yucatan (Figure 3.3). In this work, the authors grouped Agave fructans into three major groups containing principally two different fructan types (independently of the group), graminans and agavins (neoseries fructans), agavins being the most abundant type (Mancilla-Margalli and López 2006). *A. tequilana* Weber blue variety fructans from Jalisco were placed in group I along with *A. angustifolia* from Oaxaca and Sonora and *A. potatorum* from Oaxaca (Table 3.1).

3.3.2.2 Agave angustifolia Haw   Agave plants from the same species, such as *A. angustifolia*, but grown in distinct environments (Sonora-North and Oaxaca-South of Mexico) presented significant differences in their fructan content even though they fall in the same group structurally (Table 3.1) (Mancilla-Margalli and López 2006). In this same study, the DP, the ratio of graminans to agavins, and the contribution of branched points were reported. All these parameters differ in all groups; for example, the *Agave* species of group I have a ratio of graminans and agavins of 1:4 and presented mainly an LDP. Species within group II have a ratio of graminans and agavins of 1:2 with SDP with few branches. Finally, in group III, the proportion of graminans and agavins was 1:1 with SDP. *Dahlia variabilis* (DVS) and *Allium cepa* (AC) were used as controls. Table 3.1 clearly shows that *A. angustifolia* plants collected from different states (Sonora and Oaxaca) are in the same cluster (group I). Meanwhile, *A. tequilana* from Guanajuato was clustered in group III but plants belonging to the same species of *A. tequilana* from Jalisco were placed in group I. With these results, Mancilla-Margalli and López (2006) confirmed the structural heterogeneity that might be attributed to the plant adaptation mechanisms to survive in very inhospitable areas. Later on, the same authors suggest that, in Agave and in other plants different to the Agavaceae family, the synthesis of fructans may be influenced by the agronomic or growing region, the soil nutrients, the plant variety, the seasonal changes, the water regime, and of course the harvesting time (Dias-Tagliacozzo et al. 2004, Faustini-Cuzzuol et al. 2005, Livingston et al. 2006, Mancilla-Margalli and López 2006, Orthen and Wehrmeyer 2004, Shiomi et al. 2005, Wilson et al. 2004).

3.3.2.3 Agave potatorum Zucc. Different *Agave* species grown under the same geoclimatic conditions were classified in different groups, such was the case for *A. potatorum* and *A. cantala*, both growing in the same state of Oaxaca, as well as *A. angustifolia*, but all presenting different degrees of polymerization independent of sharing the same geoclimatic conditions. It was also shown that different abiotic conditions affect not only DP but also fructan concentration and developmental phases (Amiard et al. 2003, Itaya et al. 2002, Van den Ende et al. 2005).

3.3.2.4 Other Species Species that grow in a very humid environment such as *A. fourcroydes* shared many structural characteristics with other *Agave* species such as *A. cantala* and with crops from other genus such *Dasylirion* sp. in spite of the high water content where *A. fourcroydes* grow (Mancilla-Margalli and López 2006). Finally, it can be said that arid regions where *Agave* species grow successfully and where water availability is very limited, according to Hendry (1993), are conditions that might be responsible for the origin of fructan-storing plants.

3.4 Plant Age

In Agave plants, the main fructan function is as reserve carbohydrate, supplying the energy required during vegetative development and flowering (Mellado-Mojica and López 2012). The content and composition of fructans in *Agave tequilana* Weber blue variety in plants between 2 and 7 years of age varied in fructan content from 328 to 711 mg/g depending on the plant age; older plants presented higher values (5–7-year-old plants) (Figure 3.5). In chicory (*Cichorium intybus*), changes in their carbohydrate and fructan compositions and concentrations are mainly seen in roots throughout the growing season, in storage, and during forcing (Van den Ende et al. 1996). Therefore, several studies suggest that fructan profile variations, during the plant life cycle, occur due to differences in the activity of metabolizing fructan enzymes, as well as to the energy required for plant development.

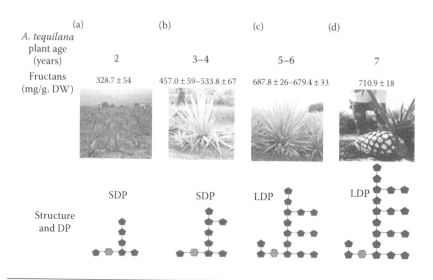

Figure 3.5 Structural characteristics and fructan contents of *Agave tequilana* at different developing stages.

Mellado-Mojica et al. (2009) found that *A. tequilana* fructans changed during the biological cycle of the plant; the highest fructan concentration was found in 8-year-old plants while the lowest was found in 4-year-old plants and a declining concentration was observed in 10-year-old plants. These differences in fructan content could also be correlated with the activities of different enzymes, allowing a possibility to propose a model that might help to explain the phenological stages for *A. tequilana* and the main fructosyltransferases involved (Figure 3.5). Fluctuations in total reducing sugars and fructose content and the DP of fructans were determined according to the plant age by the same research group (Mellado-Mojica et al. 2009). Later, Mellado-Mojica and López (2012) found interesting variations during the evaluation of soluble carbohydrates (glucose, fructose, sucrose, starch, and fructans) as well as the DP, and molecular structures of stored fructans in *A. tequilana* along its developmental cycle in the field. All these results agree well with those found by Arrizon et al. (2010), where the authors reported changes in the oligosaccharides profiles as a function of age. Younger plants (2 year old) had richer concentrations of lower-molecular-weight fructans and due to this composition, they might have good potential as dietary fibers. Matured plants (6½ year old) presented the highest fructan content with an LDP, suggesting that they might be used for tequila elaboration. In the same work, they also observed polymerization and depolymerization processes with a concomitant increasing and decreasing degree of polymerization of fructans; these variations could be associated with the physiological preparation stage of *A. tequilana* plants before they confront the flowering stage (Arrizon et al. 2010).

3.5 Analytical Tools

The knowledge of the content and molecular structure of fructans from different sources is a basic requirement for the correct classification, better understanding of their physiological functionality, and their adequate utilization in various areas, principally on health. Therefore, relevant analytical approaches for fructan characterization include chromatographic techniques such as thin layer chromatography (TLC), high-performance anion exchange chromatography combined with pulse amperometric detection (HPAEC-PAD), and gas chromatography coupled with mass spectrometry (GC-MS), besides other tools such as matrix-assisted laser desorption time-of-flight mass spectrometry (MALDI-TOF-MS), nuclear magnetic resonance (NMR), and infrared spectroscopy, among the most used. In all these cases, the calibration system and/or identification of FOS and polymers requires adequate standards with well-known structure.

3.5.1 Thin Layer Chromatography

Figure 3.6 shows a TLC separation of fructans from different Agave samples. It is clearly seen that TLC has the potential to resolve FOS of different degrees of polymerization. Solutions of *A. tequilana* fructans of different ages were analyzed on analytical silica gel plates with aluminum support and developed with an aniline–diphenylamine–phosphoric acid reagent based in acetone (Anderson et al. 2000).

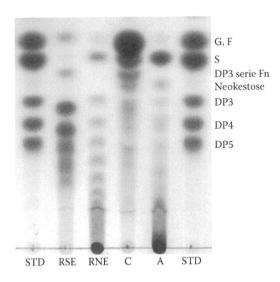

Figure 3.6 TLC of fructans from *Cichorium intybus*, *Allium cepa*, and *Agave tequilana*. From left to right: STD: standards mixture (G: glucose, F: fructose, S: sucrose, DP3: 1-kestose, DP4: 1-nystose, and DP5: 1-kestopentaose), RSE and RNE: chicory, C: onion, A: *A. tequilana*.

3.5.2 High-Performance Anion Exchange Chromatography–Pulsed Amperometric Detection

The identity of fructans can be determined by HPAEC-PAD with standards or by comparing the elution pattern of fructans of other crops under the same conditions. López and Mancilla-Margalli (2007) reported for the first time the HPAEC-PAD profiles of fructans from *A. tequilana*, *A. angustifolia*, and *A. potatorum*; they were compared with those from chicory and onion. Chicory accumulates only inulin-type fructans in its roots with β(2-1)-fructofuranosyl units and a progressive increase in DP is observed. Recently, Mellado-Mojica and López (2012) published the HPAEC-PAD profiles of *A. tequilana* Weber blue variety fructans from plants between 2 and 7 years of age and again for the first time established the characterization of Agave fructan isomers. Figure 3.7 shows a typical HPAEC of *A. tequilana* where the presence of DP3, DP4, and DP5 is very clearly distinguishable; however, after DP5, much overlapping is observed due to a large number of isomeric forms present in this species as well as in many other *Agave* species.

3.5.3 Derivatization of Fructans to Partially Methylated Alditol Acetates

This technique has allowed the characterization of fructans from different *Agave* species, mainly *A. tequilana* and *A. angustifolia*, where quantitative differences such as fructose branching abundances were the basic difference between both species. In this sense, a higher branching was found for *A. angustifolia* (peak number 8) (Figure 3.8) (López and Mancilla-Margalli 2007, López et al. 2003). This technique also permitted the characterization of *A. tequilana* fructans according to the plant age, where Mellado-Mojica and López (2012) reported the calculated molar proportion based on partially methylated alditol acetates.

3.5.4 Matrix-Assisted Laser Desorption/Ionization Time of Flight Mass Spectrometry

MALDI-TOF-MS is an ideal technique for the analysis of complex mixtures but unfortunately does not provide complete structural information. The mass spectrum for fructans from *A. tequilana* obtained by MALDI-TOF-MS

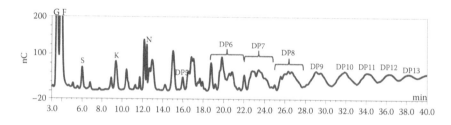

Figure 3.7 Typical HPAEC-PAD profile of fructan from *Agave tequilana* Weber blue variety. The presence of isomeric forms with the same DP is seen along the whole chromatogram.

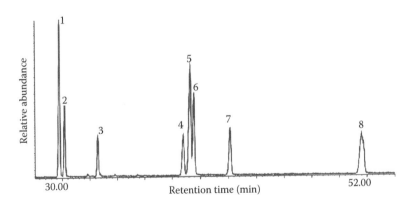

Figure 3.8 GC-MS of extracted fructans from *Agave tequilana* Weber blue variety in their partially methylated alditol acetate forms.

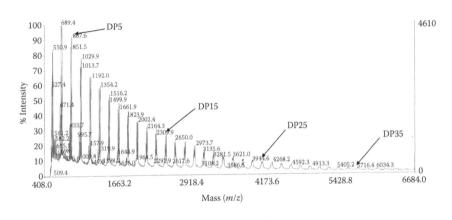

Figure 3.9 Positive ion MALDI-TOF-MS of fructans from *Agave tequilana* Weber blue variety recorded on 2,5-dihydroxybenzoic acid as the matrix.

is presented in Figure 3.9. The mass range observed falls between m/z 527 and 4739 Da and indicates fructans with a DP between 3 and 29 units, forming adducts with Na^+ (e.g., $GF_n^+ + Na^+$) (López et al. 2003). Fructans extracted from *A. tequilana* plants of different ages were analyzed with this technique (Mellado-Mojica et al. 2009).

3.5.5 Nuclear Magnetic Resonance: ^{13}C-NMR and ^1H-NMR

A sophisticated analytical tool used for complete fructan structural determination without sample preparation is NMR of ^{13}C and ^1H (Bonnett et al. 1997, Brasch et al. 1988, Liu et al. 1991, Wack and Blaschek 2006). The complex fructan structures previously observed for Agave fructans using other analytical tools were confirmed by NMR (López and Mancilla-Margalli

Table 3.2 Chemical Shifts of Anomeric Carbon Corresponding to C2 Fructose of *Agave tequilana*

	Signal δ (ppm)	Linkage Type
C2	104.06	β(2-1)-D-Fru*f*
	104.54	*t*-β-D-Fru*f*
	104.68	1,6-di-β-D-Fru*f*
	104.87	β(2-6)-D-Fru*f*

2007). Table 3.2 shows the chemical signals reported for agavins; δ 104.06 ppm was assigned to the internal-β(2-1)-D-fructofuranose β(2-1)-D-Fru*f*, which is the most intense signal. The resonance at δ 104.54 ppm corresponds to terminal-β-fructofuranose *t*-β-D-Fru*f*. The nature of branched residues 1,6-di-β-D-fructofuranose, 1,6-di-β-D-Fru*f* was confirmed with the signal at δ 104.68 ppm, whose value is similar to the assignment reported for branched residues in *Urginea maritime* (Spies et al. 1992). The internal-β-(2-6)-D-fructofuranose linkages β(2-6)-D-Fru*f* is also demonstrated by the δ 104.87 ppm resonance and confirmed by the presence of signals at δ 81.12 and 64.11 ppm due to C5 and C6, respectively, holding a substitution on O6 (Hincha et al. 2002, Sims et al. 2001). The C2-fructosyl resonance is characteristic of internal-β-D-glucopyranose *i*-β-D-Glc*p*, a neofructan, which has been reported around δ 104.5 ppm (De Bruyn and Van Loo 1991). Therefore, it is possible that resonance at δ 104.54 ppm corresponds to an overlapping resonance of both *t*-β-D-Fru*f* and *i*-β-D-Glc*p* moieties.

3.5.6 Midinfrared Spectroscopy

Midinfrared spectroscopy (MIR) is a nondestructive technique used mainly for the elucidation of molecular structures based on their functional groups (López-Medina 2006). Moreover, when MIR is coupled with a chemometric software, its potential is highly magnified. MIR-SIMCA (soft independent modeling class analogy) allowed the classification of *Agave* pines of conventional and micropropagated origins (Figure 3.10). Even if the MIR spectra of all samples were almost the same, which is logical since all have the same functional groups, plants were grouped based on their origins.

3.6 Probiotic Studies

3.6.1 Growth of Probiotic Bacteria in Fructans of Different Agave Species

3.6.1.1 Introduction Microbiota plays an important role in human health by providing a protective barrier to pathogens, producing nutrients, and maintaining the normal mucosal immunity (Salminen et al. 1998). Many factors affect the composition of the intestinal microbiota, among these factors

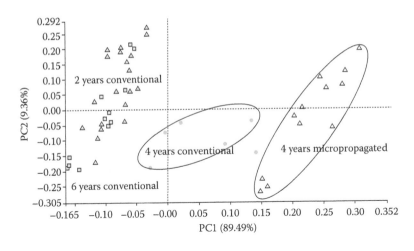

Figure 3.10 Principal component analysis (PCA) by SIMCA and midinfrared spectroscopy of *Agave* pines of different ages from conventional and micropropagated plants.

age, nutritional requirements, pH, interaction between intestinal components, the intestinal microbiota, and the presence of fermentable substrates should be mentioned. Recent advances in the field of nutrition have confirmed the considerable effect of the diet itself on the gut microbiota composition (Turnbaugh et al. 2009). Through the process of fermentation, colonic bacteria are able to produce a wide range of compounds that can have both positive and negative effects on gut physiology as well as other systemic influences. For instance, colonic bacteria produce short-chain fatty acids (SCFAs) from the metabolism of complex carbohydrates and proteins obtained from the diet (Cummings 1981, Cummings and Macfarlane 1991). A low-fiber diet and high protein intake can affect the ecosystem of the gut microbiota in a negative way. Fortunately, it can also be altered to make positive change using prebiotic fibers.

3.6.1.2 Functional Carbohydrates   Actually, the use of functional foods that promote a state of well-being, impart health benefits in general, and decrease the risk of diseases is becoming popular, as the consumer is now more health conscious. In this sense, Mussatto and Mancilha (2007) paid attention to different types of dietary carbohydrates or nondigestible carbohydrates. The latter type is characterized as dietary soluble fiber and presents important physicochemical and physiological positive effects on health. These properties include noncariogenicity, a low caloric value, and the ability to stimulate the growth of beneficial bacteria in the colon. The concept of nondigestible carbohydrates originates from the observation that the anomeric carbon atom (C1 or C2) of a monosaccharide unit of some dietary oligo- and polysaccharides has a configuration that makes their glycosidic linkages nondigestible by the hydrolytic activity of the human digestive enzymes (Roberfroid and Slavin 2000). Nondigestible carbohydrates are known to promote the growth of beneficial bacteria in the colon, mainly bifidobacteria and lactobacilli species, and are thus recognized as prebiotics. The chemical differences among these nondigestible carbohydrates include chain length, monosaccharide composition, DP, branching position and length, purity, and to mention a few.

Among the compounds used as functional foods and considered soluble fibers, fructans (fructooligosaccharides and polysaccharides), lactulose and galactooligosacharides are the most extensively known prebiotics (Mussatto and Mancilha 2007). Fructans are nonreducing carbohydrates constituted of fructosyl units generally presenting in their structure a moiety of terminal glucose. It is known that most fructans possess important physiological benefits on health. SCFAs produced by the fermentation of these carbohydrates by probiotics present a wide range of beneficial effects; for example, influencing lipid and cholesterol metabolism as well as satiety hormones, helping to normalize the immune response and increasing calcium absorption.

3.6.1.3 Prebiotic Activity of Agave Fructans A prebiotic is a selectively fermented ingredient that allows specific changes, in composition and/or activity of the gastrointestinal microbiota that confers benefits upon host well-being and health (Gibson et al. 2004). Prebiotics allow the selective growth of certain indigenous intestinal bacteria such as bifidobacteria and lactobacilli. Bacterial metabolism can result in a number of advantageous effects, including the production of vitamins, modulation of the immune system, enhanced digestion and absorption, inhibition of harmful species, and the removal of carcinogens and other toxins (Collins and Gibson 1999, Gibson and Rastall 2006).

The human intestinal flora harbors a complex microbiota containing many hundreds of different bacterial species. Although the relationship between different intestinal components and the microbiota is not clear, these microorganisms play an important role in maintaining the body's homeostasis. In terms of health, bifidobacteria and lactobacilli are among several hundred species of bacteria that colonize the large intestine known as probiotics (Gibson and Roberfroid 1995). The presence and colonization of these bacterial species are essential for the prevention of diseases and health maintenance (Rastall 2004).

Many of the physiological properties of the intestinal microbiota can be attributed to the fermentation of available substrates and specifically, the subsequent production of SCFAs, particularly acetate, propionate, and butyrate. The fermentation process is regulated by the amount and type of the substrates such as complex carbohydrates and proteins that are accessible to the bacteria present in the colonic ecosystem. The production of SCFAs is important because they have varying physiological effects in different body tissues. The study of fibers, such as prebiotics, that improve bifidobacteria and lactobacilli growth in the intestine, is necessary. The fermentation of fructans in the colon generates SCFAs, which favors the maintenance and growth of good microbiota and colonic epithelial cells (Wong et al. 2006). These complex carbohydrates have been shown to modify the species composition of the microbiota, and in various degrees, to manifest several health-promoting properties related to the regulation of glucose and lipid metabolism, laxation, prevention of colon cancer, and the enhancement of mineral absorption. Many of these effects can be linked to their digestion, fermentation, and SCFA production by bacteria in the large gut.

3.6.1.3.1 In Vitro Study Urías-Silvas and López (2009) studied *in vitro* the prebiotic potential of different *Agave* species such *A. tequilana* from Guanajuato (ATG), *A. tequilana* from Jalisco (ATJ), *A. angustifolia* from Sonora (AAS), *A. angustifolia* from Oaxaca (AAO), *A. potatorum* from Oaxaca (APO), *A. fourcroydes* from Yucatan (AFY), and *Dasylirion* sp. from Chihuahua (DSC) fructans. In this work, bifidobacteria and lactobacilli were used as probiotic strains in pure culture. The culture medium was supplemented with Agave fructans or *Dasylirion* (DSC) at a concentration of 10 g/L as the only carbon source (glucose-free), and Raftilose (RSE) and Raftiline (RNE) were used as inulin-type fructans and referred to as positive controls.

In general, the media supplemented with fructans from *Dasylirion* sp. (DSC) showed larger growth for both bacteria (Figures 3.11 and 3.12). Only for *B. breve*, DSC was not significantly different from RSE, which is reported as an excellent prebiotic. *A. tequilana* (ATG) fructans were ranked as second best and Raftilose (RSE, commercial fructans) was third on the growth of probiotics such as *B. animalis*, *B. breve*, and *B. longum*; however, this was not the case for *Lactobacillus casei*. For lactobacilli, fructans obtained from *A. cantala* (ACO) was ranked second and ATG was third. Agavins from the same *Agave* species but grown in different geographic zones showed remarkable behavior on their prebiotic effect. Fructans from *A. tequilana* (Jalisco-ATJ) turned out to be a very poor substrate when compared to the same *Agave* species that is grown in a different geographic zone (Guanajuato-ATG). The same behavior was observed for *A. angustifolia* Sonora (AAS) and from Oaxaca (AAO), AAS being a better prebiotic at least *in vitro*.

In this same study, fructans with LDP showed the least effect on the different evaluated strains. The best prebiotic soluble fiber was found in Agave fructans of SDP and with least branched structures. These results are in agreement with Santiago-García and López (2009).

Santiago-García and López (2009) evaluated the growth rate of six bifidobacteria and four lactobacilli strains with LDP and SDP fructans and mixtures of them from *Agave angustifolia*. They observed that these soluble fibers

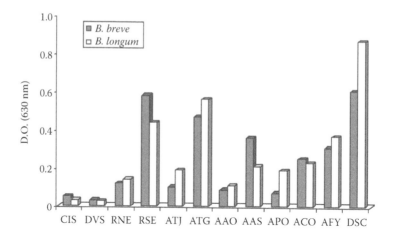

Figure 3.11 Effect of different fructans on the growth of *Bifidobacterium breve* and *B. longum* incubated anaerobically at 37°C in the presence of 10g of fructan/L. OD, optical density; CIS, *Cichorium intybus* Sigma; DVS, *Dahlia variabilis* Sigma; RNE, Raftiline; RSE, Raftilose; ATJ, *Agave tequilana*; ATG, *A. tequilana*; AAS, *A. angustifolia*; AAO, *A. angustifolia*; ACO, *A. cantala*; APO, *A. potatorum*; AFY, *A. fourcroydes*; DSC, *Dasylirion* sp.

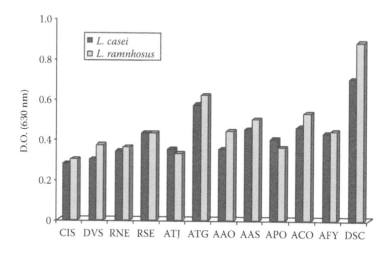

Figure 3.12 Effect of different fructans on the growth of *Lactobacillus casei* and *L. rhamnosus* incubated anaerobically at 37°C in the presence of 10g of fructan/L. OD, optical density; CIS, *Cichorium intybus* Sigma; DVS, *Dahlia variabilis* Sigma; RNE, Raftiline; RSE, Raftilose; ATJ, *Agave tequilana*; ATG, *A. tequilana*; AAS, *A. angustifolia*; AAO, *A. angustifolia*; ACO, *A. cantala*; APO, *A. potatorum*; AFY, *A. fourcroydes*; DSC, *Dasylirion* sp.

stimulated the growth of *bifidobacteria* and *lactobacilli* more efficiently than commercial inulins of the linear type (Santiago-García and López 2009). Furthermore, their fermentation revealed that mixtures of different degrees of polymerization and short fructans presented higher fermentation rates. In another *in vitro* study, the fermentation properties and prebiotic potential activity of Agave fructans from *A. tequilana* were evaluated (Gomez et al. 2010). In this study, five different commercial prebiotics were compared using 24-h pH-controlled anaerobic batch cultures inoculated with human fecal slurries. The prebiotic activity was measured by comparing bacterial changes and SCFAs production. Under the conditions of this research, Agave fructans showed a great increase in the number of bifidobacteria and lactobacilli.

With these studies, it has been shown that fructans from *Agave* spp. and *Dasylirion* sp. are able to stimulate the growth of probiotics. Prebiotic fibers with implications on health are generating great interest not only on research but also in a wide range of food applications. In this sense, a bright future awaits Agave fructans.

3.7 Mice Studies

3.7.1 Agave Fructans Impact on the Health of Mice

All fructans are considered prebiotic molecules that serve as a substrate for the gut microbiota (Kolida and Gibson 2007, López and Urías-Silvas 2007, Roberfroid 2005, Roberfroid and Delzenne 1998). A prebiotic is an ingredient selectively fermented by probiotics (bifidobacteria and lactobacilli) that induces specific changes in the composition and/or activity of the gastrointestinal microbiota, conferring benefits upon the host's well-being and health in general (Gibson and Roberfroid 1995, Gibson et al. 2004). The fermentation of fructans in the colon generates SCFAs, mostly acetate, propionate, and butyrate (Cummings and Macfarlane 1991, Gibson 1999, Topping and Clifton 2001). Some reports have established that the structure of undigested carbohydrates and the microbiota present in an ecosystem are determining factors that control fermentation in the gut (Henningsson et al. 2002). It is also known that the profiles of the production and distribution of those SCFAs in the gut are influenced not only by the type of consumed carbohydrates but also by the place where the fermentation of carbohydrates takes place, but the type of substrate may also affect the site of fermentation (Hughes and Rowland 2000). Huazano-García and López (2013) found that structural differences between inulins (chicory fructans) and agavins (Agave fructans) showed different profiles on the production of SCFAs along the whole gut (Figure 3.13). These authors fed mice with commercial inulins (Raftiline-RNE) and *Agave angustifolia* fructans (AAO) observing that mice fed with AAO produced greater amounts of SCFAs in the cecum and proximal and medial colon than those mice fed with RNE. This difference was attributed

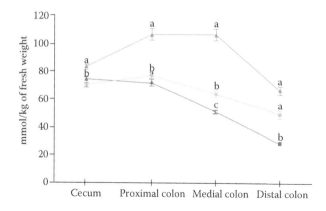

Figure 3.13 Differences in the production of short-chain fatty acids in the cecum and the three sections of the colon in mice on a standard diet (-----) or a diet supplemented with Raftiline (-----RNE-inulin) or *Agave angustifolia* (-----AAO-agavins).

to the presence of branches in the agavins, which could make the molecules more accessible to saccharolytic bacteria in colonic microbiota. This effect is important since SCFAs can interact directly or indirectly (via modification of pH) with gut cells and can participate in the control of various processes, including mucosal proliferation and inflammation, colorectal carcinogenesis, and mineral absorption (Roberfroid and Delzenne 1998).

3.7.2 Modulation of Lipid and Glucose Metabolism by Agave Fructans

The effect of fructans on lipid metabolism has been tested in rodent systems. Many studies have reported the improvement of cholesterol, triglycerides, hepatic steatosis, and plaque formation when a standard diet or high-fat diet is supplemented with fructans of the inulin type (Cani et al. 2005, Daubioul et al. 2002, Levrat et al. 1994).

Urías-Silvas et al. (2008) evaluated the potential of fructans extracted from *A. tequilana* Gto. (ATG), *Dasylirion* sp. (DSC), and commercial inulin (Raftilose-RSE) to modulate glucose and lipid metabolism in mice. These research studies reported that the diets supplemented with fructans presented a beneficial effect on the concentration of glucose and cholesterol in the mice blood. Glucose concentrations were significantly lowered by 19%, 15%, and 14% in mice fed RSE, ATG, and DSC supplemented diets, respectively, with respect to mice that were fed a standard diet. Triglycerides concentrations were reduced, with respect to mice fed a standard diet by 31%, 11%, and 7% in mice fed RSE, ATG and DSC, respectively. Cholesterol concentrations were also reduced, reaching about 20% in animals that received DSC, TEQ, and RSE diets when compared to the standard diet (Table 3.3). All these effects were attributed to the production of propionic acid, which is largely produced through the fermentation of all fructans. The high production of propionate,

Table 3.3 Concentration of Glucose, Triglycerides, and Cholesterol in Mice after the Consumption of a Standard Diet (STD) or a Diet Supplemented with: Raftilose (RSE), *Agave tequilana* (ATG), and *Dasylirion* (DSC)

Physiological Parameter	Diet							
	STD		RSE		ATG		DSC	
	Mean	SEM	Mean	SEM	Mean	SEM	Mean	SEM
Glucose*	10.36[a]	0.27	8.44[b]	0.38	8.76[b]	1.24	8.31[b]	0.39
Triglycerides*	1.40[a]	0.11	0.97[b]	0.08	1.24[ab]	0.09	1.31[b]	0.08
Cholesterol*	2.88[a]	0.12	2.40[b]	0.04	2.40[ab]	0.08	2.30[b]	0.10

Note: Mean values $n = 8$ with their standard errors of the mean for each parameter measured. Mean values with different superscript letters were significantly different ($p \leq 0.05$).

through fermentation, has been proposed as the responsible mechanism of serum and hepatic cholesterol reduction through fructans feeding in rats (Delzenne and Williams 2002).

Similar results were obtained by García-Pérez (2008) and Huazano-García and López (2013) who reported that diets supplemented with *Dasylirion* and *Agave* fructans had a beneficial effect on the concentration of glucose and cholesterol in blood from the portal vein of mice.

3.7.3 Homeostasis of the Hormones Involved in Satiety with Agave Fructans

Numerous peptides secreted by the enteroendocrine cells present along the gastrointestinal tract are involved in the regulation of energy homeostasis. For instance, glucagon-like peptide-1 (GLP-1) and ghrelin are two peptides able to modulate food intake and energy expenditure. GLP-1 is a potent insulinotropic hormone (released from intestinal L cells in response to nutrients) that lowers blood glucose, inhibits food intake, decreases glucagon secretion, and enhances β-cell neogenesis (Drucker 2006). Ghrelin is a peptide hormone released into circulation from the stomach that was first discovered as an endogenous ligand for the growth hormone secretagogue receptor (GHS-R). Ghrelin is the only known factor to increase appetite through circulation. The pattern of ghrelin release suggests that it governs feelings of hunger. Circulating ghrelin levels are increased by fasting, and usually fall after a meal. Ghrelin is often referred to as the "hunger hormone" (Kojima and Kangawa 2005).

Previous reports showed that the modulation of GLP-1 or ghrelin in rodents fed with fructans could constitute a link between the outcome of microbial fermentation in the lower part of the gut and metabolic consequences (e.g., decreased food intake, body weight and fat mass development, and improved insulin sensitivity) (Cani et al. 2004, 2006, Delmée 2006). GLP-1 (7-36) amide production occurs in different parts of the distal intestine (Orskov et al. 1989), and the site of production might influence the systemic distribution of GLP-1 (amide) through the portal vein; for this reason, Cani et al. (2004) analyzed the modulation of portal GLP-1 (7-36) amide in the sera of rats fed with a standard diet supplemented with 10% of inulins displaying different DPs, that is, oligofructose containing mainly SDP; inulin HP containing mainly LDP and synergy is a mix of both SDP and LDP. The researchers observed that inulins containing SDP (oligofructose and synergy) preferentially increased GLP-1 (7-36) amide concentration in the proximal colon and, to a lesser extent, in the medial colon. The authors suggest that an increase in proglucagon mRNA and GLP-1 levels in the proximal colon is a key event allowing fermentable inulin-type fructans to modulate food intake, body weight, and glucose homeostasis. These results are consistent with Urías-Silvas et al. (2008) who showed the increase of portal plasma GLP-1 in mice fed with *Agave tequilana* fructans from Guanajuato (ATG), *Dasylirion* sp. (DSC), and commercial inulin Raftilose (RSE) after 5 weeks with a dose of 100 g/kg. The increase in this venous compartment is physiologically relevant because glucose sensors and the terminal vagal nerve responsive to GLP-1 are located mainly in the portal vein (Burcelin et al. 2001). Interestingly, among tested fructans by Urías-Silvas et al. (2008), ATG had the most dramatic effect in increasing intestinal GLP-1 content in the proximal gut (the primary site of GLP-1 production) (Figure 3.14).

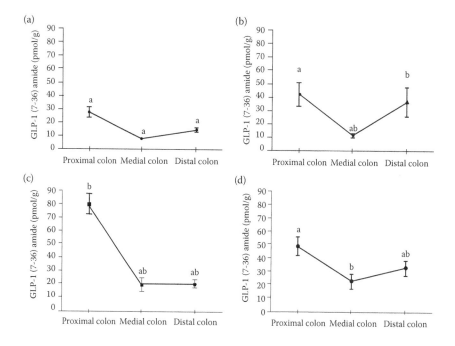

Figure 3.14 Intestinal glucagon-like peptide-1 (GLP-1) (7-36) amide concentration of mice fed (a) standard diet (STD) or diet supplemented with (b) Raftilose (RSE-inulin); (c) *Agave tequilana* (ATG); or (d) *Dasylirion* sp. (DSC). Mean values with their standard errors of the mean. Mean values with different letters were significantly different ($p \leq 0.05$).

Table 3.4 Ghrelin Concentration of Mice on a Standard Diet (STD) or on a Diet Supplemented with Raftilose (RSE), *Dasylirion* (DSC), Raftiline (RNE), and *A. angustifolia* Oax. (AAO)

	STD	RSE SDP	DSC SDP	RNE LDP	AAO LDP
Stomach (ng/mL·g of tissue)	6.90[a]	2.90[c]	3.10[c]	5.36[b]	4.38[b]

Note: Mean values with their standard errors of the mean. Mean values with different letters were significantly different ($p \leq 0.05$).

GLP-1 was the first gut peptide studied to relate events occurring in the colon due to the ingestion of fructans to modulate energy, lipids, and glucose homeostasis. However, other peptides could also be of interest such as PYY. Cani et al. (2004) showed an increase in portal GLP-1 and a decrease in serum ghrelin after oligofructose supplementation in rats; these events could participate in the satietogenic effect of oligofructose. Moreover, Djurhuus et al. (2002) demonstrated that GLP-1 (7-36) amide and ghrelin concentrations are inversely correlated after glucose ingestion. On the other hand, Lippl et al. (2004) showed that GLP-1 (7-36) amide contributes to the inhibition of ghrelin secretion in an isolated rat stomach model. Moreover, García-Pérez (2008) compared the effect of the structure and DP of two commercial fructans Raftilose (RSE) and Raftiline (RNE) derived from chicory (linear fructans) and branched fructans from *Dasylirion* sp. (DSC) and *A. angustifolia* (AAO) on ghrelin concentration in the stomach, RSE and DSC containing mainly SDP and RNE and AAO exhibiting LDP. All four fructans decreased ghrelin concentration in the stomach; nevertheless, mice fed with SDP fructans showed a lower concentration of this hormone (Table 3.4). These results match with those previously reported by Cani et al. (2004).

3.7.4 Agave Fructans on Calcium and Magnesium Absorption

Calcium levels do not depend only on its amount in the diet but also on its bioavailability. A number of nutritional factors facilitate the absorption of this mineral. Among these factors is the presence of certain complex organic acids and nondigestible but fermentable prebiotic fibers. Several mechanisms have been proposed by which these soluble fibers and other prebiotics may improve mineral absorption: (1) acidic metabolites of bacterial carbohydrate fermentation in the colon (mainly acetic, propionic, butyric, as well as lactic acid) lower the intestinal pH, solubilizing calcium and magnesium complexes (Lopez et al. 2000), thereby elevating the intestinal concentration of ionized calcium and increasing passive transport of the mineral; (2) modification of the electrical charge of calcium by the same SCFAs through the interchange of calcium–hydrogen complexes, supporting passage through the membrane. Lowering the pH and favoring the bioavailability of minerals in the large intestine is favored by this mechanism.

The beneficial effects of prebiotics on calcium absorption and bone mineralization were also demonstrated in healthy girls, adolescents, and postmenopausal women (Abrams et al. 2005, Griffin et al. 2002). In addition, many reports have also shown that fructans enhance not only intestinal calcium absorption, but bone calcium as well (Coudray et al. 2006). García-Pérez (2008) evaluated the effect of supplementing a mice diet with fructans (10%) of *Agave angustofolia* Haw. (AAO), *Dasylirion* sp. (DSC), chicory inulin (RNE and RSE as positive controls of LDP and LDP fructans, respectively) and a nonsupplemented diet (STD) on calcium and magnesium absorption in femurs. Calcium contents in femurs were significantly higher in all mice groups fed with fructan-supplemented diets presenting the highest level, the group fed with DCS diet. No difference among LDP and SDP fructans was observed. All mice groups fed with fructans increased their magnesium content; however, significant differences were observed among LDP and SDP. SDP fructans, such as DSC and RSE, had the higher magnesium contents in comparison with LDP fructans and STD group but this difference was not significant. The ingestion of all supplemented diets increased calcium and magnesium absorption in the femurs of mice. All fructans (AAO, RNE, DSC, and RSE) tended to increase calcium absorption between 23% and 25% without reaching significance ($p < 0.05$). However, only the ingestion of DSC and RSE led to a significant increment of Mg absorption in the bones. These data correlate well with previous works independently of the nature of fructans (LDP or SDP), since they all increased the calcium content in bone, which has been used as an indicator of an increased absorption of minerals. To better understand the effect of different fructans on mineral absorption, it is necessary not to overlook their calcium content but also other factors that directly impact them.

3.8 Future Potential

Agave fructans research is only at the tip of the iceberg; we deeply believe that due to their unique and complex structures, a wide range of surprises await discovery. We also believe that few of the undergoing research in different areas not only related to the impact that they might have on the metabolic syndrome but also in food applications or in the development of new and exciting food products. One of the most exciting issues to be investigated is the modulation of the microbiota of people suffering from metabolic syndromes. Based only on the scare information that we have at this point, it has been demonstrated that Agave fructans, a dietary fiber, is a very promising supplement for the control of metabolic or even in just one of components. Another even less studied aspect of Agave fructans is their presence in some of the Agave syrups, which are already in a good position in the food market.

References

Abrams, S. A., I. J. Griffin, K. M. Hawthorne et al. 2005. A combination of prebiotic short- and long-chain inulin-type fructans enhances calcium absorption and bone mineralization in young adolescents. *Am J Clin Nutr* 82:471–76.

Amiard, V., A. Morvan-Bertrand, J. P. Billard, C. Huault, F. Keller, and M. P. Prud'homme. 2003. Fructans, but not the sucrosylgalactosides, raffinose and loliose, are affected by drought stress in perennial ryegrass. *Plant Physiol* 132:2218–43.

Anderson, K., S. C. Li, and Y. T. Li. 2000. Diphenylamine–aniline–phosphoric acid reagent, a versatile spray reagent for revealing glycoconjugates on thin-layer chromatography plates. *Anal Biochem* 287:337–39.

Arrizon, J., S. Morel, A. Gschaedler, and P. Monsan. 2010. Comparison of the water-soluble carbohydrate composition and fructan structures of *Agave tequilana* plants of different ages. *Food Chem* 122:123–30.

Banguela, A. and L. Hernández. 2006. Fructans: From natural sources to transgenic plants. *Biotecnol Aplic* 23:202–10.

Bathia, I. S. and K. S. Nandra. 1979. Studies on fructosyltransferase from *Agave americana*. *Phytochemistry* 18:923–27.

Bieleski, R. L., 1993. Fructan hydrolysis drives petal expansion in ephemeral daylily flower. *Plant Physiol* 103:213–19.

Bonnett, G. D., I. M. Sims, R. J. Simpson, and A. J. Cairns. 1997. Structural diversity of fructan in relation to the taxonomy of the Poaceae. *New Phytol* 136:11–17.

Brasch, D. J., B. L. Fankhauser, and A. G. Mc Donald. 1988. A study of the glucofructofuranan from the New Zealand cabbage tree *Cordyline australis*. *Carbohydr Res* 180:315–24.

Burcelin, R., A. Da Costa, D. Drucker, and B. Thorens. 2001. Glucose competence of the hepatoportal vein sensor requires the presence of an activated glucagons-like peptide-1 receptor. *Diabetes* 50:1720–28.

Cani, P. D., C. Dewever, and N. M. Delzenne. 2004. Inulin-type fructans modulate gastrointestinal peptides involved in appetite regulation (glucagon-like peptide-1 and ghrelin) in rats. *Br J Nutr* 92:521–26.

Cani, P. D., A. M. Neyrinck, N. Maton, and N. M. Delzenne. 2005. Oligofructose promotes satiety in rats fed a high-fat diet: Involvement of glucagon-like peptide-1. *Obes Res* 13:1000–07.

Cani, P. D., C. Knauf, M. A. Iglesias et al. 2006. Improvement of glucose tolerance and hepatic insulin sensitivity by oligofructose requires a functional glucagon-like peptide 1 receptor. *Diabetes* 55:1484–90.

Chatterton, N. J. and P. A. Harrison. 2003. Fructans in crested wheatgrass leaves. *J Plant Physiol* 160:843–49.

Collins, M. D. and G. R. Gibson. 1999. Probiotics, prebiotics and synbiotics: Approaches for the nutritional modulation of microbial ecology. *Am J Clin Nutr* 69:1052–57.

Colunga-García, M. P., J. Coello-Coello, L. Espejo-Peniche, and L. Fuente-Moreno. 1993. Agave studies in Yucatan, Mexico II. Nutritional value of the inflorescence peduncle and incipient domestication. *Econ Bot* 47:328–34.

Coudray, C., C. Feillet-Coudray, E. Gueux, A. Mazur, and Y. Rayssiguier. 2006. Dietary inulin intake and age can affect intestinal absorption of zinc and copper in rats. *J Nutr* 136:117–22.

Cummings, J. H., 1981. Short chain fatty acids in the human colon. *Gut* 22:763–79.

Cummings, J. H. and G. T. Macfarlane. 1991. A review: The control and consequences of bacterial fermentation in the human colon. *J Appl Bacteriol* 70:443–59.

Daubioul, C., N. Rousseau, R. Demeure et al. 2002. Dietary fructans, but not cellulose, decrease triglyceride accumulation in the liver of obese Zucker fa/fa rats. *J Nutr* 132:967–73.

De Bruyn, A. and J. Van Loo. 1991. The identification by 1H- and 13C-NMR spectroscopy of sucrose, 1-kestose, and neokestose in mixtures present in plant extracts. *Carbohydr Res* 211:131–36.

Delmée, E., P. D. Cani, G. Gual et al. 2006. Relation between colonic proglucagon expression and metabolic response to oligofructose in high fat diet-fed mice. *Life Sci* 79:1007–13.

Delzenne, N. M. and C. M. Williams. 2002. Prebiotics and lipid metabolism. *Curr Opin Lipidol* 13:61–67.

Dias-Tagliacozzo, G. M., N. M. Itaya, M. A. Machado de Carvalho, R. C. Figueiredo-Ribeiro, and S. M. C. Dietrich. 2004. Fructans and water suppression on intact and fragmented rhizophores of *Vernonia herbacea*. *Braz Arch Biol Technol* 47:363–73.

Djurhuus, C. B., T. K. Hansen, C. Gravholt et al. 2002. Circulating levels of ghrelin and GLP-1 are inversely related during glucose ingestion. *Horm Metabol Res* 34:411–13.

Dorland, L., J. P. Kamerling, J. F. G. Vliegenthart, and M. N. Satyanarayana. 1977. Oligosaccharides isolated from *Agave vera cruz*. *Carbohydr Res* 54:275–84.

Drucker, D. J. 2006. The biology of incretin hormones. *Cell Metab* 3:153–65.

Faustini-Cuzzuol, G. R., M. A. Machado-Carvalho, L. B. Penteado-Zaidan, and P. Roberto-Furlani. 2005. Nutrient solutions for plant growth and fructan production in *Vernonia herbacea*. *Pesq Agropec Bras* 40:911–17.

García-Pérez, M. C. 2008. Efecto de los fructanos de *Dasylirion* sp. en la secreción de grelina y GLP-1 en ratones. M.Sc. Thesis CINVESTAV: México.

Gentry, H. S. 1998. *Agaves of Continental North America*, 2nd ed. Tucson, AZ: The University of Arizona Press.

Gibson, G. R. 1999. Dietary modulation of the human gut microflora using the prebiotics oligofructose and inulin. *J Nutr* 129:1438S–41.

Gibson, G. R. and M. B. Roberfroid. 1995. Dietary modulation of the human colonic microbiota: Introducing the concept of prebiotics. *J Nutr* 125:1401–12.

Gibson, G. R. and R. A. Rastall. 2006. *Prebiotics: Development and Application*. Chichester: John Wiley & Sons.

Gibson, G. R., H. M. Probert, J. V. Loo, R. A. Rastall, and M. B. Roberfroid. 2004. Dietary modulation of the human colonic microbiota: Updating the concept of prebiotics. *Nutr Res Rev* 17:259–75.

Gomez, E., K. M. Tuohy, G. R. Gibson, A. Klinder, and A. Costabile. 2010. *In vitro* evaluation of the fermentation properties and potential prebiotic activity of Agave fructans. *J Appl Microbiol* 108:2114–21.

Griffin, I. J., P. M. Davila, K. M. Harthorne, and S. A. Abrams. 2002. Non-digestible oligosaccharides and calcium absorption in girls with adequate calcium intake. *Br J Nutr* 87:187–91.

Hendry, G. A. F. 1993. The origin, distribution, and evolutionary significance of fructans. *New Phytol* 123:3–14.

Henningsson, A. M., I. M. Björck, and E. M. Nyman. 2002. Combinations of indigestible carbohydrates affect short-chain fatty acid formation in the hindgut of rats. *J Nutr* 132:3098–104.

Hincha, D. K., E. Zuther, E. M. Hellwege, and A. G. Heyer. 2002. Specific effects of fructo- and gluco-oligosaccharides in the preservation of liposomes during drying. *Glycobiology* 12:103–10.

Hincha, D. K., E. Zuther, and A. G. Heyer. 2003. The preservation of liposomes by raffinose family oligosaccharides during drying is mediated by effects on fusion and lipid phase transitions. *Biochim Biophys Acta* 1612:172–77.

Huazano-García, A. and M. G. López. 2013. Metabolism of short chain fatty acids in the colon and faeces of mice after a supplementation of diets with agave fructans. In *Lipid Metabolism*, ed. R. Valenzuela, 163–182. Rijeka: InTech.

Hughes, R. and I. R. Rowland. 2000. Stimulation of apoptosis by two prebiotic chicory fructans in the rat colon. *Carcinogenesis* 22:43–47.

Itaya, N. M., M. A. Machado de Carvahlo, and R. C. L. Figueiredo-Ribeiro. 2002. Fructosyl transferase and hydrolase activities in rizhopores and tuber roots upon growth of *Polymnia sonchifolia* (Asteraceae). *Physiol Plantarum* 116:451–59.

Kojima, M. and K. Kangawa. 2005. Ghrelin: Structure and function. *Physiol Rev* 85:495–22.

Kolida, S. and G. R. Gibson. 2007. Prebiotic capacity of inulin-type fructans. *J Nutr* 137:2503S–06.

Lasseur, B., J. Lothier, A. Djoumad et al. 2006. Molecular and functional characterization of a cDNA encoding fructan: Fructan 6G-fructosyltransferase (6G-FFT)/fructan:fructan 1-fructosyltransferase (1-FFT) from perennial ryegrass (*Lolium perenne* L.). *J Exp Bot* 57:2719–34.

Levrat, M. A., M. L. Favier, C. Moundras et al. 1994. Role of dietary propionic acid and bile acid excretion in the hypocholesterolemic effects of oligosaccharides in rats. *J Nutr* 124:531–38.

Lippl, F., F. Kircher, J. Erdmann, H. D. Allescher, and V. Schusdziarra. 2004. Effect of GIP, GLP-1, insulin and gastrin on ghrelin released in the isolated rat stomach. *Regul Pept* 119:93–98.

Liu, J., A. L. Waterhouse, and N. J. Chatterton. 1991. Proton and carbon chemicalshifts assignments for 6-kestose and neokestose from two-dimensional NMR measurements. *Carbohydr Res* 217:43–49.

Livingston, D. P. and C. A. Henson. 1998. Apoplastic sugars, fructans, fructan exohydrolase, and invertase in winter oat: Responses to second-phase cold hardening. *Plant Physiol* 116:403–08.

Livingston, D. P., R. Premakumar, and S. P. Tallury. 2006. Carbohydrate partitioning between upper and lower regions of the crown in oat and rye during cold acclimation and freezing. *Cryobiology* 52:200–08.

López-Medina, T. L. 2006. Extracción y caracterización de agavinas de *Agave tequilana* Weber var. azul de diferentes edades, B.S. Thesis.

Lopez, H. W., C. Coudray, M. A. Levrat-Verny, C. Feillet-Coudray, C. Demigné, and C. Rémésy. 2000. Fructooligosaccharides enhance mineral apparent absorption and counteract the deleterious effects of the phytic acid on mineral homeostasis in rats. *J Nutr Biochem* 11:500–08.

López, M. G. and N. A. Mancilla-Margalli. 2007. The nature of fructooligosaccharides in agave plants. In *Recent Advances in Fructooligosaccharides Research*, ed. S. Norio, B. Noureddine, and O. Shuichi, 47–67. Kerala: Research Signpost.

López, M. G. and J. E. Urías-Silvas. 2007. Agave fructans as prebiotics. In *Recent Advances in Fructooligosaccharides Research*, ed. S. Norio, B. Noureddine, and O. Shuichi, 297–310. Kerala: Research Signpost.

López, M. G., N. A. Mancilla-Margalli, and G. Mendoza-Díaz. 2003. Molecular structures of fructans from *Agave tequilana* Weber var. *azul. J Agric Food Chem* 51:7835–40.

Machado de Carvalho, M. A. and S. M. C. Dietrich. 1993. Variation in fructan content in the underground organs of *Vernonia herbecea* (Vell.) rusby at different phenological phases. *New Phytol* 123:735–40.

Mancilla-Margalli, N. A. and M. G. López. 2002. Generation of Maillard compounds from inulin during the thermal processing of *Agave tequilana* weber var. azul. *J Agric Food Chem* 50:806–12.

Mancilla-Margalli, N. A. and M. G. López. 2006. Water-soluble carbohydrates and fructan structure patterns from Agave and *Dasylirion* species. *J Agric Food Chem* 54:7832–39.

Mellado-Mojica, E. and M. G. Lopéz. 2012. Fructan metabolism in *Agave tequilana* Weber blue variety along it developmental cycle in the field. *J Agric Food Chem* 60:11704–14.

Mellado-Mojica, E., T. L. Lopéz-Medina, and M. G. Lopéz. 2009. Developmental variation in *Agave tequilana* Weber var. azul stem carbohydrates. *Dyn Biochem Biotechnol Mol Biol* 3:34–39.

Mussatto, S. I. and I. M. Mancilha. 2007. Non-digestible oligosaccharides: A review. *Carbohydr Poly* 68:587–97.

Nagaraj, V. J., D. Altenbach, V. Galati et al. 2004. Distinct regulation of sucrose: Sucrose-1-fructosyltransferase (1-SST) and sucrose: Fructan-6-fructosyltransferase (6-SFT), the key enzymes of fructan synthesis in barley leaves: 1-SST as the pacemaker. *New Phytol* 161:735–48.

Nobel, P. S., M. Castañeda, G. North, E. Pimienta-Barrios, and A. Ruiz. 1998. Temperature influence on leaf CO_2 exchange, cell viability and cultivation range of *Agave tequilana. J Arid Env* 39:1–9.

Orskov, C., M. Bersani, A. H. Johnsen, P. Hojrup, and J. J. Holst. 1989. Complete sequences of glucagon-like peptide-1 from human and pig small intestine. *J Biol Chem* 264:12826–29.

Orthen, B. and A. Wehrmeyer. 2004. Seasonal dynamics of non-structural carbohydrates in bulbs and shoots of the geophyte *Galanthus nivalis. Physiol Plantarum* 120:529–36.

Pilon-Smits, E. A. H., M. J. M. Ebskamp, M. J. Paul, M. J. Jeuken, P. J. Weisbeek, and S. C. M. Smeekens. 1995. Improved performance of transgenic fructan-accumulating tobacco under drought stress. *Plant Physiol* 107:125–30.

Pilon-Smits, E. A. H., M. J. M. Ebskamp, K. Van Dun, and N. Terry. 1999. Enhanced drought resistance in fructan-producing sugar beet. *Plant Physiol Biochem* 37:313–17.

Prud'homme, M. P., A. Morvan-Bertrand, B. Lasseur et al. 2007. *Lolium perenne*, backbone of sustainable development, source of fructans for grazing animals and potential source of novel enzymes. In *Recent Advances in Fructooligosaccharides Research*, ed. S. Norio, B. Noureddine, and O. Shuichi, 231–258. Kerala: Research Signpost.

Rastall, R. A. 2004. Bacterias in the gut: Friends and foes and how to alter the balance. *J Nutr* 134:2022–26.

Ravenscroft, N., P. Cescutti, M. A. Hearshaw, R. Ramsout, R. Rizzo, and E. M. Timme. 2009. Structural analysis of fructans from *Agave americana* grown in South Africa for spirit production. *J Agric Food Chem* 57:3995–4003.

Roberfroid, M. B. 2005. Introducing inulin type fructans. *Br J Nutr* 93:13S–25.

Roberfroid, M. B. 2007. Prebiotics: The concept revisited. *J Nutr* 137:830S–37.

Roberfroid, M. B. and N. M. Delzenne. 1998. Dietary fructans. *Annu Rev Nutr* 18:117–43.

Roberfroid, M. B. and J. Slavin. 2000. Nondigestible oligosaccharides. *Crit Rev Food Sci* 40:461–80.

Roberfroid, M., J. Van Loo, and G. Gibson. 1998. The bifidogenic nature of chicory inulin and its hydrolysis products. *J Nutr* 128:11–19.

Ruiz-Corral, J. A., E. Pimienta-Barrios, and J. Zañudo-Hernández. 2002. Optimal and marginal regions for the cultivation of *Agave tequilana* on the Jalisco State. *Agrociencia* 36:41–53.

Salminen, S., C. Bouley, M. C. Boutron-Ruault et al. 1998. Functional food science and gastrointestinal physiology and function. *Brit J Nutr* 80:147–71.

Sánchez-Marroquín, A. and P. H. Hope. 1953. Agave juice: Fermentation and chemical composition studies of some species. *J Agric Food Chem* 1:246–49.

Santiago-García, P. A. and M. G. López. 2009. Prebiotic effect of Agave fructans and mixtures of different degrees of polymerization from *Agave angustifolia* Haw. *Dyn Biochem Biotechnol Mol Biol* 3:52–58.

Shiomi, N., N. Benkeblia, S. Onodera, and N. Kawazoe. 2005. Fructooligosaccharides changes during maturation in inflorescences and seeds of onion (*Allium cepa* L. 'W202'). *Canadian J Plant Sci* 86:269–78.

Sims, I. M., A. J. Cairns, and R. H. Furneaux. 2001. Structure of fructans from excised leaves of New Zealand flax. *Phytochemistry* 57:661–68.

Spies, T., W. Praznick, A. Hofinger, F. Altmann, E. Nitsch, and R. Wutka. 1992. The structure of the fructan sinistrin from *Uriginea maritime*. *Carbohydr Res* 235:221–30.

Spollen, W. G. and C. J. Nelson. 1994. Response of fructan to water deficit in growing leaves of tall fescue. *Plant Physiol* 106:329–36.

Srinivasan, M. and I. S. Bathia. 1953. The carbohydrates of *Agave vera cruz* Mill. *Biochem J* 55:286–89.

Srinivasan, M. and I. S. Bathia. 1954. The carbohydrates of *Agave vera cruz* Mill. 2. Distribution in the stem and pole. *Biochem J* 56:256–59.

Tamura, K., A. Kawakami, Y. Sanada, K. Tase, T. Komatsu, and M. Yoshida. 2009. Cloning and functional analysis of a fructosyltransferase cDNA for synthesis of highly polymerized levans in timothy (*Phleum pratense* L.). *J Exp Bot* 60:893–905.

Thomas, H. and A. P. James. 1999. Partitioning of sugars in *Lolium perenne* (perennial ryegrass) during drought and on rewatering. *New Phytol* 118:35–48.

Topping, D. L. and P. M. Clifton. 2001. Short-chain fatty acids and human colonic function: Roles of resistant starch and nonstarch polysaccharides. *Physiol Rev* 81:1031–64.

Turnbaugh, P. J., V. K. Ridaura, J. J. Faith, F. E. Rey, R. Knight, and J. F. Gordon. 2009. The effect of diet on the human gut microbiome: A metagenomic analysis in humanized gnotobiotic mice. *Sci Transl Med* 6:1–19.

Turner, L. B., A. J. Cairns, I. P. Armstead et al. 2006. Dissecting the regulation of fructan metabolism in perennial ryegrass (*Lolium perenne*) with quantitative trait locus mapping. *New Phytol* 169:45–58.

Urías-Silvas, J. E. and M. G. López. 2009. *Agave* spp. and *Dasylirion* sp. fructans as a potential novel source of prebiotics. *Dyn Biochem Biotechnol Mol Biol* 3:59–65.

Urías-Silvas, J. E., P. D. Cani, E. Delmeé, A. Neyrinck, M. G. López, and N. M. Delzenne. 2008. Physiological effects of dietary fructans extracted from *Agave tequilana* Gto. and *Dasylirion* spp. *Br J Nutr* 99:254–61.

Valluru, R. and W. Van den Ende. 2008. Plant fructans in stress environments: Emerging concepts and future prospects. *J Exp Bot* 59:2905–16.

Van den Ende, W., A. Mientiens, H. Speleers, A. A. Onuchoa, and A. Van Laere. 1996. The metabolism of fructans in roots of *Cichorium intybus* during growth, storage and forcing. *New Phytol* 132:555–63.

Van den Ende, W., M. Yoshida, S. Clerens, R. Vergauwen, and A. Kawakami. 2005. Cloning, characterization and functional analysis of novel 6-kestose exohydrolases (6-KEHs) from wheat (*Triticum aestivum*). *New Phytol* 166:917–32.

Van den Ende, W., M. Coopman, S. Clerens et al. 2011. Unexpected presence of graminan- and levan-type fructans in the evergreen frost-hardy *Eudicot Pachysandra terminalis* (Buxaceae): Purification, cloning, and functional analysis of a 6-SST/6-SFT enzyme. *Plant Physiol* 155:603–14.

Van Loo, J., P. Coussement, L. De Leenheer, H. Hoebregs, and G. Smits. 1995. On the presence of inulin and oligofructose as natural ingredients in the western diet. *Crit Rev Food Sci Nutr* 35:525–52.

Van Waes, C., J. Baert, L. Carlier, and E. Van Bockstaele. 1998. A rapid determination of the total sugar content and the average inulin chain length in roots of chicory (*Cichorium intybus* L.). *J Sci Food Agric* 76:107–10.

Vereyken, I. J., V. Chupin, R. A. Demel, S. C. M. Smeekens, and B. De Kruijff. 2001. Fructans insert between the headgroups of phospholipids. *Biochim Biophys Acta* 1510:307–20.

Vijn, I. and S. Smeekens. 1999. Fructan: More than a reserve carbohydrate? *Plant Physiol* 120:351–60.

Wack, M. and W. Blaschek. 2006. Determination of the structure and degree of polymerisation of fructans from *Echinacea purpurea* roots. *Carbohydr Res* 341:1147–53.

Wang, N. and P. Nobel. 1998. Phloem transport of fructans in the crassulacean acid metabolism species *Agave deserti*. *Plant Physiol* 116:709–14.

Wiemken, A., M. Frehner, F. Keller, and W. Wagner. 1986. Fructan metabolism, enzymology and compartmentation. *Curr Top Plant Biochem Physiol* 5:17–37.

Wilson, R. G., J. A. Smith, and C. D. Yonts. 2004. Chicory root yield carbohydrate composition influenced by cultivar selection, planting, and harvest date. *Crop Sci* 44:748–52.

Wong, J. M., R. D. de Souza, C. W. C. Kendall, A. Emam, and D. J. Jenkings. 2006. Colonic health: Fermentation and short chain fatty acids. *J Clin Gastroenterol* 40:235–43.

CHAPTER 4

Fructooligosaccharides in *Allium* Species

Chemistry and Nutrition

NOUREDDINE BENKEBLIA

Contents

4.1   Introduction   75
4.2   History of *Allium* Species   76
4.3   History of Fructooligosaccharides and Fructans   77
4.4   Diet and Edible *Allium* Species   78
4.5   Fructooligosaccharides of *Allium* Species   79
     4.5.1   Chemistry   79
     4.5.2   Structural Composition   79
     4.5.3   FOS Occurrence in Edible *Allium* Species   81
4.6   Biosynthesis Pathways of FOS in *Allium* Species   85
4.7   Mechanism of Hydrolysis of FOS   86
4.8   Biotechnology and Breeding of High-FOS *Allium* Species   89
4.9   Putative and Potential Health Benefits of FOS   90
     4.9.1   FOS and Cancer Prevention   91
     4.9.2   FOS and Lipids Metabolism   92
     4.9.3   Prebiotic Effects of FOS   93
     4.9.4   Action of FOS on Mineral Absorption   94
     4.9.5   Actions of FOS on Glycemia and Insulinemia   94
4.10   Concluding Remarks and Future Directions   95
References   96

4.1 Introduction

From the simple and valued sentence of Hippocrates "Let food be your medicine," we started to learn that fibers, including fructans and fructooligosaccharides (FOS), are more than roughage. The fibers are in fact all around us, in fruits, vegetables, whole grains, breads and cereals, beans, and other legumes, but still majority of people have trouble getting even minimal amounts of fibers in their daily diets because of many reasons such as feeding customs, life style, and even some personal beliefs.

In the quest for healthy diet, many people have turned to targeted diet and eating styles, and are acquiring knowledge that many available foods in groceries and markets contain different kinds of fibers. Because science and medicine have been evolving considerably these last few decades, it has been established that eating a balanced diet with fruits, vegetables, and grains is the only way to get the complete benefits from fibers. Moreover, one important step is also educating ourselves about the foods we eat so we can make the often small changes in our diet that add up to feeling better and living longer, and then meeting the aforementioned statement of Hippocrates.

Recently, there has been a lot of attention paid to the carbohydrate portion of the diet. The word "fiber" has become a rallying point for people looking for ways to combat cardiovascular disease (CVD) and several types of intestinal cancer. However, other carbohydrates are also getting a lot of publicity. FOS are a carbohydrate that many feel should become a greater portion of the diet.

Despite the fact that scientific evidence has approved many health claims related to fructans and FOS, including a lowered risk of heart disease and cancer, ongoing research is discovering more and more benefits of eating these carbo-polymers; the typical consumer in developed countries eats only 10–15 g of fiber per day, which is less than half the recommended amount (Farnworth 1993). On the other hand, the ancestry of cultivated *Allium* species is not definitely established because one difficulty in the identification of its wild progenitor is the sterility of the cultivars. However, this fact did not deter passionate people and scientists from researching the history of both *Allium* species and fructans. This chapter describes the same in detail.

4.2 History of *Allium* Species

Prehistoric remains of cultivated plants are often extremely helpful to the reconstruction of their botanical evolvement and evolution as well as their history. This concept is true especially for long-living seed crops, for example, cereals and trees, but much less so for many species such as the onion bulb. Because *Allium* species are small and leave no archaeologic evidence, they have little chance of long preservation, which is also behind their exact origin, which still remains mysterious. However, *Allium* species are probably considered to be one of the world's oldest cultivated vegetables and they were much reported upon. It is presumed that our predecessors discovered and consumed wild *Allium* species long before farming or writing was invented. Onion and garlic could probably be the first cultivated crops due to their growing versatility, long storage time, and portability. They could be dried and preserved for times when food was scarce. The Chinese have cultivated *Allium* species in gardens for 5000 years, and they have been referenced in the ancient Vedic writings of India. *Allium* species can be traced back as far as 3500 BC in Egypt, where they served as an object of worship. The onion symbolized eternity to the Egyptians who buried the root vegetable alongside Pharaohs. In medicine, *Allium* species have a variety of medicinal properties. Early American settlers used wild onion to treat colds, coughs, and asthma, and to repel insects. In Chinese medicine, *Allium* species have also been used to treat angina, coughs, bacterial infections, and breathing problems.

At the present time, the *Allium* family has over 600 species distributed all over Europe, North America, Northern Africa and Asia. Edible *Allium* species that belong to the liliaceous family are onions (*Allium cepa*), garlic (*Allium sativum*), leek (*Allium porum*), chive (*Allium schoenoprasum*), scallion (called also Welsh onion, green onion, spring onion) (*Allium fistulosum*), and shallot (*Allium oschaninii*), each differing in taste, form, and color, but having close ties as far as biochemical, phytochemical, and nutraceutical content is concerned. As an example of their cropping importance, world onion production is steadily increasing so much so that the onion is now the second most important horticultural crop after tomatoes. Besides their remarkable medicinal powers, *Allium* species are generally consumed for their flavors, while their nutritive values have been appreciated only recently (Fenwick and Hanley 1990, Shiomi et al. 2007). Carbohydrates in *Allium* species account for a major portion of their dry matter, contributing as much as 65–80% of the dry weight. The principal components of the nonstructural carbohydrates are glucose, fructose, sucrose, and a series of FOS (fructosyl polymers) with degrees of polymerization (DP) up to c.a. 12 (Benkeblia et al. 2002, Brewster 1990, Darbyshire 1978, Suzuki and Cutcliffe 1989).

4.3 History of Fructooligosaccharides and Fructans

FOS, as fructan molecules, have a history spanning two centuries, and review articles have reported some historical aspects, including general history on fructans research (Meier and Reid 1982, Pollock and Cairns 1991, Pontis and Del Campillo 1985). Prior to the contemporary science of fructans and FOS, ancient peoples were using fructan-containing plants not only as a source of food, but also for feed and medicine. Two of the most used and oldest vegetables are onions and garlic, which were widely used by the Pharaoh in their rituals and these two plants have been considered two of numerous symbols of religious rites. Nevertheless, the modern history of fructans began with their discovery by the scientist Rose (1804), and this history saw considerable development at the turn of the past century when the scientist Edelman proposed a mechanism concerning their metabolism in higher plants. More recently, fructans and FOS research has seen considerable progress, in particular with the boom of molecular biology tools. Thus, the scope of fructans and FOS research has been moving from basic to applied science. At the present time, fructans and FOS are not only considered food ingredients but also foods in themselves, and are found in more than 500 food products resulting in a significant daily consumption. Because the science of nutrition itself has changed, FOS are now considered functional foods, which is a new concept (Duggan et al. 2002, Roberfroid 2002). In addition, they are nowadays used as a feed additive in poultry in the United States and Japan. The history of FOS concerning their safety and health benefits continues to pique the interest of scientists who every day discover their potential as whole food and as ingredients.

4.4 Diet and Edible *Allium* Species

At the turn of the past century and the development of many diseases related to food and diet, interest in the potential health benefits of fruits and vegetables, including edible *Allium* species, mainly onion and garlic, has started to rise; yet these interests have origins in antiquity, and are one of the earliest documented examples of plants used for the maintenance of health and treatment of diseases (Block 1985, Griffiths et al. 2002, Khan 1996, Rivlin 2001). Edible *Allium* species formed an important part of the daily diet of the people of ancient Egypt, and the Pharaohs fed them to the working class involved in heavy labor, such as in building pyramids (Moyers 1996). The Jewish slaves in Egypt were fed *Allium*, apparently to give them strength and increase their productivity. In ancient Greece, edible *Allium* species were associated with strength and work capacity, and garlic formed an important part of the military diet (Moyers 1996). *Allium* species were considered by the Romans as an aid to strength and endurance, and were fed to both soldiers and sailors and were part of a ship's manifest when it set out to sea (Green and Polydoris 1993). In ancient Chinese civilization, *Allium* species were evidently and frequently used in combination therapy as medicinal agents (Woodward 1996), while also forming a part of the daily diet, particularly when consumed together with raw meat (Khan 1996).

During the middle ages, knowledge of the therapeutic use of plants was gained, and *Allium* species were thought to have medicinal properties and were grown in monasteries (Khan 1996). With the onset of the Renaissance, attention was increasingly paid in Europe and America to the medical uses of *Allium* species, such as other aromatic plants. Thus, onion and garlic became two of the major plants and the ruling class began to adopt the former and not to restrict its consumption to the working class. Moreover, contemporary research tends to validate many of the earlier views concerning the efficacy of *Allium* species, while also seeking to elucidate the mechanisms behind the actions of the major components of onion and garlic such as FOS.

4.5 Fructooligosaccharides of *Allium* Species

4.5.1 Chemistry

From the chemical and structural points of view, the fructooligosaccharide polymers (FOS), also known as fructans, are polyfructosylsucroses of varying molecular size built on a sucrose starter unit and are biochemically designated by 1^F (1-β-D-fructofuranosyl)$_n$ sucrose oligomers, where n may vary from 0 to 15. Instead, FOS are considered carbohydrates with a very low DP in comparison to other poly-carbohydrates and consequently have low molecular weight (Yun 1996). As shown in Figure 4.1, FOS consist of a sucrose molecule to which other molecules of fructose have been added, although the term FOS is somewhat ambiguous since the number of fructose moieties added varies. Indeed, major researchers agree with the concept that FOS have a polymerized chain if n varies from 1 to c.a. 12 units of fructose, while longer chains are considered as inulin polymers (inulin-type fructans). On the other hand, FOS have also been variously defined and have been considered as polymers that include anything from 2 to 20 monosaccharide units. However, according to IUB-IUPAC terminology, the dividing point between oligo- and poly-fructooligosaccharides is 10.

4.5.2 Structural Composition

Because FOS polymers of *Allium* species, as well as other fructan types, are complex and their structures vary, the nomenclature is not simple. At the beginning of fructan science, the nomenclatures for FOS proposed by Lewis (1993) and Waterhouse and Chatterton (1993) were first used in the literature to illustrate the chemical structures of FOS and fructans. Nevertheless, from a purely chemical point of view, some controversies and discrepancies were raised in the scientific references concerning this nomenclature. However, in a recent paper, it has been suggested that FOS are a common name for only fructose with a low DP (oligomers) that are mainly composed of FOS shown in Table 4.1 and Figure 4.2 (Yun 1996).

Consequently, the simple structured FOS are "inulin-type," which consist of β(1-2)-linked fructose residues and these FOS are found in almost all fructan-containing plants. Moreover, in liliaceous plants, including *Allium* species, for example, onion and garlic, a second and different type of FOS has been found in their tissues and was named the "inulin neo-series." These types of FOS have two β(1-2)-linked fructose chains attached to the sucrose starter unit. One chain is linked to the carbon 1 [C1] of the fructose residue (as is also the case of inulin-type), and the other to the carbon 6 [C6] of the glucose residue (Figure 4.2).

However, the analytical and structural studies carried out on the structures of the FOS and fructans were characterized by a relative lack of data. Indeed, in most studies, chemical and/or enzymatic methods have been used

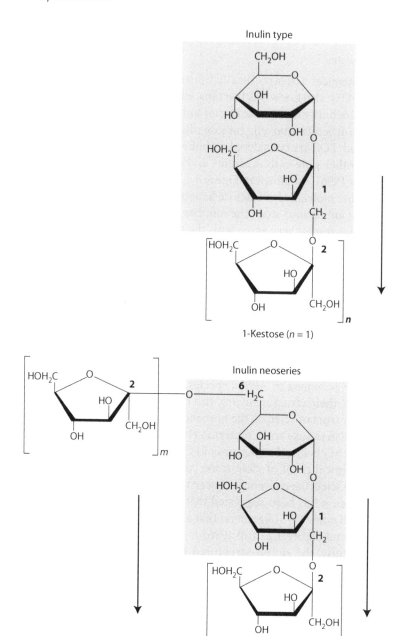

Figure 4.1 Molecular structures of the different types of fructooligosaccharides found in higher plants.

Table 4.1 Nomenclature of Fructooligosaccharide Oligomers Adopted by the Scientific Literature

Common Name	Polymer Name	Structural Name
1-Kestose	GF$_2$ or 1-kestotriose	1^F-β-D-fructofuranosylsucrose
Nystose	GF$_3$ or 1,1-kestotetraose	1^F (1-β-D-fructofuranosyl)$_2$ sucrose
1^F-Fructofuranosyl nystose	GF$_4$ or 1,1,1-kestopentaose	1^F (1-β-D-fructofuranosyl)$_3$ sucrose

to determine and deduce many highly polymerized FOS, although techniques used for analyses did not allow a good and reliable separation and identification of higher polymerized FOS. Two decades ago, new techniques for the separation and the determination of the structural composition of the different FOS in onions, as well as other plants, have been developed. Shiomi et al. (1997) separated different FOS of onion bulbs using high-performance anion exchange chromatography and pulsed amperometric detection (HPAEC–PAD) technique, while Stahl et al. (1997) used simultaneous matrix-assisted laser desorption ionization–mass spectrometry (MALDI–MS) and HPAEC methods and obtained similar results as shown in Table 4.2. These results have also been confirmed later by Benkeblia et al. (2005).

4.5.3 FOS Occurrence in Edible Allium Species

The occurrence and the distribution of FOS in some *Allium* species was first discovered in 1894 as reported by Archbold (1940), and almost all the investigation carried out focused mainly on onion bulbs, very few on garlic, while none referenced to leek, shallot, or chives. The content, distribution, and structure of the FOS of *Allium* species have been first investigated by Bacon (1959) and Darbyshire and Henry (1978, 1981) during the 1970s. Later, FOS content and distribution were the subject of vast and numerous investigations (Benkeblia et al. 2004, Campbell et al. 1997, Jaime et al. 2001, O'Donoghue et al. 2004, Shiomi et al. 1997), which contributed to the elucidation of their structures and properties. Advanced and modern analytical technologies also led to an ideal separation and identification of the different FOS found in onion bulbs (Table 4.2 and Figure 4.3) (Benkeblia et al. 2005).

As a result of these analytical methodologies used to elucidate the structural composition of FOS, it was also found that this composition varies, although slightly, with the type of *Allium* (dry onion, green onion), cultivar (sweet or pungent cultivar), dry matter content (high or low DM), and stage of maturity (Benkeblia 2005, Brewster 1994). It was also reported that the content of the FOS increases from the outer (old) to the inner (young) scales (Darbyshire and Henry 1978) (Figure 4.4), and the content of low-DP FOS is correlated to that of dry matter (DM < 10%) (Darbyshire and Steer 1990);

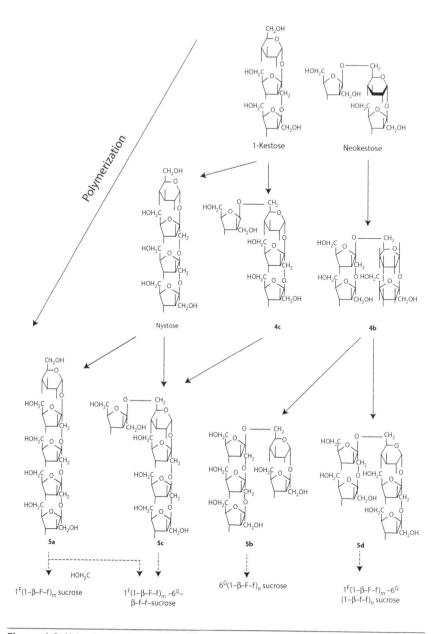

Figure 4.2 Molecular structures of the different fructooligosaccharides found in onion and other edible *Allium* species.

however, in high-dry-matter onion bulbs, the maximum DP varies largely and ranges between 10 and 15 (Darbyshire 1978, Ernst et al. 1998).

In garlic, only a few studies investigated the presence and the structural chemistry of the different FOS. First, Das and Das (1978) studied the structure of the fructans in garlic bulbs and suggested that FOS are linear and

Table 4.2 Structural Composition of the Different Fructooligosaccharides of Onion Bulb Separated by HPAEC

Common Name	Structural Name
1-Kestose (3a)	1^F-β-D-fructofuranosylsucrose
Neokestose (3b)	6^G-β-D-fructofuranosylsucrose
Nystose (4a)	1^F (1-β-D-fructofuranosyl)$_2$ sucrose
4b	6^G (1-β-D-fructofuranosyl)$_2$ sucrose
4c	1^F, 6^G-di-β-D-fructofuranosyl sucrose
5a	1^F (1-β-D-fructofuranosyl)$_3$ sucrose
5b	6^G (1-β-D-fructofuranosyl)$_3$ sucrose
5c	1^F (1-β-D-fructofuranosyl)$_2$–6^G-β-D-fructofuranosyl sucrose
5d	1^F-β-D-fructofuranosyl–6^G (1-β-D-fructofuranosyl)$_2$ sucrose
6a	1^F (1-β-D-fructofuranosyl)$_4$ sucrose
6b	6^G (1-β-D-fructofuranosyl)$_4$ sucrose
6c	1^F (1-β-D-fructofuranosyl)$_3$–6^G-β-D-fructofuranosyl sucrose
6d$_1$	1^F-β-D-fructofuranosyl–6^G (1-β-D-fructofuranosyl)$_3$ sucrose
6d$_2$	1^F (1-β-D-fructofuranosyl)$_2$–6^G (1-β-D-fructofuranosyl)$_2$ sucrose
7a	1^F (1-β-D-fructofuranosyl)$_5$ sucrose
7	1^F (1-β-D-fructofuranosyl)$_m$–6^G (1-β-D-fructofuranosyl)$_n$ sucrose ($m + n = 5$)
8	1^F (1-β-D-fructofuranosyl)$_m$–6^G (1-β-D-fructofuranosyl)$_n$ sucrose ($m + n = 6$)
9x	1^F (1-β-D-fructofuranosyl)$_m$–6^G (1-β-D-fructofuranosyl)$_n$ sucrose ($m + n \geq 7$)

Source: Benkeblia, N. et al. 2002. *Int J Food Sci Technol* 37:169–76.

belong to the inulin-type series, that is, linear chains without branching. Later, other results have shown that isolated and analyzed fructans of garlic belong to the inulin neo-series type, and Baumgartner et al. (2000) isolated fructans of high molecular weight, and studied their structure by enzymatic, chemical, and NMR spectroscopy, confirming their structural composition as belonging to the "inulin neo-series" type.

Surprisingly, except for the limited data on carbohydrate content reported by some researchers as shown in Table 4.3, we did not come across any reference reporting upon the structural composition of the nonstructural carbohydrates or the FOS found in leeks, shallots, or other edible *Allium* species. This shortage is probably due to many reasons, such as their limited importance in the general diet as compared to onions and garlic, and their limitations with regard to storage and consumption, while onion and garlic can be stored for months, and it is well known that their carbohydrates play a major role in their longevity of storage (Darbyshire and Henry 1978, Rutherford and Wittle 1984).

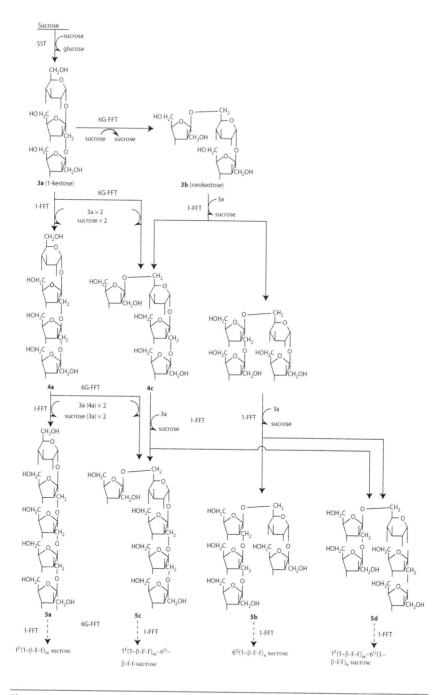

Figure 4.3 (Continued)

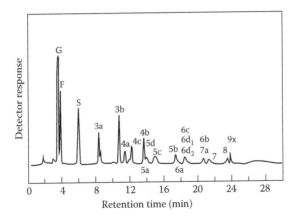

Figure 4.4 Distribution of fructooligosaccharides in onion bulbs. (Adapted from Darbyshire, B. and R. J. Henry. 1978. *New Phytol* 81:29–34.)

4.6 Biosynthesis Pathways of FOS in *Allium* Species

So far, the biosynthesis pathway of FOS in *Allium* species was studied mainly in onion tissue, which is considered a "model pathway" in FOS biosynthesis in liliaceous plants. It was demonstrated that FOS biosynthesis and polymerization are localized in the vacuoles of the cells (Frehner et al. 1984, Wagner and Wiemken 1986).

In liliaceous plants, because particular branched types "inulin neo-series" of FOS are produced, three enzymes are required (Pollock and Cairns 1991, Shiomi 1989, Wagner and Wiemken 1986, Wiemken et al. 1995) (Figure 4.5). The sucrose:sucrose 1-fructosyltransferase (1-SST, EC 2.4.1.99) initiates FOS synthesis by catalyzing the transfer of a fructosyl residue from one sucrose molecule to another sucrose molecule, resulting in the formation of the first trisaccharide 1-kestose (1^F-β-D-fructofuranosylsucrose or G1-2F1-2F). After that, the fructan:fructan 1-fructosyltransferase (1-FFT, EC 2.4.1.100)

Figure 4.3 (Continued) Separation of neutral soluble carbohydrates of onion bulbs by high-performance anion exchange chromatography and pulsed amperometric detection (HPAEC–PAD). **G**: glucose; **F**: fructose; **S**: sucrose; 1^F-β-D-fructofuranosylsucrose (**3a**, 1-kestose); 6^G-β-D-fructofuranosylsucrose (**3b**, neokestose); 1^F (1-β-D-fructofuranosyl)$_2$ sucrose (**4a**, nystose); 6^G (1-β-D-fructofuranosyl)$_2$ sucrose (**4b**); 1^F, 6^G-di-β-D-fructofuranosyl sucrose (**4c**); 1^F (1-β-D-fructofuranosyl)$_3$ sucrose (**5a**); 6^G (1-β-D-fructofuranosyl)$_3$ sucrose (**5b**); 1^F (1-β-D-fructofuranosyl)$_2$–6^G-β-D-fructofuranosyl sucrose (**5c**); 1^F-β-D-fructofuranosyl–6^G (1-β-D-fructofuranosyl)$_2$ sucrose (**5d**); 1^F (1-β-D-fructofuranosyl)$_4$ sucrose (**6a**); 6^G (1-β-D-fructofuranosyl)$_4$ sucrose (**6b**); 1^F (1-β-D-fructofuranosyl)$_3$–6^G-β-D-fructofuranosyl sucrose (**6c**); 1^F-β-D-fructofuranosyl–6^G (1-β-D-fructofuranosyl)$_3$ sucrose (**6d$_1$**); 1^F (1-β-D-fructofuranosyl)$_2$–6^G (1-β-D-fructofuranosyl)$_2$ sucrose (**6d$_2$**); 1^F (1-β-D-fructofuranosyl)$_5$ sucrose (**7a**); 1^F (1-β-D-fructofuranosyl)$_m$–6^G (1-β-D-fructofuranosyl)$_n$ sucrose (**7**, $m + n = 5$)1^F (1-β-D-fructofuranosyl)$_m$–6^G (1-β-D-fructofuranosyl)$_n$ sucrose (**8**, $m + n = 6$); 1^F (1-β-D-fructofuranosyl)$_m$–6^G (1-β-D-fructofuranosyl)$_n$ sucrose (**9x**, $m + n ≥ 7$).

Table 4.3 Distribution of Fructooligosaccharides in Edible *Allium* Species

	FOS (mg g⁻¹ FW)	DPᵃ	Reference
Bunching onion	—	—	—
Chinese chive	<0.1	—	Campbell et al. (1997)
Garlic	3.9	3 ~ 5	Campbell et al. (1997)
Garlic, powder	1.7	3 ~ 5	Campbell et al. (1997)
Leek	0.9	2 ~ 4	Campbell et al. (1997)
Onion, welsh	1.1	3 ~ 5	Campbell et al. (1997)
Onion, white	3.1	3 ~ 5	Campbell et al. (1997)
Onion, yellow	26.3	3 ~ 12	Stahl et al. (1997), Benkeblia et al. (2004)
Onion, red	27.1	3 ~ 12	Brewster (1990)
Onion, powder	47.7	3 ~ 5	Campbell et al. (1997)
Shallot	8.5	—	Campbell et al. (1997)

ᵃ Degree of polymerization.

elongates the chain initiating the formation of inulin-type FOS (linear FOS). A second enzyme, the fructan:fructan 6G-fructosyltransferase acts on the linear FOS and links one fructosyl residue by (2 → 6) initiating the formation of inulin neo-series FOS (branched FOS). It was initially thought that these two enzymes are two distinct proteins. Indeed, the involvement of two different enzymatic proteins (6G-FFT and 1-FFT) has been established in other vegetables, that is, asparagus; however, recent proteomic and genomic studies carried out on 6G-FFT and 1-FFT activities have demonstrated that both activities in onion bulbs are assigned to a single and unique enzymatic protein (Fujishima et al. 2005, Ritsema 2003), and the production of FOS was studied by their activity *in vitro* (Figure 4.6).

Biochemically, the first enzyme 1-SST was purified and well characterized from onion seeds (Shiomi et al. 1985) and bulb tissues (Henry and Darbyshire 1980). The second enzyme was also purified and characterized. It was classified as fructan:fructan 6G-fructosyltransferase (EC 2.4.1.243, 6G-FFT 47), and was recently included in the IUBMB enzyme nomenclature (http://www.chem.qmul.ac.uk/iubmb/enzyme/EC2/4/1/243.html).

4.7 Mechanism of Hydrolysis of FOS

When fructan-containing plants are harvested after complete maturity, FOS are no longer exported to meristematic cells (bulbs) or storage organs (tubers and rhizomes) and photosynthesis normally ceases (Lang 1996, Nilsson 2000). The harvesting may result in a change in the allocation of carbon with new sources (areas of carbohydrate supply) and sinks (areas of carbohydrate

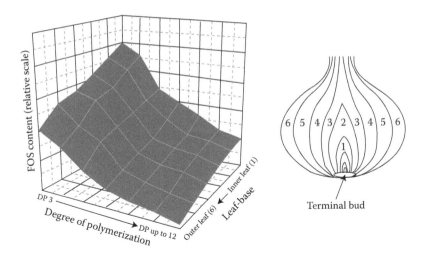

Figure 4.5 Pathway of the enzymatic synthesis of fructooligosaccharides in liliaceous plants (SST, sucrose:sucrose 1-fructosyltransferase; 1-FFT, fructan:fructan 1^F-fructosyltransferase; 6G-FFT, fructan:fructan 6^G-fructosyltransferase).

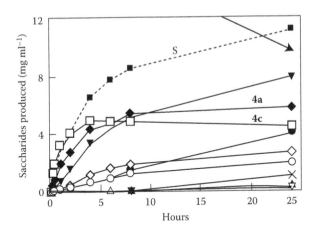

Figure 4.6 Production of tetrasaccharides and other oligosaccharides from 1-kestose by onion fructosyl-transferase: ■ sucrose; ▲ 1-kestose (**3a**); ▼ neokestose (**3b**); ◆ nystose (**4a**); ● 6^G (1-β-D-fructofuranosyl)$_2$ sucrose (**4b**); □ [1^F, 6^G–di-β-D-fructofuranosyl sucrose] (**4c**); △ [1^F (1-β-D-fructofuranosyl)$_3$ sucrose] (**5a**); ▽ [6^G (1-β-D-fructofuranosyl)$_3$ sucrose] (**5b**); ◇ [1^F (1-β-D-fructofuranosyl)$_2$–6^G-β-D-fructofuranosyl sucrose] (**5c**); ○ [1^F-β-D-fructofuranosyl–6^G (1-β-D-fructofuranosyl)$_2$ sucrose] (**5d**); × [6^G (1-β-D-fructofuranosyl)$_4$ sucrose] (**6**); + 1^F (1-β-D-fructofuranosyl)$_m$–6^G (1-β-D-fructofuranosyl)$_n$ sucrose ($m + n = 5$). (From Fujishima, M., H. Sakai, K. Ueno et al. 2005. *New Phytol* 165:513–24.)

demand), resulting in a redirection of metabolism (Lang 1996, Mohr and Schopfer 1995). At maturity, fructan-accumulating organs are supposed to be in "dormancy" and this physiological stage may be linked to the metabolic changes following this source-to-sink transition, when dormant organs are preparing to sprout again (Espen et al. 1999). From a purely physiological point of view, dormant bulbs are still metabolically active, although at greatly reduced levels. However, it is well-established that the duration of dormancy varies among growing years and among cultivars, and depends on atmospheric and environmental conditions (Asega and Carvalho 2004, Lang 1987, Le Nard and De Hertogh 1993). During the storage of fructan-containing bulbs, FOS are hydrolyzed to low-DP FOS, then disaccharides, and finally to monosaccharides. This hydrolysis usually takes place early in the first few weeks following harvesting with little further change during the first few weeks of dormancy. However, after a prolonged period, and when sprouting starts, a considerable increase in the amount of reducing sugars (i.e., fructose and glucose) can occur (Rutherford 1981).

The enzyme responsible for the hydrolysis of fructans in *Allium* species, as well as fructan-containing plants, is fructan 1-exohydrolase (FEH, EC 3.2.1.80), and it is localized in vacuoles of the protoplasts (Darwen and Johnn 1989, Wagner and Wiemken 1986). Although a large number of fructan-degrading enzymes have been identified from bacteria, fungi, and plants (Van den Ende et al. 2002), the FEHs of higher plants, which have been characterized up to date, exhibit a strong preference for either the β-2-1 or the β-2-6 linkage but were not completely specific for one type of linkage and many showed some ability to hydrolyze sucrose (Bonnett and Simpson 1993, Henson 1989).

FEH hydrolyzes fructan molecules at the terminal, nonreducing fructosyl-residue (exolytic attack), thus releasing free fructose. Initially, two FEH activities (hydrolases A and B) were found in *Helianthus tuberosus* tubers. Later, other FEHs were purified from oats (Edelman and Jefford 1964) and Jerusalem artichoke (Henson and Livingston 1996, Marx et al. 1997) while FEH from chicory has been purified (Claessens et al. 1990, De Roover et al. 1999, Van den Ende et al. 2002), cloned, and well biochemically characterized (Van den Ende et al. 2000, 2001). However, the detection of FEH activity can be limited in crude or partially purified enzyme preparations by contaminating invertase (EC 3.2.1.26) (Simpson et al. 1991) and very little is known about the regulation of its activity, which is of considerable interest because the vacuole is also the site of fructan synthesis and storage.

Despite the advances in FOS hydrolysis and enzymes involved in their hydrolysis, few investigations focus on the FEHs in onion bulbs during the dormancy and the postdormancy (Benkeblia et al. 2005). It seems that the activity of 1-FEH seems to be under strict control because of the evidence of seasonal variation. It was also noted that a degrading activity of 1-kestose, which showed patterns closely reflecting 1-FEH activity, was independent of temperatures, and a similar variation of 1-FEH activity in the rhizophores of *Vermonia herbacea* was reported (Asega and Carvalho 2004), although this plant is biologically different from bulbs and *Allium* species.

However, in a recent work, another fructan-hydrolyzing activity was reported and was assigned to another enzyme named 1-kestose hydrolyze (1-KHE). This was recently highlighted in onions (1-kestose hydrolase) (Benkeblia et al. 2005) and wheat (6-kestose hydrolase) (Van den Ende et al. 2005). This recent finding of these two highly specialized enzymes is probably behind the lack of their studies in vegetable crops, mainly liliaceous.

The different results confirm the claim that saccharides produced by the hydrolysis and low-DP FOS (DP 3-4) play a role in the balance of the catabolism of FOS during the dormancy period and the regrowth stage. This balance maintains a specific level of monosaccharides (glucose and fructose), avoiding their accumulation. They also probably exert a feedback effect by inducing the synthesis activities (1-FFT and 6G-FFT), which help to maintain this balance.

4.8 Biotechnology and Breeding of High-FOS *Allium* Species

To date, most of the emphasis of plant biotechnology programs has been devoted to large-market commodity crops, including some *Allium* species— mainly garlic—which are used in food industries as condiment or additives. Essential oils derived from *Allium* species, in particular from garlic and onions, are used in food industries and pharmacology, and some flavonoids and anthocyanins extracted from the outer scales of colored onions are also used as additives and health promotion (Addy and Stuart 1983, Okuda 1993, Shahidi and Naczk 1995). The potential for vegetable biotechnology to revolutionize biological sciences has been well established, in scientific literature as well as in the public forum. Biotechnological tools offer the opportunities to not only modify the expression of a single gene but also to introduce new genes into plants from species that are often sexually incompatible, and desirable (or undesirable) characteristics can be promoted (or inhibited) or characteristics not normally present in the tissue can be made to be expressed. Moreover, biotechnology is also proposed as an important complement to conventional plant-breeding procedures in different crops species (Poehlman and Sleper 1995). Since crop qualities have become increasingly important in the present market economy, a high amount of consideration is given, in breeding for improved quality, to the physical and chemical characteristics of the crops harvested that affect its (i) nutritional value, (ii) processing, and (iii) utilization in the diet.

In *Allium* species, the objectives of biotechnology and breeding for their improvement are still under discussion, in the experimental stages, and are directed toward the enhancement of fructan content. The principal use of *Allium* species is for the fresh market, dehydration, or other minor uses.

Likewise, other utilization would be expected such as a source of short-chain FOS, which could be extracted from onions and garlic. However, before moving to this step, it is necessary to breed specific onion and garlic cultivars, which are required to have two main characteristics: (i) high fructan content and high dry matter to have acceptable yield; and (ii) very low pungency or sulfur compounds behind the odor of *Allium* species, which are considered the "sole break" to their large industrial utilization. In this study (McCallum et al. 2006), the carbohydrate composition of onion bulbs was evaluated in progeny from crosses between high-dry-matter storage onion varieties and sweet, low-dry-matter varieties.

4.9 Putative and Potential Health Benefits of FOS

With the problems related to health and human evolution to a higher life quality, it was observed that the last two decades had an increased demand for healthy and nutritious food products because consumers have and still are being better educated and are generally more demanding (Deliza et al. 2003). This fact contributes to a continuous need for new food products, and a more differentiated food product assortment (Linneman et al. 1999). This attitude has led to the fact that the development of healthy foods is rated as the most important area of research by a large majority of the interviewed companies, while developing natural foods is considered rather close but of less concern (Katz 2000). Presently, the methods of production are a matter of increasing concern to many consumers because of the ingredients (presence of chemicals, additives, GMO, etc.), which are considered as one of the most important factors themselves. Although food products meet their nutritional requirements, it is unlikely to be accepted by consumers if they do not like one or more quality attributes (Deliza et al. 2003).

Generally, it is recommended to eat an average of 400 g of fruits and vegetables per day, and scientific advances linking diet and health have fostered unprecedented attention on the role of nutrition in health promotion and disease prevention. This is unfortunate as considerable evidence indicates that adequate fruit and vegetable consumption has a role in preventing many chronic diseases, including heart diseases, stroke, and several cancers (Appel et al. 1997, Block and Patterson 1992, Bornet et al. 2002, Cherbut 2002, Flamm et al. 2001, Hertog et al. 1996, Johnsen et al. 2003, Joshipura et al. 1999, Ness and Powles 1997, Olsen and Gudmand-Heyer 2000, WCRF-AICR 1997). Because of the increasing interest of consumers in diet food, and also because FOS are not yet being marketed widely throughout the world as food ingredients or additives, cultivated crops remain the main source of FOS such as bananas, wheat, barley, asparagus, and the Jerusalem artichoke (Mitsuoka et al. 1987, Spiegel et al. 1994, Tashiro et al. 1992). In *Allium* species, onions and garlic are considered the major source of FOS since FOS constitute 25–35% of total nonstructural carbohydrates, while leeks and shallots are a minor source (Campbell et al. 1997, Van Loo et al. 1995). Thus, FOS are presently produced industrially and used as food ingredients, while in Japan they are considered as food and are found in more than 500 food products, including soft drinks, cookies, cereals, and candies, resulting in significant daily consumption (Spiegel et al. 1994, Tomomatsu 1994).

Surprisingly, *Allium* species were consumed mainly for their flavor and used as condiments, while the fructan-containing foods have been consumed because of availability, low cost, and personal preference rather than for any specific effect on nutrition and health. In fact, the use of FOS in the human diet has increased since the initial commercial production of a specific oligofructan (Neosugar®) in Japan in 1983. The benefits of adding FOS to the human diet were first reported by the NSG (Neosugar Study Group) at a series of conferences held in Japan to highlight research with Neosugar in 1982, 1983, and 1984. The reports linked biochemical–nutritional–health changes in humans resulting from eating Neosugar, and these results were confirmed later by Buddington et al. (1996). Although this history started with Neosugar, it has become evident that many of the conclusions could be extended to other FOS.

FOS have shown numerous physiological actions in human nutrition (Roberfroid 1999, Scheppach et al. 2001), and these physiological effects are the basis for associating FOS intake with reduced diseases and prevention. Tomomatsu (1994) has enumerated some health benefits attributed to oligosaccharides:

- Encourage the proliferation of bifidobacteria and reduce detrimental bacteria
- Reduce toxic metabolites and detrimental enzymes
- Prevent pathogenic and autogenous diarrhea
- Prevent constipation
- Protect liver function
- Reduce serum cholesterol
- Reduce blood pressure
- Have an anticancer effect
- Produce nutrients

4.9.1 FOS and Cancer Prevention

From the clinical point of view, we do not exactly know how the FOS exert their beneficial effects and the suggested ways are not certain yet. However, increase in the numbers of beneficial bacteria in the lower intestine and changes in the pH of the intestinal contents, together with increases in enzyme levels that may be related to the detoxification of carcinogens in the diet, have all been cited as reasons for increases in the FOS levels in the diet.

The effects of nutrition on tumor incidence and growth were and are still a subject of priority interest (Roberfroid 1991, Williams and Dickinson 1990), and among the most frequently investigated dietary compounds and fibers, the nondigestible carbohydrates (NDO) play a major role in nutritional prevention (Roberfroid 1991, Witte et al. 1996). FOS were used in various experimental models to study their cancer-risk-reducing capacity (for details, see Chapter 16).

4.9.2 FOS and Lipids Metabolism

Lipids, such as cholesterol, triglycerides, and fatty acids, are fat and fat-like substances stored in tissues by the mammal organism and used as a source of "energy" by the body, or are found in the bloodstream. The levels of lipid in the organism can be an important measure and indicator of health; for example, a person who has high cholesterol has an increased risk of heart disease and stroke. They are also an important part of cell structure and other biological functions in the body. However, high levels of low density lipoproteins (LDL)-cholesterol, and other abnormal lipids (fats), are risk factors for CVD, and can lead to clogging of the arteries, an increased risk of heart attack and ischemic stroke.

Many attempts have been made by controlling triacylglycerol (TAG) concentrations through the modification of dietary habits (Delzenne and Kok 2001, Delzenne and Williams 2002). The hypotriglyceridemic effect of FOS, as well as other nondigestible carbohydrates, has been described both in humans (Canzi et al. 1992, Glore et al. 1994, Jackson et al. 1999, Letexier et al. 2003) and animals (de Deckere et al. 1995, Delzenne et al. 2002, Overton et al. 1994, Tokunaga et al. 1996). In fact, almost all studies were carried out on inulin or HP-inulin, and none concerned short-chain FOS and lipid metabolism in healthy men. On the other hand, the daily addition of 10 g inulin to the diet significantly resulted in lower plasma TAG levels, supporting that fructans influence the formation and/or degradation of TAG-rich lipoprotein (Appel et al. 1997). Letexier et al. (2003) also reported that the addition of HP-inulin has a beneficial effect on plasma lipids by decreasing hepatic lipogenesis and plasma TAG concentrations. Indeed, this effect is likely to result from a decrease in the hepatic synthesis of triglycerides acid (TGA) rather than from high catabolism of TGA-rich lipoproteins.

Unfortunately, the mechanisms behind the serum-lipid lowering effects of FOS remain still unclear and have to be elucidated (Delzenne and Williams 1999). In fact, the liver plays a key role in TAG-rich lipoprotein homeostasis and because newly synthesized fatty acids are preferentially channeled into very low density lipoproteins (VLDL), the lipogenic activity of the liver is a key factor for the hepatic TAG-VLDL output (Gibbons 1990). The SCFA (short-chain fatty acids) produced by fermentation decrease circulatory cholesterol concentrations either by inhibiting hepatic cholesterol synthesis or by redistributing cholesterol from plasma to the liver. Consequently, cholesterol would also be utilized to a greater extent for de novo bile acid synthesis. These combined actions are proposed as contributing mechanisms to decreasing circulating cholesterol concentrations (St-Onge et al. 2000). Furthermore, fatty acid synthase (FAS), among the key enzymes that control lipogenesis, is the most sensitive to nutrients and hormones (Girard et al. 1997). Thus, it is proposed that decreased lipogenesis in the liver is a key event in the reduction of VLDL-triglyceride secretion in fructan-fed rats, and the activities of many enzymes for example, acetyl CoA carboxylase, FAS, malic enzyme, ATP citrate lyase, and G-6-P 1-deshydrogenase, are decreased by 50% (Delzenne and Kok 2001).

4.9.3 *Prebiotic Effects of FOS*

A prebiotic is defined as "a nondigestible food component or an ingredient that beneficially affects the host organism by selectively stimulating the growth and/or activity of one or a number of bacteria in the colon" (Gibson and Roberfroid 1995). Thus, any modification by prebiotics of the composition of the colonic microflora leads to the predominance of a few of the potentially health-promoting bacteria, especially, but not exclusively, *Lactobacillus* sp. and *Bifidobacterium* sp. (Gibson and Roberfroid 1995). The only prebiotic for which sufficient data has been reported thereby allowing an evaluation of its possible classification as "functional food ingredients" are the inulin-type FOS or fructans, which include native inulin or short-chain FOS, enzymatically hydrolyzed inulin or oligofructose, and synthetic FOS (Roberfroid and Delzenne 1998, Roberfroid et al. 1998).

The large bowel is by far the most colonized region of the gastrointestinal tract, with c.a. 10^{12} bacteria per gram of gut content. Through the fermentation process, colonic bacteria, most of which are anaerobes, produce a wide variety of compounds that may affect the gut as well as systemic physiology. Thus, the fermentation of carbohydrates upon reaching the large bowel produces short-chain carboxylic acids, mainly acetate, propionate and butyrate, and lactate, which allows the host to salvage part of the energy of nondigestible oligosaccharides and that may play a role in regulating both cell division and cellular metabolism. In addition to their selective effects on bifidobacteria and lactobacilli, FOS influence many aspects of bowel function through fermentation, and are mildly laxative (Cummings et al. 1997). Indeed, FOS constitute a carbon source for microbial flora of bowel and the ability of bifidobacteria to utilize FOS was well-demonstrated (Biedrzycka and Bielecka 2004, Bouhnik et al. 2004, Marx et al. 2000, Mitsuoka 1996, Tannock et al. 2004). These works also reported that the majority of *Bifidobacterium* strains fermented all FOS and even low polymerized inulin. Biedrzycka and Bielecka (2004) claimed that the results of *in vitro* studies indicate the specificity of *Bifidobacterium* except *B. bifidum* to utilize short-chain FOS and oligofructose, but not HP-inulin. However, according to Van Laere et al. (1997), the main factors affecting the susceptibility of FOS to fermentation are chemical structure, DP, and possible linear or branched structure, as well as solubility in water. Generally, FOS with short chain length, unbranched nature, and high solubility in water are well and preferentially fermented. Nevertheless, discrepancies in the capability of different *Bifidobacterium* species to metabolize FOS may be due to the differences in the expression of fructan-hydrolyzing enzymes, since the latter have not been extensively investigated.

In food technology and processing, inulin and inulin-type fructans are the unique oligosaccharides used in food technologies. They are used as sugar substitutes and texture and foam stabilizer or for improving mouth palatability in miscellaneous products such as fermented dairy products, desserts and ice creams, bakery products and spreads, and infant formulas, while inulin is used as fat replacers (Cummings and Roberfroid 1997).

4.9.4 Action of FOS on Mineral Absorption

Contrary to the fact that nondigestible carbohydrates have been accused of causing an impairment in the small intestine absorption of minerals (Ellegård et al. 1997), van den Heuvel et al. (1999a,b) demonstrated that the amount of Ca, Mg, and Fe ions recovered in the ileostomate over a period of 3 days is significantly modified after supplementing the diet with 15 g per day of these fructans. Later, a vast number of studies were carried out on the effects of FOS and mineral absorption and reviewed by Scholz-Ahrens et al. (2001) and Scholz-Ahrens and Schrezenmeir (2002a); the scientific evidence claimed that FOS enhance mineral absorption is based on both animal (Coudray et al. 2003, Flickinger et al. 2003, Ohta et al. 1995, Scholz-Ahrens and Schrezenmeir 2002b) and human experiments (Coudray et al. 1997, Griffin et al. 2002, Tahiri et al. 2003). Coudray et al. (2003) studied the effects of different chain length and the types of branching on intestinal absorption and the balance of calcium and magnesium in rats and their results showed that all tested fructans studied seem to have similar activity by increasing absorption and/or balance of Ca and Mg. However, the combination of oligofructose and HP-inulin showed synergistic effects on intestinal calcium absorption and balance. In humans, van den Heuvel et al. (1999b) reported that 15 g of oligofructose per day stimulates fractional calcium absorption in male adolescents. Tahiri et al. (2003) noted that short-chain FOS may positively influence calcium absorption in the late postmenopausal phase in women. Moreover, Griffin et al. (2002) also noted that calcium absorption is increased by a combination of oligofructose + inulin in a girl at or near menarche.

In fact, the hypotheses most frequently proposed to explain the enhancing effect of FOS on mineral absorption are: osmotic effect; acidification of the colonic content due to fermentation and production of short-chain carboxylic acids; and the formation of calcium and magnesium salts of these acids and the hypertrophy of the colon wall (Coudray et al. 1997, Younes et al. 1996). However, according to Ohta et al. (1995), different mechanisms may be involved in the increased absorption of calcium and magnesium, the former being absorbed mostly in the cecum and the latter mostly in the colon.

4.9.5 Actions of FOS on Glycemia and Insulinemia

The effects of FOS on glycemia and insulinemia are not yet fully understood, and the nondigestible oligosaccharides for which published data are available on the effects related to glucose are inulin-type fructans (Rumessen et al. 1990, Yamashita et al. 1984). Besides that, available data on the effects of FOS on glucose and insulin concentrations are sometimes contradictory; these effects also may depend on physiological (fasting compared to postprandial or disease (diabetes) conditions (Alles et al. 1999, Delzenne and Kok 2001, Roberfroid 2000). Moreover, other nondigestible carbohydrates are known to modify the kinetics of absorption of carbohydrates, thus decreasing the incidence of glycemia and insulinemia (Leclère et al. 1994). The effects of inulin-type fructans on glycemia and insulinemia are not fully understood, and available data are sometimes contradictory, indicating that these effects may depend on physiological or disease conditions. Luo et al. (1996) reported that chronic ingestion of short-chain FOS (20 g per day for 4 weeks) did not modify fasting plasma glucose and insulin in healthy humans, even if it lowered basal hepatic glucose production. However, in diabetic subjects taking 8 g per day of short-chain FOS for 14 days leads to a decrease in fasting blood glucose (Yamashita et al. 1984).

4.10 Concluding Remarks and Future Directions

In conclusion, and after reviewing their occurrence, chemistry, and health benefits, it is presently admitted that the FOS of *Allium* species, as well as the FOS of other vegetables, fit well within the current concept of the class of dietary ingredients and could be labeled as "functional foods" since their vast health benefits are continuously appreciated. These dietary carbohydrates make up a large family of miscellaneous compounds with different physiological effects and diverse nutritional properties that deserve the attention of nutritionists. Because they are indigestible oligosaccharides, they need particular interest and may, in the next decade, be one of the most fascinating functional food ingredients. In addition to having nutritional properties, which may justify their classification as "functional food ingredients," FOS and fructans are low-energy carbohydrates, and have interesting technological properties in food product development, although these properties depend on their molecular structure, especially their DP, which determines their physical and chemical properties.

Likely due to their specific properties, FOS—for which a wide range of scientific observations are already available and which demonstrate an array of potential health benefits—affect several physiological, biochemical, and bacterial functions and contribute to reduce the risk of many diseases. Thus, they may contribute in a significant way to well-being by their specific effects on several physiological functions. However, bearing in mind their superior functional properties, such as the bioavailability of minerals, prebiotic affects and modulation of colonic microflora, the improvement in gastrointestinal physiology, the metabolism of lipids, or prevention of some cancers, some further basic research on their real utilization in the human diet are needed.

Having increasingly improved technical tools, such as genetics and molecular biology, the methodology can be reversed, showing the consequences under the administration of FOS. Moreover, to justify claims of enhanced function or reduction in the risk of disease, most of the available information must be confirmed in humans in relevant nutrition studies focusing on well-validated endpoints. The results of such studies will be of much value if they are based on sound mechanistic hypotheses. In human nutrition and natural therapy, changes in the composition of the colonic microbiota, the modulation of the metabolism of TAG, modulation of insulinemia, improved bioavailability of dietary calcium, and negative modulation of colon carcinogenesis are the most promising areas for further research and data acquisition.

References

Addy, N. D. and D. A. Stuart 1983. Impact of biotechnology on vegetable processing. *Food Technol* 40:64–6.

Alles, M. S., N. M. de Roos, J. C. Bakx, E. van de Lisdonk, P. L. Zock, and J. G. A. J. Hautvast. 1999. Consumption of fructooligosaccharides does not affect blood glucose and serum lipid concentrations in patients with type2 diabetes. *Am J Clin Nutr* 69:64–9.

Appel, L. J., T. J. Moore, E. Obarzanek et al. 1997. A clinical trial of the effects of dietary patterns on blood pressure. *New Engl J Med* 336:1117–24.

Archbold, H. K. 1940. Fructosans in the monocotyledons. A review. *New Phytol* 39:185–219.

Asega, A. F. and M. A. M. Carvalho. 2004. Fructan metabolising enzymes in rhizophores of *Vernonia herbacea* upon excision of aerial organs. *Plant Physiol. Biochem* 42:313–9.

Bacon, J. S. D. 1959. The trisaccharides fraction of some monocotyledons. *Biochem J* 73:507–14.

Baumgartner, S., T. G. Dax, W. Praznik, and H. Falk. 2000. Characterisation of the high-molecular weight fructan isolated from garlic (*Allium sativum* L.). *Carbohydr Res* 328:177–83.

Benkeblia, N. 2005. Effect of cultivar type on fructooligosaccharides (FOS) content and distribution in onion bulbs (*Allium cepa* L.). *Allium Improv Newslett* 16:24–31.

Benkeblia, N., S. Onodera, and N. Shiomi. 2004. Effect of gamma irradiation and temperature on fructans (fructo-oligosaccharides) of stored onion bulbs (*Allium cepa* L.). *Food Chem* 87:377–82.

Benkeblia, N., S. Onodera, and N. Shiomi. 2005. Variation in 1-fructo-exohydrolase (1-FEH) and 1-kestose-hydrolysing (1-KH) activities and fructo-oligosaccharides (FOS) status in onion bulbs. Influence of temperature and storage time. *J Sci Food Agric* 85:227–34.

Benkeblia, N., P. Varoquaux, N. Shiomi, and H. Sakai. 2002. Storage technology of onion bulbs c.v. Rouge Amposta: Effect of irradiation, maleic hydrazide and carbamate isopropyl, *N*-phenyl (CIP) on respiration rate and carbohydrates. *Int J Food Sci Technol* 37:169–76.

Biedrzycka, E. and M. Bielecka. 2004. Prebiotic effectiveness of fructans of different degrees of polymerization. *Trends Food Sci Technol* 15:170–5.

Block, E. 1985. The chemistry of garlic and onion. *Sci Am* 252:114–9.

Block, J., B. Patterson, and A. Subar. 1992. Fruits, vegetables and cancer prevention: A review of the epidemiological evidence. *Nutr Cancer* 18:1–29.

Bonnett, G. D. and R. J. Simpson. 1993. Fructan hydrolyzing activities from *Lolium rigidum* Gaudin. *New Phytol* 123:443–51.

Bornet, R. J., F. Brouns, Y. Tashiro, and V. Duvillier. 2002. Nutritional aspects of short-chain fructooligosaccharides: Natural occurrence, chemistry, physiology and health implications. *Digest Liver Dis* 34 (Suppl. 2):S111–20.

Bouhnik, Y., L. Raskine, G. Simoneau et al. 2004. The capacity of nondigestible carbohydrates to stimulate fecal bifidobacteria in healthy humans: A double-bind, randomized, placebo-controlled, parallel-group, dose-response relation study. *Am J Clin Nutr* 80:1658–64.

Brewster, J. L. 1990. Onions and allied crops. In *Onion and Allied Crops*, eds. J. L. Brewster, and H. D. Rabinowitch, 63–102. Boca Raton: CRC Press.

Brewster, J. L. 1994. *Onion and Allied Crops*. Wallingford: CABI Publisher.

Buddington, R. K., C. H. Williams, S. C. Chen, and S. A. Witherly. 1996. Dietary supplement of neosugar alters fecal flora and decreases activities of some reductive enzymes in human subjects. *Am J Clin Nutr* 63:709–16.

Campbell, J. M., L. L. Bauer, G. C. Fahey, A. J. C. L. Hogarth, B. W. Wolf, and D. E. Hunter. 1997. Selected fructooligosaccharides (1-kestose, nystose, and 1^F-β-fructofuranosylnystose) composition of foods and feeds. *J Agric Food Chem* 45:3076–82.

Canzi, E., F. B. Brighenti, M. C. Casiraghi, E. Del Puppo, and A. Ferrari. 1992. Prolonged consumption of inulin ready-to-eat breakfast cereals: Effects on intestinal ecosystem, bowel habits and lipid metabolism. In *COST 92*, ed. European Union, 280–284. Brussels: EU Publication.

Cherbut, C. 2002. Inulin and oligofructose in the dietary fiber concept. *Brit J Nutr* 87 (Suppl. 2):S159–62.

Claessens, G., A. Van Laere, and M. De Proft. 1990. Purification and properties of an inulinase from chicory roots (*Cichorium intybus* L.). *J Plant Physiol* 136:35–9.

Coudray, C., J. Bellanger, C. Castiglia-Delavaud, C. Rémésy, M. Vermorel, and Y. Rayssiguier. 2003. Effects of inulin-type fructans of different chain length and type of branching on intestinal absorption and balance of calcium and magnesium in rats. *Eur J Nutr* 42:91–8.

Coudray, C., J. Bellanger, C. Castiglia-Delavaud, C. Rémésy, M. Vermorel, and Y. Rayssiguier. 1997. Effect of soluble or partly soluble dietary fibers supplementation on absorption and balance of magnesium, iron and zinc in healthy young men. *Eur J Clin Nutr* 51:375–80.

Cummings, J. H. and M. B. Roberfroid. 1997. A new look at dietary carbohydrate: Chemistry, physiology and health. *Eur J Clin Nutr* 51:417–42.

Cummings, J. H., M. B. Roberfroid, H Andersson et al. 1997. A new look at dietary carbohydrate: Chemistry, physiology and health. *Eur J Clin Nutr* 51:417–23.

Darbyshire, B. and R. J. Henry. 1981. Differences in fructan content and synthesis in some *Allium* species. *New Phytol* 87:49–56.

Darbyshire, B. and R. J. Henry. 1978. The distribution of fructans in onions. *New Phytol* 81:29–34.

Darbyshire, B. and B. T. Steer. 1990. Carbohydrate biochemistry. In *Onions and Allied Crops, Vol. 3: Biochemistry, Food Science, and Minor Crops*, eds. H. D. Rabinowitch, and J. L. Brewster, 1–16. Boca Raton: CRC Press.

Darbyshire, D. 1978. Changes in the carbohydrate content of onion bulbs stored for various times at different temperatures. *J Hort Sci* 53:195–201.

Darwen, C. W. E. and P. Johnn. 1989. Localization of the enzyme of fructan metabolism in vacuoles isolated by a mechanical method from tubers of Jerusalem artichoke (*Helianthus tuberosus* L). *Plant Physiol* 89:658–63.

Das, N. N. and A. Das. 1978. Structure of the D-fructan isolated from garlic (*Allium sativum*) bulbs. *Carbohydr Res* 64:155–67.

de Deckere, E. A., W. Kloots, and J. M. van Amelsvoort. 1995. Both raw and retrograded starch decrease serum triacylglycerol concentration and fat accretion in the rat. *Brit J Nutr* 73:287–98.

Deliza, R., A. Rosenthal, and A. L. S. Silva. 2003. Consumer attitude towards information on non-conventional technology. *Trends Food Sci Technol* 14:43–9.

Delzenne, N. M. and N. Kok. 2001. Effects of fructans-type prebiotics on lipid metabolism. *Am J Clin Nutr* 73 (Suppl.):456S–8.

Delzenne, N. M. and C. M. Williams. 2002. Prebiotics and lipid metabolism. *Curr Opin Lipidol* 13:61–7.

Delzenne, N. M., C. Daubioul, A. Neyrinck, M. Lasa, and H. S. Taper. 2002. Inulin and oligofructose modulate lipid metabolism in animals: Review of biochemical events and future prospects. *Brit J Nutr* 87 (Suppl. 2):S255–9.

Delzenne, N. M. and C. Williams. 1999. Actions of non-digestible carbohydrates on blood lipids in humans and animals. In *Colonic Microbiota, Nutrition and Health*, eds. G. Gibson, and M. Roberfroid, 213–232. Amsterdam: Kluwer Academic Press.

De Roover, J., A. Van Laere, M. De Winter, J. W. Timmermans, and W. Van den Ende. 1999. Purification and properties of a second fructan exohydrolase from the roots of *Cichorium intybus*. *Physiol Plant* 106:28–34.

Duggan, C., J. Gannon, and W. A. Walker. 2002. Protective nutrients and functional foods for the gastrointestinal tracts. *Am J Clin Nutr* 75:789–808.

Edelman, J. and T. G. Jefford. 1964. The metabolism of fructose polymers in plants. 4. β-fructofuranosidases of tubers of *Helianthus tuberosus*. *Biochem J* 93:148–61.

Ellegård, L., H. Andersson, and I. Bosaeus. 1997. Inulin and oligofructose do not influence the absorption of cholesterol, or the excretion of cholesterol, Ca, Mg, Zn, Fe, or bile acids but increases energy excretion in ilestomy subjected. *Eur J Clin Nutr* 41:1–5.

Ernst, M. K., N. J. Chatterton, P. A. Harrison, and G. Matitschka. 1998. Characterization of fructan oligomers from species of the genus *Allium cepa* L. *J Plant Physiol* 153:53–60.

Espen, L., S. Morgutti, A. Abruzzese et al. 1999. Changes in the potato (*Solanum tuberosum* L.) tuber at the onset of dormancy and during storage at 23°C and 3°C. I. Biochemical and physiological parameters. *Potato Res* 42:189–201.

Farnworth, E. R. 1993. Fructans in human and animal diet. In *Science and Technology of Fructans*, eds. M. Suzuki, and N. J. Chatterton, 257–272. Boca Raton: CRC Press.

Fenwick, G. R. and A. B. Hanley. 1990. Chemical composition. In *Onion and Allied Crops*, eds. J. L. Brewster, and H. D. Rabinowitch, 17–31. Boca Raton: CRC Press.

Flamm, G., W. Glinsman, D. Kritchevsky, L. Prosky, and M. Roberfoid. 2001. Inulin and oligofructose as dietary fiber: A review of the evidence. *Crit Rev Food Sci Nutr* 45:353–62.

Flickinger, E. A., J. Van Loo, and C. Fahey. 2003. Nutritional responses to the presence of inulin and oligofructose in the diets of domesticated animals: A review. *Crit Rev Food Sci Nutr* 43:19–60.

Frehner, M., F. Keller, and A. Wiemken. 1984. Localization of fructan metabolism in the vacuoles isolated from protoplasts of Jerusalem artichoke tubers (*Helianthus tuberosus* L). *J Plant Physiol* 116:197–208.

Fujishima, M., H. Sakai, K. Ueno et al. 2005. Purification and characterization of a fructosyltransferase from onion bulbs and its key role in the synthesis of fructo-oligosaccharides *in vivo*. *New Phytol* 165:513–24.

Gibbons, G. F. 1990. Assembly and secretion of hepatic very-low-density lipoprotein. *Biochem J* 268:1–13.

Gibson, G. R. and M. B. Roberfroid. 1995. Dietary modulation of the human colonic microflora: Introducing the concept of prebiotics. *J Nutr* 125:1401–12.

Glore, V., D. van Treeck, A. Knehans, and M. Guild. 1994. Soluble fibers and serum lipids: A literature review. *J Am Diet Assoc* 94:425–36.

Girard, J., P. Ferré, and F. Foufell. 1997. Mechanism by which carbohydrates regulate expression of genes for glycolytic and lipogenic enzymes. *Annu Rev Nutr* 17:325–52.

Griffin, I. J., P. M. Davila, and S. A. Abrams. 2002. Non-digestible oligosaccharides and calcium absorption in girls with adequate calcium intakes. *Brit J Nutr* 87 (Suppl.2):S187–91.

Griffiths, G., L. Trueman, T. Crowther, B. Thomas, and B. Smith. 2002. Onions—A global benefits to health. *Phytother Res* 16:603–15.

Green, O. C. and N. G. Polydoris. 1993. *Garlic, Cancer and Heart Diseases: Review and Recommendations*, 21–41. Chicago: GN Communications.

Henry, R. J. and B. Darbyshire. 1980. Sucrose:sucrose fructosyltransferase, and fructan:fructan fructosyltransferase from *Allium cepa*. *Phytochemistry* 19: 1017–20.

Henson, C. A. 1989. Purification and properties of barley stem fructan exohydrolase. *J Plant Physiol* 134:186–91.

Henson, C. A. and D. P. Livingston III. 1996. Purification and characterization of an oat fructan exohydrolase that preferentially hydrolases β-2,6-fructans. *Plant Physiol* 110:639–44.

Hertog, M. G., G. B. Bueno de Mesquita, A. Fehily, P. M. Sweetnam, P. C. Elwood, and D. Kroumhout. 1996. Fruit and vegetable consumption and cancer mortality in the Caerphilly study. *Epidemiol Biomarkers Prev* 5:673–7.

Jackson, K. G., G. R. L. Taylor, A. M. Clohessy, and C. M. Williams. 1999. The effect of the daily intake of inulin on fasting lipid, insulin and glucose concentrations in middle-aged men and women. *Brit J Nutr* 82:23–30.

Jaime, L., M. A. Martín-Cabrejas, E. Mollá, F. J. López-Andréu, and R. M. Esteban. 2001. Effect of storage on fructan and fructo-oligosaccharide of onion (*Allium cepa* L.). *J Agric Food Chem* 49:982–8.

Johnsen, S. P., K. Overvad, C. Stripp, A. Tjonneland, S. E. Husted, and H. T. Sorensen. 2003. Intake of fruit and vegetable and the risk of ischaemic stroke in a cohort of Danish men and woman. *Am J Clin Nutr* 78:57–64.

Joshipura, K. J., A. Ascherio, J. Mansun et al. 1999. Fruit and vegetable intake in relation to risk of ischaemic stroke. *J Am Med Assoc* 282:1233–9.

Katz, F. 2000. Research priorities more toward healthy and safe. *Food Technol* 54:42–4.

Khan, G. 1996. History of garlic. In *Garlic: The Science and Therapeutic Application of Allium sativum and Related Species*, eds. H. P. Koch, and L. D. Lawson, 5–36. New York: Williams & Wilkins.

Lang, A. 1996. *Plant Dormancy: Physiology, Biochemistry and Molecular Biology.* Wallingford: CABI Publisher.

Lang, G. A. 1987. Dormancy: A new universal terminology. *HortScience* 22:817–20.

Leclère, C. J., M. Champ, J. Boillot et al. 1994. Role of viscous guar gums in lowering the glycemic response after slid meal. *Am J Clin Nutr* 59:914–21.

Le Nard, M. and A. A. De Hertogh. 1993. Bulb growth and development and flowering. In *The Physiology of Flower Bulbs*, eds. A. A. De Hertogh, and M. Le Nard, 29–42. Amsterdam: Elsevier.

Letexier, D., F. Diraison, and M. Beylot. 2003. Addition of inulin to a moderate high-carbohydrate diet reduces hepatic lipogenesis and plasma triacylglycerol concentrations in humans. *Am J Clin Nutr* 77:559–64.

Lewis, D. H. 1993. Nomenclature and diagrammatic representation of oligomeric fructans—A paper for discussion. *New Phytol* 124:583–94.

Linneman, A. R., G. Meerdink, M. T. G. Meulenberg, and W. M. F. Jongen. 1999. Consumer-oriented technology development. *Trends Food Sci Technol* 9: 409–14.

Luo, J., S. W. Rizkala, C. Alamowitch et al. 1996. Chronic consumption of short-chain fructooligosaccharides in healthy subjects decreased basal glucose production but had not effect on insulin-stimulated glucose metabolism. *Am J Clin Nutr* 63:939–45.

Marx, S. P., S. Winkler, and W. Hartmeier. 2000. Metabolization of β-(2,6)-linked fructo-oligosaccharides by different bifidobacteria. *FEMS Microbiol Lett* 182:163–9.

Marx, S. P., J. Nösberger, and M. Frehner. 1997. Seasonal variation of fructo-β-fructosidase (FEH) activity and characterization of a β-(2-1)-linkage specific FEH from tubers of Jerusalem artichoke (*Helianthus tuberosus*). *New Phytol* 135:267–77.

McCallum, J., A. Clarke, M. Pither-Joyce et al. 2006. Genetic mapping of a major gene affecting onion bulb fructan content. *Theor Appl Genet* 112:958–67.

Meier, H. and J. S. Reid. 1982. Reserve polysaccharides other than starch in higher plants. In *Encyclopedia of Plant Physiology*, eds. F. A. Loewus, and W. Tanner, 418–471. Berlin: Springer Verlag.

Mitsuoka, T. 1996. Intestinal flora and human health. *Asia Pacific J Clin Nutr* 5:2–9.

Mitsuoka, T., H. Hidaka, and T. Eida. 1987. Effects of fructo-oligosaccharides on intestinal microflora. *Nahrung* 31:427–36.

Mohr, H. and P. Schopfer. 1995. *Plant Physiology*. 4th Edition. Berlin: Springer-Verlag.

Moyers, S. 1996. *Garlic in Health, History, and World Cuisine*. St Petersburg: Suncoast Press.

Ness, A. R. and J. W. Powles. 1997. Fruits and vegetables, and cardiovascular disease: A review. *Int J Epidemiol* 26:1–13.

Nilsson, T. 2000. Postharvest handling and storage of vegetables. In *Fruit and Vegetable Quality (An Integrated View)*, eds. R. L. Shewfelt, and B. Brückner, 96–121. Lancaster: Technomic Publishing.

O'Donoghue, E. M., S. D. Somerfield, M. Shaw et al. 2004. Evaluation of carbohydrates in Pukekohe, Longkeeper and Grano cultivars of *Allium cepa*. *J Agric Food Chem* 52:5383–90.

Ohta, A., M. Ohtsuki, S. Baba, T. Takizawa, T. Adachi, and S. Kimura. 1995. Effects of fructooligosaccharides on the absorption of iron, calcium and magnesium in iron-deficiency anemic rats. *J Nutr Sci Vitaminol* 41:281–91.

Okuda, T. 1993. Natural polyphenols as antioxidants and their potential use in cancer prevention. In *Plant Phenomena*, ed. A. Scalbert, 221–236. Paris: INRA Publications.

Olsen, M. and. E. Gudmand-Heyer. 2000. Efficacy, safety, and tolerability of fructooligosaccharides in the treatment of irritable bowel syndrome. *Am J Clin Nutr* 72:1570–5.

Overton, P., N. Furlonger, J. Beety, J. Chakraborty, J. A. Tredger, and L. M. Morgan. 1994. The effects of dietary sugar-beet fiber, guar gum on lipid metabolism in Wistar rats. *Brit J Nutr* 72:385–95.

Poehlman, J. M. and D. A. Sleper. 1995. *Breeding Field Crops*. Ames: Iowa State Publishing.

Pollock, C. J. and A. J. Cairns. 1991. Fructan metabolism in grasses and cereals. *Annu Rev Plant Physiol Plant Mol Biol* 42:77–101.

Pontis, H. G., and E. Del Campillo. 1985. Fructan. In *Biochemistry of Storage Carbohydrates in Green Plants*, eds. P. M. Dey, and R. A Dixon, 205–227. London: Academic Press.

Ritsema, T., J. Joling, and S. Smeekens. 2003. Patterns of fructan synthesized by onion fructan: Fructan 6G–fructosyltransferase expressed in tobacco BY2 cells—Is fructan:fructan 1-fructosyltrasferase needed in onion? *New Phytol* 160:61–7.

Rivlin, R. S. 2001. Historical perspectives on the use of garlic. *J Nutr* 131 (Suppl.):951S–4.

Roberfroid, M. 1991. Dietary modulation of experimental neoplastic development: Role of fat fiber content and caloric intake. *Mut Res* 259:351–62.

Roberfroid, M. B. 2000. Fructo-oligosaccharides: Benefit for gastrointestinal functions. *Curr Opin Gastroenterol* 16:173–7.

Roberfroid, M. B. 2002. Functional foods: Concepts and application to inulin and oligofructose. *Brit J Nutr* 87 (Suppl. 2):S139–43.

Roberfroid, M. B. and N. Delzenne. 1998. Dietary fructans. *Annu Rev Nutr* 18:117–43.

Roberfroid, M. B., J. A. E. Van Loo, and G. R. Gibson. 1998. The bifidogenic nature of chicory inulin and its hydrolysis products. *J Nutr* 128:11–29.

Rumessen, J., S. Bode, O. Hamberg, and E. Gudmand-Hoyer. 1990. Fructans of Jerusalem artichoke: Intestinal transport, absorption, fermentation, and influence on blood glucose, insulin, and C-peptide response in healthy subjects. *Am J Clin Nutr* 52:675–80.

Rutherford, P. P. 1981. Some biochemical changes in vegetables during storage. *Ann Appl Biol* 98:538–41.

Rutherford, P. P. and R. Wittle. 1984. Methods predicting the long term storage of onions. *J Hort Sci* 59:537–43.

Scheppach, W., H. Luehrs, and T. Menzel. 2001. Beneficial health effects of low-digestible carbohydrate consumption. *Brit J Nutr* 85 (Suppl. 1):S23–30.

Scholz-Ahrens, K. and J. Schrezenmeir. 2002a. Inulin, oligofructose and mineral metabolism—Experimental data and mechanism. *Brit J Nutr* 87 (Suppl.2):S179–86.

Scholz-Ahrens, K. and J. Schrezenmeir. 2002b. Effect of oligofructose on dietary calcium on repeated calcium and phosphorus balances, bone mineralization and tubular structure in ovariectomized rats. *Brit J Nutr* 88:365–77.

Scholz-Ahrens, K., G. Schaafsma, E. G. M. H. van den Heuvel, and J. Schrezenmeir. 2001. Effects of prebiotics on mineral absorption. *Am J Clin Nutr* 73 (Suppl.):459S–64.

Shahidi, F. and M. Naczk. 1995. *Food Phenolics: Source, Chemistry and, Effects and Application*. Lancaster: Technomic Publishing.

Shiomi, N. 1989. Properties of fructosyltransferases involved in the synthesis of fructan in liliaceous plants. *J Plant Physiol* 134:151–5.

Shiomi, N., N. Benkeblia, and S Onodera. 2007. *Recent Advances in Fructooligosaccharides Research*. Kerala: Research Signpost Publisher.

Shiomi, N., H. Kido, and S. Kiriyama. 1985. Purification and properties of sucrose:sucrose 1F-β-D-fructosyltransferase in onion seeds. *Phytochemistry* 24:695–8.

Shiomi, N., S. Onodera, and H. Sakai. 1997. Fructo-oligosaccharide content and fructosyltransferase activity during growth of onion bulbs. *New Phytol* 136:105–13.

Simpson, R. J., R. P. Walker, and C. J. Pollock. 1991. Fructan exohydrolase activity from leaves of *Lolium temulentum* L. *New Phytol* 119:499–507.

Spiegel, J. E., R. Rose, P. Karabell, V. H. Franks, and D. F. 1994. Schmitt. Safety and benefits of fructooligosaccharides as food ingredients. *Food Technol* 1:85–9.

Stahl, B., A. Linos, M. Karas, F. Hillenkamp, and M. Steup. 1997. Analysis of fructans from higher plants by matrix-assisted laser desorption/ionization mass spectrometry. *Anal Biochem* 246:195–204.

St-Onge, M. P., E. R. Farnworth, and P. J. H. 2000. Jones. Consumption of fermented and nonfermented dairy products: Effects on cholesterol concentrations and metabolism. *Am J Clin Nutr* 71:674–81.

Suzuki, M. and J. A. Cutcliffe. 1989. Fructans in onion bulbs in relation to storage life. *Can J Plant Sci* 69:1327–33.

Tahiri, M., J. C. Tressol, J. Arnaud et al. 2003. Effect of short-chain fructooligosaccharides on intestinal calcium absorption and calcium status in postmenopausal women: A stable-isotope study. *Am J Clin Nutr* 77:449–57.

Tannock, G. W., K. Munro, R. Bibiloni et al. 2004. Impact of consumption of oligosaccharide-containing biscuits on the fecal microbiota of humans. *Appl Environ Microbiol* 70:2129–36.

Tashiro, Y., T. Eida, and H. Hidaka. 1992. Distribution and quantification of fructooligosaccharides in food materials. *Sci Rep Meiji Seiki Kaisha* 31:35–40.

Tokunaga, T., T. Oku, and N. Hosoya. 1996. Influence of chronic intake of a new sweetener fructooligosaccharides (neosugar) on growth and gastrointestinal function of the rat. *J Nutr Sci Vitaminol* 32:111–21.

Tomomatsu, H. 1994. Health effects of oligosaccharides. *Food Technol* 10:61–5.

Van den Ende, W., A. Michiels, J. De Roover, and A. Van Laere. 2002. Fructan biosynthetic and breakdown enzymes in dicots evolved from different invertases. Expression of fructan genes throughout chicory development. *Scientific World J* 2:1273–87.

Van den Ende, W., A. Michiels, D. Van Wonterghem, S. P. Clerens, J. De Roover, and A. J. Van Laere. 2001. Defoliation induces fructan 1-exohydrolase II in witloof chicory roots. Cloning and purification of two isoforms, fructan 1-exohydrolase IIa and fructan 1-exohydrolase IIb. Mass fingerprint of the fructan 1-exohydrolase II enzymes. *Plant Physiol* 126:1186–95.

Van den Ende, W., A. Michiels, J. De Roover, P. Verhaert, and A. Van Laere. 2000. Cloning and functional analysis of chicory root fructan 1–exohydrolase I (1-FEH I): A vacuolar enzyme derived from a cell-wall invertase ancestor? Mass fingerprint of the 1-FEH I enzyme. *Plant J* 124:447–56.

Van den Ende, W., M. Yoshida, S. Clerens, R. Vergauwen, and A. Kawakami. 2005. Cloning, characterization and functional analysis of novel 6-kestose exohydrolases (6-KEHs) from wheat (*Triticum aestivum*). *New Phytol* 166:917–32.

van den Heuvel, E. G. M. H., G. Schaafsma, T. Muys, and W. van Dokkun. 1999a. Nondigestible oligosaccharides do not interfere with calcium and nonheme-iron absorption in young, healthy men. *Am J Clin Nutr* 67:445–51.

van den Heuvel, E. G. M. H., T. Muys, W. van Dokkun, and G. Schaafsma. 1999b. Oligofructose stimulates calcium absorption in adolescents. *Am J Clin Nutr* 69:544–8.

Van Laere, K. M. J., M. Bosveld, H. A. Schols, C. Beldman, and A. G. J. Voragen. 1997. Fermentative degradation of plant cell wall derived oligosaccharides by intestinal bacteria. In *Proceedings of the International Symposium on Non Digestible Oligosaccharides: Healthy Food for the Colon?* ed. R. Hartemink, 37–46. Wageningen: Wageningen Pers Publisher.

Van Loo, J., P. Coussement, L. De Leentheer, H. Hoebregs, and G. Smits. 1995. On the presence of inulin and oligofructose as natural ingredients in the western diet. *Crit Rev Food Sci Nutr* 35:525–52.

Wagner, W. and A. Wiemken. 1986. Properties and subcellular localization of fructan hydrolase in the leaves of barley (*Hordeum vulgare* L. cv. Gerbel). *J Plant Physiol* 123:429–39.

Wagner, W., A. Wiemken, and P. Matile. 1986. Regulation of fructan metabolism in leaves of barley (*Hordeum vulgare* L. cv. Gerbel). *Plant Physiol* 81:444–7.

Waterhouse, A. L., and N. J. Chatterton. 1993. Glossary of fructan terms. In *Science and Technology of Fructans*, eds. M. Suzuki, and N. J. Chatterton, 1–7. Boca Raton: CRC Press.

WCRF-AICR (World Cancer Research Fund-American Institute of Cancer Research). 1997. Food, nutrition and the prevention of cancer: A global perspective, WCRF International London. http://www.dietandcancerreport.org (accessed: 23 August, 2013).

Wiemken, A., N. Sprenger, and T. Boller. 1995. Fructan—An extension of sucrose by sucrose. In *International Symposium on Sucrose Metabolism*, eds. H. G. Pontis, G. L. Salerno, and E. J. Echeverria, 179–189. Rockville: American Society of Plant Physiologist (ASPP) Publications.

Williams, C. M. and J. W. Dickinson. 1990. Nutrition and cancer. Some biochemical mechanism. *Nutr Res Rev* 3:45–100.

Witte, J. S., M. P. Longnecker, C. L. Bird, E. R. Lee, H. D. Frank, and R. W. Haile. 1996. Relation of vegetable, fruit, and grain consumption to colorectal adenomatous polyps. *Am J Epidemiol* 144:1015–25.

Woodward, P. W. 1996. *Garlic and Friends: The History, Growth and Use of Edible Alliums*. Melbourne: Hyland House Publisher.

Yamashita, K., K. Kawai, and K. Itakara. 1984. Effect of fructo-oligosaccharides on blood glucose and serum lipids in diabetic subjects. *Nutr Res* 4:961–6.

Younes, H., C. Demigné, and C. Rémésy. 1996. Acidic fermentation in the caecum increases absorption of calcium and magnesium in the large intestine of the rat. *Brit J Nutr* 75:301–14.

Yun, J. W. 1996. Fructooligosaccharides—Occurrence, preparation, and application. *Enz Microbiol Technol* 19:107–17.

CHAPTER 5

Potato Starches

Properties, Modifications, and Nutrition

NOUREDDINE BENKEBLIA

Contents

5.1   Introduction   105
5.2   History of Starch   106
5.3   Potato Starch   107
    5.3.1   Production   107
    5.3.2   Properties and Biochemistry   108
5.4   Structural Features of Potato Starch Granules   110
5.5   Starch Modification   110
    5.5.1   Physical Modifications   111
    5.5.2   Chemical Modifications   113
5.6   Amylases and Enzymatic Actions and Modifications of Potato
    Starch   117
    5.6.1   α-Amylases   118
    5.6.2   β-Amylase   119
    5.6.3   Glucoamylase   120
    5.6.4   Cyclodextrin Glycosyltransferase   120
    5.6.5   α-Glucanotransferases   121
5.7   Potato Starches, Diet, and Health   122
5.8   Perspectives and Conclusions   122
References   123

5.1 Introduction

Roots, tubers, and other plant parts utilize two fundamentally different strategies for the storage of carbohydrates in vegetative tissues, as an energy source. Thus, starch, sucrose, or other sucrose derivatives such as oligo- and poly-fructosyl sucrose—also called fructo-oligosaccharides and fructans, respectively—are the major hydrocarbons involved in this process. In plants, these carbohydrates are metabolized in different ways. While sucrose and fructans (which are generally soluble) are synthesized and accumulated in vacuoles, starch (which is insoluble) is stored in plastids. In most species, starch is predominantly utilized for diurnal carbon storage in leaves, and studies have shown that the biosynthesis of starch is regulated to provide this energetic substrate for utilization through the dark period (Smith and Stitt 2007). Moreover, mechanisms controlling starch synthesis in heterotrophic sink tissues such as potato tubers have also been elucidated and are well-understood (Tiessen et al. 2002, 2003).

Structurally, starch is composed mainly of two glucose polymers, namely, amylose and amylopectin. Both amylose and amylopectin have a $\beta(1 \rightarrow 4)$-linked D-glucan backbone. Amylose is composed of a linear chain of varying numbers of glucose units depending on the plant source, but the average length varies between 500 and 2000 glucose units, with a molecular weight ranging from 10^5 to 10^6 g/mole. Amylopectin is extensively branched by $(1 \rightarrow 6)$ linkage due to the occasional linkage with glucose resulting in a more massive molecule but with linear chain lengths of only 25–30 glucose units, and a molecular weight ranging from 2×10^7 to 50×10^7 g/mole (Buleon and Colonna 1998, Swinkels 1985, Zobel 1988).

However, starch has a variable composition depending on its origin or the plant species. The variation is on the amylose-to-amylopectin ratio, and the degree and type of crystallinity. These two properties considerably affect the properties and processability of both amylose and amylopectin (Wang et al. 1998).

5.2 History of Starch

Although the history of starch and its use is not well-recorded, there are many examples of its early use in industries. Around 4000 BC, strips of Egyptian papyrus were stuck together with a starchy adhesive; and in 170 BC, Cato described a process of separating starch from grain by Romans. Later, around 312 AD, starch was shown to provide resistance to ink penetration in Chinese paper, and by the sixteenth century, starch was being widely used in Western Europe, primarily in the textile industry and linen as a stiffener.

Over millennia, starch was used for numerous domestic and industrial applications. However, scientific research on starch started in 1716 when Antonie van Leeuwenhoek (1632–1723) observed starch microscopically as discrete granules. Afterwards, the use of starch expanded in the early nineteenth century when its conversion into sugars by acid hydrolysis was discovered. However, it was more than a century before the nature and the true molecular structure of the basic monomeric unit was established. Only after this was it possible to clarify the nature of the glycosidic linkages in starch (Seetharaman and Bertoft 2012). In 1804, Edme-Jean Baptiste Bouillon-Lagrange (1805) first reported the production of dextrin, and in 1811, Kirchoff (1815) reported that sugar could be produced from potato starch by hydrolysis with acid, thus bringing into being the first modified starches and starch sweeteners.

The word "starch" also has different origins. First, it is thought that the word "starch" derives from Middle English "sterchen", meaning to stiffen because it was first used for this purpose. The Latin word "amylum" and the Greek "amylon," which means "not ground at a mill," have also contributed to starch terminology. Furthermore, starch granules from *Typha* (cattails, bull-rushes) as flour have been identified from grinding stones in Europe dating back to 30,000 years ago (Anonymous 2013a).

5.3 Potato Starch

5.3.1 Production

Besides starch consumed directly from fresh roots and tubers, more than 70 M tonnes of starch are produced per year worldwide since 2010, with ca 40% used by the manufacturing industry and 60% (most of it as glucose syrups) used in food industries.

Today, the most refined starch found in commercial starches is obtained from potato, corn, wheat, and tapioca. However, other crop sources are used to a lesser extent, such as rice, sweet potato, sago, and mung bean, although more than 50 types of plants are nowadays used to extract starch. The final yield of starch depends to a great extent on the starch content of fresh potatoes, which is correlated with potato density. This yield would be determined by the following equation of estimation:

$$\text{Starch (\% dry matter)} = \left[\frac{\dfrac{Wo}{(Wo - Wu)} - 1.015}{0.0046} \right]$$

where Wo = weight of the potato sample at 18°C and Wu = weight of the sample immersed in clean water.

The refining of starch starts during the raw material intake where the damage to the tuber should be minimal, and loose dirt, sand, and gravel are removed. During extraction, cooling is recommended to reduce microbial growth that can break down protein, causing an off-flavor. Rasping is the first step in starch extraction, and it consists of the opening of the tuber cells and the release of starch granules. The obtained slurry is a mixture of pulp (cell walls), fruit juice, and starch. Immediately after rasping, sulfur dioxide (SO_2) gas or sodium bisulfite solution ($NaHSO_3$) is added to prevent browning of the cell juice. Starch is then extracted *via* extractors (rotating conical sieves) and concentrated. The concentrate is refined to purify the crude starch milk

Table 5.1 Composition and Size Distribution (μm) of Starch Granules of Refined Potato Starch

Constituents	Analysis	Size Distribution (μm)	%
Starch, dry substance	80%	87–140	3
Water	20%	53–87	24
Ash	0.3%	38–53	34
Sand	0.02%	28–38	17
Protein	0.09%	22–28	9.1
Phosphorus	0.07%	17–22	7.7
Calcium, Ca	0.03%	13–17	3.3
Iron, Fe	3 ppm	10–13	0.9
Cold water soluble	0.1%	8–10	0.5
		6–8	0.2
		0–6	2.0

(suspension) and remove residual fruit juice and impurities. The concentrate is finally dried and sifted with a fine sieve with a specific composition and physical granulometry (Table 5.1). However, untreated starch requires heat to thicken or gelatinize. When a starch is precooked (annealing; see details in the sections below), it can then be used to thicken instantly in cold water, and this is referred to as a pregelatinized starch (Anonymous 2013b).

5.3.2 Properties and Biochemistry

The functional characteristics of starch follow from the basic physicochemical properties of the granules (Alvani et al. 2011). The size and distribution of starch granules is very important for specific applications and even basic physical characteristics (Kulp and Lorenz 1981, Zobel 1988). The quality of starch granules to a great extent depends critically on the characterization of the physicochemical properties of starch during the growth (Cottrell et al. 1995, Liu et al. 2003), on the genotype (Cottrell et al. 1995), and on the harvesting date of the tubers (Noda et al. 2009).

As an example, the small granule size of starch makes it very suitable for applications like laundry sizing of fine fabrics and for skin cosmetics, and this starch is obtained from rice whose granules average 5.5 μm, while potato granules size averages 36 μm (Jane et al. 1994). The most important properties of starch are gelatinization and swelling.

Starch gelatinization is a process by which the organized granule structure is disrupted, and this process is often considered the first step in the application of starch treatments (Zobel 1984). The phenomena of gelatinization are known but the different methods used to determine this gelatinization process are still difficult to establish, thus not allowing a precise and common definition. Discrepancies exist between the different studies carried out to interpret gelatinization thermograms obtained by differential scanning calorimetry (DSC)

(Eberstein et al. 1980, Evans and Haisman 1982, Hoseney et al. 1986, Maurice 1986, Shiotsubo and Takahshi 1984), and often gelatinization is considered as a melting process. However, it was found that identification of the transitions using x-ray diffraction was considered critical to understanding starch gelatinization, and complementary x-ray data showed that some transitions are caused by the melting of crystalline V-type amylose–lipid complexes (Kugimiya et al. 1980, Zobel et al. 1988). Later, Svensson and Eliasson (1995) compared potato and cereal starches by WAXS (wide-angle x-ray scattering) and noted that the crystalline properties are strongly affected by the amount of water available during gelatinization, but the subcellular cereal starches is more stable to water than the subcell of potato tuber starches. Moreover, potato starch DSC characteristics did not correlate with amylose, intrinsic viscosity, or water binding when the thermal properties and some physicochemical properties of starch from 42 potato genotypes were compared by Kim et al. (1995); the amylose content of starches was reported to be negatively correlated to the onset and the minimum temperatures peak of gelatinization (Fredriksson et al. 1998).

The swelling power (SP) of native potato starch granules was studied by Hoover and Hadziyev (1981) and x-ray diffraction analysis proved that complexes were true clathrates (inclusion) compounds. The presence of clathrates in granules decreased SP up to 10 times, and granule size, amylose content, or heat of gelatinization alone did not seem significantly correlated with the SP (Yune and Yeh 2001).

The highest swelling ability is mainly due to its higher content of phosphate groups (Galliard and Bowler 1987). Tester and Morrison (1990) attributed this property to amylopectin, and claim that it is the consequence of the repelling action of phosphate groups on one another, thus weakening the interchain bonds and increasing their hydration capacity (Singh et al. 2003) (Table 5.2). The swelling of starch is caused by its sensitivity to water mainly

Table 5.2 Amylose and Phosphorus Content of 10 Potato Starches

Cultivar	Amylose (α-Glucan Basis, %)	Phosphorus (mg/100 g, db)
Brodick	29.05 ± 0.13	57.38 ± 0.59
Desiree	25.51 ± 0.05	52.90 ± 0.26
Inca Sun	26.23 ± 0.19	52.59 ± 0.32
Kara	27.04 ± 0.20	64.50 ± 0.46
Maris Piper	27.06 ± 0.20	58.04 ± 0.29
Mayan Gold	25.23 ± 0.18	66.20 ± 0.45
Pentland Crown	26.91 ± 0.10	59.48 ± 0.25
Pentland Dell	26.54 ± 0.06	62.05 ± 0.25
Pentland Javelin	27.97 ± 0.12	65.76 ± 0.34
Record	28.10 ± 0.06	65.02 ± 0.33

Source: Adapted from Alvani, K. et al. 2011. *Food Chem* 125:958–65.

due to the presence of the hydroxyl groups of the glucose units, which yield a high hygroscopicity; therefore, starch granules rapidly adapt their moisture content to the surrounding water resulting in dramatic changes in the physical properties with changes in the moisture content (Stading et al. 2001).

5.4 Structural Features of Potato Starch Granules

Starch granules are complex structures consisting of crystalline and amorphous areas, and amylose and amylopectin molecules are arranged in particular ways. In the structural organization of the granules, the branched and short chain amylopectin has a double helical conformation and forms the crystalline lamellae (crystallites). One part of this double helix with the crystallites forms the semicrystalline-ordered part of the starch granule, while the other part of the double helix is disordered, forming the amorphous part, which is thought to be composed of chains of amylopectin and amylose (Blanshard 1987, French 1984). Therefore, the starch granule seems to be structured by alternating layers of semicrystalline and amorphous material (Imberty and Perez 1988, Perez and Imberty 1996, Pérez et al. 2009).

Oostergetel and van Bruggen (1993) have proposed a three-dimensional (3D) model describing the crystallite arrangement in potato starch granules, which the total size varies between 15 and 75 μm (Perez and Bertoft 2010). The authors give the following description: the short chains in the amylopectin form double helices of ca 5 nm long, and are crystallized into lamellae of 5 nm thickness, which alternate with the amorphous layers containing α(1,6) branching points. The crystalline lamellae have cavities, and the double helices forming the lamellae are packed in polymorph structures of B type.

Observation using high-resolution noncontact atomic force microscopy (nc-AFM) studied the surface and revealed some details of the starch granule nanostructure. Oblong nodules with a diameter of ca 20–50 nm were observed at the surface of the potato starch granules. The same size particles were precipitated by ethanol from gelatinized potato starch suspensions. After multiple freezing and thawing, the eroded potato granule surface revealed an internal lamellar structure, and these findings are in agreement with those reported, suggesting the structural elements in the crystalline region of the starch granule (Szymońska and Krok 2003).

5.5 Starch Modification

The properties and inherent characteristics of native starches are, to the extent possible, exploited by food processors to meet specific needs. However, these native properties do not currently function adequately in the entire range of food products. The modern food industry with its enormous variety of food products requires that starch be able to tolerate a wide range of processing, handling, and storage. Therefore, these needs are met by modifying native starches by chemical and physical methods (Bemiller 1997, Rutenberg and Solarek 1984, Whistler et al. 1984).

5.5.1 Physical Modifications

Annealing and heat–moisture treatment are two hydrothermal treatments that modify the physicochemical properties of starch without destroying its granular structure. These two treatments involve incubation of the starch granules in excess water/intermediate water content (annealing) or at low moisture levels (heat–moisture treatment) during a certain period of time, at a temperature above the glass transition temperature but below the gelatinization temperature, respectively. These hydrothermal treatments significantly impact the physicochemical properties of starch such as granule morphology, crystallinity, as well as the double-helix content, the amount and appearance of amylose–lipid complexes, the gelatinization and pasting, the swelling power and solubility, the gel properties, and finally susceptibilities to acid and enzymatic hydrolysis of the modified or treated starch granules (Jacobs and Delcour 1998).

5.5.1.1 Pregelatinization The most important and used physical method of starch modification is "pregelatinization"; most pregelatinized starches are also called pregels or instant starches. This treatment has the most processing, and is a recent development in the technology of physically modified starches that have similar features and uses in food applications to those chemically modified.

Pregelatinized starches are not paste-forming products in cold water and partially or totally soluble in cold water (Colonna et al. 1984), but they disperse easily and absorb more water than native starches, form a gel at room temperature, and are less prone to deposit (Powell 1965). Moreover, pregelatinized starches are easily digested by the human amylolytic enzymes (Englyst and Cummings 1985). The classic model of pregelatinization is a slow heating of the granules in slightly agitated water in excess, and this promotes imbibition, swelling, and polymer release (Leach 1965, Maarschalk 1997). Other methods such as extrusion, spray-drying, and drum-drying followed by drying, which promote fast starch gelatinization, are also used to modify starches that may have long-term stability and quick preparation. As a result, most pregelatinized starches existing in the market have lost their granular integrity; however, instant starches marketed as cold-water swelling (CWS) types are unique because they have been modified by a process that maintains granular integrity and are generally used as thickeners in foods that receive minimal heat processing (Meng and Rao 2005).

5.5.1.2 Heat Treatment and Annealing Although less common as a starch modification technique, heat treatment is also considered an interesting physical modification process. Under controlled application of heat/moisture conditions, starch granules maintain their features and properties without any damage to the starch granules with respect to size, shape, or birefringence. This technique also improves the viscosity and stability when starch granules are subsequently gelatinized and pasted (Stute 1992), and heat–moisture-treated potato starch influences its physical properties (Eerlingen et al. 1997) and digestibility (rate) *in vivo* as well (Lee et al. 2012).

Two types of heat treatment processes are used. The first one is called "heat–moisture" and the second one is called "annealing," and both cause a physical modification of starch but with the particular ability to not gelatinize or cause any damage to the granular integrity, or birefringence loss (Stute 1992). The heat–moisture treatment involves heating starch at a temperature above its gelatinization point but with insufficient moisture to cause gelatinization. Investigation showed that this heat treatment does not change the potato granule size and shape, but at 95°C the x-ray diffraction intensities decrease and the x-ray patterns of starches become more cereal-like (Hoover and Vasanthan 1993, Kawabata et al. 1994, Li and Yeh 2001, Lim et al. 2001). These authors also reported that the swelling factor decreases and amylose leaching is more pronounced in potatoes. The DSC of the heat-treated starch potato samples shows pronounced changes in broadening of the gelatinization temperature range and a shifting of the endothermal transition toward higher temperatures, as well as a decrease in gelatinization enthalpy. Hoover and Vasanthan (1999) indicated that heat–moisture-treated gelatinized starch features are influenced by the interaction between leached starch components (amylose–amylose, amylose–amylopectin, amylose–amylopectin), the granule remnants, and leached amylose and amylopectin.

Annealing of starch involves heating a slurry of granular starch at a temperature below its gelatinization point for prolonged periods of time, and after this treatment, annealed granules of starch show an enhanced viscosity profile.

Annealing of potato starches also affects the physicochemical properties of the granules with a relationship between (native and modified) physical properties and the extent of phosphorylation (Muhrbeck and Svensson 1996). On the other hand, annealing leads to a slowing down of the initial swelling and cooperative melting of the granules; however, it does not alter the stability of the most perfect crystallites (Jacobs et al. 1998). Annealing increases the gelatinization temperatures of potato starches where the magnitude of change depends on the initial gelatinization temperatures (Alvani et al. 2012), and the susceptibility of potato starches to acid or enzymatic hydrolysis decreases upon annealing (Hoover and Vasanthan 1993). It was also reported that the amount of amylose leached from the granules is not linked to viscosity changes, and less amylose is leached from the granules of annealed potato starches (Jacobs et al. 1995). However, the magnitude of changes in gelatinization transition temperature (GTT) increases with the increase in annealing moisture content, but the swelling factor (SF), amylose leaching (AML), and gelatinization temperature range (GTR) decrease on annealing (Hoover and Vasanthan 1993). Vermeylen et al. (2006) studied potato starch annealing at different temperatures and heat–moisture treated (HNT), and noted that both annealing and HMT increase the DSC gelatinization temperatures, suggesting that the stacked lamellae, present in native and annealed starches, are disrupted in the HMT process.

Methods of cooking can also affect the amount and profile of resistant starch in potato and hence the glycemic index in food systems (Gracia-Alonso and Goñi 2000, Kingman and Englyst 1994, Mishra et al. 2008).

5.5.2 Chemical Modifications

The chemical modification of starches consists of the treatment of native starch with approved chemicals, and this modification leads to some changes in functionality of native starches. The chemical reactions primarily involve reactions associated with the hydroxyl groups of the starch polymer. Derivatization (where, in most cases, the efficiency is >70%) via ether or ester formation, oxidation of the hydroxyl groups to carbonyl or carboxylic groups, and hydrolysis of glycosidic bonds are some of the major mechanisms of chemical modification. These reactions are run in an aqueous appropriate chemical medium of 3/7 to 4.5/5.5 starch/water ratio, and this suspension of starch in water, typically 30–45% solids (by weight), is under proper agitation, temperature, and pH. At the end of the reaction, starch is brought to the desired pH by a neutralizing chemical, and then purified by washing with water and then recovered as a dry powder.

5.5.2.1 Crosslinking

The technique of crosslinking is likely the most common chemical modification technique used for the derivatization of starch by using a bi- or polyfunctional chemical reagent that reacts with at least two different hydroxyl groups of the same or different starch polymers. This crosslinking controls granular swelling and produces starches that tolerate high temperature, high shear, and acidic conditions.

Crosslinked starches are typically produced by mixing an alkaline granular starch slurry (pH 7.5–12, at 3/7 to 4.5/5.5 w/v) and a crosslinking reagent, often in the presence of salt. The most used and approved chemicals are phosphorus oxychloride ($POCl_3$), sodium trimetaphosphate ($Na_3P_3O_9$), and mixes of adipic anhydride (2,7-oxepanedione, hexahydrooxepin-2,7-dione, oxepane-2,7-dione) and acetic anhydride ($C_4H_6O_3$). After the reaction is complete, the pH of the reaction is adjusted to neutral, and the solution is filtered, washed, and dried (Rutenberg and Solarek 1984, Whistler et al. 1984). However, some results show that the optimal crosslinking reaction is obtained at a pH range of 9.0–9.5, a temperature of 35°C, and a reaction time of 2 h (Luo et al. 2009).

Phosphorus oxychloride is commonly used to produce crosslinked starch esters, and depending upon the extent of crosslinking, the di-starch phosphate that is generated produces starch with improved viscosity, stability, and process tolerance.

Sodium trimetaphosphate is less used than phosphorus oxychloride, although the product of this crosslinking reaction is chemically similar (distarch phosphate, by ester linkage). Although this chemical modification requires much more time, modified starches have the same properties as those of phosphorus oxychloride crosslinked starches.

A mixed reagent of adipic and acetic anhydride is also used to create organic ester linkages in starches that are relatively stable under conditions of neutral pH, but under extreme pH, these crosslinks are less stable than ether or inorganic ester linkages, and that is why the mixed anhydride reaction is conducted at a pH less than 9.

However, the distinguishing factors that affect the efficiency of the modification are the starch source, amylose-to-amylopectin ratio, granule morphology, and the type and concentration of the chemical reagents. Therefore, a good preparation of modified starches with desirable properties and degree of substitution can be achieved by selecting a suitable modifying agent, as well as the native starch sources (Singh et al. 2007).

Other chemicals have been used to produce crosslinked potato starch. Kim and Lee (2002) used epichlorohydrin (C_3H_5ClO) at different concentrations, and noted that the molar degree of crosslinking of the crosslinked starch increased proportionally with the increase in epichlorohydrin concentration, and the x-ray diffraction pattern and scanning electron microscopy showed that this crosslinking did not affect the crystallinity or granular shape of starch.

5.5.2.2 Substitution (Stabilization)   As discussed above, starch paste viscosity tends to change and this viscosity and textural change can be extreme for certain types of amylose-containing starches. Starches can form rigid gels, caused by the reassociation of amylose molecules, and this reassociation of starch polymers is called retrogradation. To prevent or at least minimize this, starch is stabilized by substituting specific monofunctional chemical groups called "blocking groups" along the polymer backbone, such as acetyl or hydroxypropyl groups. Stabilization leads to lowering of the gelatinization temperature and prevents the retrogradation of starches after cooking, and such starch is particularly useful for refrigerated and frozen foods (Rutenberg and Solarek 1984).

5.5.2.2.1 Starch Esters   So far, acetylation (esterification) is the most common method of starch modification, where acetyls replace hydroxyl groups in the native starch with acetyl groups. Although acetylated starches are commercially produced by using acetic acid (CH_3COOH), acetic anhydride ($C_4H_6O_3$), ketene (R'R''C=C=O), vinyl acetate ($CH_3COOCH=CH_2$), or a combination of these reagents, acetic anhydride is the most used (Kruger and Rutenberg 1967). Typically, starch acetate containing 0.5–2.5% acetyl groups is mostly used in foods, particularly crosslinked acetylated starch, which is used as a thickener because of its stability and clarity. Although the extent of change in these properties depends on the acetic anhydride concentration, acetic-anhydride-acylated potato starches have high acetyl (%), degree of substitution (DS), swelling power, solubility, and light transmittance than native starches (Singh et al. 2004a), and the change in these functional properties also depends on the source and the granule morphology of native starch (Singh et al. 2004b).

5.5.2.2.2 Starch Octenylsuccinates   For most starches used in food industries, the degree of monosubstitution is low; therefore, the chemical modification has little impact on the overall hydrophilic property of polymers. Nevertheless, upon substitution of starch with 1-octenylsuccinic anhydride (OSA, $C_{12}H_{18}O_3$), or succinic anhydride ($C_4H_4O_3$), a hydrophobic moiety is introduced into the polymer and a new class of starch product is created. Although OSA modification causes little change in the crystalline pattern of potato starch (Hui et al. 2009), OSA-treated starch has a similar pasting property to that of other monosubstituted starch derivatives, but significantly higher cool paste viscosity (CPV) and gelatinization temperature, with slightly lower swelling volumes (SV) at a high degree of substitution (DS) as compared to native starch, although the magnitude of changes in physical properties of OSA-modified starches depends not only on their DS but also on the botanical origin of the native starches (Bao et al. 2003).

OSA-treated starches are effective as emulsion stabilizers, as stabilizing agents in products such as beverages and salad dressings, as a flavor-encapsulating agent, as clouding agents, and as a processing aid. One key application of OSA-treated starch is the replacement of gum arabic in systems that require emulsion stabilization and/or encapsulation (Hedges 1992).

5.5.2.2.3 Starch Phosphates   Starch phosphates are ester derivatives of phosphoric acid, and unlike crosslinked starch, they are produced by using monofunctional reagents such as sodium orthophosphate (NaH_2PO_4) and sodium tripolyphosphate ($Na_5P_3O_{10}$) (Solarek 1986).

Starch phosphates have been reported to give clear pastes of high consistency, with good freeze–thaw stability and emulsifying properties (Lloyd 1970, Nierle 1969). Pastes of starch phosphate derivatives usually have improved clarity, low-temperature stability, and emulsifying properties. Starch phosphates have been recommended for salad dressing applications as a means to improve the stability of vinegar and vegetable oil emulsions (Solarek 1986).

5.5.2.2.4 Starch Ethers   Hydroxypropylated starch has brought a new dimension to the food industry because of its improved functional characteristics as compared to other types of substituted starch products. On these polymers, amylose is modified to a greater extent than amylopectin, while the modification of amylopectin occurs close to branch points, likely because the amorphous regions are more accessible to the modifying reagent (Kavitha and BeMiller 1998).

Studies were carried out on some physicochemical, morphological, thermal, and rheological properties of different cultivars potato starches. Results showed that treated starches showed higher swelling power, solubility, solubility in dimethyl sulfoxide (DMSO), and paste clarity than native starches. Light transmittance (LT) of treated starches remains stable during refrigerated storage, while the LT of native starches decreases, and scanning electron microscopy (SEM) showed that treated starch granules have different shape and size than native starch granules. Moreover, the phase transitions associated with the gelatinization of starches showed lower gelatinization parameters among the hydroxypropylated starches, whereas the native starches did not possess freeze–thaw stability (Kaur et al. 2004, Perera and Hoover 1999).

Pastes of hydroxypropylated starch have improved clarity, greater viscosity, reduced syneresis, and freeze–thaw stability, and when crosslinked, freeze–thaw stability during prolonged storage periods is also further enhanced. Therefore, crosslinked, hydroxypropylated starches are perhaps the most commonly used modified starches in the food industry (Gunaratne and Corke 2007).

5.5.2.3 Conversion   For applications that utilize high starch content, such as candies and food coatings, the practice is to use starches that have been converted, and this conversion process results in starch products that contain reduced-molecular-weight polymers and exhibit very reduced viscosity. There are different methods of starch conversion; however, the most common are acid hydrolysis, oxidation, pyroconversion, and enzyme conversion (see Section 5.3). The properties of converted starches can vary widely depending on the starch source used and the conversion process such as time and method used (acid, oxidant, heat, or combinations).

Although recorded as early as 1811 for the production of sugars and syrups (Kirchoff 1815), acid hydrolysis of starches for the commercial production of acid-converted starches began in the 1900s, with a primary objective to reduce the hot viscosity of starch pastes giving starches than can be easily dispersed without excessive thickening when at high concentrations.

The chemistry of the conversion process involves the acid-catalyzed hydrolysis of α-1,4 and α-1,6 glycosidic linkages using mainly hydrochloric (HCl) and sulfuric (H_2SO_4) acids. The hydrolysis occurs preferentially in the amorphous regions of the starch granules that will have a more crystalline structure. Although the molecular masses of both amylose and amylopectin of the granular potato starch decrease (van Soest et al. 1995), acid hydrolysis degrades mainly amylose and long amylopectin chains, resulting in increasing the proportion of short chains (Kim et al. 2012).

Different methods are used to measure the extent of hydrolysis; however, in the starch industry, an empirical scale referred to as water fluidity (WF) is used. It refers to the reciprocal of viscosity and ranges from 0 (unmodified or native starch) to 100 (water viscosity) and in potato starches, the strongest gelling ability occurs at a WF value ranging from 60 to 70 (Chiu and Solarek 2009).

Oxidation and bleaching of starch are also used to modify starch properties. Under controlled conditions, starch for food industries can be modified using oxidation agents such as sodium hypochlorite (NaClO), or bleaching agents such as hydrogen peroxide (H_2O_2), ammonium persulfate [$(NH_4)_2S_2O_8$], calcium hypochlorite [$Ca(ClO)_2$], potassium permanganate ($KMnO_4$), or sodium chlorite [$Na(ClO_2)$]. Oxidized starches are often used in batters and bread for coating a wide variety of foodstuffs.

When potato starch is oxidized by hydrogen peroxide, the molecular weight decreases with the degree of oxidation, and is dependent on the catalyst used (Tolvanen et al. 20013). Rheological measurements also reveal that when the molecular weight of the moderately oxidized starch is high, a firm gel is obtained with 25% starch concentration, and the more the oxidized starch content in the carbonyl groups, the higher the gelatinization temperature (Parovuori et al. 1995). On the other hand, bleaching is mainly used for corn starch and the goal is to improve the whiteness of the starch powder by oxidizing the impurities such as carotene, xanthophyll, and related pigments.

In pyroconversion, also referred to as dextrinization, starch products are prepared by dry roasting of acidified starch, and are referred to as pyrodextrins. The reaction of dextrinization of potato starch with gaseous hydrogen chloride was first described by Smith and Morris (1944). Although extensive literature exists on pyroconversion or dextrinization of corn and some cereal starches, we did not find a referral paper reporting on potato starch and this conversion. However, depending upon the reaction conditions (e.g., pH, moisture, temperature, and treatment duration), pyroconversion produces a range of products that vary in viscosity, cold-water solubility, color, reducing sugar content, and stability (Chinnaswamy and Hanna 1988, Wankhede and Umadevi 1982). Moreover, pyrodextrins have typically low viscosity, good film-forming ability, and high solubility in water. These pyrodextrins are widely used in the coating of foods and can replace more costly gums, and the special high-viscosity dextrins are also used as fat replacers in bakery and dairy products (Lucca and Tepper 1994).

5.6 Amylases and Enzymatic Actions and Modifications of Potato Starch

The history of modern enzyme technology and engineering began in 1874 when Christian Hansen, a Danish chemist, produced rennet by extracting dried calf's stomach with saline solution, and this was probably the first commercially available enzyme used for industrial purposes. By using enzymes, wide and various ranges of products can be produced for the starch industry, and these products can be obtained by enzyme engineering through controlled product formation (Pandey et al. 2000). Enzymatic modifications of starch remain an active area in the functional modified starches. These modifications offer the possibilities to tailor very specific properties because of the specificity of enzyme attacking and the selective modification of targeted applications (Benjamin et al. 2013, Holló et al. 1983).

Historically, starch-based products have been hydrolyzed by fermentation processes to produce sugars, which can be further converted into alcohol, and amylases and other enzymes have been used commercially for many years to modify starch. In the 1950s, amylase from fungi was used to manufacture specific syrups containing a range of sugars, which could not be produced by acid hydrolysis. The real turn in the history of starch enzymology was in the 1960s when glucoamylase was used to completely break down starch into glucose. In a few years, glucose production was reorganized and enzyme hydrolysis was used instead of acid hydrolysis because of many advantages such as greater yield, higher degree of purity, and easier crystallization. There are many enzymes that hydrolyze the glycosidic linkages in starch polymers. Amylases hydrolyze primarily the α-1,4 linkages, and another group of debranching enzymes specifically cleaves the α-1,6 linkages at the branch points in starch polymers (Kruger and Lineback 1987, Teague and Brumm 1992).

5.6.1 α-Amylases

A number of starch-converting enzymes belong to a single family of α-amylases (or glycosyl hydrolases). α-Amylases share a number of common characteristics such as structure, hydrolysis or formation of glycosidic bonds in the α conformation, and a number of conserved amino acid residues in the active site. To date, 25 3D structures of a few members of the α-amylase family have been determined using protein crystallization and x-ray crystallography. These help to better understand the interactions between the substrate or product molecule, since ca 21 different reaction and product specificities are found in α-amylases (van der Maarel et al. 2002).

α-Amylase (EC 3.2.1.1) is a common endoenzyme extracted from many sources, including fungi, bacteria, mammals, and cereals (Muralikrishna and Nirmala 2005, Pandey et al. 2000, Petrova et al. 2013, Thoma et al. 1971), and their mode of action, properties, and degradation products differ depending on their source (Kulp 1975). α-Amylase can neither hydrolyze the α-1,6 glycosidic bonds that form the branch points in amylopectin, nor sever the α-1,4 glycosidic bonds close to the branching point. Starch annealing also increases the accessibility of α-amylase to the amorphous as well as the crystalline regions to effect significant changes in gelatinization properties during enzyme hydrolysis (O'Brien and Wang 2008). Native granules of potato starch show a high resistance to α-amylase, but with heating to 60°C, the digestibility increases although there is no noticeable increase in the measured viscosity (Farhat et al. 2001). However, a recent study showed that during the initial stage of the reaction, enzymatic hydrolysis of native potato starches is mainly affected by the particle size of the granules, although the surface area and particle size also affect the initial rate at which native starch is digested by the debranching enzymes (Jung et al. 2013). The x-ray diffraction method and DSC used to study the effects of enzyme hydrolysis on the physicochemical properties of potato showed that the highest percentage of hydrolysis depends on the origin of the α-amylase. The enzymatic treatment decreases the degree of crystallinity of A-type crystals starches, while B- and C-types are weakened when hydrolysis is run at 60°C and completely disappeared at 100°C. Moreover, the gelatinization endotherm decreases for samples with a low degree of crystallization and disappears in samples with the amorphous stage (Gorinstein and Lii 1992).

After hydrolysis, residues of potato starch have lower apparent amylose contents and higher resistant starch contents. The gelatinization enthalpy, peak viscosity, and breakdown values of the residues markedly decrease, although the final viscosity values did not show much change. Furthermore, chain length distribution of debranched amylopectin from the residues indicates that the relative portion of short chain in the residue decreases and more molecules with intermediate chain length (DP 16–31) are found (Jiang and Liu 2002). The liquefying action of α-amylase is higher when it is combined with cyclomaltodextrin glucanotransferase (CGTase) and the concentration of glucose and maltose is higher after hydrolysis (Moreno et al. 2004).

5.6.2 β-Amylase

β-Amylase (EC 3.2.1.2) plays a central role in the complete degradation of starch to metabolizable or fermentable sugars, and it finds considerable application, together with starch debranching enzymes, in the production of high-maltose syrups. β-Amylase is an exoenzyme that specifically removes one maltose unit at a time from the nonreducing end of a starch molecule by hydrolyzing every other α-1,4 glycosidic linkage. The activity stops when the α-1,6 bond of amylopectin is reached or before it reaches the α-1,6 bond if there is an insufficient number of glucose units for it to react, thus yielding to what is called β-limit dextrin.

One enzymatic characteristic that has been used to distinguish the two forms of amylase is the dissimilarity of the end products of amylolytic hydrolysis (Bilderback 1973, Jacobsen et al. 1970, Tanaka and Akazawa 1970). α-Amylase is insensitive to high temperatures and heavy metal ions, requires Ca^+ ion, and is deactivated at lower pH, whereas β-amylase is sensitive to high temperatures and heavy metal ions, does not require Ca^+, and is more stable at lower pH. On the other hand, β-amylase hydrolyzes soluble starch or amylose, yields only maltose as an end product. The hydrolysis of soluble starch or amylose by α-amylase occurs randomly, releasing a large amount of oligosaccharides or dextrins. The dextrin is then hydrolyzed, yielding a large quantity of maltose and little glucose and maltotriose (Akazawa 1965). Therefore, the hydrolysis by α- or β-amylase would yield essentially similar end products. However, in cases where further hydrolysis of maltose by α-amylase is rate-limiting and depends on the concentration of the enzyme and pH (Tanaka and Akazawa 1970), little or no glucose would be expected. A few studies have reported on the activity of β-amylase on potato starch. One study reported that pure potato amylose is hydrolyzed by β-amylase at a steadily declining rate, without velocity changes until 100% of maltose has been formed. However, in case "denaturation" of the amylose occurs, there is a break in the progress curve and the hydrolysis is incomplete, and the shorter the molecular chains, the more slowly they are hydrolyzed (Hopkins et al. 1948). Recently, a bacterial hyper-thermostable β-amylase being fully active at 121°C for 15 min was used on raw and gelatinized native potato starches, and results showed that saccharification and maltose production were somewhat higher when compared to others observed on other different starches (Poddar et al. 2011).

5.6.3 Glucoamylase

Glucoamylase (EC 3.2.1.3), also known as γ-amylase, glucan 1,4-α-glucosidase, amyloglucosidase, exo-1,4-α-glucosidase, lysosomal α-glucosidase or 1,4-α-D-glucan glucohydrolase (Tateno et al. 2007), is an exoenzyme that removes glucose units from the nonreducing end of starch molecules. In addition to cleaving the last α-(1-4)-glycosidic linkages at the nonreducing end of amylose and amylopectin yielding glucose, glucoamylase also cleaves the α-(1-6)-glycosidic linkages (Tateno et al. 2007), and unlike the other forms of amylases, γ-amylase is best active in acidic environments (Kumar and Satyanarayana 2009). However, hydrolysis of the α-1,4 linkages is considerably faster than that of the α-1,6 bonds, and eventually if the glucoamylase activity lasts long enough, an entire starch molecule is completely converted into glucose, regardless of the extent of branching.

5.6.4 Cyclodextrin Glycosyltransferase

Some α-amylases catalyze transfer reactions in addition to hydrolysis, and cyclodextrin glycosyltransferase (CDGTase, EC 2.4.1.19) is therefore used for the production of cyclodextrins. It has been observed that the α-amylases capable of transferring glycoside residues are also those that generate low-molecular-weight products from their action on starch (i.e., saccharifying α-amylases) (Uitdehaag et al. 1999). CDGTs have been used to investigate the structure of amylopectins of potato starch (Bender et al. 1982) because they act on starch or starch derivatives, and the resulting product is a circular ring of glucose units linked by α-1,4 bonds (Hedges 1992). On potato starch, the optimum pH for the formation of γ-cyclodextrin ranges from 7 to 10 and the optimum temperature is 60°C, while the addition of ethanol to the reaction mixture enhances the formation of γ-cyclodextrin. With soluble starch or potato starch as a substrate, CDGTs produce a considerable amount of γ-cyclodextrin at the initial stage of the reaction. The amount of β-cyclodextrin increases gradually with time (Fujita et al. 1990), and the addition of polar organic solvents affects the yield and the type of cyclodextrins produced (Blackwood and Bucke 2000).

CDGTases from bacterial sources are being used in the commercial preparation of cyclodextrins, which usually contain six (α-cyclodextrin), seven (β-cyclodextrin), or eight (γ-cyclodextrin) glucose units. Cyclodextrins are used commercially to form inclusion complexes with a wide variety of molecules.

5.6.5 α-Glucanotransferases

As described in the previous sections, numerous starch-degrading enzymes are used in food industrial sectors to produce sweeteners, different concentrated syrups, and many other products and ingredients. However, during the last two decades other enzymes acting on starch have been raising the interests of scientists. The two enzymes that have received considerable attention are the branching α-glucanotransferases (EC 2.4.1.18) and the 4-α-glucanotransferase (EC 2.4.1.25). This interest is due to the fact that instead of catalyzing the hydrolysis of starch, they remodel parts of the amylose and amylopectin molecules by cleaving and reforming the α-1,4- and the α-1,6-glycosidic bonds, generating novel starch derivatives (van der Maarel and Leemhuis 2013).

AGTases belong to the superfamily of glycoside hydrolases (GHs, see www. cazy.org), and act on substrates with a number of consecutive α-1,4-glycosidic linkages such as amylose, amylopectin, and maltodextrins (Murakami et al. 2006, Stam et al. 2006, Zona et al. 2004). By far, the GH13 family is the largest one and contains numerous hydrolases such as α-amylase that have a central role in starch degradation. These catalyze the formation of a glycosidic bond that has the same anomeric configuration as the bond cleaved in the substrate, and that is why they are considered as α-retaining enzymes, and depending on the reaction catalyzed, three types of AGTase enzymes are distinguished: the 4-α-glucanotransferase (4αGT; EC 2.4.1.25) (Kaper et al. 2004), the cyclodextrin glucanotransferase (CGTase, EC 2.4.1.19, see description above) (Leemhuis et al. 2010), and the branching enzyme (BE; EC 2.4.1.18) (Boyer and Preiss 1977). As AGTases use polymeric substrates, the products can be a cyclic product, α-, β-, and γ-cyclodextrins with 6, 7, or 8 α-1,4-linked anhydroglucose residues, and linear products. (Kaper et al. 2004, Terada et al. 1999).

All the enzymes described above are, to an extent, used to modify starch and starch products. The most widely used enzymatic modification of starch is the conversion of starch to maltodextrins, corn syrups, sweeteners, and sugars (glucose and dextrose), and a wide range of these products are found. However, the extent of starch conversion is always monitored as the reaction proceeds, and besides the fundamental and technical conditions, it is typically admitted that the longer the conversion time, the lower the viscosity of the resultant product and the higher the reducing sugar content. Depending on the enzymes employed and the reaction conditions run, it is possible to commercially hydrolyze starch entirely to dextrose or to other other conversion products. In general, the change of DE (dextrose equivalent) leads to the change of the functional attributes such as hygroscopicity, solubility, sweetness, viscosity, gelling, and water-binding properties.

5.7 Potato Starches, Diet, and Health

The digestion of starch has been largely discussed and two main hypotheses were proposed. The first hypothesis stipulates that all starch is hydrolyzed and absorbed more slowly than simple sugar saccharides. Several studies *in vitro* and *in vivo* have shown that the physical form of food is the probably major determinant of the digestion rate of both starches and sugars (Wahlqvist et al. 1978, Wong and O'Dea 1983). On the other hand, a second assumption stipulates that starch is completely hydrolyzed and absorbed within the small intestine. Presently, it is admitted that the extent of starch digestion within the small intestine varies and depends again on the physical form, and part of this starch escapes digestion and enters the colon (Englyst et al. 1992). High-molecular-weight (high-MW) amylose is preferentially digested rather than amylose content alone and that MW is associated with resistance of starch to digestion in the upper gut of humans (Zhou et al. 2010).

Probiotics (principally lactic acid bacteria; LAB) may assist in lowering many diseases, and resistant starch (RS), as high-amylose starch prebiotic, can assist in promoting colonization, as a prebiotic and synbiotic. This starch also exerts its synbiotic action through the adhesion of the bacteria to the granule surface, and assists in recovery from infectious diarrhea in man and animals (Topping et al. 2003), by exerting mild laxative properties, predominantly through the stimulation of biomass excretion (Cummings et al. 1996).

5.8 Perspectives and Conclusions

Because potato starch and its derivatives have a long history of use in the human diet, the main issues to address was to understand the starch granule structure, and how the polymers of these granules can be modified to obtain the desired properties to satisfy food industries and consumers. The potato starch industry, even though small as compared to other industries, is however a very innovative and versatile sector in both food and nonfood applications. Because potato starch, raw and/or modified, has a large potential in the field of bio-based chemistry, much more is done to understand and modify starches to adapt to the new market demands by developing new starch products. Starches also present a versatility and heterogeneity of application in the food industry. This starch industry is related to agro-food sectors; the major challenge for starch scientists is to develop new starch products because the use of these products as food and ingredients is usually not based on their nutritional value but on their functional value, which can be modified.

Although much has been done on starch, still much needs to be done to: (i) characterize the different products that can be obtained by different modifying methods; (ii) develop new methodologies in modifying starch; and (iii) describe the different uses of the developed products in the food industry.

References

Akazawa, T. 1965. Starch, inulin, and other reserve polysaccharides. In *Plant Biochemistry*, eds. J. Bonner and J. E. Varner, 258–297. New York: Academic Press.

Alvani, K., X. Qi, and R. F. Tester. 2012. Gelatinisation properties of native and annealed potato starches. *Starch-Stärke* 64:297–303.

Alvani, K., X. Qi, R. F. Tester, and C. E. Snape. 2011. Physico-chemical properties of potato starches. *Food Chem* 125:958–65.

Anonymous. 2013a. http://www.aaf-eu.org/history/ (accessed: June 17, 2013).

Anonymous. 2013b. History of starch: Starch or amylum is a carbohydrate consisting of glucose units. http://www.meckey.com/history-of-starch/ (accessed: June 23, 2013).

Bao, J., J. Xing, D. L. Phillips, and H. Corke. 2003. Physical properties of octenyl succinic anhydride modified rice, wheat, and potato starches. *J Agric Food Chem* 51:2283–7.

Bemiller, J. N. 1997. Starch modification: Challenges and prospects. *Starch-Stärke* 49:127–31.

Bender, H., R. Siebert, and A. Stadler-Szöke. 1982. Can cyclodextrin glycosyltransferase be useful for the investigation of the fine structure of amylopectins?: Characterisation of highly branched clusters isolated from digests with potato and maize starches. *Carbohydr Res* 110:245–59.

Benjamin, S., R. B. Smitha, V. N. Jisha et al. 2013. A monograph on amylases from *Bacillus* spp. *Adv Biosci Biotechnol* 4:227–41.

Bilderback, D. E. 1973. A simple method to differentiate between α- and β-amylase. *Plant Physiol* 51:594–5.

Blackwood, A. D. and C. Bucke. 2000. Addition of polar organic solvents can improve the product selectivity of cyclodextrin glycosyltransferase: Solvent effects on CGTase. *Enzyme Microb Tech* 27:704–8.

Blanshard, J. M. V. 1987. Starch granule structure and function: A physicochemical approach. In *Starch: Properties and Potential*, ed. T. Galliard, 16–54. New York: John Wiley & Sons.

Bouillon-Lagrange, E. J. B. 1805. Analyse de la glucine. *Ann Chem France* 56:24–36.

Boyer, C. and J. Preiss. 1977. Biosynthesis of bacterial glycogen. Purification and properties of the *Escherichia coli* α-1,4-glucan: α-1,4-glucan 6-glycosyltansferase. *Biochemistry* 16:3693–9.

Buleon, A. and P. Colonna. 1998. Starch granules: Structure and biosynthesis. *Int J Biol Macromol* 23:85–112.

Chinnaswamy, R. and M. A. Hanna. 1988. Expansion, color and shear strength properties of com starches extrusion-cooked with urea and salts. *Starch-Stärke* 40:186–90.

Chiu, C. W. and D. Solarek. 2009. Modification of starches. In *Starch: Chemistry and Technology*. 3rd Edition, ed. J. BeMiller and R. Whistler, 629–655. Amsterdam: Elsevier.

Colonna, P., J. J. Doublier, J. P. Melcion, F. Monredon, and C. Mercier. 1984. Extrusion cooking and drum drying of wheat starch, part I, physical and macromolecular modifications. *Cereal Chem* 61:538–43.

Cottrell, J. E., C. M. Duffus, L. Paterson, and G. R. Mackay. 1995. Properties of potato starch: Effects of genotype and growing conditions. *Phytochemistry* 40:1057–64.

Cummings, J. H., E. R. Beatty, S. M. Kingman, S. A. Bingham, and H. N. Englyst. 1996. Digestion and physiological properties of resistant starch in the human large bowel. *Brit J Nutr* 75:733–47.

Eberstein, K., R. Hopcke, G. Konieczny-Janda, and R. Stute. 1980. DSC investigations on starches, Part 1. Feasibility of thermoanalytical methods to characterize starches. *Starke* 32:397–404.

Eerlingen, R. C., H. Jacobs, K. Block, and J. A. Delcour. 1997. Effects of hydrothermal treatments on the rheological properties of potato starch. *Carbohydr Res* 297:347–56.

Englyst, H. M. and J. H. Cummings. 1985. Digestion of the polysaccharides of some cereal foods in the human small intestine. *Am J Clin Nutr* 42:778–87.

Englyst, H. N., S. M. Kingman, and J. H. Cummings. 1992. Classification and measurement of nutritionally important starch fractions. *Eur J Clin Nutr* 46 (Suppl. 2):S33–50.

Evans, I. D. and D. R. Haisman. 1982. The effect of solutes on the gelatinization temperature range of potato starch. *Stärke* 34:224–31.

Farhat, I. A., J. Protzmann, A. Becker, B. Vallès-Pàmies, R. Neale, and S. E. Hill. 2001. Effect of the extent of conversion and retrogradation on the digestibility of potato starch. *Starch-Stärke* 53:431–6.

Fredriksson, H., J. Silverio, R. Andersson, A. C. Eliasson, and P. Aman. 1998. The influence of amylose and amylopectin characteristics on gelatinization and retrogradation properties of different starches. *Carbohydr Polym* 35:119–23.

French, D. 1984. Organization of starch granules. In *Starch: Chemistry and Technology*, ed. R. L. Whistler, J. N. BeMiller, and E. F. Paschall, 183–247. San Diego: Academic Press.

Fujita, Y., H. Tsubouchi, Y. Inagi, K. Tomita, A. Ozaki, and K. Nakanishi. 1990. Purification and properties of cyclodextrin glycosyltransferase from *Bacillus* sp. AL-6. *J Ferment Bioeng* 70:150–4.

Galliard, T. and P. Bowler. 1987. Morphology and composition of starch. In *Starch Properties and Potential*, ed. T. Galliard, 55–78. Chichester: John Wiley & Sons.

Gorinstein, S. and C. Y. Lii. 1992. The effects of enzyme hydrolysis on the properties of potato, cassava and amaranth starches. *Starch-Stärke* 44:461–6.

Gracia-Alonso, A. and I. Goñi. 2000. Effect of processing on potato starch: *In vitro* availability and glycaemic index. *Starch-Stärke* 52:81–4.

Gunaratne, A. and H. Corke. 2007. Functional properties of hydroxypropylated, crosslinked, and hydroxypropylated cross-linked tuber and root starches. *Cereal Chem* 84:30–7.

Hedges, A. R. 1992. Cyclodextrin: Production, properties, and application. In *Starch Hydrolysis Products*, ed. F. W. Schenck and R. E. Hebeda, 319–333. New York: VCH Publishers.

Holló, J., E. Laszlo, and A. Hoschke. 1983. Enzyme engineering in starch industry. *Starch-Starke* 35:169-75.

Hoover, R. and D. Hadziyev. 1981. Characterization of potato starch and its monoglyceride complexes. *Starch-Stärke* 33:290–300.

Hoover, R. and T. Vasanthan. 1993. The effect of annealing on the physicochemical properties of wheat, oat, potato and lentil starches. *J Food Biochem* 17:303–25.

Hoover, R. and T. Vasanthan. 1999. Effect of heat-moisture treatment on the structure and physicochemical properties of cereal, legume, and tuber starches. *Carbohydr Res* 252:33–53.

Hopkins, R. H., B. Jelinek, and L. E. Harrison. 1948. The action of β-amylase on potato amylose. *Biochem J* 43:32–8.

Hoseney, R. C., K. J. Zeleznak, and D. A. Yost. 1986. A note on the gelatinization of starch. *Starke* 38:407–9.

Hui, R., Q. H. Chen, M. L. Fu Mg, Q. Xu, and G. Q. He. 2009. Preparation and properties of octenyl succinic anhydride modified potato starch. *Food Chem* 114:86–9.

Imberty, I. and S. Perez. 1988. A revisit to the three-dimensional structure of B-type starch. *Biopolymers* 27:1205–21.

Jane, J. L., T. Kasemsuwan, S. Leas, H. Zobel, and J. F. Robyt. 1994. Anthology of starch granule morphology by scanning electron microscopy. *Starch-Stärke* 46:121–9.

Jacobs, H. and J. A. Delcour. 1998. Hydrothermal modifications of granular starch, with retention of the granular structure: A review. *J Agric Food Chem* 46:2895–905.

Jacobs, H., N. Mischenko, M. H. J. Koch, R. C. Eerlingen, J. A. Delcour, and H. Reynaers. 1998. Evaluation of the impact of annealing on gelatinisation at intermediate water content of wheat and potato starches: A differential scanning calorimetry and small angle x-ray scattering study. *Carbohydr Res* 306:1–10.

Jacobs, H., R. C. Eerlingen, W. Clauwert, and J. A. Delcour. 1995. Influence of annealing on the pasting properties of starches from varying botanical sources. *Cereal Chem* 72:480–7.

Jacobsen, J. V., T. G. Scandalios, and J. E. Varner. 1970. Multiple forms of amylase induced by gibberellic acid in isolated barley aleurone layers. *Plant Physiol* 45:367–71.

Jiang, G. and Q. Liu. 2002. Characterization of residues from partially hydrolyzed potato and high amylose corn starches by pancreatic α-amylase. *Starch-Stärke* 54:527–33.

Jung, K. H., M. J. Kim, S. H. Park et al. 2013. The effect of granule surface area on hydrolysis of native starches by pullulanase. *Starch-Stärke* 65:848–53.

Kaper, T., M. J. E. C. van der Maarel, G. J. Euverink, and L. Dijkhuizen. 2004. Exploring and exploiting starch-modifying amylomaltases from thermophiles. *Biochem Soc T* 32:279–82.

Kaur, L., N. Singh, and J. Singh. 2004. Factors influencing the properties of hydroxypropylated potato starches. *Carbohydr Polym* 55:211–23.

Kavitha, R. and J. N. BeMiller. 1998. Characterization of hydroxypropylated potato starch. *Carbohydr Polym* 37:115–21.

Kawabata, A., N. Takase, E. Miyoshi, S. Sawayama, T. Kimura, and K. Kudo. 1994. Microscopic observation and x-ray diffractometry of heat/moisture-treated starch granules. *Starch-Stärke* 46:463–9.

Kim, M. and S. J. Lee. 2002. Characteristics of crosslinked potato starch and starch-filled linear low-density polyethylene films. *Carbohydr Polym* 50:331–7.

Kim, Y. S., D. P. Wiesenborn, P. H. Orr, and L. A. Grant. 1995. Screening potato starch for novel properties using differential scanning calorimetry. *J Food Sci* 60:1060–5.

Kima, H. Y., D. J. Park, J. Y. Kim, and S. T. Lim. 2012. Preparation of crystalline starch nanoparticles using cold acid hydrolysis and ultrasonication. *Carbohydr Polym* 98(1):295–301.

Kingman, S. M. and H. N. Englyst. 1994. The influence of food preparation methods on the *in vitro* digestibility of starch in potatoes. *Food Chem* 49:181–6.

Kirchoff, G. S. C. 1815. Über die zukerlbildung beim malzen des getreides beim bebrühen seines mehl mit kochendem wassel. *J Chem Phys Schweigger's Nürnberg* 14:389–98.

Kruger L. H. and D. R. Lineback. 1987. Carbohydrate-degrading enzymes. In: *Enzymes and their Roles in Cereal Chemistry*, eds. J. E. Kruger, D. R. Lineback, and S. E. Stauffer, 117–39. St-Paul: American Association of Chemical Society.

Kruger, L. H. and M. W. Rutenberg. 1967. Production and uses of starch acetates. In *Starch: Chemistry and Technology* Vol. II, ed. R. L. Whistler, J. N. BeMiller, and E. F. Paschall, 369–401. New York: Academic Press.

Kugimiya, B. M., J. W. Donovan, and R. Y. Wong. 1980. Phase transitions of amylose-lipid complexes in starches: A calorimetric study. *Stärke* 32:265–70.

Kulp, K. 1975. Carbohydrases. In *Enzymes in Food Processing*. 2nd edition. ed. G. Reed, 53–122. New York: Academic Press.

Kulp, K. and K. Lorenz. 1981. Heat-moisture of starch. 1. Physico-chemical properties. *Cereal Chem* 58:46–8.

Kumar, P. and T. Satyanarayana. 2009. Microbial glucoamylases: Characteristics and applications. *Crit Rev Biotechnol* 29:225–55.

Leach, H. W. 1965. Gelatinization of starch. In *Starch Chemistry and Technology*, Vol. I, ed. R. L. Whistler and E. F. Paschall, 289–307. New York: Academic Press.

Lee, C. J., Y. Kim, S. J. Choi, and T. W. Moon. 2012. Slowly digestible starch from heat-moisture treated waxy potato starch: Preparation, structural characteristics and glucose response in mice. *Food Chem* 133:1222–9.

Leemhuis, H., R. M. Kelly, and L. Dijkhuizen. 2010. Engineering of cyclodextrin glucanotransferases and the impact for biotechnological applications. *Appl Microbiol Biotechnol* 85:823–35.

Li, J. Y. and A. I. Yeh. 2001. Relationships between thermal, rheological characteristics and swelling power for various starches. *J Food Eng* 50:141–8.

Lim, S. T., E. H Chang, and H. J. Chung. 2001. Thermal transition characteristics of heat–moisture treated corn and potato starches. *Carbohydr Polym* 46:107–15.

Liu, Q., E. Weber, V. Currie, and R. Yada. 2003. Physicochemical properties of starches during potato growth. *Carbohydr Polym* 51:213–22.

Lloyd, N. E. 1970. Starch esters. U.S. patent 3-539-551.

Lucca, P. A. and B. J. Tepper. 1994. Fat replacers and the functionality of fat in foods. *Trends Food Sci Technol* 5:12–9.

Luo, F. X., Q. Huang, X. Fu, L. X. Zhang, and S. J. Yu. 2009. Preparation and characterisation of crosslinked waxy potato starch. *Food Chem* 115:563–8.

Maarschalk, K. V. D. V., H. Vromans, W. Groenendijk, G. K. Bolhuis, and C. F. Lerk. 1997. Effect of water on deformation and bonding of pregelatinized starch compacts. *Eur J Pharm Biopharm* 44:253–60

Maurice, T. L. 1986. Thermomechanical analysis of starch. *Cereal Food World* 31:584–9.

Meng, Y. and M. A. Rao. 2005. Rheological and structural properties of cold-water-swelling and heated cross-linked waxy maize starch dispersions prepared in apple juice and water. *Carbohydr Polym* 60:291–300.

Mishra, S., J. Monro, and D. Hedderley. 2008. Effect of processing on slowly digestible starch and resistant starch in potato. *Starch-Stärke* 60:500–7.

Moreno, A., G. Saab-Rincón, R. I. Santamaría, X. Soberón, and A. López-Munguía. 2004. A more efficient starch degradation by the combination of hydrolase and transferase activities of α-amylase and cyclomaltodextrin glucanotransferase. *Starch-Stärke* 56:63–8.

Muhrbeck, P. and E. Svensson. 1996. Annealing properties of potato starches with different degrees of phosphorylation. *Carbohydr Polym* 31:263–7.

Murakami, T., T. Kanai, H. Takata, T. Kuriki, and T. Imanaka. 2006. A novel branching enzyme of the GH-57 family in the hyperthermophilic archaeon *Thermococcus kodakaraensis* KOD1. *J Bacteriol* 188:5915–24.

Muralikrishna, G. and M. Nirmala. 2005. Cereal α-amylases—An overview. *Carbohydr Polym* 60:163–73.

Nierle, W. 1969. The influence of the manufacturing conditions on the properties of phosphated corn starches and their application. *Starke* 21:13–8.

Noda, T., S. Tsuda, M. Mori et al. 2009. The effect of harvest dates on the starch properties of various potato cultivars. *Food Chem* 86:119–25.

O'Brien, S. and Y. J. Wang. 2008. Susceptibility of annealed starches to hydrolysis by α-amylase and glucoamylase. *Carbohydr Polym* 72:597–60.

Oostergetel, G. T. and E. F. J. van Bruggen. 1993. The crystalline domains in potato starch granules are arranged in a helical fashion. *Carbohydr Polym* 21:7–12.

Pandey, A., P. Nigam, C. R. Soccol, V. T. Soccol, D. Singh, and R. Mohan. 2000. Advances in microbial amylases. *Biotechnol Appl Biochem* 31:135–52.

Parovuori, P., A. Hamunen, P. Forssell, K. Autio, and K. Poutanen. 1995. Oxidation of potato starch by hydrogen peroxide. *Starch-Stärke* 47:19–23.

Perera, C. and R. Hoover. 1999. Influence of hydroxypropylation on retrogradation properties of native, defatted and heat-moisture treated potato starches. *Food Chem* 64:361–75.

Perez, S. and E. Bertoft. 2010. The molecular structures of starch components and their contribution to the architecture of starch granules: A comprehensive review. *Starch-Stärke* 62:389–420.

Perez, S. and A. Imberty. 1996. Structural features of starch. *Carbohydr Eur* 15:17–21.

Pérez, S. P. M. Baldwin, and D. J. Gallant. 2009. Structural features of starch granules. In *Starch: Chemistry and Technology*, ed. J. BeMiller and R. Whistle, 149–192. New York: Academic Press.

Petrova, P., K. Petrov, and G. Stoyancheva. 2013. Starch-modifying enzymes of lactic acid bacteria—Structures, properties, and applications. *Starch-Stärke* 65:34–47.

Poddar, A., R. Gachhui, and S. C. Jana. 2011. Saccharification of native starches by hyperthermostable β-amylase from Bacillus subtilis DJ5 and optimization of process condition for higher production of maltose. *Int J Appl Biotechnol Biochem* 1:221–30.

Powell, E. L. 1965. Production and uses of pre-gelatinized starches. In *Starch Chemistry and Technology*, ed. R. L. Whistler and E. F. Paschall, 523–547. New York: Academic Press.

Ruan H., Q. H. Chen, M. L. Fu, Q. Xu, and G. Q. He. 2009. Preparation and properties of octenyl succinic anhydride modified potato starch. *Food Chem* 114:81–86.

Rutenberg, M. W. and Solarek, D. 1984. Starch derivatives: Production and uses. In *Starch: Chemistry and Technology*, ed. R. L. Whistler, J. N. BeMiller, and E. F. Paschall, 311–388. New York: Academic Press.

Seetharaman, K. and E. Bertoft. 2012. Perspectives on the history of research on starch. Part I: On the linkages in starch. *Starch-Stärke* 64:677–82.

Shiotsubo, T. and Takahshi, K. 1984. Differential thermal analysis of potato starch gelatinization. *Agric Biol Chem* 48:9–17.

Singh, J., L. Kaur, and O. J. McCarthy. 2007. Factors influencing the physico-chemical, morphological, thermal and rheological properties of some chemically modified starches for food applications—A review. *Food Hydrocolloid* 21:1–22.

Singh, J., L. Kaur, and N. Singh. 2004b. Effect of acetylation on some properties of corn and potato starches. *Starch-Stärke* 56:586–601.

Singh, N., D. Chawla, and J. Singh. 2004a. Influence of acetic anhydride on physico-chemical, morphological and thermal properties of corn and potato starch. *Food Chem* 86:601–8.

Singh, N., N. S. Sodhi, M. Kaur, and S. K. Saxena. 2003. Physiochemical, morphological, thermal, cooking, and textural properties of chalky and translucent rice kernels. *Food Chem* 82:433–9.

Smith, A. and M. Stitt. 2007. Coordination of carbon supply and plant growth. *Plant Cell Environ* 30:1126–49.

Smith, L. T. and S. G. Morris. 1944. Dextrinization of potato starch with gaseous hydrogen chloride. *Ind Eng Chem* 36:1052–4.

Solarek, D. B. 1986. Phosphorylated starches and miscellaneous inorganic esters. In *Modified starches: Properties and Uses*, ed. O. B. Wurzburg, 97–112. Boca Raton: CRC Press.

Stading, M., A. Rindlav-Westling, and P. Gatenholm. 2001. Humidity-induced structural transitions in amylose and amylopectin films. *Carbohydr Polym* 45:209–17.

Stam, M. R., E. G. J. Danchin, C. Rancurel, P. M. Coutinho, and B. Henrissat. 2006. Dividing the large glycoside hydrolase family 13 into subfamilies: Towards improved functional annotations of α-amylase-related proteins. *Protein Eng Des Sel* 19:555–62.

Stute, R. 1992. Hydrothermal modification of starches: The difference between annealing and heat/moisture treatment. *Starch-Staerke* 44:205–14.

Svensson, E. and A. C. Eliasson. 1995. Crystalline changes in native wheat and potato starches at intermediate water levels during gelatinization. *Carbohydr Polym* 26:171–76.

Swinkels, J. J. M. 1985. Composition and properties of commercial native starches. *Starch-Staerke* 37:1–5.

Szymońska, J. and F. Krok. 2003. Potato starch granule nanostructure studied by high resolution non-contact AFM. *Int J Biol Macromol* 33:1–7.

Tanaka, Y. and T. Azakawa. 1970. α-Amylase isozymes in gibberellic acid-treated barley half-seeds. *Plant Physiol* 46:586–91.

Tateno, T., H. Fukuda, and A. Kondo. 2007. Production of L-lysine from starch by *Corynebacterium glutamicum* displaying γ-amylase on its cell surface. *Appl Microbiol Biotechnol* 74:1213–20.

Teague, W. M. and P. J. Brumm. 1992. Commercial enzymes for starch hydrolysis products. In *Starch Hydrolysis Products*, ed. F. W. Schenck and R. E. Hebeda, 45–78. New York: VCH Publishers.

Terada, Y., K. Fujii, T. Takaha, and S. Okada. 1999. *Thermus aquaticus* ATCC 33923 amylomaltase gene cloning and expression and enzyme characterization: Production of cycloamylose. *Appl Environ Microbiol* 65:910–5.

Tester, R. F. and W. R. Morrison. 1990. Swelling and gelatinization of cereal starches.1. Effects of amylopectin, amylose and lipids. *Cereal Chem* 67:551–7.

Thoma, J. A., J. E. Spradlin, and S. Dygert. 1971. Plant and animal amylases. In: *The Enzymes, Vol. V: Hydrolysis (Sulfate Esters, Carboxyl Esters, Glycosides) and Hydration*, ed. P. D. Boyer, 115–189. New York: Academic Press.

Tiessen, A., J. H. M. Hendriks, M. Stitt et al. 2002. Starch synthesis in potato tubers is regulated by post-translational redox modification of ADP-glucose pyrophosphorylase: A novel regulatory mechanism linking starch synthesis to the sucrose supply. *Plant Cell* 14:2191–213.

Tiessen, A., K. Prescha, A. Brandscheid et al. 2003. Evidence that SNF1-related kinase and hexokinase are involved in separate sugar-signalling pathways modulating post translational redox activation of ADP-glucose pyrophosphorylase in potato tubers. *Plant J* 35:490–500.

Tolvanen, P., A. Sorokin, P. Mäki-Arvela, D. Y. Murzin, and T. Salmi. 2013. Oxidation of starch by H_2O_2 in the presence of iron tetrasulfophthalocyanine catalyst: The effect of catalyst concentration, pH, solid–liquid ratio, and origin of starch. *Ind Eng Chem Res* 52:9351–8.

Topping, D. L., M. Fukushima, and A. R. Bird. 2003. Resistant starch as a prebiotic and synbiotic: State of the art. *Proc Nutr Soc* 62:171–6.

Uitdehaag, J. C. M., R. Mosi, K. H. Kalk et al. 1999. X-ray structures along the reaction pathway of cyclodextrin glycosyltransferase elucidate catalysis in the amylase family. *Nat Struct Biol* 6:432–6.

van der Maarel, M. J. E. C. and H. Leemhuis. 2013. Starch modification with microbial alpha-glucanotransferase enzymes. *Carbohydr Polym* 93:116–21.

van der Maarel, M. J. E. C., B. van der Veen, J. C. M Uitdehaag, H. Leemhuis, and L. Dijkhuizen. 2002. Properties and applications of starch-converting enzymes of the α-amylase family. *J Biotechnol* 94:137–55.

van Soest, J. J. G., K. Benes, and D. De Wi. 1995. The influence of acid hydrolysis of potato starch on the stress-strain properties of thermoplastic starch. *Starch-Stärke* 47:429–34.

Vermeylen, R., B. Goderis, and J. A. Delcour. 2006. An x-ray study of hydrothermally treated potato starch. *Carbohydr Polym* 64:364–75.

Wahlqvist, M. L., E. G. Wilmshurst, C. R. Murton, and E. Richardson. 1978. Effect of chain length on glucose absorption and the related metabolic response. *Am J Clin Nutr* 31:1998–2001.

Wang, T. L., T. Y. Bogracheva, and C. L. Hedley. 1998. Starch: As simple as A, B, C? *J Exp Bot* 49:481–502.

Wankhede, D. B. and S. Umadevi. 1982. Preparation and some physicochemical properties of pyrodextrins of ragi, wheat, jowar and rice starches. *Starch-Stärke* 34:162–5.

Whistler, R. L., J. N. BeMiller, and E. F. Paschall. 1984. *Starch: Chemistry and Technology*. 2nd Edition. New York: Academic Press.

Wong, S. and K. O'Dea. 1983. Importance of physical form rather than viscosity in determining the rate of starch hydrolysis in legumes. *Am J Clin Nutr* 37:66–70.

Zhou, Z., D. L. Topping, M. K. Morell, and A. R. Bird. 2010. Changes in starch physical characteristics following digestion of foods in the human small intestine. *Brit J Nutr* 104:573–81.

Zobel, H. F. 1984. Starch gelatinization and mechanical properties of starch pastes. In: *Starch: Chemistry and Technology*, eds. R. L. Whistler, J. N. Bemiller, and E. F. Paschall, 285–309. Orlando: Academic Press.

Zobel, H. F. 1988. Molecules to granules—A comprehensive starch review. *Starch-Stärke* 40:44–50.

Zobel, H. F., S. N. Young, and L. A. Rocca. 1988. Starch gelatinization: An x-ray diffraction study. *Cereal Chem* 65:443–6.

Zona, R., F., Chang-Pi-Hin, M. J., O'Donohue, and S. Janecek. 2004. Bioinformatics of the glycoside hydrolase family 57 and identification of catalytic residues in amylopullulanase from *Thermococcus hydrothermalis. Eur J Biochem* 271:2863–72.

CHAPTER **6**

Potential of the Filamentous Fungi from the Brazilian Cerrado as Producers of Soluble Fibers

RITA DE CÁSSIA L. FIGUEIREDO-RIBEIRO, KELLY SIMÕES,
MAURÍCIO B. FIALHO, ROSEMEIRE A. B. PESSONI,
MARCIA R. BRAGA, and MARÍLIA GASPAR

Contents

6.1 Introduction   131
6.2 Brazilian Cerrado as a Potential Source of Filamentous Fungi   132
6.3 Production of Fructo-Oligosaccharides by Fungal Enzymes   134
6.4 Biotechnological Applications and Perspectives   140
Acknowledgments   145
References   145

6.1 Introduction

In recent years, the concept that food is not only required for energy and nutrition supply but also to provide health, prevent diseases, and maintain physical and mental well-being has been introduced to consumers. As a consequence, the demand for functional foods has increased in the last few decades. One class of functional food that has received special attention are the soluble fibers, which include carbohydrates such as fructose-based polymers (fructans) and its oligomers (DP 2-10) named fructo-oligosaccharides (FOS).

The interest in FOS and fructans as food ingredients has increased due to their prebiotic and health-enhancing properties. FOS are not digested in the small intestine and have low caloric value, noncariogenicity, and anticarcinogen effects (Velázquez-Hernández et al. 2009). Other properties reported for these compounds are the decreasing levels of phospholipids, triglycerides, and cholesterol, increase of calcium and magnesium absorption, and the stimulation of bifidobacterial growth in the human colon (Mussatto and Mancilha 2007, Yun 1996). In addition, fructans can improve the organoleptic properties of several food products such as dairy, bakery, cereals and cereal bars, infant formulas, beverages, confectionery, and ice cream. FOS are easily incorporated into foods, are stable at high and at freezing temperatures, improve the texture, humectancy, and mouth feel, and can be used as sugar and fat replacer. The combination of FOS with high-intensity sweeteners provides a balanced sweetness profile and masks the aftertaste of aspartame or acesulfame k (Crittenden and Playne 1996, Niness 1999, Patel and Goyal 2011, Yun 1996).

The large number of patents (from 2001 to 2009) related to FOS production and their applications highlight their importance in food and nutrition (Lafraya et al. 2011). Therefore, the development of efficient biotechnological procedures for the synthesis of FOS is of considerable economic interest to the food and pharmaceutical industries (Singh and Singh 2010) and their production from sucrose has gained special attention.

Different classes of FOS are produced from sucrose by microbial β-fructofuranosidases (invertases and inulinases) or by fructosyltransferases (Sangeetha et al. 2005) as shown in Figure 6.1. In the inulin type, the fructosyl unit is β-2,1 linked to the fructosyl moiety of the terminal sucrose at the reducing end forming the trisaccharide 1-kestose, whereas in levan-type fructans, the fructosyl unit is β-2,6 linked to the terminal sucrose forming the trisaccharide 6-kestose. In neolevan-type, the trisaccharide precursor is the neokestose, in which the fructosyl unit is β-2,6 linked to the glucosyl moiety of sucrose. Biotechnologically, invertases with transfructosylation activity have been used to produce FOS at higher concentrations of sucrose (Rustiguel et al. 2011). On the other hand, inulinases target the β-2,1 linkage of inulin by both exo- and endo-action. Exo-inulinases release fructose as the main end product, whereas endo-inulinases produce mainly short-chain FOS and a minor proportion of monosaccharides.

The vegetation of the Brazilian Cerrado has a number of native plants accumulating inulin-type fructans and their rhizosphere has been revealed as a source of microbes able to produce FOS by the hydrolysis of fructans or through biosynthesis using sucrose as a substrate (Figueiredo-Ribeiro et al. 2007).

6.2 Brazilian Cerrado as a Potential Source of Filamentous Fungi

The Cerrado is the second largest biome of Brazil, representing 21% of the national territory, surpassed in area only by the Amazonian forest, and is considered a biodiversity hotspot. The term "Cerrado" is commonly used to designate a set of ecosystems (savanna, grasslands, and gallery forests)

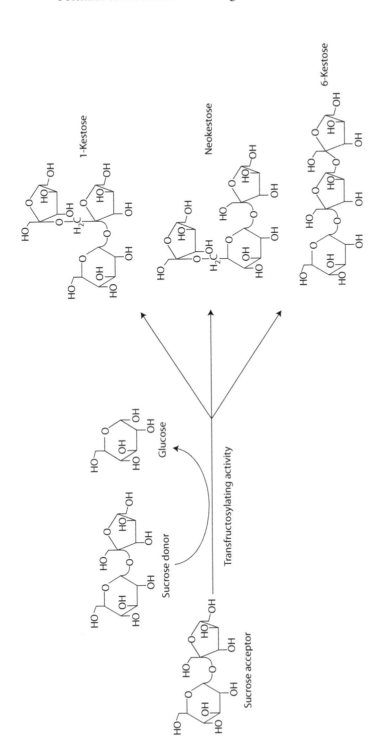

Figure 6.1 Different fructan structures produced by enzymes with transfructosylating activity on sucrose.

characterized by a well-defined dry season (Batalha 2011, Coutinho 2002). The Cerrado vegetation is composed of an array of drought- and fire-adapted plant species, predominantly the herbaceous ones (Mantovani and Martins 1988). The most representative species belong to the Asteraceae family, and about 60% of them store large amounts of inulin-type fructans in their underground organs (Figueiredo-Ribeiro et al. 1986, Tertuliano and Figueiredo-Ribeiro 1993). The rhizosphere of these Asteraceae species is a zone with high exudation of carbohydrates and intense microbial activity due to the presence of bacteria and filamentous fungi able to produce fructan-metabolizing enzymes (Cordeiro-Neto et al. 1997, Vullo et al. 1991).

As a consequence of the commercial interest for FOS produced by the enzymatic activity of microbial inulinases and invertases and the wide environmental diversity of plants and microbes in the tropics, we focused our work on the isolation of filamentous fungi from the rhizosphere of Asteraceae species from the Cerrado, aiming at future applications of such microorganisms for several purposes, particularly as alternative sources for FOS production. Using inulin as the sole carbon source, Cordeiro Neto et al. (1997) isolated 50 species of filamentous fungi from the rhizosphere of *Calea platylepsis*, *Vernonia cognata*, *V. herbacea*, *Viguiera discolor*, and *V. aff-robusta*, native Asteraceae species from the Brazilian Cerrado, many of them able to produce extracellular inulinases. The characterization of some of these enzymes, particularly related to their affinities to different substrates and capability of producing FOS, has been performed by our group (Pessoni et al. 1999, 2007).

6.3 Production of Fructo-Oligosaccharides by Fungal Enzymes

FOS can be produced as the result of the activity of fructan-producing enzymes (fructosyltransferases FTases) or fructan-hydrolyzing enzymes (inulinases and levanases), FTases cleave the glycosidic bond of sucrose and use the energy released to link the free fructosyl moiety to either sucrose or longer fructose-containing molecules producing FOS (Sangeetha et al. 2005). However, a limited amount of sucrose can be converted into FOS when FTases are used, because of the inhibition of enzyme activity by glucose also released as product from this reaction (Mussatto et al. 2009). The physiological significance of FOS production from sucrose by microorganisms is uncertain. It has been suggested that these sugars might confer tolerance to osmotic stress and nutrient deprivation (Velázquez-Hernández et al. 2009). When sucrose is hydrolyzed to glucose and fructose, the osmotic concentration of the medium increases due to the increased number of molecules released. In contrast, the osmolarity of the medium does not change when sucrose is transformed into FOS, suggesting the role of these molecules as osmoprotectants. In addition, microorganisms able to produce FOS may have advantages against competitor microbes able to use only sucrose as substrate since FOS are much less susceptible to microbial hydrolysis (Yoshikawa et al. 2006).

Microbial β-fructofuranosidases (inulinases, levanases, and invertases) are enzymes generally secreted opportunistically into the environment, which are able to hydrolyze oligo- and polymeric fructans. They are included in the GH-32, GH-68, and GH-100 families of glycosidases according to the CAZY database (http://www.cazy.org) (Cantarel et al. 2009) based on sequence similarity and they also share conserved domains (Naumoff 2001). Exo-inulinases (EC 3.2.1.80) cleave β-2,1 linkages sequentially starting from the nonreducing end of inulin and split off terminal fructosyl units, yielding fructose as the main product. Endo-inulinases (EC 3.2.1.7), on the other hand, act randomly on the inulin chain and hydrolyze internal linkages yielding FOS of different sizes. Inulinases can also, to some extent, hydrolyze sucrose. Because of the overlapping substrate specificity between inulinases and invertases, the distinction between both enzymes is sometimes difficult and controversial (Singh and Singh 2010).

In an assay to evaluate the ability of some filamentous fungi isolated from the rhizosphere of Asteraceae of the Cerrado to hydrolyze sucrose (15 g L^{-1}), *Neocosmospora vasinfeca* and *Paecilomyces lilacinum* demonstrated a lesser ability to deplete sucrose from the medium after 5 days of culture when compared to other fungal isolates (Figure 6.2). However, the analyses of the culture filtrates of *N. vasinfecta* by high-performance anion exchange chromatography (HPAEC/pulsed amperometric detector (PAD)) evidenced the presence of oligofructans with the predominance of the trisaccharide 1-kestose, an intermediate of the synthesis of larger fructan chains (Figure 6.3b). The presence of FOS produced by *N. vasinfecta* was confirmed by thin layer chromatography using kestose-specific reagent, as found in the culture filtrates and mycelia (Figure 6.3c).

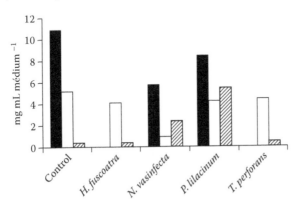

Figure 6.2 Sugar concentration (mg mL^{-1}) in a liquid medium after 5 days culture of filamentous fungi isolated from the rhizosphere of Asteraceae from Cerrado supplemented with 15 g L^{-1} sucrose: *Humicola fuscoatra*, *Neocosmospora vasinfecta*, *Paecilomyces lilacinus*, and *Tiarospora perforans*. Total sugar (■), fructose content (□), and reducing sugar (▨). Control refers to the concentration of sugars in the medium before fungal inoculation.

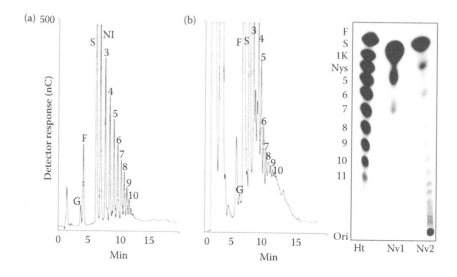

Figure 6.3 HPAEC/PAD profiles of fructo-oligosaccharides. (a) *Helianthus tuberosus* (standard, Ht). (b) Culture filtrates of *Neocosmospora vasinfecta* (Nv) after 5 days culture on sucrose-containing media. (c) Thin-layer chromatography of FOS present in culture filtrates (Nv1) and mycelia (Nv2) of *Neocosmospora vasinfecta*. G—glucose; F—fructose; S—sucrose; 1-K—1-kestose; Nys—nystose; NI—not identified; numbers indicate degree of polymerization.

In contrast, FOS were not detected in the culture filtrates of *H. fuscoatra* grown in sucrose. However, when these culture filtrates were incubated with inulin, increased amount of sucrose and oligofructans were detected in the reaction mixture, suggesting the presence of endo-inulinase activity in these cultures (Figure 6.4a and b). The endo-inulinase activity of *H. fuscoatra* was fairly low when compared to the endo-inulinase activity from *Penicillium janczewskii* (URM 3511), isolated from the rhizosphere of *V. herbacea*. Incubation of culture filtrates from *P. janczewskii* with commercial inulin resulted in increased FOS production after 10 min of incubation at 55°C, pH 5.0 (Figure 6.5). The endo-inulinases secreted by *P. janczewskii* remain uncharacterized, but two exo-inulinases and one invertase were purified by our group from the extracellular medium of this fungus when it was cultured in inulin extracted from rhizophores of *V. herbacea* or in sucrose as carbon sources (Pessoni et al. 1999, 2007). More recently, a different strain of *P. janczewskii* (URM 3361), also isolated from the rhizosphere of *V. herbacea*, showed distinct enzymatic activity in the culture medium as compared to the strain URM 3511 of the same fungus. *P. janczewskii* URM 3361 secretes enzymes with a low affinity for inulin (Zaninette et al., unpublished data), but seems to produce β-fructofuranosidases that are able to synthesize short-chain FOS when grown in sucrose (Figure 6.6).

The assignment of a particular enzyme as a β-fructofuranosidase or as a fructosyltransferase is based on the ratio of transferase to hydrolase activity,

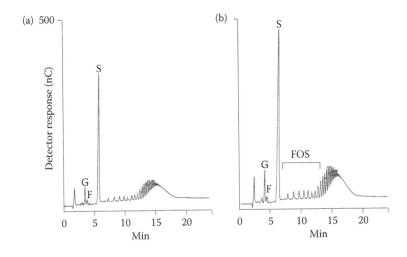

Figure 6.4 HPAEC/PAD profiles of carbohydrates produced by the enzymatic assays of cultured filtrates from *Humicola fuscoatra* and inulin from *Vernonia herbacea* as substrate. (a) 0 min and (b) 60 min. G—glucose; F—fructose; S—sucrose; FOS—fructo-oligosaccharides.

especially at low substrate concentrations. In fact, only a few of these enzymes have a transfructosylating activity significantly high for the industrial production of FOS.

The enzymatic production of β-2,6-linked FOS has been scarcely studied, although their presence has been reported in various food products (Marx et al. 2000). The synthesis of 6-kestose at high sucrose concentrations by an invertase from *Saccharomyces cerevisiae* was firstly reported by Straathof et al. (1986). After that, 1-kestose, neokestose, and 6-kestose were detected in the fructan syrup obtained by a levansucrase from *Zymomonas mobilis* (Bekers et al. 2002).

The microbiota of the Cerrado soil is also a source of enzymes for 6-FOS synthesis as reported by Fialho et al. (2013), using a new strain of *Gliocladium virens* (strain 3333). This naturally occurring soil filamentous fungus is a saprophyte and a mycoparasite, and was one of the first to be registered as a commercial biological control agent against soil-borne plant pathogens. In the Brazilian Cerrado, *G. virens* occurs simultaneously with other filamentous fungi in the rhizosphere of *V. herbacea*. Although many of these fungi have been reported to produce extracellular inulinases (Cordeiro Neto et al. 1997, Pessoni et al. 1999, 2007), this activity was not detected in *G. virens* when neither inulin nor sucrose was used as the carbon source. Instead, *G. virens* was able to produce FOS in the sucrose-based medium (Pessoni et al. 2009).

The influence of different nitrogen sources on FOS production by *G. virens* was also investigated. Culture media containing complex sources of nitrogen, such as corn and yeast extracts, increased fungal biomass and extracellular

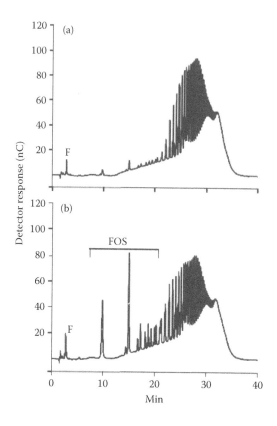

Figure 6.5 HPAEC/PAD profiles of FOS produced from chicory inulin by endo-inulinase activity of *Penicillium janczewskii* (URM3511) culture filtrates. (a) 0 min and (b) 10 min. F—fructose; FOS—fructo-oligosaccharides.

proteins, especially when supplemented with peptone (Pessoni et al. 2009). However, while FOS production by *G. virens* was unaffected by the nitrogen source, the concentration of the carbon source had dramatic effects on the FOS yield. The production of biomass, extracellular proteins, and inulin-type FOS (1-kestose, nystose, and [1]F-fructofuranosylnystose) by *G. virens* was lower in a medium containing 3 g L^{-1} sucrose than in a medium containing 30 g L^{-1} sucrose (Pessoni et al. 2009), which was also confirmed by Fialho et al. (2013). However, instead of inulin-type FOS, levan-type FOS were produced in high sucrose concentrations. The differences in FOS composition observed between the studies of Pessoni et al. (2009) and Fialho et al. (2013) highlighted the physiological performance of the fungal strain. Chromosomal abnormalities and polymorphisms in fungi after long-term preservation have been reported by several authors (Ryan and Smith 2004) and could explain the differences in *G. virens* behavior concerning the type of FOS synthesized after the culture preservation (Fialho et al. 2013).

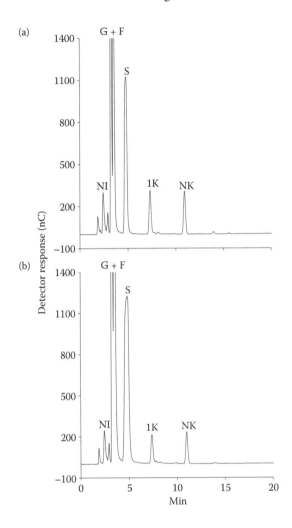

Figure 6.6 HPAEC/PAD profiles of 2-day culture filtrates from *Penicillium janczewskii* (URM 3361) indicating FOS production. (a) Medium containing 3% of sucrose as carbon source, and (b) 10% of sucrose. G—glucose; F—fructose; S—sucrose; 1-K—1-kestose; NK—neokestose; NI—not identified.

The highest production of 6-kestose (3 g L^{-1}) by *G. virens* occurred after 6 days of cultivation in 150 g L^{-1} sucrose, ca. 10- to 100-fold higher than in media containing lower sucrose concentrations (Fialho et al. 2013). Unlike *G. virens*, the thermophilic fungus *Sporotrichum thermophile* produced the highest level of 6-kestose (~1.6 g L^{-1}) at 250 g L^{-1}. At 150 g L^{-1}, the fungus produced only ca. 0.5 g L^{-1} of 6-kestose (Katapodis et al. 2004), one-sixth of the amount produced by *G. virens* grown in the same sucrose concentration.

According to Maiorano et al. (2008), sucrose is preferably hydrolyzed and used for mycelial growth, but at high concentrations, the excess of sucrose is generally converted into FOS due to the upregulation of β-fructofuranosidases with transfructosylating activity.

G. virens growing in sucrose concentrations higher than 150 g L^{-1} (300 and 400 g L^{-1}) resulted in increased fungal biomass; however, the amounts of extracellular proteins and FOS were unaffected (Fialho et al. 2013). Limitation of FOS production when the sucrose concentration exceeds a certain level has already been reported for *S. thermophile* (Katapodis et al. 2004), *Rhodotorula* sp. (Alvarado-Huallanco and Filho 2011), and *Xanthophyllomyces dendrorhous* (Linde et al. 2012), and might be related to the osmotic stress caused by the high sugar concentration.

The optimal pH and temperature for the hydrolytic activity of *G. virens* culture filtrates were 5.0°C and 30°C, respectively (Pessoni et al. 2009). Culture filtrates incubated in low sucrose concentration (10 g L^{-1}) presented high hydrolytic activity (94.5 U per mg of protein); however, no transfructosylating activity was detected (Figure 6.7a). Conversely, at a high sucrose concentration (200 g L^{-1}), the synthesis of 6-kestose and traces of neokestose (Figure 6.7b) were observed by Fialho et al. (2013), indicating that the production of FOS by *G. virens* is probably catalyzed by β-fructofuranosidases (invertases) that primarily hydrolyze sucrose to glucose and fructose, but at high sucrose concentrations may exhibit reverse hydrolysis. By this enzymatic reaction, the α (2,1) linkage of sucrose is cleaved, releasing glucose and transferring the fructosyl group to a sucrose acceptor molecule.

Many fungal species are known to produce enzymes involved in the biosynthesis of FOS but currently β-fructofuranosidases and fructosyltransferases from *Aspergillus* sp. and *Aureobasidium* sp. are the main commercial sources of inulin-type FOS (Ghazi et al. 2007, Sangeetha et al. 2005). The enzymatic synthesis of levan and neolevan-type FOS, such as 6-kestose and neokestose, respectively, by *G. virens* (Fialho et al. 2013) is uncommon in yeasts and filamentous fungi (Linde et al. 2009), being of great interest since these FOS have enhanced stability and prebiotic activity when compared to the typical inulin-type FOS.

6.4 Biotechnological Applications and Perspectives

Although FOS are found in rye, wheat, banana, asparagus, onion, garlic, jerusalem artichoke, and tomato, among other vegetables, the concentration of FOS found in these sources is too low to exert any beneficial effect (Sangeetha et al. 2005, Yun 1996), and extraction procedures to obtain these compounds from these plants are not economically viable. Since FOS production on an industrial scale is desirable, microbial enzymatic systems can provide a cost-effective and convenient alternative to this. Different enzymatic processes, which produce slightly different end products, can be employed: synthesis from sucrose by fructosyltransferases or by β-fructofuranosidases with high transfructosylating activity and controlled enzymatic hydrolysis of inulin by

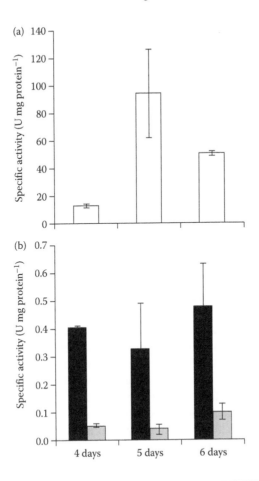

Figure 6.7 Enzymatic activity of *Gliocladium virens* culture filtrates obtained after 4, 5, and 6 days of growth in a medium containing 150 g L^{-1} sucrose. Hydrolyzing activity (10 g L^{-1} sucrose for 30 min at 40°C) (a) and transfructosylating activity (200 g L^{-1} sucrose for 24 h at 40°C) (b). Values are means of three replicates (±SD). Glucose (□), 6-kestose (■), and neokestose (▨). (From Fialho, M. B. et al. 2013. *Mycoscience* 54:198–205. With permission.)

the action of endo-inulinases (Antošová et al. 2008, Katapodis et al. 2004, Sangeetha et al. 2005, Singh and Singh 2010, Vega-Paulino and Zúniga-Hansen 2012).

The action mechanism of transfructosylating enzymes depends of the organism used as source of enzyme, plant, or microorganism. While in plants a series of enzymes act together, most of the microorganisms synthesize FOS employing only one enzyme. In addition, generally, enzymes derived from microorganisms are more thermostable in comparison to those derived from plants, a convenient feature for biotechnological applications (Yun 1996).

The process of FOS production from sucrose by transfructosylating activity generates 1-kestose (GF2), 1-nystose (GF3), and 1-fructofuranosyl nystose (GF4), in which one, two, and three fructose units are bound to sucrose, respectively (Yun 1996). The transfructosylation process can be more advantageous than the inulin hydrolysis since by using the first one it is possible to synthesize FOS of either a defined chain length or desired composition mixture, by modulating the reaction time (Nemukula et al. 2009). A typical reaction mixture on mass basis is as follows: 65% FOS, 25% glucose, 5% fructose, and 5% sucrose (Sangeetha et al. 2004). After a chromatographic step for purification, the commercial product usually presents 95% of FOS (37% 1-kestose, 53% nystose, and 10% 1-fructofuranosyl nystose) and 5% of sucrose and monosaccharides (Bornet et al. 2002).

In spite of the fact that a large number of microbial producers of β-fructofuranosidases and β-fructosyltransferases have been reported, only a few species of filamentous fungi (mainly *Aspergillus* and *Aureobasidium* genera) have received particular attention and have been reported as a good enzyme producer for industrial application (Patel et al. 1994, Sangeetha et al. 2005, Yun et al. 1993). For instance, *Aspergillus niger* ATCC20611 was selected as the most suitable strain for FOS production (Hidaka et al. 1988). The β-fructofuranosidase of this fungus catalyzes almost exclusively transfructosylation reaction in 50% (w/v) sucrose solution, yielding 55–60% (w/w) FOS (Singh and Singh 2010). Thus, high concentration of sucrose is required for efficient transfructosylation. The enzymatic synthesis route to FOS production using β-fructofuranosidase from *A. niger* ATCC20611 was first developed by Meiji Seika Kaisha Ltd. (Japan) to launch the commercial product Meioligo®. Then, this company also established a joint venture with Beghin-Meiji Industries (France) to produce FOS marketed as Actilight®, and also with GTC Nutrition (USA) to produce FOS under the trade name NutraFlora®. In 1987, Jung et al. reported the existence of an enzyme from *Aureobasidium pullulans* with industrial potential for FOS production, which originated another industrial process employed by Cheil Foods and Chemicals Co. (South Korea). It consists of a continuous process using immobilized cells of *A. pullulans* entrapped in calcium alginate beads (Yun et al. 1990).

Conventionally, FOS are produced in a two-step process, in which the first one consists of the microbial production of β-fructofuranosidases, and the second step consists of a reaction of the extracted enzymes with sucrose as the substrate (Mussatto et al. 2009, Sangeetha et al. 2005). This second step can be developed by two different methods: batch systems with soluble enzymes or continuous systems using immobilized enzymes or whole cells (Figure 6.8). Since unwanted hydrolytic activity is also present, leading to fructose and glucose as by-products, FOS yield is relatively low. As glucose inhibits FTases activity (Mussato et al. 2009, Yun 1996), its elimination can increase the production of FOS. For this purpose, membrane and chromatographic separation, and the use of mixed enzyme system, including glucose oxidase, can be

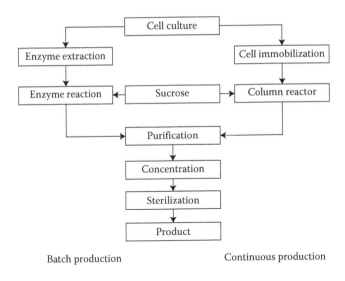

Batch production   Continuous production

Figure 6.8 Industrial processes for the production of fructo-oligossacharides. (Adapted from Yun, J. W. 1996. *Enzyme Microb Tech* 19:107–17.)

employed to produce high-content FOS (up to 98%) (Sangeetha et al. 2005, Yun 1996).

In general, food-grade oligosaccharides are not pure products but mixtures containing oligosaccharides of different degrees of polymerization, unreacted sucrose, and monosaccharides. However, most manufacturers produce different types of commercial products. Higher-grade products contain purer FOS mixtures with lower levels of contaminating sugars often removed by membrane or chromatographic procedures, as commented above. The absence of simple sugars lowers cariogenicity and caloric value, and allows the oligosaccharides to be included in diabetic foods (Crittenden and Playne 1996, 2002).

The second approach used for the production of FOS is the controlled hydrolysis of inulin extracted from chicory roots by endo-inulinases, which act randomly cleaving the β-2,1 linkages of inulin. As result, a mixture of FOS similar to that obtained by transfructosylation of sucrose is produced (Franck 2002, Sangeetha et al. 2005). However, unlike the FOS produced by FTases, not all the β-2,1-linked fructosyl chains carry a terminal glucose moiety. Furthermore, the FOS mixture produced from inulin hydrolysis contains longer (DP 2-7) chains compared to that obtained from sucrose by the transfructosylation process (DP 3-5) (Rastall 2010). By this method, FOS yield ranges from 60% to 86% under optimal hydrolysis conditions.

The main FOS producers are Orafti Active Food Ingredients (USA) who make inulin-derived products from chicory roots under the trade name Raftilose®, an inulin-derived product produced by partial enzymatic hydrolysis of chicory inulin. It contains mainly FOS (950 g kg^{-1}) with a DP ranging from 3 to 7 (average DP of 4). Similar inulin-hydrolyzed products on the market are Fibrulose® (Cosucra Groupe Warcoing, Belgium) and Inulin FOS® (Jarrow Formulas, USA) (Singh and Singh 2010).

FOS are the ingredients of the future that meet the needs of the food industry today and are on the leading edge of the emerging trend toward functional foods (Singh and Singh 2010). In the industrial production of FOS, a few types of β-fructofuranosidases are used. The production of enzymes involved in FOS synthesis can be enhanced by strain development and genetic manipulation (Shin et al. 2004). Genes that encode extra- or intracellular FTases have been isolated from bacteria, fungi, and plants (Alméciga-Díaz et al. 2011, and references there in); they retain eight motifs highly conserved in the glycoside hydrolase 32 (GH32) family. These genes have been expressed in genetically modified bacteria, yeast, molds, and plants, allowing the production of recombinant FTases with similar or even better fructosyltransferase activity than that observed in native enzymes, increasing FOS production (Alméciga-Díaz et al. 2011).

Alméciga-Díaz et al. (2011) conducted a computational analysis of reported sequences for FTases from a diverse source of organisms. The authors focused their analyses on domain A, which contains highly conserved sequence located in the active site of GH32 and GH68 members. FTases from fungi were grouped in two clades (VIa and VIb), having a catalytic residue (Asp) highly conserved in both. The main difference between these clades was the presence of a Cys immediately after the Asp residue in clade VIb sequences, while an Asn residue was observed in clade VIa members. These changes in the active site could have significant effect on enzyme activity, and could explain part of the difference in the yield of FOS production among fungi strains (Alméciga-Díaz et al. 2011).

Fungi FTases genes have been isolated mainly from *Aspergillus* strains, although a database mining analysis identified FTase-related sequences in *Gibberella zeae*, *Magnaporthe grisea*, and *Ustilago maydis* genomes (Yuan et al. 2006).

Considering that the molecular studies on β-fructofuranosidases have been focused particularly in the *Aspergillus* model, information about the sequences of genes encoding these fungal enzymes is still limited. Since the filamentous fungi isolated from the rhizosphere of plants from the Brazilian Cerrado are an important source of enzymes for the production of FOS either by synthesis from sucrose or by the hydrolysis of inulin, the large-scale sequencing of these microorganisms will allow the finding of new models of FOS production. Sequence analyses may enhance the possibility to unravel the mode of action of these enzymes and improve FOS production and to increase the understanding of fructan metabolism in fungi for further biotechnological applications, mainly in those microorganisms that present fructan-hydrolyzing and transfructosylation activities.

Acknowledgments

This research was supported by FAPESP (The State of São Paulo Research Foundation 2005/04139-7 and 2012/16332-0), PNADB/CAPES (National Plan for Botany Development—454/2010), and by CNPq (National Council for Scientific and Technological Development). M.B.F. and K.S thank CNPq and FAPESP for the postdoctoral fellowships, and M.R.B. and R.C.L.F-R. thank CNPq for the researcher fellowships. The authors thank Dr. M.A.M. Carvalho for the critical revision and helpful comments on the manuscript.

References

Alméciga-Díaz, C. J., A. M. Gutierrez, I. Bahamon, A. Rodríguez, M. A. Rodríguez, and O. F. Sánchez. 2011. Computational analysis of the fructosyltransferase enzymes in plants, fungi and bacteria. *Gene* 484:26–34.

Alvarado-Huallanco, M. B. and F. M. Filho. 2011. Kinetic studies and modelling of the production of fructooligosaccharides by fructosyltransferase from *Rhodotorula* sp. *Cat Sci Tec* 1:1043–50.

Antošová M., V. Illeová, M. Vandáková, A. Družkovská, and M. Polakovič. 2008. Chromatographic separation and kinetic properties of fructosyltransferase from *Aureobasidium pullulans. J Biotechnol* 135:58–63.

Batalha, M. A. 2011. The Brazilian cerrado is not a biome. *Biota Neotrop* 11:21–4.

Bekers, M., J. Laukevics, D. Upite et al. 2002. Fructooligosaccharide and levan producing activity of *Zymomonas mobilis* extracellular levansucrase. *Process Biochem* 38:701–6.

Bornet, F. R., F. Brouns, Y. Tashiro, and V. Duvillier. 2002. Nutritional aspects of short-chain fructooligosaccharides: Natural occurrence, chemistry, physiology and health implications. *Digest Liver Dis* 34:S111–S20.

Cantarel, B. L., P. M. Coutinho, C. Rancurel, T. Bernard, V. Lombard, and B. Henrissat. 2009. The carbohydrate-active enzymes database (CAZy): An expert resource for glycogenomics. *Nucleic Acids Res* 37:D233–D38.

Cordeiro-Neto, F., R. A. B. Pessoni, and R. C. L. Figueiredo-Ribeiro. 1997. Fungos produtores de inulinases isolados da rizosfera de Asteráceas herbáceas do Cerrado (Moji-Guaçu, SP, Brasil). *Rev Bras Cienc Solo* 21:149–53.

Coutinho, L. M. 2002. O bioma do cerrado. In *Eugen Warming e o cerrado brasileiro: um século depois*, ed. A. L. Klein, 77–92, São Paulo: Editora Unesp.

Crittenden, R. G. and M. J. Playne. 1996. Production, properties and applications of food-grade oligosaccharides. *Trends Food Sci Tech* 7:353–61.

Crittenden, R. G. and M. J. Playne. 2002. Purification of food-grade oligosaccharides using immobilized cells of *Zymomonas mobilis. Appl Microbiol Biot* 58:297–302.

Fialho, M. B., K. Simões, C. A. Barros, R. A. B. Pessoni, M. R. Braga, and R. C. L. Figueiredo-Ribeiro. 2013. Production of 6-kestose by the filamentous fungus *Gliocladium virens* as affected by sucrose concentration. *Mycoscience* 54:198–205.

Figueiredo-Ribeiro, R. C. L., S. M. C. Dietrich, E. P. Chu, M. A. M. Carvalho, C. C. J. Vieira, and T. T. Graziano. 1986. Reserve carbohydrates in underground organs of native Brazilian plants. *Rev Bras Bot* 9:159–66.

Figueiredo-Ribeiro, R. C. L., M. A. M. Carvalho, R. A. Pessoni, M. R., Braga, and S. M. C. Dietrich. 2007. Inulin and microbial inulinases from the Brazilian cerrado:

Occurrence, characterization and potential uses. In *Functional Ecosystems and Communities*, ed. J. T. Silva, 42–48. Kenobe: Global Science Books Ltd.

Franck, A. 2002. Technological functionality of inulin and oligofructose. *Br J Nutr* 87:S287–S91.

Ghazi, I., L. Fernandez-Arrojo, H. Garcia-Arellano, F. J. Plou, and A. Ballesteros. 2007. Purification and kinetic characterization of a fructosyltransferase from *Aspergillus aculeatus*. *J Biotechnol* 128:204–11.

Hidaka, H., M. Hirayama, and N. Sumi. 1988. A fructo-oligosaccharide producing enzyme from *Aspergillus niger* ATCC 20611. *Agr Biol Chem* 52:1181–87.

Jung, K. H., J. Y. Lim, S. J. Yoo, J. H. Lee, and M. Y. Yoo. 1987. Production of fructosyltransferase from *Aureobosidium pullulans*. *Biotechnol Lett* 9:703–8.

Katapodis, P., E. Kalogeris, D. Kekos, and B. J. Macris. 2004. Biosynthesis of fructooligosaccharides by *Sporotrichum thermophile* during submerged batch cultivation in high sucrose media. *Appl Microbiol Biotechnol* 63:378–82.

Lafraya, A., J. Sanz-Aparicio, J. Polaina, and J. Marín-Navarro. 2011. Fructooligosaccharide synthesis by mutant versions of *Saccharomyces cerevisiae* invertase. *Appl Environ Microbiol* 77:6148–57.

Linde, D., I. Macias, L. Fernández-Arrojo, F. J. Plou, A. Jiménez, and M. F. Lobato. 2009. Molecular and biochemical characterization of a beta-fructofuranosidase from *Xanthophyllomyces dendrorhous*. *Appl Environ Microbiol* 75:1065–73.

Linde, D., B. Rodríguez-Colinas, M. Estévez, A. Poveda, F. J. Plou, and F. M. Lobato. 2012. Analysis of neofructooligosaccharides production mediated by the extracellular β-fructofuranosidase from *Xanthophyllomyces dendrorhous*. *Bioresour Technol* 109:123–30.

Maiorano, A. E., R. M. Piccoli, E. S. da Silva, and M. F. A. Rodrigues. 2008. Microbial production of fructosyltransferases for synthesis of prebiotics. *Biotechnol Lett* 30:1867–77.

Mantovani, W. and F. R. Martins. 1988. Variações fenológicas das espécies de cerrado da reserva biológica de Mogi-Guaçu, São Paulo. *Rev Bras Bot* 11:101–12.

Marx, S. P., S. Winkler, and W. Hartmeier. 2000. Metabolization of beta-(2,6)-linked fructose-oligosaccharides by different bifidobacteria. *FEMS Microbiol Lett* 182:163–9.

Mussatto, S. I. and I. M. Mancilha. 2007. Non-digestible oligosaccharides: A review. *Carbohyd Polym* 68:587–97.

Mussatto, S. I., C. Aguilar, L. R. Rodrigues, and J. A. Teixeira. 2009. Colonization of *Aspergillus japonicus* on synthetic materials and application to the production of fructooligosaccharides. *Carbohyd Res* 344:795–800.

Naumoff, D. G. 2001. Beta-fructosidase superfamily: Homology with some alpha-L-arabinases and beta-D-xylosidases. *Proteins* 42:66–76.

Nemukula, A., T. Mutanda, B. S. Wilhelmi, and C. G. Whiteley. 2009. Response surface methodology: Synthesis of short chain fructooligosaccharides with a fructosyltransferase from *Aspergillus aculeatus*. *Bioresour Technol* 100:2040–5.

Niness, K. R. 1999. Inulin and oligofructose: What are they? *J Nutr* 129:1402S–6S.

Patel, V., G. Saunders, and C. Bucke. 1994. Production of fructooligosaccharides by *Fusarium oxysporum*. *Biotechnol Lett* 16:1139–44.

Patel, S. and A. Goyal. 2011. Functional oligosaccharides: Production, properties and applications. *World J Microb Biot* 27:1119–28.

Pessoni, R. A. B., R. C. L. Figueiredo-Ribeiro, and M. R. Braga. 1999. Extracellular inulinases from *Penicillium janczewskii*, a fungus isolated from the rhizosphere of *Vernonia herbacea* (Asteraceae). *J Appl Microbiol* 87:141–7.

Pessoni, R. A. B., M. R. Braga, and R. C. L. Figueiredo-Ribeiro. 2007. Purification and properties of exo-inulinases from *Penicillium janczewskii* growing on distinct carbon sources. *Mycologia* 99:493–503.

Pessoni, R. A. B., K. Simões, M. R. Braga, and R. C. L. Figueiredo-Ribeiro. 2009. Effects of substrate composition on growth and fructo-oligosaccharide production by *Gliocladium virens*. *DBPBMB* 3:96–101 (Special Issue 1), Proceedings of the 6th International Fructan Symposium (IFS), Hokkaido, Japan, July 2008.

Rastall, R. A. 2010. Functional oligosaccharides: Application and manufacture. *Ann Rev Food Sci Technol* 1:305–39.

Rustiguel, C. B., A. H. C. Oliveira, H. F. Terenzi, J. A. Jorge, and L. H. S. Guimarães. 2011. Biochemical properties of an extracellular β-D-fructofuranosidase II produced by *Aspergillus phoenicis* under solid-sate fermentation using soy bran as substrate. *Electron J Biotechnol* 14. http://dx.doi.org/10.2225/vol14-issue2-fulltext-1

Ryan, M. J. and D. Smith. 2004. Fungal genetic resource centres and the genomic challenge. *Mycol Res* 108:1351–62.

Sangeetha, P. T., M. N. Ramesh, and S. G. Prapulla. 2004. Production of fructooligosaccharides by fructosyl transferase from *Aspergillus oryzae* CFR 202 and *Aureobasidium pullulans* CFR 77. *Process Biochem* 39:753–8.

Sangeetha, P. T., M. N. Ramesh, and S. G. Prapulla. 2005. Recent trends in the microbial production, analysis and application of fructooligosaccharides. *Trends Food Sci Technol* 16:442–57.

Shin, H. T., S. Y. Baig, S. W. Lee et al. 2004. Production of fructo-oligosaccharides from molasses by *Aureobasidium pullulans* cells. *Bioresour Technol* 93:59–62.

Singh, R. S. and R. P. Singh. 2010. Fructooligosaccharides from inulin as prebiotics. *Food Technol Biotech* 48:435–50.

Straathof, A. J. J., A. P. G. Kieboom, and H. van Bekkum. 1986. Invertase catalyzed fructosyl transfer in concentrated solutions of sucrose. *Carbohydr Res* 146:154–9.

Tertuliano, M. F. and R. C. L. Figueiredo-Ribeiro. 1993. Distribution of fructose polymers in herbaceous species of Asteraceae from the cerrado. *New Phytol* 123:741–9.

Vega-Paulino, R. J. and M. E. Zúniga-Hansen. 2012. Potential application of commercial enzyme preparations for industrial production of short-chain fructooligosaccharides. *J Mol Catal B Enzym* 76:44–51.

Velázquez-Hernández, M. L., V. M. Baizabal-Aguirre, A. Bravo-Patino, M. Cajero-Juarez, M. P. Chavez-Moctezuma, and J. J. Valdez-Alarcon. 2009. Microbial fructosyltransferases and the role of fructans. *J Appl Microbiol* 106:1763–78.

Vullo, D., C. E. Coto, and F. Sineriz. 1991. Characteristics of an inulinases produced by *Bacillus subtilis* 430A, a strain isolated from the rhizosphere of *Vernonia herbacea* (Vell Rusby). *Appl Environ Microbiol* 57:2392–4.

Yoshikawa, J., S. Amachi, H. Shinoyama, and T. Fujii. 2006. Multiple β-fructofuranosidases by *Aureobasidium pullulans* DSM2404 and their roles in fructooligosaccharide production. *FEMS Microbiol Lett* 265:159–63.

Yuan, X. L., C. Goosen, H. Kools et al. 2006. Database mining and transcriptional analysis of genes encoding inulin-modifying enzymes of *Aspergillus niger*. *Microbiology* 152:3061–73.

Yun, J. W. 1996. Fructooligosaccharides—Occurrence, preparation and application. *Enzyme Microb Tech* 19:107–17.

Yun, J. W., K. H. Jung, J. W. Oh, and J. H. Lee. 1990. Semibatch production of fructo-oligosaccharides from sucrose by immobilized cells of *Aureobasidium pullulans*. *Appl Biochem Biotech* 24/25:299–308.

Yun, J. W. and S. K. Song. 1993. The production of high content fructo-oligosaccharides from sucrose by the mixed-enzyme system of fructosyltransferase and glucose oxidase. *Biotechnol Lett* 15:573–6.

Zaninette, F., G.A.L.M. Rocha, M.B.F. Fialho, R. A. B. Pessoni, M. R. Braga, R. L. Figueiredo-Ribeiro, and K. Simões. Unpublished, manuscript in drafting. Extracellular β-fructofuranosidases produce 1-kestose and neo-kestose when *Penicillium janczewskii* is cultured on sucrose.

CHAPTER 7

Polysaccharides from Mushrooms

A Natural Source of Bioactive Carbohydrates

ANA VILLARES

Contents

7.1 Introduction 150
7.2 Isolation and Characterization of Polysaccharides from
 Fungal Material 151
   7.2.1 Extraction 151
   7.2.2 Structural Characterization 153
7.3 Structural Features of Polysaccharides Extracted
 from Mushrooms 154
7.4 Physical Properties 157
   7.4.1 Molecular Weight 157
   7.4.2 Solubility 157
   7.4.3 Rheological Properties 158
7.5 Prevention of Common Diseases 160
   7.5.1 Tumor Therapy 161
   7.5.2 Cardiovascular Disease 162
   7.5.3 Antiviral Activity 162
   7.5.4 Antimicrobial Activity 163
7.6 Health Regulations 163
7.7 Conclusions 164
Acknowledgments 164
References 164

7.1 Introduction

Mushrooms have been consumed since ancient times due to their excellent sensory properties, including their unique aroma and taste. Nowadays, the amount of consumed mushrooms has risen greatly, and spans a large number of species. Owing to the emerging new technologies in cultivation, harvest, postharvest, processing, and storage treatments, the consumption of several fungal species has spread worldwide and it is possible throughout the year.

Mushrooms are not only consumed worldwide due to their sensory characteristics, but they have also attracted much attention owing to their healthy properties. Mushrooms can be considered as a healthy food since they have high protein and fiber content, with considerable levels of vitamins and minerals, and a low amount of fat (Barros et al. 2007, Manzi et al. 2001). Furthermore, mushrooms have become attractive as a functional food and as a material for the development of drugs and nutraceuticals, a phenomenon that has been ascribed to the presence of a wide range of bioactive molecules, such as β-glucans, polyphenols, phytosterols, terpenes, and so on. Mushrooms seem to be involved in immunomodulating therapies (Wasser 2002), and have proved to be effective as anti-inflammatory, antioxidant, antitumor, or as antiviral and antibacterial agents (Dore et al. 2007, García-Lafuente et al. 2010, Moro et al. 2012).

Among the biologically active substances present in mushrooms, polysaccharides have attracted much attention mainly due to their excellent properties as immunomodulating agents, and also because of their antioxidant, anti-inflammatory, or antitumor activities, among others. Several polysaccharides have been isolated from fungal material. Generally, these carbohydrates are β-glucans, that is to say, polymers formed by glucose units bound by β-glycosidic linkages; although it is also possible to find other monomer units such as in mannans, composed of mannose monomers, or in galactans, consisting of galactose, and so on (Smiderle et al. 2008). When all the monosaccharides composing the carbohydrate are of the same type, the polymer is called a homopolysaccharide or homoglycan; however, if more than one type of monosaccharide is present within the structure, they are called heteropolysaccharides or heteroglycans. Thus, heteropolysaccharides formed by different sugars (Chen et al. 2008, Smiderle et al. 2008) and polysaccharide–protein complexes (Gonzaga et al. 2005) can also be found in certain mushrooms.

The structural features, such as the monomer nature, the linkage type and position, as well as the number and position of the branches occurring within the polymer chain would strongly influence the three-dimensional arrangement and, in addition to the molecular size, would determine the polysaccharide behavior (Bohn and BeMiller 1995). Similarly, the physical properties, such as solubility, viscosity, or gelation, among others, may influence the biological activity since the bioavailability may be considerably modified (Muralikrishna 2007, Sletmoen 2008). Therefore, the elucidation of the molecular structure and physical properties of the polysaccharides occurring in mushrooms are very important issues in terms of predicting the biological behavior.

7.2 Isolation and Characterization of Polysaccharides from Fungal Material

7.2.1 Extraction

Polysaccharide extraction involves the separation of the carbohydrates from the fungal material. Conventional extraction methods usually involve stirring the sample into aqueous solutions. Samples are subjected to successive extractions to increase the yield (da Silva et al. 2008). Generally, water at room temperature, boiling water, or even aqueous NaOH or KOH solutions (2% w/v) are employed. Once the residue is separated by centrifugation, polysaccharides are precipitated with ethanol in a 2:1 ratio (v/v).

In some cases, water or basic aqueous solutions are not strong enough for separating water-insoluble polysaccharides so that acidic solutions may be employed. Several acids, including acetic, formic, hydrochloric, and phosphoric acids, have been tested in the process for the isolation of water-insoluble β-(1-3)-glucans (Muller et al. 1997).

Conventional solvent extraction techniques use large quantities of toxic organic solvents, which are generally laborious, and possess low selectivity and/or low extraction yields. Furthermore, sometimes, conventional extraction can expose the extracts to excessive heat, light, and oxygen, and requires long extraction times, which may favor the activity of glucan-degrading enzymes. During the extraction, several bioactive compounds may be easily lost due to ionization, hydrolysis, and oxidation. Therefore, sophisticated techniques, such as pressurized liquid extraction (PLE), ultrasound-assisted extraction, or microwaves, may be a good strategy for isolating polysaccharides. Table 7.1 reviews the main techniques and required conditions used for the extraction of polysaccharides from mushrooms.

PLE is an emerging technique that presents important advantages over traditional extraction. PLE can be viewed as an environmentally friendly method because low solvent quantities are used, generally water, in a shorter period of time, the method is automated and involves retaining the sample in an oxygen- and light-free environment. A pressure of 10.1 MPa for 70 min at 28°C was the optimal condition for the isolation of α-(1 $\rightarrow$ 4) and β-(1 $\rightarrow$ 6) glucans from *Lentinus edodes* mushrooms (Lo et al. 2007). Similarly, other authors described the isolation of β-(1 $\rightarrow$ 3)-glucans from seaweeds at 150°C for 20 min (Santoyo et al. 2010).

Supercritical fluid extraction provides a good strategy to isolate polysaccharides since the technique uses carbon dioxide as the extraction solvent due to its excellent properties: CO_2 is environment friendly, has a relatively high, liquid-like density, low viscosity, and high diffusivity. This special solvent

Table 7.1 Techniques and Operating Conditions for the Extraction of Polysaccharides from Mushrooms

Technique	Operating Conditions	Mushroom	Reference
Pressurized liquid extraction	10.1 MPa; 28°C; 70 min	*Lentinus edodes*	Lo et al. (2007)
Supercritical fluid extraction	35 MPa; 10 kg/h CO_2 flow rate; 25°C; 4 h	*Ganoderma lucidum*	Fu et al. (2009)
Ultrasonic-assisted extraction	Ultrasonic power 230 W; 70°C; 62 min; ratio of water volume to material 30 mL/g	*Agaricus bisporus*	Tian et al. (2012)
Microwave-assisted extraction	Microwave power 400 W; 74.64°C; 29.37 min; ratio of water to material 32.7:1	*Agaricus blazei*	Zhang et al. (2011c)
Microwaves hyphenated with ultrasounds	Ultrasonic power 50 W; microwave power 284 W; 701 s; water/solid ratio 11.6:1	*Ganoderma lucidum*	Huang and Ning (2010)

is effective both at dissolving materials and at penetrating solid matrices. During supercritical carbon dioxide (SC-CO_2) extraction, the temperature is relatively low and organic solvents are excluded; so, decomposition of the active components is avoided. In addition, during the dynamic process, fresh supercritical CO_2 flows through materials continuously and the mass transfer is intensive, which may result in a satisfactory performance. This technique was used to isolate carbohydrates from *Ganoderma lucidum* at the following optimum conditions: pressure 35 MPa, temperature 25°C, time 4 h, and CO_2 flow rate 10 kg/h (Fu et al. 2009).

Ultrasonic-assisted extraction (UAE) is an expeditious, inexpensive, and efficient alternative to conventional extraction techniques and, in some cases, even to supercritical fluid and microwave-assisted extraction (MAE). The separation of polysaccharides from black fungus was performed at an ultrasonic power of 350 W, a ratio of water to sample 5, and 35 min of extraction time at 90°C (Jiangwei 2011). Similarly, polysaccharides from *Agaricus bisporus* mushrooms were extracted at the following conditions: ultrasonic power 230 W, temperature 70°C for 62 min, and a ratio of water volume to the raw material weight of 30 mL/g (Tian et al. 2012). UAE was also employed for the extraction of water-soluble polysaccharides from *Boletus edulis* mycelia. Carbohydrates were separated at 56°C, 1:55 of ratio of dried mycelia to water, and time contact of 8.4 min (Chen et al. 2012).

An alternative approach to the traditional extraction methods is MAE. This technique is widely used in the isolation of bioactive compounds since it uses reduced amounts of the solvent and provides a rapid sample preparation. Microwaves have been employed for the extraction of polysaccharides from *Agaricus blazei* Murrill (Zhang et al. 2011c). The optimum conditions were microwave power 400 W, extraction time 29.37 min, temperature 74.64°C, and a water-to-material ratio of 32.7:1. In the case of *Cordyceps militaris*, the optimal conditions to obtain the highest polysaccharide yield were microwave power of 744.8 W for 4.2 min and a solution-to-solid ratio of 31.1 mL/g (Song 2009). Similarly, three polysaccharide fractions were separated from *Lycoris aurea* (Ru et al. 2009).

Microwaves can be hyphenated with other techniques, such as ultrasound-assisted extraction, to reduce extraction time, increase efficiency, and to save energy. The experimental results confirm that the hyphenated ultrasonic-/microwave-assisted extraction (UMAE) of polysaccharides had great potential and efficiency as compared to traditional hot-water extraction. The coupled method was used for the separation of polysaccharides from *Lycium barbarum* at the following operating conditions: microwave power of 500 W for 10 min, ultrasonication at 50°C for 30 min, and pH 9.0 (Dong et al. 2011). Regarding polysaccharides from *G. lucidum*, the optimal extraction conditions were ultrasonic power of 50 W, microwave power of 284 W, extraction time of 701 s and water/solid ratio of 11.6:1 (Huang 2010). Polysaccharides were also separated from *Inonotus obliquus* by UMAE at 90 W microwave power, 40 kHz ultrasonic frequency, and the solid/water ratio was 1:20 (w/v) for 19 min (Chen et al. 2010).

7.2.2 Structural Characterization

Structural analysis of polysaccharides requires the determination of different molecular features, such as molecular mass, chain composition, configuration and conformational isomers, the sequence of monosaccharide residues, the presence and position of branches, and the presence of interglycosidic linkages. Nowadays, there is a wide range of characterization techniques available to obtain structural details of polysaccharides.

Molecular size is generally determined by size-exclusion chromatography (SEC) by comparison with standard materials. Other techniques, such as electrophoresis, are less used for this purpose.

Monosaccharide composition may be studied by acid hydrolysis of the polysaccharides and subsequent analysis of the resultant sugars by high-performance liquid chromatography (HPLC) or, after derivatization, by gas chromatography (GC) (Blakeney et al. 1983).

The presence and position of branches can be elucidated by the formation of derivatives, such as partially methylated alditol acetates, trimethylsilyl, acetyl, trifluoroacetyl, methaneboronate, acetal, or a combination of them, and the subsequent analysis can be elucidated by gas chromatography coupled with mass spectrometry (GC–MS) (Bernardo et al. 1999). MS is a useful technique that requires low sample amounts (picograms or less) and not a high purity of polysaccharides. Although structural analysis by MS can be performed on many underivatized olygosaccharides and glycoconjugates, O-methylated polysaccharides are still preferred to increase the stability of ions and sensitivity of MS detection. GC–MS gives information regarding the position of glycosidic linkage, the occurrence of branches, and monosaccharide composition in complex carbohydrates.

Nuclear magnetic resonance (NMR) is a nondestructive technique that can theoretically perform almost a full structural analysis of underivatized complex carbohydrates. NMR is a powerful tool for obtaining information about the pattern of branching, the monosaccharide composition, anomeric configuration (α or β), and so on (Agrawal 1992). Two-dimensional (2D) NMR techniques are gaining much importance in structural elucidation including correlated spectroscopy (COSY), rotating frame Overhauser enhancement spectroscopy (ROESY), nuclear Overhauser effect spectroscopy (NOESY), heteronuclear multiple quantum coherence (HMQC), and heteronuclear multiple bond coherence (HMBC).

Other techniques are also used for the structural characterization of polysaccharides, for instance, infrared spectroscopy, multiangle laser light scattering (Kulicke 1997), or x-ray crystallography (Jelsma 1975).

7.3 Structural Features of Polysaccharides Extracted from Mushrooms

Edible mushrooms represent an excellent source of bioactive carbohydrates since they can be easily included in the diet, thus avoiding the isolation and purification processes required for the inedible species. The β-(1 → 3),(1 → 6)-linked glucans are widely known; however, other different structural patterns have also been found in polysaccharides isolated from mushrooms. In this field, the polysaccharide lentinan from *L. edodes* has attracted much interest. Lentinan is composed of (1 → 3)-linked D-glucopyranosyl units with branches at O-6, displaying a triple-helical conformation (Zhang et al. 2011b). Other bioactive carbohydrates have also been isolated from this mushroom; for instance, a heteropolysaccharide consisting of a fucomannogalactan with a main chain of (1 → 6)-linked α-D-galactopyranosyl units branched at O-2 (Carbonero et al. 2008a).

The most studied polysaccharide from *Ganoderma* spp. mushrooms is ganoderan. It is composed of a backbone structure of β-(1 → 3)-linked D-glucose residues with side chains at O-6 consisting of single β-(1 → 6)-linked D-glucopyranose residues. Furthermore, a linear water-insoluble β-(1 → 3)-D-glucan has been extracted from the fruit body of *G. lucidum* (Wang and Zhang 2009b) as well as a water-soluble (1 → 6)-linked glucan with (1 → 4) branches at O-4 (Dong et al. 2012), or a heteropolysaccharide composed of 1,4-linked α-D-glucopyranosyl and 1,6-linked β-D-galactopyranosyl residues with branches at O-6 of glucose and O-2 of galactose residues (Bao et al. 2002). A mixed polysaccharide composed of glucose, galactose, and rhamnose was also isolated from *G. lucidum* (Pan et al. 2012). More complex structures showing antioxidant properties, such as a protein-bound polysaccharide, have also been isolated from the genus *Ganoderma*, specifically from *G. atrum* (Chen et al. 2008).

The genus *Agaricus* has been widely studied. Hence, several polysaccharides have been found in the cell walls of *A. bisporus*. The fractions contained the mucilage fraction composed of glucose and galactose, a second fraction with a xylomannan associated with the glucan, and several fractions of glucans showing different attachment sites (Bernardo et al. 1999). The *A. bitorquis* mushrooms contained a water-soluble β-(1 → 3)-linked glucan (Nandan et al. 2008), and a glucan–protein complex was isolated from *A. blazei* mushrooms by extraction with water at 100°C for 5 h. The glucan moieties showed both α and β linkages, of which β is more abundant (Gonzaga et al. 2005).

The genus *Pleurotus* has also been investigated; for instance, pleuran, isolated from *P. ostreatus*, consists of a backbone of (1 → 3)-linked D-glucan on every fourth residue, being substituted at O-6 with single D-glucopyranosyl groups (Karacsonyi 1994). The occurrence of different structural patterns between polysaccharides from the *Pleurotus* species has been previously observed, for instance, a linear α-(1 → 3)-linked D-glucan has been isolated from *P. ostreatus* and *P. eryngii* (Synytsya et al. 2009). Hot aqueous extraction of the basidiocarps of the mushroom *P. sajor-caju* provided a gel-like glucan showing a branched structure with a β-(1 → 3)-linked Glcp main chain, substituted at O-6 by single unit β-Glcp side chains, on an average of two to every third residue of the backbone (Carbonero et al. 2012). Furthermore, the mushroom *P. florida* has shown different types of glucans, which are a water-soluble αβ-polysaccharide consisting of a main chain of α-(1 → 3)-linked D-glucan partially substituted at O-3 and O-6 by β-D-glucose (Santos-Neves et al. 2008) and a water-insoluble (1 → 3), (1 → 6)-linked β-D-glucan (Rout et al. 2008). Other complex carbohydrates have been found in the genus *Pleurotus*; for instance, a 3-O-methylated α-galactan (Carbonero et al. 2008b), and a partially 3-O-methylated α-(1 → 4)-linked D-galactan and D-mannan (Rosado et al. 2002).

A β-(1 → 3)-linked D-glucan with single unit glucosyl branches attached at O-6 of every third backbone residue has been isolated from *Hericium erinaceus* (Dong et al. 2006). Heteropolysaccharides have also been isolated from this mushroom; thus, an α-(1 → 6)-linked D-galactopyranosyl with rhamnose and glucose branches at O-2 has been described (Jia et al. 2004).

A water-soluble neutral polysaccharide was extracted from *Auricularia auricula-judae* consisting of a β-(1 → 3)-D-glucan with two β-(1 → 6)-D-glucosyl residues for every three main chain glucose residues, showing a comb-branched structure (Xu 2012). A water-soluble αβ-glucan was obtained from the fruiting bodies of the edible mushroom *Auricularia polytricha* (Song 2012). The backbone contained α-(1 → 6)-D-glucopyranosyl and β-(1 → 6)-D-glucopyranosyl residues, partially substituted at O-3 of the β-D-glucopyranosyl residues by side chains of α-(1 → 4)-D-Glcp and terminated with nonreducing end α-D-Glcp.

Polysaccharides from *Calocybe indica* have received attention due to their immunoenhancing properties. Homopolysaccharides composed of glucose have been isolated from this mushroom, for instance, a water-soluble αβ-(1 → 4),(1 → 6)-glucan (Mandal et al. 2012), and a water-insoluble β-(1 → 3),(1 → 4)-glucan (termed calocyban) as well as β-(1 → 6)-linked glucan with α-(1 → 4)-type branches (Mandal et al. 2010). Mixed polysaccharides were also found in this mushroom and the structural analysis revealed that they were composed of α-(1 → 3)-linked galactose, β-(1 → 4),(1 → 6)-linked glucose, and fucose branches (Mandal et al. 2011).

Among the wild mushrooms, some fungi, such as *Boletus erythropus*, have also shown to be water-soluble β-glucans (Chauveau et al. 1996). The structural elucidation showed that the polysaccharides are composed of (1 → 3)-linked glucose units with branches at O-6. One novel polysaccharide was extracted from the wild mushroom *Boletus speciosus* Forst harvested in China at an elevation of 3400 m. The polysaccharide was composed of α-(1 → 4)-linked mannopyranose residues with α-galactopyranosyl branches at O-6 (Ding 2012).

The genus *Cantharellus cibarius* has been scarcely studied and only a glycan composed of the α-(1 → 6)-linked fucose and α-(1 → 2,6)-linked mannose units was found (Grass et al. 2011).

Medicinal mushrooms have been traditionally consumed due to their excellent properties, which are due to the presence of different types of polysaccharides. Hence, a polysaccharide isolated from *Geastrum saccatum*, consisting of a β-linked glucopyranosyl residue attached to a protein, has shown antioxidant and anti-inflammatory activities (Dore et al. 2007). Other mushrooms, for instance, *Flammulina velutipes*, contain complex carbohydrates. This fungus showed a polysaccharide composed of a 6-O-substituted galactopyranosyl main chain, partially substituted at O-2 by 3-O-D-mannopyranosyl-L-fucopyranosyl, α-D-mannopyranosyl, and, in a minor proportion, by α-L-fucopyranosyl groups (Smiderle et al. 2008). Similarly, to edible species, the moiety (1 → 3),(1 → 6)-linked D-glucose has also been found in several medicinal fungi. The polysaccharides have been fully characterized and some of them even have a descriptive name. For instance, the glucan isolated from *Schizophyllum commune* is termed schizophyllan and this polysaccharide is composed of β-(1 → 3)-linked glucose units with one β-(1 → 6)-glucose side group for every three main chain residues (Numata et al. 2006). Other mushrooms, such as *Sparassis crispa* or *Phellinus linteus* (Park et al. 2009), have also shown to possess β-D-glucans with different linkage patterns depending on the fungal species. Water-insoluble (1 → 3)-linked glucans have also been found in *Termitomyces eurhizus* (Chakraborty et al. 2006) as well as (1 → 6)-linked polysaccharides from *Termitomyces robustus* (Bhanja et al. 2012) or glucan–protein complexes from *Termitomyces microcarpus* (Chandra et al. 2009). In addition, polysaccharides showing mixed bounds, such as α-(1 → 4)-β-(1 → 3), are present in *T. microcarpus* (Chandra et al. 2007).

7.4 Physical Properties

Physical properties, such as water solubility, viscosity, and gelation properties, appear to be important determinants of the bioavailability and the physiological action in the gastrointestinal tract. Most of the studies on the physical properties of polysaccharides have been performed on the β-glucans from cereals, although the polysaccharides isolated from mushrooms are gaining more importance and nowadays, the number of studies is increasing significantly.

7.4.1 Molecular Weight

Estimates of the molecular weights (MWs) of polysaccharides vary depending on the method used. Water-soluble β-glucans from mushrooms have shown MWs within the range of 105–106 Da. Size-exclusion chromatography combined with multiangle laser light scattering (SEC-LLS) is commonly employed for the measurement of molecular size. Thus, polysaccharides from *A. auricula-judae* presented an MW of $2.15 \cdot 10^6$ Da (Xu 2012), carbohydrates from *G. lucidum* $1.24 \cdot 10^5$ Da (Wang et al. 2009a), and from *Pleurotus tuber-regium* $3.14 \cdot 10^5$ Da (Tao 2006). Similar techniques coupled with different detectors, such as refractive index (HPLC-RI), demonstrated that the polysaccharides from *C. indica* showed an MW of $2 \cdot 10^5$ Da (Mandal et al. 2011), the spores from *G. lucidum* $1.26 \cdot 10^5$ Da (Bao et al. 2001), and a carbohydrate isolated from the fruiting bodies of *Pleurotus sajor-caju* $9.75 \cdot 10^5$ Da (Carbonero et al. 2012).

7.4.2 Solubility

Water solubility of polysaccharides is strongly dependent on the type of linkage occurring within the chain. Generally, blocks of adjacent bonds of the same type, for instance, β-(1 → 3) or β-(1 → 4), may exhibit a tendency for interchain aggregation via strong hydrogen bonds and, consequently, may contribute to the stiffness of the molecules in solution and the lower solubility. Long blocks of contiguous β-(1 → 4) or β-(1 → 3) associate in a cellulose-like manner and cause insolubility. Curdlan and other β-(1 → 3)-linked glucans are insoluble in water, alcohols, and most organic solvents but dissolve in dilute bases (0.25 M NaOH), dimethylsulfoxide (DMSO), formic acid, and certain aprotic reagents (McIntosh 2005). Polysaccharides linked by repeating units of (1 → 3),(1 → 6)-linked glucose generally possess a very stiff, rod-like, triple-helical conformation in aqueous solutions. Three helical strands are held together and stabilized by strong interchain hydrogen bonds. Several conditions may disrupt the triple helix, such as high concentrations of DMSO (above 87%), heat ($T > 135°C$), or the addition of sodium hydroxide ([NaOH] > 0.2 mol/L) so that the triple helices dissociate almost completely into single chains and the solubility increases.

The presence of different linkages within the structure breaks up the regularity of the sequence and makes the molecule more soluble and flexible.

The irregular spacing in the β-glucan chain is responsible for the nonordered overall conformation of the polysaccharide and hence, the chains are unable to align closely over extended regions, increasing the water solubility of the polysaccharide. Nevertheless, the presence of a repeating pattern alternating linkages, such as three consecutive cellotriosyl residues, may constitute a conformationally stable motif. This ordered domain might impose some conformational regularity on the β-glucan chain, and consequently, a higher degree of organization of the polymer in solution and, therefore, lower solubility (Storsley et al. 2003).

The occurrence of different monosaccharides within the chain may modulate the solubility; for instance, the xylan backbone is relatively flexible because it is supported by only one hydrogen bond between two adjacent xylose residues and it aggregates into insoluble complexes, stabilized by intermolecular hydrogen bonding. The presence of different monosaccharides, for instance, arabinosyl substituents, appears to prevent this aggregation, and stiffens the molecules by maintaining the xylan backbone in a more extended conformation (Muralikrishna 2007).

7.4.3 Rheological Properties

Several factors, for instance, the overall MW, asymmetrical conformation, degree of polymerization, and spatial arrangement of the side chains along the backbone, will influence the behavior of polysaccharides in solution. The viscosity of polysaccharides in solution has a characteristic behavior. Generally, a viscosity enhancement is observed when the concentration of β-glucan increases in water solutions. Figure 7.1 shows a representative plot of viscosity (η) as a function of shear rate (γ) for β-glucan solutions in water.

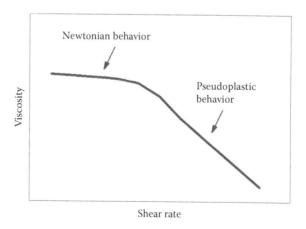

Figure 7.1 Representative plot of viscosity (η) as a function of shear rate (γ) for β-glucan solutions in water.

This curve may be modified depending on the conditions, such as polymer concentration or temperature.

The shear rate dependence of viscosity exhibits a linear plateau or Newtonian behavior at the low shear rate region and non-Newtonian pseudoplastic behavior with a shear-thinning zone at high shear rates (Doublier 1995). The pseudoplastic behavior is due to disruption of molecular entanglements between β-glucan chains by the applied high shear, while at low shear rates, the viscosity remains unchanged. The time at low shear rates is sufficient for the formation of new entanglements between different chain patterns to compensate the disentanglement caused by the shear flow. Differently, at high shear rates, the rate of reentanglement is much slower than the rate of disruption and, consequently, the viscosity decreases (Vaikousi 2004).

Polysaccharides are capable of forming three-dimensional gels or viscous solutions. Gelation of polysaccharides is widely used for achieving a desired texture in foods such as jellies, aspics, tarts, and puddings. A gel is defined as a soft, solid, or solid-like material consisting of two or more components, one of which is a liquid, present in substantial quantity (Almdal et al. 1993). Gel-forming polysaccharides must have a moderately irregular structure that allows partial but not overall association, which could cause precipitation or insolubility. Solid-like gels are further defined in terms of the dynamic mechanical properties. A gel is rheologically characterized by the storage modulus nearly independent of the angular frequency G'_p (plateau modulus), the dynamic storage modulus, G', and the loss modulus G'' (Clark 1987).

The plateau modulus G'_p, nearly frequency independent, is associated with the number of cross-links in the network structure. The larger G'_p is, the smaller the entanglement molar mass and, therefore, the higher the cross-link density, which determines the rigidity of the gel. G'_p is predominantly dependent on the concentration and not on the molar mass, although a low molar mass reduces the mechanical stress that is required for disrupting the gel (Mitchell 1980). Therefore, to improve gel strength, it is more effective to increase the concentration than the molar mass.

Solid–gel transformations are also characterized by the storage modulus, G', accessible via rheological oscillatory time experiments. The logarithm of G' as a function of time generally proved to be sigmoidally shaped for barley β-glucans but differs with concentration and molar mass. The slope of log $G'(t)$ at the turning point may be chosen as a measure of gelation rate, namely, elasticity increment (IE) (Bohm and Kulicke 1999). Figure 7.2 shows a representative plot of the storage modulus (G') as a function of time for β-glucan solutions in water.

The gelation rate generally declines with decreasing concentration and increasing molar mass. The polysaccharide concentration determines the segment density in solution and hence the probability of contact between the coils, which is a basic requirement for three-dimensional network formation.

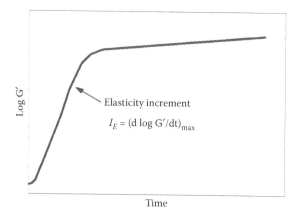

Figure 7.2 Representative plot of storage modulus (G′) as a function of time for β-glucan solutions in water. (From *Carbohydr Res* 315:302–311, Bohm, N. and W. M. Kulicke. Rheological studies of barley (1→3)(1→4)-betaglucan in concentrated solution: Mechanistic and kinetic investigation of the gel formation, Copyright 1999, with permission from Elsevier.)

The molar mass influence can be explained by the higher mobility of shorter chains (Doublier 1995).

Denatured chains can be renatured by two different molecular processes consisting of the collapse of the random coil chains to a more compact conformation and the formation of aggregates, both processes conducted by interchain hydrogen bonding. Depending on the polysaccharide nature, the renaturation process may include the formation of several forms, such as globular, linear, circular, or even more complicated multichain clusters (Kitamura et al. 1996).

7.5 Prevention of Common Diseases

Mushrooms have been known for their medicinal properties for ages. In modern terms, they can be viewed as functional foods since they provide several health benefits due to the bioactive compounds they contain. In this field, polysaccharides from mushroom have received much attention due to their demonstrated healthy properties. Polysaccharides are responsible for a wide range of biological activities, of which, the most studied is the modulation of the immune system. In this field, polysaccharides from mushrooms showing a β-linkage have demonstrated to boost the human immune system and to modulate the immunological response under certain circumstances; so, they are commonly termed as host defense potentiators or biological response modifiers (BRMs). As a result of the activation of the host's immune system, these polysaccharides show significant antitumor, antiviral, and antimicrobial activity, among other effects.

7.5.1 *Tumor Therapy*

Polysaccharides from fungi have been widely employed in tumor therapies due to their properties as immunological enhancers. The mechanisms of antitumor action of polysaccharides are not completely clear; it is believed that the mitogenic activity of fungal polysaccharides involves several immune responses through the activation of specific immune cells to enhance a variety of cellular functions. These include the activation of macrophages, T lymphocytes, and natural killer cells (NK), which are able to secrete inflammatory mediators and cytokines such as the α tumor necrosis factor (TNF-α), γ interferon (IFN-γ), or 1β interleukin (IL-1β). Polysaccharides can also depress the E-selectin protein and gene expressions, which inhibit tumoral cell-to-cell adhesion (Yue et al. 2012). Other mechanisms include antiproliferative effects, apoptosis induction, and differentiation of the tumoral cells as well (Wang et al. 2012).

Research studies have demonstrated that polysaccharides isolated from different mushrooms genera are capable of providing antitumoral activity, for instance, *Agaricus, Calocybe, Ganoderma, Grifola, Inonotus, Lentinus, Phellinus, Pholiota, Pleurotus*, and so on (Hsieh 2011, Hu 2012, Lee 2011, Lo et al. 2011, Selvi et al. 2011, Wang et al. 2012, Yue et al. 2012, Zhang et al. 2011a). (1 → 6),(1 → 3)-linked polysaccharides isolated from *Agaricus brasiliensis* induced the production of various cytokines from both murine splenocytes and bone marrow-derived dendritic cells in the presence of exogenous granulocyte–macrophage colony-stimulating factor. The mechanism of action seemed to involve the receptor dectin-1 for 1,3-β-glucan (Yamanaka et al. 2012). A water-soluble polysaccharide purified from *Inonotus obliquus* had not only shown antitumor activity *in vivo*, but it also enhanced the immune response of tumor-bearing mice, and the lymphocyte proliferation while it increased the production of TNF-α (Fan et al. 2012).

Lentinan, the polysaccharide isolated from *L. edodes*, has been used in the combined treatment of patients with advanced or recurrent gastric or colorectal cancer. The study was carried out with 89 patients of stomach cancer, and the results showed that the life span increased in 80 days when 2 mg of intravenous lentinan per week was used (Chihara et al. 1987, Ochiai et al. 1992). Similarly, the life span increased in 106 days in patients with breast cancer when similar doses of lentinan were used (Taguchi et al. 1982). In a similar study, carried out with 30 patients of breast cancer, the combination of lentinan with chemoendocrine therapy was more effective than chemoendocrine therapy alone on the improvement of hormonal parameters such as serum levels of oestradiol, follicle-stimulating hormone, luteinizing hormone, and prolactin. The use of lentinan permitted to reduce the dose of epirubicin (EPIR) in breast cancer patients, and that combination therapy of lentinan and low-dose EPIR was more effective for the enhancement of the host defense activity (Kosaka 1995). The combination of lentinan and interleukin-2 (IL-2) showed a synergistic effect in the reduction of lung metastasis colony numbers (85%). The experimental results suggested that the life-prolonging effect of the combination of lentinan and IL-2 was mediated by antigen-specific T cells and that the combination of pre- and postoperative therapy with lentinan and IL-2 may be effective to prevent cancer recurrence and metastasis after surgical resection (Hamuro et al. 1994).

7.5.2 Cardiovascular Disease

Cardiovascular diseases (CVD) are among the main important causes of death in developed countries. Cardiovascular diseases have a multifactorial etiology and the pathogenesis of arterial forms of CVD is associated with atherosclerosis. Several potential risk biomarkers related to CVD have been identified, such as lipid and lipoprotein metabolism (low-density lipoprotein [LDL] and high-density lipoprotein [HDL] cholesterol and triacylglycerol amounts), the hemostatic function, the oxidative damage, the homocysteine metabolism, and blood pressure (Mensink et al. 2003). Polysaccharides from mushrooms have demonstrated to protect against cardiovascular diseases and their complications. In this field, the administration of black fungus polysaccharides had significantly enhanced myocardium and blood antioxidant enzyme activities and reduced lipid peroxidation levels in high-fat mice (Jiangwei 2011). At the intestinal level, β-glucans reduced the absorption of cholesterol and long-chain fatty acids and, furthermore, these polysaccharides downregulated the genes involved in lipogenesis and lipid transport (Drozdowski et al. 2010). Male rats were fed with 2% cholesterol and 1% β-glucan-type extracellular polysaccharide isolated from *Volvariella volvacea* showed a significant reduction in the levels of serum total cholesterol, LDL-cholesterol, and liver total cholesterol whereas there were no significant changes in the levels of serum triacylglycerol, HDL-cholesterol, and liver total lipids (Cheung 1996). Similarly, the administration of polysaccharides from *A. auricula* showed a remarkable hypocholesterolemic effect and an increase in the level of HDL cholesterol in mice fed with a cholesterol-enriched diet (Chen et al. 2011). The polysaccharide fraction from *Pleurotus nebrodensis* mushrooms has demonstrated to decrease systolic blood pressure in spontaneously hypertensive rats (Miyazawa 2008). The effect of a hot-water extract from *Cordyceps sinensis* was evaluated in mice on a cholesterol-free diet and mice on a cholesterol-enriched diet. The serum total cholesterol of all mice groups decreased after polysaccharide administration. Among the mice fed with the cholesterol-enriched diet, the HDL cholesterol level increased but decreased the very-low-density lipoprotein (VLDL) and LDL cholesterol levels (Koh et al. 2003).

7.5.3 Antiviral Activity

Different carbohydrate extracts from *L. edodes* mushrooms have been tested for their antiviral activity against poliovirus type 1 (PV-1) and bovine herpes virus type 1 (BoHV-1). Results showed that the polysaccharides were effective and they acted on the initial processes of the replication of both strains of the virus (Rincao et al. 2012). Regarding human immunodeficiency virus (HIV) treatment, there is not actually a wide number of studies involving polysaccharides from mushrooms. A study was carried out with 88 HIV-positive patients with CD4 levels of 200–500 cells/mm. The patients were treated with a combination of the polysaccharide lentinan from *L. edodes* and didanosine (ddI). The combination caused significant increases in CD4 levels up to 38 weeks, whereas ddI alone was significant at the 5% level at 14 weeks (Gordon et al. 1995).

7.5.4 Antimicrobial Activity

The ability of polysaccharides from mushrooms to modulate the immune response makes them potential candidates as antimicrobial agents. A water-soluble polysaccharide isolated from the mushroom substrate was tested to study the antibacterial activity against *Escherichia coli*, *Staphylococcus aureus*, and *Sarcina lutea*. The antibacterial activity of the polysaccharide against *E. coli* was the strongest, whereas it was the weakest against *S. lutea*. On the other hand, the combined intranasal application of lentinan (at a dose of 1 mg/kg) followed by the administration of *Calmette-Guerin bacillus* (BCG) produced high levels of alveolar macrophage activation. Pretreatment with lentinan enhanced the local immunohistological response to BCG in the lung and reduced the generalized side effects (Drandarska et al. 2005).

7.6 Health Regulations

As commented upon in the previous section, several healthy effects have been found for diets rich in cereals containing β-glucan-type polysaccharides, for instance, the reduction of cholesterol levels and the regulation of blood glucose concentration. For this reason, in 1997, the U.S. Food and Drug Administration (FDA) approved a health claim for the use of soluble fiber from oats for reducing the risk of coronary heart disease. It was concluded that the β-glucan-type polysaccharides are primarily responsible for the association between the consumption of oat foods and the observed lowering of blood cholesterol levels. FDA passed a unique ruling that allowed oat bran to be registered as the first cholesterol-reducing food at a dosage of 3 g β-glucan per day, with a recommendation of 0.75 g of β-glucan per serving. In 2005, a similar health claim for the whole-grain barley and barley-containing products was also approved. The health claim informs about the relationship between the consumption of β-glucan from barley and the reduction of the risk of coronary heart disease in terms of lowering serum cholesterol.

Many pharmaceutical substances and preparations have been developed based on certain components from mushrooms; however, polysaccharides from mushrooms have been less studied than those from cereals and, recently, new regulations can be found regarding these materials. Most mushroom-derived preparations find use not as pharmaceuticals but as a novel class of products by a variety of names: dietary supplements, functional foods, nutraceuticals, phytochemicals, mycochemicals, biochemopreventives, and so on. Actually, several types of medicinal preparations are available in the market; the problem is that mushroom-based products are so diverse that there is a serious need for improving quality and legal control. In 2011, the European Food Safety Authority (EFSA) approved that extracts from *L. edodes* containing β-glucan-type polysaccharides could be used as food ingredients in processed meals. The regulation did not note the healthy properties of such types of polysaccharides; it only describes the safety properties of the extracts from *L. edodes*. Nevertheless, the excellent results from clinical studies suggest that the use of polysaccharides from mushrooms as healthy supplements will be soon approved.

7.7 Conclusions

Mushrooms can be considered as a source of dietary fiber and bioactive polysaccharides. Carbohydrates from different species of fungus have been isolated and characterized throughout. The β-$(1 \to 3),(1 \to 6)$-linkage pattern has attracted much attention and this structural feature has been observed in several polysaccharides, for instance, lentinan from *L. edodes*, pleuran from *Pleurotus* spp. mushrooms, or ganoderan from *G. lucidum*. More complex structures have been also isolated from different mushrooms and, besides their physical properties, they have received a great deal of interest in recent years due to their healthy properties such as the enhancement of the immune response, the antitumoral effect, the anti-inflammatory property, or the antioxidant activity, among others.

Acknowledgments

The author is grateful to Ministerio de Ciencia e Innovación and INIA (projects RTA2009-00049 and AT07-003) for financial support to this work.

References

Agrawal, P. K. 1992. NMR spectroscopy in the structural elucidation of oligosaccharides and glycosides. *Phytochemistry* 31:3307–3330.

Almdal, K., J. Dyre, S. Hvidt, and O. Kramer. 1993. What is a gel? *Makromolekulare Chemie—Macromol Symp* 76:49–51.

Bao, X. F., J. N. Fang, and X. Y. Li. 2001. Structural characterization and immunomodulating activity of a complex glucan from spores of *Ganoderma lucidum*. *Biosci Biotechnol Biochem* 65:2384–2391.

Bao, X. F., X. S. Wang, Q. Dong, J. N. Fang, and X. Y. Li. 2002. Structural features of immunologically active polysaccharides from *Ganoderma lucidum*. *Phytochemistry* 59:175–181.

Barros, L., P. Baptista, L. M. Estevinho, and I. C. F. R. Ferreira. 2007. Effect of fruiting body maturity stage on chemical composition and antimicrobial activity of *Lactarius* sp. mushrooms. *J Agric Food Chem* 55:8766–8771.

Bernardo, D., C. G. Mendoza, M. Calonje, and M. Novaes-Ledieu. 1999. Chemical analysis of the lamella walls of *Agaricus bisporus* fruit bodies. *Curr Microbiol* 38:364–367.

Bhanja, S. K., C. K. Nandan, S. Mandal et al. 2012. Isolation and characterization of the immunostimulating beta-glucans of an edible mushroom *Termitomyces robustus* var. *Carbohydr Res* 357:83–89.

Blakeney, A. B., P. J. Harris, R. J. Henry, and B. A. Stone. 1983. A simple and rapid preparation of alditol acetates for monosaccharide analysis. *Carbohydr Res* 113:291–299.

Bohm, N. and W. M. Kulicke. 1999. Rheological studies of barley $(1\rightarrow3)(1\rightarrow4)$-beta-glucan in concentrated solution: Mechanistic and kinetic investigation of the gel formation. *Carbohydr Res* 315:302–311.

Bohn, J. A. and J. N. BeMiller. 1995. $(1\rightarrow3)$-beta-D-glucans as biological response modifiers: A review of structure–functional activity relationships. *Carbohydr Polym* 28:3–14.

Carbonero, E. R., A. H. P. Gracher, D. L. Komura et al. 2008a. *Lentinus edodes* heterogalactan: Antinoreceptive and anti-inflammatory effects. *Food Chem* 111:531–537.

Carbonero, E. R., A. H. P. Gracher, M. C. C. Rosa et al. 2008b. Unusual partially 3-O-methylated alpha-galactan from mushrooms of the genus *Pleurotus*. *Phytochemistry* 69:252–257.

Carbonero, E. R., A. C. Ruthes, C. S. Freitas et al. 2012. Chemical and biological properties of a highly branched beta-glucan from edible mushroom *Pleurotus sajorcaju*. *Carbohydr Polym* 90:814–819.

Clark, A. H. and S. B. Rossmurphy. 1987. Structural and mechanical properties of biopolymer gels. *Adv Polym Sci* 83:57–192.

Chakraborty, I., S. Mondal, D. Rout, and S. S. Islam. 2006. A water-insoluble $(1 \rightarrow 3)$-beta-D-glucan from the alkaline extract of an edible mushroom *Termitomyces eurhizus*. *Carbohydr Res* 341:2990–2993.

Chandra, K., K. Ghosh, A. K. Ojha, and S. S. Islam. 2009. A protein containing glucan from an edible mushroom, *Termitomyces microcarpus* (var). *Nat Prod Commun* 4:553–556.

Chandra, K., K. Ghosh, S. K. Roy et al. 2007. A water-soluble glucan isolated from an edible mushroom *Termitomyces microcarpus*. *Carbohydr Res* 342:2484–2489.

Chauveau, C., P. Talaga, J. M. Wieruszeski, G. Strecker, and L. Chavant. 1996. A water-soluble beta-D-glucan from *Boletus erythropus*. *Phytochemistry* 43:413–415.

Chen, G., Y.-C. Luo, B.-P. Ji et al. 2011. Hypocholesterolemic effects of *Auricularia auricula* ethanol extract in ICR mice fed a cholesterol-enriched diet. *J Food Sci Technol* 48:692–698.

Chen, W., W.-P. Wang, H.-S. Zhang, and Q. Huang. 2012. Optimization of ultrasonic-assisted extraction of water-soluble polysaccharides from *Boletus edulis* mycelia using response surface methodology. *Carbohydr Polym* 87:614–619.

Chen, Y., X. Gu, S.-Q. Huang et al. 2010. Optimization of ultrasonic/microwave assisted extraction (UMAE) of polysaccharides from *Inonotus obliquus* and evaluation of its anti-tumor activities. *Int J Biol Macromol* 46:429–435.

Chen, Y., M. Y. Xie, S. P. Nie, C. Li, and Y. X. Wang. 2008. Purification, composition analysis and antioxidant activity of a polysaccharide from the fruiting bodies of *Ganoderma atrum*. *Food Chem* 107:231–241.

Cheung, P. C. K. 1996. The hypocholesterolemic effect of extracellular polysaccharide from the submerged fermentation of mushroom. *Nutr Res* 16:1953–1957.

Chihara, G., J. Hamuro, Y. Y. Maeda et al. 1987. Antitumor and metastasis–inhibitory activities of lentinan as an immunomodulator: An overview. *Cancer Detect Prev* 1:423–443.

da Silva, M. D. C., E. K. Fukuda, A. F. D. Vasconcelos et al. 2008. Structural characterization of the cell wall D-glucans isolated from the mycelium of *Botryosphaeria rhodina* MAMB-05. *Carbohydr Res* 343:793–798.

Ding, X., Y.-L. Hou, and W.-R. Hou. 2012. Structure elucidation and antioxidant activity of a novel polysaccharide isolated from *Boletus speciosus* Forst. *Int J Biol Macromol* 50:613–618.

Dong, Q., L. M. Jia, and J. N. Fang. 2006. A beta-D-glucan isolated from the fruiting bodies of *Hericium erinaceus* and its aqueous conformation. *Carbohydr Res* 341:791–795.

Dong, J.-Z., Z.-C. Wang, and Y. Wang. 2011. Rapid extraction of polysaccharides from fruits of *Lycium barbarum* L. *J Food Biochem* 35:1047–1057.

Dong, Q., Y. Wang, L. Shi et al. 2012. A novel water-soluble beta-D-glucan isolated from the spores of *Ganoderma lucidum*. *Carbohydr Res* 353:100–105.

Dore, C., T. C. G. Azevedo, M. C. R. de Souza et al. 2007. Antiinflammatory, antioxidant and cytotoxic actions of beta-glucan-rich extract from *Geastrum saecatum* mushroom. *Int Immunopharmacol* 7:1160–1169.

Doublier, J. L. and P. J. Wood. 1995. Rheological properties of aqueous solutions of (1–3)(1–4)-beta-D-glucan from oats (*Avena sativa* L). *Cereal Chem* 72:335–340.

Drandarska, I., V. Kussovski, S. Nikolaeva, and N. Markova. 2005. Combined immunomodulating effects of BCG and lentinan after intranasal application in guinea pigs. *Int Immunopharmacol* 5:795–803.

Drozdowski, L. A., R. A. Reimer, F. Temelli et al. 2010. Beta-glucan extracts inhibit the *in vitro* intestinal uptake of long-chain fatty acids and cholesterol and down-regulate genes involved in lipogenesis and lipid transport in rats. *J Nutr Biochem* 21:695–701.

Fan, L., S. Ding, L. Ai, and K. Deng. 2012. Antitumor and immunomodulatory activity of water-soluble polysaccharide from *Inonotus obliquus*. *Carbohydr Polym* 90:870–874.

Fu, Y.-J., W. Liu, Y.-G. Zu et al. 2009. Breaking the spores of the fungus *Ganoderma lucidum* by supercritical CO_2. *Food Chem* 112:71–76.

García-Lafuente, A., C. Moro, A. Villares et al. 2010. Mushrooms as a source of anti-inflammatory agents. *Anti-Inflamm Anti-Allergy Agents Med Chem* 9:125–141.

Gonzaga, M. L. C., N. Ricardo, F. Heatley, and S. D. Soares. 2005. Isolation and characterization of polysaccharides from *Agaricus blazei* Murill. *Carbohydr Polym* 60:43–49.

Gordon, M., M. Guralnik, Y. Kaneko et al. 1995. A phase II controlled study of a combination of the immune modulator, lentinan, with didanosine (DDI) in HIV patients with CD4 cells of 200–500/mm(3). *J Med* 26:193–207.

Grass, J., M. Pabst, D. Kolarich et al. 2011. Discovery and structural characterization of fucosylated oligomannosidic N-glycans in mushrooms. *J Biol Chem* 286:5977–5984.

Hamuro, J., F. Takatsuki, T. Suga, T. Kikuchi, and M. Suzuki. 1994. Synergistic antimetastatic effects of lentinan and interleukin-2 with preoperative and postoperative treatments. *Jpn J Cancer Res* 85:1288–1297.

Hsieh, T.-C. and J. M. Wu. 2011. Suppression of proliferation and oxidative stress by extracts of *Ganoderma lucidum* in the ovarian cancer cell line OVCAR-3. *Int J Mol Med* 28:1065–1069.

Hu, Q., H. Wang, and T. B. Ng. 2012. Isolation and purification of polysaccharides with anti-tumor activity from *Pholiota adiposa* (Batsch) P. Kumm. (higher basidiomycetes). *Int J Med Mushrooms* 14:271–284.

Huang, S.-Q. and Z.-X. Ning. 2010. Extraction of polysaccharide from *Ganoderma lucidum* and its immune enhancement activity. *Int J Biol Macromol* 47:336–341.

Jelsma, J. and D. R. Kreger. 1975. Ultrastructural observations on (1→3)-beta-D-glucan from fungal cell-walls. *Carbohydr Res* 43:200–203.

Jia, L. M., L. Liu, Q. Dong, and J. N. Fang. 2004. Structural investigation of a novel rhamnoglucogalactan isolated from the fruiting bodies of the fungus *Hericium erinaceus*. *Carbohydr Res* 339:2667–2671.

Jiangwei, M., Q. Zengyong, and X. Xia. 2011. Optimisation of extraction procedure for black fungus polysaccharides and effect of the polysaccharides on blood lipid and myocardium antioxidant enzymes activities. *Carbohydr Polym* 84:1061–1068.

Karacsonyi, S. and L. Kuniak. 1994. Polysaccharides of *Pleurotus ostreatus*—Isolation and structure of pleuran, an alkali-insoluble beta D-glucan. *Carbohydr Polym* 24:107–111.

Kitamura, S., T. Hirano, K. Takeo et al. 1996. Conformational transitions of schizophyllan in aqueous alkaline solution. *Biopolymers* 39:407–416.

Koh, J. H., J. M. Kim, U. J. Chang, and H. J. Suh. 2003. Hypocholesterolemic effect of hot-water extract from mycelia of *Cordyceps sinensis*. *Biol Pharm Bull* 26:84–87.

Kosaka, A., T. Suga, and A. Yamashita. 1995. Dose reductive effect of lentinan on the epirubicin therapy for breast cancer patients. *Int J Immunother* 11:143–151.

Kulicke, W. M., A. I. Lettau, and H. Thielking. 1997. Correlation between immunological activity, molar mass, and molecular structure of different (1→3)-beta-D-glucans. *Carbohydr Res* 297:135–143.

Lee, K. H., C. H. Cho, and K.-H. Rhee. 2011. Synergic anti-tumor activity of gamma-irradiated exo-polysaccharide from submerged culture of *Grifola frondosa*. *J Med Plants Res* 5:2378–2386.

Lo, T. C.-T., F.-M. Hsu, C. A. Chang, and J. C.-H. Cheng. 2011. Branched alpha-(1,4) glucans from *Lentinula edodes* (L10) in combination with radiation enhance cytotoxic effect on human lung adenocarcinoma through the toll-like receptor 4 mediated induction of THP-1 differentiation/activation. *J Agric Food Chem* 59:11997–12005.

Lo, T. C. T., H. H. Tsao, A. Y. Wang, and C. A. Chang. 2007. Pressurized water extraction of polysaccharides as secondary metabolites from *Lentinula edodes*. *J Agric Food Chem* 55:4196–4201.

Mandal, E. K., K. Maity, S. Maity et al. 2012. Chemical analysis of an immunostimulating (1 → 4)-, (1 → 6)-branched glucan from an edible mushroom, *Calocybe indica*. *Carbohydr Res* 347:172–177.

Mandal, E. K., K. Maity, S. Maity et al. 2011. Structural characterization of an immunoenhancing cytotoxic heteroglycan isolated from an edible mushroom *Calocybe indica* var. APK2. *Carbohydr Res* 346:2237–2243.

Mandal, S., K. K. Maity, S. K. Bhunia et al. 2010. Chemical analysis of new water-soluble (1 → 6)-, (1 → 4)-alpha, beta-glucan and water-insoluble (1 → 3)-, (1 → 4)-beta-glucan (calocyban) from alkaline extract of an edible mushroom, *Calocybe indica* (Dudh Chattu). *Carbohydr Res* 345:2657–2663.

Manzi, P., A. Aguzzi, and L. Pizzoferrato. 2001. Nutritional value of mushrooms widely consumed in Italy. *Food Chem* 73:321–325.

McIntosh, M., B. A. Stone, and V. A. Stanisich. 2005. Curdlan and other bacterial (1 → 3)-beta-D-glucans. *Appl Microbiol Biotechnol* 68:163–173.

Mensink, R. P., A. Aro, E. Den Hond et al. 2003. PASSCLAIM—Diet-related cardiovascular disease. *Eur J Nutr* 42:6–27.

Mitchell, J. R. 1980. The rheology of gels. *J Texture Stud* 11:315–337.

Miyazawa, N., M. Okazaki, and S. Ohga. 2008. Antihypertensive effect of *Pleurotus nebrodensis* on spontaneously hypertensive rats. *J Oleo Sci* 57:675–681.

Moro, C., I. Palacios, M. Lozano et al. 2012. Anti-inflammatory activity of methanolic extracts from edible mushrooms in LPS activated RAW 264.7 macrophages. *Food Chem* 130:350–355.

Muller, A., H. Ensley, H. Pretus et al. 1997. The application of various protic acids in the extraction of (1 → 3)-beta-D-glucan from *Saccharomyces cerevisiae*. *Carbohydr Res* 299:203–208.

Muralikrishna, G. and M. Rao. 2007. Cereal non-cellulosic polysaccharides: Structure and function relationship—An overview. *Crit Rev Food Sci Nutr* 47:599–610.

Nandan, C. K., P. Patra, S. K. Bhanja et al. 2008. Structural characterization of a water-soluble beta-(1–6)-linked D-glucan isolated from the hot water extract of an edible mushroom, *Agaricus bitorquis*. *Carbohydr Res* 343:3120–3122.

Numata, M., S. Tamesue, T. Fujisawa et al. 2006. Beta-1,3-glucan polysaccharide (schizophyllan) acting as a one-dimensional host for creating supramolecular dye assemblies. *Org Lett* 8:5533–5536.

Ochiai, T., K. Isono, T. Suzuki et al. 1992. Effect of immunotherapy with lentinan on patients survival and immunological parameters in patients with advanced gastric-cancer—Results of a multicenter randomized controlled-study. *Int J Immunotherap* 8:161–169.

Pan, D., L. Wang, C. Chen et al. 2012. Structure characterization of a novel neutral polysaccharide isolated from *Ganoderma lucidum* fruiting bodies. *Food Chem* 135:1097–1103.

Park, H. G., Y. Y. Shim, S. O. Choi, and W. M. Park. 2009. New method development for nanoparticle extraction of water-soluble beta-(1 → 3)-D-glucan from edible mushrooms, *Sparassis crispa* and *Phellinus linteus*. *J Agric Food Chem* 57:2147–2154.

Rincao, V. P., K. A. Yamamoto, N. M. Pontes Silva Ricardo et al. 2012. Polysaccharide and extracts from *Lentinula edodes*: Structural features and antiviral activity. *Virol J* 9 (37):1–6.

Rosado, F. R., E. R. Carbonero, C. Kemmelmeier et al. 2002. A partially 3-O-methylated (1 → 4)-linked alpha-D-galactan and alpha-D-mannan from *Pleurotus ostreatoroseus* Sing. *FEMS Microbiol Lett* 212:261–265.

Rout, D., S. Mondal, I. Chakraborty, and S. S. Islam. 2008. The structure and conformation of a water-insoluble (1–3), (1–6)-beta-D-glucan from the fruiting bodies of *Pleurotus florida*. *Carbohydr Res* 343:982–987.

Ru, Q. M., L. R. Zhang, J. D. Chen, Z. M. Pei, and H. L. Zheng. 2009. Microwave-assisted extraction and identification of polysaccharide from *Lycoris aurea*. *Chem Nat Compd* 45:474–477.

Santos-Neves, J. C., M. I. Pereira, E. R. Carbonero et al. 2008. A novel branched alpha beta-glucan isolated from the basidiocarps of the edible mushroom *Pleurotus florida*. *Carbohydr Polym* 73:309–314.

Santoyo, S., M. Plaza, L. Jaime et al. 2010. Pressurized liquid extraction as an alternative process to obtain antiviral agents from the edible microalga *chlorella vulgaris. J Agric Food Chem* 58:8522–8527.

Selvi, S., P. Umadevi, S. Murugan, and G. J. Senapathy. 2011. Anticancer potential evoked by *Pleurotus florida* and *Calocybe indica* using T-24 urinary bladder cancer cell line. *Afr J Biotechnol* 10:7279–7285.

Sletmoen, M. and B. T. Stokke. 2008. Review: Higher order structure of (1,3)-beta-D-glucans and its influence on their biological activities and complexation abilities. *Biopolymers* 89:310–321.

Smiderle, F. R., E. R. Carbonero, G. L. Sassaki, P. A. J. Gorin, and M. Iacomini. 2008. Characterization of a heterogalactan: Some nutritional values of the edible mushroom *Flammulina velutipes*. *Food Chem* 108:329–333.

Song, G. and Q. Du. 2012. Structure characterisation of a alpha beta-glucan polysaccharide from *Auricularia polytricha*. *Nat Prod Res* 26:1963–1970.

Song, J.-F., D.-J. Li, and C.-Q. Liu. 2009. Response surface analysis of microwave-assisted extraction of polysaccharides from cultured *Cordyceps militaris*. *J Chem Technol Biotechnol* 84:1669–1673.

Storsley, J. M., M. S. Izydorczyk, S. You, C. G. Biliaderis, and B. Rossnagel. 2003. Structure and physicochemical properties of beta-glucans and arabinoxylans isolated from hull-less barley. *Food Hydrocolloids* 17:831–844.

Synytsya, A., K. Mickova, I. Jablonsky et al. 2009. Glucans from fruit bodies of cultivated mushrooms *Pleurotus ostreatus* and *Pleurotus eryngii*: Structure and potential prebiotic activity. *Carbohydr Polym* 76:548–556.

Taguchi, T., O. Abe, K. Enomoto et al. 1982. Life-span prolongation effect of lentinan on patients with advanced or recurrent breast-cancer. *Int J Immunopharmacol* 4:271–271.

Tao, Y. and L. Zhang. 2006. Determination of molecular size and shape of hyperbranched polysaccharide in solution. *Biopolymers* 83:414–423.

Tian, Y., H. Zeng, Z. Xu et al. 2012. Ultrasonic-assisted extraction and antioxidant activity of polysaccharides recovered from white button mushroom (*Agaricus bisporus*). *Carbohydr Polym* 88:522–529.

Vaikousi, H., C. G. Biliaderis, and M. S. Izydorczyk. 2004. Solution flow behavior and gelling properties of water-soluble barley (1 → 3,1 → 4)-beta-glucans varying in molecular size. *J Cereal Sci* 39:119–137.

Wang, G., L. Dong, Y. Zhang et al. 2012. Polysaccharides from *Phellinus linteus* inhibit cell growth and invasion and induce apoptosis in HepG2 human hepatocellular carcinoma cells. *Biologia* 67:247–254.

Wang, J., L. Zhang, Y. Yu, and P. C. K. Cheung. 2009a. Enhancement of antitumor activities in sulfated and carboxymethylated polysaccharides of *Ganoderma lucidum*. *J Agric Food Chem* 57:10565–10572.

Wang, J. G. and L. Zhang. 2009b. Structure and chain conformation of five water-soluble derivatives of a beta-D-glucan isolated from *Ganoderma lucidum*. *Carbohydr Res* 344:105–112.

Wasser, S. P. 2002. Medicinal mushrooms as a source of antitumor and immunomodulating polysaccharides. *Appl Microbiol Biotechnol* 60:258–274.

Xu, S., X. Xu, and L. Zhang. 2012. Branching structure and chain conformation of water-soluble glucan extracted from *Auricularia auricula-judae*. *J Agric Food Chem* 60:3498–3506.

Yamanaka, D., R. Tada, Y. Adachi et al. 2012. *Agaricus brasiliensis*-derived beta-glucans exert immunoenhancing effects via a dectin-1-dependent pathway. *Int Immunopharmacol* 14:311–319.

Yue, L., H. Cui, C. Li et al. 2012. A polysaccharide from *Agaricus blazei* attenuates tumor cell adhesion via inhibiting E-selectin expression. *Carbohydr Polym* 88:1326–1333.

Zhang, L., C. Fan, S. Liu et al. 2011a. Chemical composition and antitumor activity of polysaccharide from *Inonotus obliquus*. *J Med Plants Res* 5:1251–1260.

Zhang, Y. Y., S. Li, X. H. Wang, L. N. Zhang, and P. C. K. Cheung. 2011b. Advances in lentinan: Isolation, structure, chain conformation and bioactivities. *Food Hydrocolloids* 25:196–206.

Zhang, Z., G. Lv, H. Pan, L. Shi, and L. Fan. 2011c. Optimization of the microwave-assisted extraction process for polysaccharides in Himematsutake (*Agaricus blazei* Murrill) and evaluation of their antioxidant activities. *Food Sci Technol Res* 17:461–470.

CHAPTER 8

Polysaccharides from Medicinal Mushrooms for Potential Use as Nutraceuticals

IOANNIS GIAVASIS

Contents

8.1	Introduction	171
8.2	Types and Sources of Bioactive Mushroom Polysaccharides	173
8.3	Production of Bioactive Mushroom Polysaccharides	179
8.4	Medicinal Properties of Mushroom Polysaccharides	185
	8.4.1 Immunostimulating and Antitumor Properties	186
	8.4.2 Antioxidant Properties	188
	8.4.3 Antimicrobial Properties	190
	8.4.4 Hypolipidemic, Hypoglycemic, and Prebiotic Properties	191
8.5	Applications of Mushroom Bioactive Polysaccharides in Functional Foods and Nutraceuticals	193
8.6	Conclusions	195
	References	196

8.1 Introduction

Mushrooms have been used for centuries in Asian and other traditional cuisine and traditional medicines due to their culinary and medicinal properties, but their properties remained unknown to the wide scientific community for a long time. In the last few decades, a large amount of research has focused on the types, sources, biosynthesis, and medicinal properties and applications of many mushrooms, mainly members of the Basidiomycetes family. The most common active ingredients in these higher fungi are their extracellular, intracellular, or cell wall polysaccharides, which exhibit immunostimulating, antitumor, antimicrobial, anti-inflammatory, antioxidant, prebiotic, hypogly-cemic, and hypocholesterolemic effects. In the last few years, some of these mushrooms or their biopolymers have been commercialized in pharmaceuti-cal applications, but their application in food and nutraceuticals is still at an early stage. However, the fact that many of these mushrooms are edible (and thus nontoxic) as well as tasty makes them, or their polysaccharides, poten-tially ideal ingredients for the formulation of novel functional foods and nutra-ceuticals. However, their biological properties might be affected after addition to food, due to food processing and/or interaction with food ingredients. This chapter describes the most important and studied types and sources of bio-active mushroom polysaccharides, the biosynthesis and bioprocess condi-tions used for the production/cultivation in solid or liquid media, the relation between molecular/structural characteristics and bioactivity, their medicinal properties, and their existing or potential applications in human nutrition.

Microbial polysaccharides excreted or contained in the cell wall of bac-teria, yeast, and fungi are long known to possess biological properties that promote human health, largely because they serve as dietary fiber, but few of them have been utilized to formulate novel drugs or nutraceuticals (Giavasis 2013, Giavasis and Biliaderis 2006). For centuries, a large number of medici-nal mushrooms have been consumed in the Far East (China, Japan, Korea, and other countries where they are native), as part of a healthy diet and as a traditional cure for several diseases, since they can stimulate a general, non-specific positive immune response, which is at the core of the holistic cura-tive approach of traditional Asian medicine (Wasser 2002). In the last few decades, scientific research has focused on exploring the properties of several higher fungi, which produce a variety of bioactive polysaccharides in order to bridge the gap between traditional practice and the development of novel standardized, commercial functional foods, and nutraceuticals (Chang and Wasser 2012). This research has revealed that many of the members of the Basidiomycetes family (as well as some of the Ascomycetes family) are able to produce immunomodulating, hepatoprotective, antimicrobial, prebiotic, antioxidant, hypoglycemic, and hypolipidemic substances, which are usu-ally β-glucans, or heteropolysaccharides, or proteoglucans (although other bioactive ingredients such as terpenes, sterols, phenols, and flavonoids also exist in many higher fungi) (Chang and Wasser 2012, Giavasis 2013, Mizuno and Nishitani 2013, Wasser 2011). These macromolecules are often described with the general term "biological response modifiers" (BRMs) due to their multiple biological effects and their indirect or nonspecific modes of action, which trigger several immune responses and potentiate the curative proper-ties of the human body (Giavasis and Biliaderis 2006, Sullivan et al. 2006, Wasser 2002).

The bioactive polysaccharides from edible mushrooms in particular (in comparison to nonedible fungi) are very interesting and useful ingredients for the formulation of functional foods and nutraceuticals, since they are already consumed as part of the traditional diet in Asian or South American countries, without any toxicological concerns. For instance, Lingzhi, Maitake, Shiitake, oyster, or other mushrooms deliver medicinal biopolymers that can be and have been adopted as the basis of novel nutraceuticals, in order to boost the immune system, act as anticancer or antiageing ingredients, reduce the side effects of chemotherapy/radiotherapy, protect against viral infections, reduce blood sugar and cholesterol, and stimulate the growth of probiotic bacteria (Giavasis 2013, Stachowiak and Reguła 2012, Wasser 2002, Xu 2001). However, despite the discovery of many medicinal mushrooms and the identification of their bioactive polysaccharides, only a handful of functional food products exist where these polysaccharides are utilized. This is probably because there are several concerns regarding the application of these important molecules in final food products, such as the molecular and structural diversity of the biopolymers that can be produced from the same fungus (which may affect the expression of pharmaceutical properties), the appropriate concentration of biopolymer that needs to be applied in nutraceuticals in order to express a health effect without inferring any toxic effects, the unstable quantity, quality, and availability of these mushroom polysaccharides, the impact of the purification process and food processing on the bioactivity of the biopolymers, and their production costs (Cho et al. 1999, Falch et al. 2000, Giavasis 2013, Maji et al. 2013, Wasser 2011, Zhang et al. 2011). Therefore, some of the issues that need attention and further investigation before the broad adoption of these biopolymers by the industry are the structure–function relationships of these polysaccharides (Falch et al. 2000, Giavasis and Biliaderis 2006, Maji et al. 2013), the standardization of the production/cultivation process and the purification process, the development of cost-effective strategies for controlled and stable productivity (e.g., by the cultivation of the fungal mycelium in bioreactors, which could shorten production time significantly and allow optimization and control of environmental process conditions) (Kim et al. 2002, Lee et al. 2004, Tang and Zhong 2003) and the conduction of more toxicological and clinical studies in humans, which will support the health claims that can be linked to the consumption of bioactive mushrooms polysaccharides as nutraceuticals (Aleem 2013, Jeurink et al. 2008, Zhou et al. 2005). Below, the issues already mentioned will be addressed and the most recent developments will be summarized regarding the types, properties, production process, and the utilization of medicinal mushroom polysaccharides as sources for novel functional foods.

8.2 Types and Sources of Bioactive Mushroom Polysaccharides

Lentinus (or *Lentinula*) *edodes*, also known as the Shiitake mushroom, is one of the most common, popular, and well-studied medicinal and edible mushrooms in China and Japan, which produces a β-glucan known as lentinan. Lentinan contains a backbone of β-(1,3)-ᴅ-glucose residues to which β-(1,6)-ᴅ-glucose side groups are linked via glycosidic linkages (there is one branch to every third main chain unit) and has an average molecular weight of around 500 kDa, but may range from 400 to 800 kDa (Ganeshpurkar et al. 2010, Giavasis 2013, Ooi and Liu 2000, Thakur and Singh 2013). It is one of the most well-studied immunomodulating polysaccharides and has been used in commercial pharmaceutical applications (Giavasis 2013, Lakhanpal and Rana 2005). Glycoproteins have also been extracted from cultured mycelia of *L. edodes*. Among them, KS-2 is an α-mannan peptide known to have antitumor properties (Bisen et al. 2010, Lakhanpal and Rana 2005).

Schizophyllan (also called sizofiran) is similar to lentinan β-(1,3)-ᴅ-glucan with β-(1,6) branches, which is excreted by cultured mycelia of the edible fungus *Schizophyllum commune*. It has a lower molecular weight as compared to lentinan (in the range of 100–200 kDa) and acquires a triple helical conformation in solutions. Schizophyllan is also well-studied for its anticancer, antiviral, and other health effects, which have led to its utilization in industrial pharmaceutical applications, as an adjunct cancer therapy, together with conventional drugs (Ganeshpurkar et al. 2010, Giavasis 2013, Giavasis and Biliaderis 2006, Thakur and Singh 2013, Wasser 2002). The chemical structure (basic repeating unit) of lentinan and schizophyllan and the fruiting bodies of the producer mushrooms are depicted in Figure 8.1.

Hot water extracts or dry powders of *Ganoderma lucidum* (known as the Lingzhi mushroom in China, or Reishi mushroom in Japan, which means "supernatural mushroom") have also been used in traditional Asian medicine for over 2000 years, due to their immunostimulating, antiageing, and antioxidant properties (Bao et al. 2002, Eo et al. 2000, Wasser 2002). *G. lucidum* is an important medicinal mushroom of the Basiodiomycetes family, which produces a number of bioactive polysaccharides. The most typical is called ganoderan. It is a β-(1,3)-glucan with β-(1,6)-glucose branches at C-6, with a variable molecular weight and degree of branching, especially when isolated from the water extracts of the fruiting body. The equivalent glucan isolated from filtrates/centrifugates of liquid-cultured mycelia has a molecular weight of $1.2-4.4 \times 10^6$ Da (Bao et al. 2002, Ganeshpurkar et al. 2010, Giavasis 2013, Wasser 2002). In addition to these, *G. lucidum* also produces several other heteroglucans and proteoglucans with immunostimulating activity, most of which are isolated from water extracts of the fruiting bodies. This variety of isolated biopolymers is quite common among bioactive polysaccharides from mushroom fruiting bodies, which can be a problem with regard to the production of commercial purified and standardized ingredients for drugs and nutraceuticals (Giavasis and Biliaderis 2006, Wasser 2002, Wasser 2011). Ye et al. (2010) studied the structure and

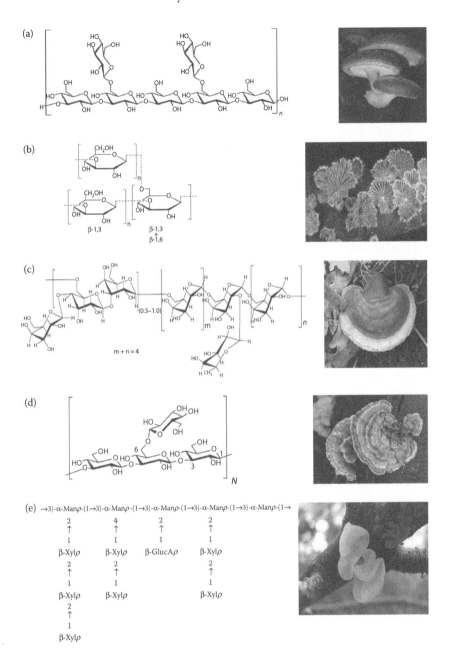

Figure 8.1 Chemical structures of polysaccharide repeating units (up) and the corresponding fruiting bodies (down) of (a) lentinan from *Lentinus edodes*, (b) schizophyllan from *Schizophyllum commune*, (c) the polysaccharide moiety of a *Ganoderma lucidum* proteoglycan, (d) the exopolysaccharide from *Coriolus (Trametes) versicolor*, and (e) the acidic heteroglycan from *Tremella mesenterica*.

composition of a complex polysaccharide moiety of a proteoglucan from
G. lucidum fruiting bodies. This had a main chain of 1,6-α-galactopyranoside,
1,2,6-trisubstituted-α-galactopyranoside, 1,3-disubstituted-β-glucopyranoside,
and 1,4,6-trisubstituted-β-glucopyranoside groups, with branches of
1-β-glucopyranoside and 1-α-fucopyranoside residues, and a relative molecular weight of 1.12×104 Da (Figure 8.1).

A close relative of *G. lucidum*, *Ganoderma tsugae* produces water-soluble
and alkali-soluble antioxidant polysaccharides (Tseng et al. 2008), as well
as water-soluble antitumor protein–heteropolysaccharide complexes with
a mean molecular weight of ~62–82 kDa (Peng et al. 2005). It also yields
(1,3)-β-D-glucans and (1,4)-α-D-glucans with antitumor properties, after
submerged cultivation of the mycelium (Peng et al. 2005).

Another popular and tasty edible mushroom with bioactive polysaccharides is *Pleurotus ostreatus* (oyster mushroom), which forms pleuran, an
insoluble β-(1,3/1,6)-D-glucan that exhibits immunostimulating and anticancer properties, especially after solubilization of the carboxymethylated
derivatives (Bergendiova et al. 2011, Synytsya et al. 2009). Both *P. ostreatus*
and *P. eryngii* produce a water-soluble branched 1,3/1,6-β-D-glucan, a linear
alkali-soluble 1,3-α-D-glucan, and an insoluble glucan originating from the
cell wall, which may serve as a prebiotic dietary fiber and source of nutraceuticals (Paulik et al. 1996, Synytsya et al. 2009). Similar glucans with pharmaceutical potential are found in other *Pleurotus* species, such as *P. florida*,
P. tuber-regium, and *P. pulmonarius* (Bergendiova et al. 2011, Synytsya et al.
2009, Zhang et al. 2001).

Agaricus blazei, or *Agaricus brasiliensis*, as it was recently reclassified,
is another well-studied edible medicinal mushroom that originates from
Brazil, where it is called Piedade mushroom, medicinal mushroom (cogumelo medicinal), sun mushroom (cogumelo do sol), or God's mushroom
(cogumelo de Deus) (Largeteau et al. 2011). It yields several antitumor polysaccharides contained in its fruiting body (Giavasis and Biliaderis 2006,
Wasser 2002) such as a β-(1,6)/β-(1,3) glucan, an acidic β-(1,6)/α-(1,3) glucan, and an acidic β-(1,6)/α-(1,4) glucan. Unlike most mushroom glucans
that are characterized by a β-(1,3)-linked backbone, *A. blazei* glucans have
a main chain of β-(1,6) glycopyranose (Giavasis 2013, Mizuno 2002, Wasser
2002). Interestingly, the structure of these glucans can be influenced by the
maturity stage of the fruiting bodies as a higher proportion of β-(1,3) and
α-(1,4) glycosidic bonds are found in glucans from the most mature mushrooms (compared to immature ones) (Camelini et al. 2005). The fruiting
body also contains an antitumor water-soluble proteoglucan with a molecular weight of 380 kDa, which has an α-(1,4)-glucopyranoside main chain
and β-(1,6) glucopyranoside branches at a ratio of 4:1 (Fujimiya et al. 1998,
Mizuno 2002, Wasser 2002). In addition, two immunostimulating heteroglucans have been isolated from *A. blazei* fruiting bodies, which are composed of glucose, galactose and mannose, one of which contains glucose and

ribose, and a xyloglucan (Giavasis and Biliaderis 2006). When the mycelium is cultivated in liquid cultures, *A. blazei* excretes an extracellular antitumor proteoglucan of very high molecular weight (1000–10,000 kDa), which is composed of mannose, glucose, galactose, and ribose groups (Mizuno 2002, Tsuchida et al. 2001).

Grifolan is also an important immunostimulating gel-forming β-(1,3)-D glucan with β-(1,6) glucosidic linkages at every third glucose residue, which is contained in the fruiting bodies of the edible fungus *Grifola frondosa* (Maitake mushroom) (Boh and Berovic 2007). In submerged cultures, *G. frondosa* produces extracellular antioxidant proteoglucans of high molecular weight (770–1650 kDa) and a protein content of 6–27%, depending on the composition of the fermentation medium as well as proteoglucans of lower molecular weight (around 500 kDa) in the cultured mycelia (Lee et al. 2003). Cui et al. (2007) have also reported the isolation of a low-molecular-weight (21 kDa) antitumor heteropolysaccharide extracted from the mycelia of submerged cultures of *G. frondosa*.

Krestin, or polysaccharide-K (PSK), is one of the most successful therapeutic mushroom polysaccharides (or polysaccharopeptide as it is often referred to) that have been marketed as anticancer drugs (in combination with chemotherapy) and nutraceuticals. It derives from the edible mushroom *Coriolous versicolor* (also known as *Trametes versicolor*) (Hobbs 2004). Ooi and Liu (2000) reported that it is a low-molecular-weight (94,000 Da) proteoglucan containing 25–38% protein residues. PSK has a main chain of β-(1,4)-glucopyranoside, with β-(1,6)-glucopyranosidic lateral chains at every fourth glucose unit. The major monosaccharide is glucose, but other sugar residues are also present, such as mannose, fucose, xylose, and galactose. The proteinaceous residue consists predominantly of acidic amino acids (glutamic and aspartic) and neutral amino acids (valine, leucine) (Ooi and Liu, 2000). However, other studies revealed that three fractions of different molecular weights can be extracted from the mushroom fruiting bodies, namely, a high-molecular-weight fraction (1200 kDa) with only 4.1% protein content, a medium-molecular-weight fraction (150 kDa), and a low-molecular-weight fraction (15 kDa), the latter having the highest proportion of protein. From these three fractions, the highest immunostimulatory activity was attained with the high-molecular-weight fraction, which contained glucose and arabinose moieties at a ratio of 4.3:1.0 (Jeong et al. 2004).

In addition, two similar polysaccharide–protein complexes (PSPC), but of lower molecular weight, one intracellular (28 kDa) and one extracellular (15 kDa), have been isolated from mycelia and liquid culture filtrates, respectively, of *Coriolus* (or *Trametes*) *versicolor* (Ooi and Liu 2000). In another study with submerged cultures of *C. versicolor*, two extracellular proteoglucans were identified, one of very high molecular weight (4100 kDa) and one of very low molecular weight (2.6 kDa) with a protein content of 2–3.6% (Rau et al. 2009). The main polysaccharide chain in the biopolymers is very similar to schizophyllan as it is composed of β-(1,3)/β-(1,6)-linked D-glucose molecules, except that it does not adopt a triple helix conformation like schizophyllan (Figure 8.1) (Rau et al. 2009).

Another source of therapeutic (immunomodulatory and antidiabetic) polysaccharides are the edible medicinal *Tremmella* mushrooms (*T. mesenterica, T. fuciformis, T. auriantica, T. auriantialba,* and *T. cinnabarina*), which form a group of unusual jelly mushrooms of very high polysaccharide content (60–90% of the fruiting body, in contrast to 10–30% in other mushrooms) (Lo et al. 2006, Reshetnikov et al. 2000). *Tremella* polysaccharides are acidic with a pH of 5.1–5.6 in aqueous solutions as they are composed of a linear backbone of α-(1,3)-D-rhamnose, with side groups of xylose and glucuronic acid (Figure 8.1) (De Baets and Vandamme 2001, Khondkar 2009, Lo et al. 2006, Reshetnikov et al. 2000). Extracellular acidic heteroglycans from filtrates of *Tremella* species have also been studied; these are characterized by an α-(1 → 3)-mannan backbone with β-linked side chains and contain xylose, arabinose, mannose, galactose, glucose, and glucuronic acid residues (Khondkar 2009).

Cordyceps mushrooms belonging to the *Ascomycetes* group of fungi also have a long history of applications in traditional Chinese medicine. *Cordyceps sinensis* is a fungal parasite on the larvae of Lepidoptera and grows slowly to form a worm-like fruiting body. It produces several medicinal biopolymers that differ depending on whether they are isolated from fruiting bodies or cultured mycelia, the cultivation/fermentation conditions, the substrate used, and the purification method that is followed (Zhong et al. 2009). Polysaccharides extracted from the fruiting bodies or mycelia of *C. sinensis, C. militaris,* and other *Cordyceps* species exhibit antitumor, antiviral, and antioxidant activity (Khan et al. 2010). Wu et al. (2011) studied the antioxidant properties of a polysaccharide isolated from the fruiting bodies of *C. militaris,* which was composed mainly of mannose, glucose, and galactose in a molar ratio of 1.35:8.34:1.00, and linked by α-glycosidic linkages. Several highly branched galactomannans have been purified from fruiting bodies of *C. sinensis.* Their main chain contains predominantly (1,2)-α-D-mannopyranose groups, with branches of (1,3)-, (1,5)-, and (1,6)-linked D-galactofuranose and (1,4)-D-galactopyranose residues (Nie et al. 2013a). Also, a water-soluble protein–galactomannan complex from *C. sinensis* was reported, which has an estimated molecular weight of 23 kDa (Nie et al. 2013a). In addition, from extracts of cultured mycelia of *C. sinensis,* a 210 kDa polysaccharide with antioxidant and hypoglycemic properties was obtained that contained glucose, mannose, and galactose in a ratio of 1:0.6:0.75 (Li et al. 2003, 2006).

Chen et al. (2008) have extracted and characterized a hypolipidemic polysaccharide from fruiting bodies of the edible mushroom *Auricularia auricula* (AAP), which was found to contain 42.5% total carbohydrate, 19.6% uronic acids, 15.8% sulfate groups, 1.7% total nitrogen, and 20.3% ash. The neutral sugar components were mainly rhamnose, xylose, glucose, and smaller amounts of mannose, galactose, and arabinose. In another study, an antithrombotic polysaccharide was obtained from alkali extracts of *A. auricula* fruiting bodies, which had a molecular weight of 160 kDa and was composed mainly of mannose, glucose, glucuronic acid, and xylose, without having any sulfate esters (Yoon et al. 2003).

Other less studied but still interesting polysaccharides from medicinal mushrooms with biological activities that could be exploited as the basis for novel nutraceuticals include the immunostimulatory and hypoglycemic heteroglycans from the edible *Hericium erinaceus* (Lakhanpal and Rana 2005, Mizuno 1998), the antitumor glucans from the bitter mushroom *Phellinus linteus* (Kim et al. 2004), the antitumor and hypoglycemic heteroglycans from the culinary *Morchella esculenta* (Duncan et al. 2002, Lakhanpal and Rana 2005), the immunostimulatory heteroglycans from *Flammulina velutipes* mycelium (the edible Enokitake mushroom) (Yin et al. 2010), and several others (Ooi and Liu 2000, Zhang et al. 2007).

8.3 Production of Bioactive Mushroom Polysaccharides

In the past, the consumption of mushrooms was limited in most countries (with the exception of China), and was based on the individual collection of wild mushrooms. In the last few decades, the industrial cultivation of mushrooms has increased rapidly, with China having a leading role in the worldwide production, followed by Italy, the United States, and several European countries (the European Union is the second worldwide producer) (Table 8.1) (F.A.O. 2013). This increase has been parallel to the increasing acknowledgment by scientists and consumers of the multiple dietary and health benefits of mushroom consumption (Stachowiak and Reguła 2012, Wasser 2002).

At the same time, there seems to be a shortage of commercial, industrialized polysaccharides from medicinal mushrooms, despite the extensive literature on their therapeutic properties, which is partly due to the fact that many of these fungi only grow as wild mushrooms in forests and are hard to cultivate in farms. But even for medicinal mushrooms that have been successfully cultivated as fruiting bodies in large scale, there are several concerns that limit their industrial exploitation for bioactive polysaccharide production, such as the long period of growing into mature fruiting bodies, the high purification costs, the erratic quality, and the limited availability. Furthermore, some scientists have raised the issue of the potential toxicity of mushrooms found in urban and industrial areas that may contain elevated levels of heavy metals or radioactive elements that the mushrooms can accumulate from the soil (Stachowiak and Reguła 2012, Vetter 2004, Vinichuk et al. 2010). These disadvantages could be overcome by the cultivation of the mycelia in fermentors (bioreactors) under controlled and sterile

Table 8.1 Worldwide Production of Mushrooms in the Years 1991, 2001, and 2011

	Production (Tons)		
Country	1991	2001	2011
Australia	24,394	39,394	49,696
Belgium	20,592[a]	40,500	41,556
Canada	53,020	86,357	78,930
China	775,000	2,660,000	5,000,000
France	198,500	196,254	115,669
Germany	56,000	63,000	62,000
India	4000	30,000	40,600
Indonesia	8000	25,500	45,851
Iran	6387	19,000	37,664
Ireland	39,000	68,000	67,063
Italy	79,536	72,900	761,858
Japan	78,000	66,100	60,180
The Netherlands	165,000	275,000	304,000
Poland	101,500	110,000	198,235
Republic of Korea	13,181	21,251	30,574
Spain	29,693	109,605	148,000
UK	123,300	92,600	69,300
USA	338,760	376,980	390,902
Vietnam	9000	16,000	21,957

Source: Data from FAO—Food and Agriculture Organization of the United Nations, 2011.

[a] Belgium-Luxemburg.

conditions, which shortens the production time from months to only a few days or a couple of weeks at the most, allows a close quality and process control, eliminates potential problems of toxicity and contamination, and offers practically unlimited quantity and constant, all-year-round availability, and usually entails lower purifications costs. Another potential advantage of some fungal fermentation processes is that the exopolysaccharides that are secreted to the process medium are more uniform in type, composition, and structure and easier to standardize as a commercial product, in comparison to the high diversity of polysaccharides that can be isolated from extracts of fruiting bodies (Donot et al. 2012, Giavasis and Biliaderis 2006, Lee et al. 2004, Wasser 2002). For all these reasons, the study of fungal physiology and the optimization of the fermentation conditions and the downstream processing for achieving a maximal bioactive polysaccharide production become critical factors for their commercial utilization (Giavasis 2013, Giavasis and Biliaderis 2006, McNeil and Harvey 2006). However, for several higher fungi, the submerged cultivation of mycelia is not feasible, or results in very low yields of biomass and biopolymer, thus the cultivation of mushroom fruiting bodies is the only option for their commercial production (Chang 1993).

With regard to the large-scale cultivation of edible and/or medicinal mushrooms, nonectomycorrhizal mushrooms (without roots) can be grown on wood, straw, sawdust, or other cellulosic material (e.g., *Lentinus*, *Pleurotus*, *Auricularia*, *Tremella*, *Hericium*), animal manure (e.g., *Agaricus*), or soil (e.g., *Morchella*). On the contrary, ectomycorrhizal mushrooms (with roots under the ground) are very hard to cultivate artificially (Chang 1993). The artificial cultivation of mushrooms takes place on the appropriate substrate either in open farms, where mushroom productivity is limited by uncontrolled environmental conditions, such as temperature, moisture, and aeration, or in beds or sterile plastic bags of compost substrate, which are placed in indoor chambers where environmental conditions (pH, temperature, humidity, aeration) can be controlled, at the expense of energy. This process is of course very slow as it takes from several weeks up to 8–10 months until the fungal mycelia become mature fruiting bodies (Chang 1993). It is also susceptible to contamination by other fungi or bacteria that cause mushroom rot, or to pathogenic parasites and mites (Largeteau et al. 2011).

The isolation process of bioactive mushroom polysaccharides from mature fruiting bodies involves hot water or the alkali extraction of dried mushrooms, filtration, ethanol precipitation, and the removal of impurities (e.g., proteins, starch, and oligosaccharides) from the filtrate enzymatically or by a phenolic or other reagent, dialysis, and lyophilization (Synytsya et al. 2009, Zhang et al. 2007). If a higher purity is desired (e.g., for strictly pharmaceutical applications), gel permeation, ion-exchange, or affinity chromatography can be implemented, depending on the nature of the biopolymer (Zhang et al. 2007). A proposed process for the isolation and purification of different fractions of mushroom polysaccharides is depicted in Figure 8.2. Other processing methods such as ultrasonication have been proposed in order to enhance extraction yields of mushroom polysaccharides, by facilitating the disruption of the mushroom cell wall, the reduction of particle size, and the solubility of the biopolymers (Yang et al. 2011).

As concerns the fermentative or submerged culture of mycelia for the production of bioactive polysaccharides, several process parameters have to be taken into account in order to achieve high polysaccharide yields, such as the optimal pH, temperature, aeration, agitation, and process medium composition (Elisashvili 2012, Giavasis and Biliaderis 2006, Kim et al. 2002).

For instance, several mushroom polysaccharides are optimally synthesized at low pH, such as grifolan at pH 5.5 (Lee et al. 2004) and ganoderan at pH 4–4.5 (Yang and Liau 1998), or via a gradual pH drop from 5 to 4 in the absence of pH control (Kim et al. 2002). In contrast, Shu et al. (2004) observed that there was an increase in polysaccharide formation by *A. blazei* as the process pH increased from 4 to 7; however, at a low pH, a higher molecular weight (and biological activity) of the glucans was attained. According to

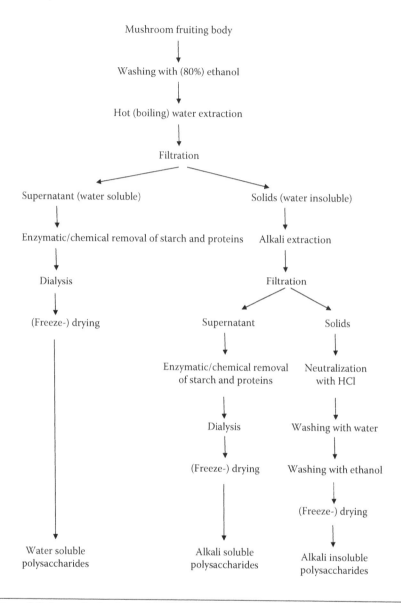

Figure 8.2 Proposed extraction and purification process for the isolation of water-soluble, alkali-soluble, and insoluble fractions of mushroom polysaccharides. (Adapted from Synytsya, A. et al. 2009. *Carbohydr Polym* 76:548–556.)

Fan et al. (2007), the optimum pH for exopolysaccharide production from *A. brasiliensis* was 6.1.

The optimum temperature for the growth of mycelia and polysaccharide production by medicinal fungi is usually around 30°C as in the case of *Ganoderma lucimum* (Yang and Liau, 1998) and *A. brasiliensis* (Fan et al.

2007), although for some fungal biopolymers such as grifolan from *G. frondosa*, a process temperature of 25°C has been proposed (Lee et al. 2004).

An agitation rate of 150 rpm was found to be the most preferable for the production of *G. lucidum* polysaccharide in shake flasks. Higher agitation may improve mixing, but high shear stress has a detrimental effect on the size and growth of mycelia and the synthesis of polysaccharides (Yang and Liau 1998). Fungal morphology is in fact a very important factor in submerged fungal cultures and polysaccharide production. Generally, as the culture grows, the morphology changes from a loose mycelium to unicellular pellets, the latter being associated with the maximum production of polysaccharides. In the case of *G. lucidum* polysaccharides, the pellet size was becoming more compact and small during a 13-day fermentation, at the end of which a maximum exopolysaccharide concentration of 5.7 g/L was obtained (Wagner et al. 2004).

Small–medium pellet size was also associated with an increased production of schizophyllan. Specifically, Shu et al. (2005) applied a pellet size control device in a bubble column fermentor where the pellet size of *S. commune* was reduced from 20.5 to 12.3 mm, causing an increase in schizophyllan yield and maximum concentration. However, at lower pellet size, schizophyllan production dropped, despite the increased specific growth rate of the smaller mycelia pellets (Shu et al. 2005).

Although all fungi are obligate aerobic organisms and an adequate aeration is expected to be necessary for submerged fungal cultures, it has been reported that low dissolved oxygen (DO) in the bioreactor, or even DO limitation, can stimulate the biosynthesis of schizophyllan or other fungal glucans, despite limiting cell growth (Rau et al. 1992). This can be attributed to the presence of oxygen-sensitive biosynthetic enzymes, or to a metabolic shift from catabolism and cell growth to glucan biosynthesis under growth-limiting conditions. Shu et al. (2005) tested the effect of different aeration rates upon schizophyllan production (0.05, 0.1, 0.2, 0.5 vvm) and observed that the maximum yield and polysaccharide concentration was achieved at the lowest aeration rate (0.05 vvm). This is a very low aeration rate and differs greatly from the high aeration rates usually applied for the production of bacterial polysaccharides (Borges et al. 2008, Giavasis et al. 2006). Similarly, low DO levels seem to favor exopolysaccharide production by *G. lucidum*, at the expense of cell growth (Tang and Zhong 2003). Lee et al. (2004) observed that the aeration rate had a great impact on the fungal morphology of *G. frondosa*, with low aeration favoring compact cell pellets and a high aeration rate leading to more freely suspended mycelia. This can probably explain the detrimental effect of high aeration for many mushroom polysaccharides, as described above. However, in the case of *G. frondosa*, the optimal morphology for exopolysaccharide production was that of loose mycelia hairy clumps (Lee et al. 2004) and an optimal aeration rate of 1.16 vvm was proposed.

The optimal medium composition for the production of bioactive polysaccharides via submerged cultures differs depending on each fungi and each polysaccharide. Generally, a glucose-based medium is used, although in many cases, a medium based on other sugars or potato extract has led to higher biopolymer yields (Kim et al. 2002). A phosphorous source such as phosphate salts, and a nitrogen source such as peptone, yeast extract, or ammonium salts are used to facilitate biomass growth, but high C/N ratios are usually required, so that nitrogen limitation can halt cell growth at some point during the fermentation and stimulate polysaccharide synthesis (Giavasis 2013). Kumari et al. (2008) noticed that sucrose was the most preferable sugar for schizophyllan production, while organic nitrogen sources such as beef or yeast extract gave rise to high biopolymer synthesis in comparison to inorganic nitrogen sources. For the production of exopolysaccharides of *A. brasiliensis*, glucose (at a relatively low concentration of 10 g/L) and yeast extract were the most suitable carbon and nitrogen sources, respectively (Fan et al. 2007), while the synthesis of exopolysaccharides by *G. lucidum* was optimal when using a medium containing complex carbon and nitrogen sources, namely, potato dextrose broth, peptone, and malt extract (Kim et al. 2002).

The presence of vegetable oils has been reported to enhance the production of fungal biomass and polysaccharide in liquid cultures (Hsieh et al. 2008, Huang et al. 2009), possibly because the assembly of polysaccharides generally takes place via the accumulation of sugar monomers to lipid carriers of the cytoplasmic membrane, where they are subsequently polymerized (Giavasis 2013, Sutherland 1990, Whitfield and Valvano 1993); thus the presence of lipids in the fermentation medium may facilitate this metabolic process. More specifically, Huang et al. (2009) reported a doubling of the mycelia biomass concentration and a ~50% increase in exopolysaccharide production by *G. lucidum* after addition of 2% corn oil in the process medium. Even more interesting was the fact that oil addition also changed fungal morphology, since the fungal pellets changed from spherical to oval, became darker inside, with apparent oil micelles adsorbed on the cell membrane, while the decay of pellets at the late stages of the fermentation was prevented after the addition of corn oil (Huang et al. 2009). Hsieh et al. (2008) reported an increase in biomass concentration in submerged cultures of *G. frondosa*, after the addition of several plant oils (olive, safflower, sunflower, and soybean oil) or surfactants such as Tween 80 or Span 80. However, the production of exopolysaccharide was only stimulated by olive oil, especially at 1% concentration. Taking into account the fact that some bioactive polysaccharide may be isolated from the mycelia (cell wall polysaccharides) while others from the fermentation medium (exopolysaccharides), these results show that one can design the appropriate medium composition according to the type of polysaccharides that need to be isolated.

In contrast to bacterial polysaccharides where genetic or biochemical engineering has been implemented to improve strains and productivity, such approaches are very scarce among mushroom polysaccharides, probably due to the unexplored complex genome of such higher fungi, while information on basic biosynthetic routes is limited to a few industrial fungal biopolymers such as pullulan and scleroglucan, which do not derive from mushrooms (Cheng et al. 2011, Elisashvili 2012, Giavasis 2013, Schmid et al. 2011).

Another issue that must be taken into account with regard to the submerged cultures of fungal mycelia is the potential biosynthesis of fungal glucanases or other lyases that can degrade the biopolymer. Such fungal lyases have been described for pullulan production (Manitchotpisit et al. 2011); however, little is known about the biosynthesis of lyases during the submerged cultivation for the production of bioactive mushroom polysaccharides. Interestingly, Minato et al. (1999) found that lentinan glucanases are produced during the storage of *L. edodes* mushroom, so it is possible that such enzymes are also synthesized in liquid cultures, resulting in a decrease in biopolymer concentration. During the storage of *L. edodes* mushrooms for 7 days at 20°C, lentinan content dropped from 12.8 mg/kg of dry weight to 3.7 mg/kg, while at 5°C storage, the degradation was slower, resulting in a decrease of lentinan content to 9.3 mg/kg (Minato et al. 1999).

The isolation process of medicinal fungal polysaccharides from liquid cultures differs among cell wall polysaccharides, exopolysaccharides, and endopolysaccharides. For the isolation of exopolysaccharides, the downstream processing usually begins with the inactivation of cells and undesirable enzymes by heating. This also enables a better dissociation and separation of exopolysaccharides from the cell membrane. Hot alkali treatment or sonication can be applied to facilitate the separation of biopolymers from the cells (Morin 1998, Wang et al. 2010). Exopolysaccharides are separated from the biomass by filtration or centrifugation, precipitated by the addition of alcohol and further purified (if necessary) by ultrafiltration, gel permeation/ion-exchange chromatography, or dialfiltration. The final product is obtained after vacuum during spray-drying or freeze-drying (Donot et al. 2012, Fan et al. 2012, Giavasis and Biliaderis 2006, Wang et al. 2010). In the case of biopolymers from the mycelial cell wall, a hot water or alkali extraction process is followed, which is similar to the one applied to mushroom fruiting bodies (as described above). Intracellular bioactive polysaccharides, for example, those from *G. lucidum* cells, are obtained after enzymatic, chemical, thermal, or ultrasonic cell lysis in order for the biopolymer to be released from the cytoplasm, and the rest of the separation process is analogous to the one described above for extracellular biopolymers (Habijanic et al. 2001, Liu et al. 2012).

8.4 Medicinal Properties of Mushroom Polysaccharides

Medicinal mushroom polysaccharides act as BRMs, that is, they can alter and enhance immune responses against cancer cells, bacteria and viruses, inflammation, and oxidative stress via an indirect, nonspecific mechanism that potentiates and alerts the human immune system. At the same time, they may act as dietary fibers with hypolipidemic, hypoglycemic, antiatherogenic, or prebiotic properties (Giavasis 2013, Kim et al. 2006, Mizuno and Nishitani 2013, Stachowiak and Reguła 2012, Wasser 2002).

Apart from dose dependence, these properties are closely related to the physicochemical and structural characteristics of each biopolymer, that is, composition of sugar monomers, molecular weight, type of side chains and the degree of branching, presence of a triple or double helix or random coil, presence of peptide–protein complexes and sulfate groups, and solubility. Generally, it has been observed that water solubility (often associated with short side chains and a low degree of branching) and a medium or large molecular weight usually leads to high immunomodulating activity, although low-molecular-weight bioactive polysaccharides have also been described (Bohn and BeMiller 1995, Giavasis 2013, Giavasis and Biliaderis 2006, Kim et al. 2006, Kulicke et al. 1997, Mizuno and Nishitani 2013, Sletmoen and Stokke 2008, Wasser 2002). Furthermore, the downstream and purification process followed for these biopolymers (filtration or water/alkali extraction alcohol/acetone precipitation of the polysaccharide, gel filtration, etc.), as well the drying method used for the formulation of the final product may affect their structural and functional characteristics (Giavasis 2013, Giavasis and Biliaderis 2006, Fan et al. 2012).

Below, the most recent findings on the medicinal properties of mushroom polysaccharides will be summarized, with reference to structure–function relationships and the mode of action.

8.4.1 Immunostimulating and Antitumor Properties

There is now a large volume of *in vitro* studies with human cell lines, as well as a fair amount of clinical studies that explore and verify the immunomodulatory effects of mushroom polysaccharides, especially in relation to their antitumor properties. In these studies, the active substances are mostly used in pure form (polysaccharide solution given intravenously, intraperitoneally, or orally) or sometimes in crude form (i.e., digested as dried mycelia/fruiting bodies), but since these mushrooms contain several medicinal ingredients, only studies on the application of pure polysaccharides can lead to safe conclusions on the bioactivity of specific molecules and their mode of action. At the same time, the incorporation of such biopolymers in functional foods and nutraceuticals may alter their functionality, and clinical studies based on the consumption of therapeutic biopolymers via food and nutraceuticals are needed to establish their medicinal properties in functional foods.

Lentinan and schizophyllan are two of the most well-studied mushroom glucans and many researchers underline their immunostimulating properties (stimulation of secretion of tumor necrosis factor-α (TNF-α) by human monocytes and activation of macrophages, or platelet hemopoietic activity), and specifically their effects against gastric, breast, lung, cervical, or colorectal cancer, especially when combined with conventional (synthetic) antitumor drugs (chemotherapy) or radiotherapy, although they usually do not exhibit a direct tumor-killing capacity. Moreover, they can prevent metastasis and minimize the side effects of chemotherapy and radiotherapy upon the healthy tissue (Chang and Wasser 2012, Giavasis 2013, Ikekawa 2001, Lo et al. 2011, Stachowiak and Reguła 2012). Clinical studies on the therapeutic effects of lentinan showed that it improves the survival of patients with advanced gastric cancer significantly, when it is used in combination with standard chemotherapy (compared to chemotherapy alone) (Oba et al. 2009). These β-glucans exhibit no toxicity to humans even at high dosages, and are more effective when administered in the early stages of cancer treatment. Their bioactivity has been connected to the high molecular weight of these β-glucans and the presence of a triple helix conformation (Falch et al. 2000, Giavasis and Biliaderis 2006, Lo et al. 2011, Sletmoen and Stokke 2008). Both these mushroom glucans are poorly absorbed in the intestine after oral intake, so in most clinical or animal trials, they are injected intrapleurally, intraperitoneally, or intravenously (Chan et al., 2009, Giavasis 2013).

The glucans from *G. frondosa* and *T. versicolor* have also been used in clinical trials where they increased the survival rate and survival time on patients suffering from different types of cancer, especially when supplied in combination with chemotherapy or when administered after surgery, in order to prevent metastasis (Lindequist et al. 2005, Stachowiak and Reguła 2012).

In a phase I/II trial of a polysaccharide extract from *G. frondosa* administered orally to breast cancer patients, it was observed that the intake of the polysaccharide preparation increased cytokine production (IL-2, TNF-α, and IL-10) by immune cells by over 50% compared to a control group (Deng et al. 2009).

Krestin (also known as PSK), the medicinal biopolymer extracted from *T. versicolor*, is used in Asia as a complementary cancer treatment due to its immunostimulating, antimetastatic, and direct antitumor effects (Kobayashi et al. 1995). Krestin was also shown to have TLR2-agonist activities and to stimulate dendritic cells (DC) and T cells in murine models of breast cancer, where it significantly inhibited cancer growth (Lu et al. 2011). Similarly, in *in vitro* studies of mice with prostate cancer, PSK enhanced mRNA expression of interferon-γ (IFN-γ) compared to the control, and when used in combination with docetaxel drug it increased the survival rate of white blood cells and induced splenic natural killer (NK) cell cytolytic activity (Wenner et al. 2012). In clinical studies with crude preparation of *T. versicolor* dry mushroom powder given to women with breast cancer after standard chemotherapy and radiotherapy, up to 9 g/day appeared to be safe and tolerable in the postprimary treatment and could improve the immune status in the immunocompromised patients (Torkelson et al. 2012). However, clinical studies with purified polysaccharides of *Trametes (Coriolus) versicolor* were not conducted in this study.

Ganoderan is another fungal biopolymer that has been used as adjuvant cancer therapy, as it increases the cytotoxic effect of chemotherapy and enhances the immune responses in patients with prostate cancer (Mahajna et al. 2009, Vannucci et al. 2013, Yuen and Gohel 2005). *G. lucidum* polysaccharides and proteoglucans are also reported to prolong the survival of mice with Lewis carcinoma, to increase the excretion of TNF-α and IFN-γ in blood serum in a dose-dependent manner, to stimulate the expression of macrophages and T-cell immunity, to facilitate the recovery of splenic and lymphokine NK cells in immunosuppressed mice, and to exhibit prophylactic activity toward chemically injured macrophages (Ganeshpurkar et al. 2010, Nie et al. 2013b, Stachowiak and Reguła 2012, You and Lin 2002, Yuen and Gohel 2005).

The glucans and proteoglucans from *A. blazei* have been very effective against different types of sarcomas and carcinomas in mice, in stimulating the excretion of IFN-γ, and also capable of suppressing allergic reactions (antiallergic immunomodulation) (Firenzuoli et al. 2008, Mizuno and Nishitani 2013). The *A. blazei* proteoglucans activate a number of immune system cells (macrophages, interferons, T cells, and NK cells) in order to halt the multiplication, metastasis, and recurrence of cancer cells (Fujimiya et al. 1998, Lakhanpal 2005).

Water or methanolic extracts of *P. ostreatus* β-glucans can induce apoptosis in human prostate cancer and suppress the proliferation of human breast and colon cancer cells (Asaduzzaman and Mousumi 2012). Similarly, the β-glucans from the fruiting body extracts of *P. tuber-regium* exhibit antiproliferative activity against several human cancer cell lines (Zhang et al. 2001), while the proteoglucan extracts from the sclerotia of the same mushroom were found to activate innate immune cells such as macrophages, and T-helper cells *in vivo* (in mice) in order to destroy tumor cells (Wong et al. 2011).

The antitumor and immunomodulatory polysaccharides from other medicinal mushroom exhibit a similar mode of action (Ooi and Liu, 2000, Zhang et al. 2007). This action is a combination of mechanisms that include a mitogenic activity of soluble glucans, stimulation of NK cells, T cells, DCs, neutrophils, and monocytes, enhanced phagocytosis, and excretion of cytokines (Chan et al. 2009, Giavasis 2013, Mizuno and Nishitani 2013, Wasser 2002). A simplified illustration of the immunostimulatory mechanisms of fungal glucans and proteoglucans is shown in Figure 8.3.

8.4.2 Antioxidant Properties

Polysaccharides extracted from *G. lucidum, T. versicolor, L. edodes, P. linteus,* and *Agaricus* mushrooms have reducing power abilities and chelating properties and can inhibit lipid oxidation or reduce oxidative stress. This effect

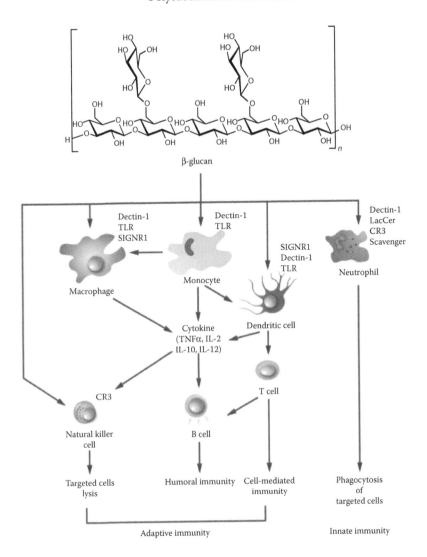

Figure 8.3 Postulated mechanisms of immunostimulatory fungal β-glucans: β-glucans are attached to membrane receptors of the immune cells (such as dectin, TLR) and subsequently activate macrophages, monocytes DCs, NK cells, B cells, T cells, and neutrophils, while they can also stimulate the excretion of cytokines, such as tumor necrosis factor (TNF)-α and interleukins (ILs). This immunostimulation may be either an innate or adaptive immune response. (Adapted from Chan, G. C. F., W. K. Chan, and D. M. U. Sze. 2009. *J Hematol Oncol* 2:25–36.)

was correlated with the presence of a β-glucan and a phenolic (mainly tyrosine and ferrulic acid) moiety bound to the β-glucan main chain by covalent bonds (Giavasis 2013, Kozarski et al. 2011, Yu et al. 2009). Although the phenolic compounds present in *G. lucidum* fruiting bodies and mycelia are the compounds with the highest antioxidant activity, *G. lucidum* polysaccharides also exhibit free radical-scavenging properties, reducing power and inhibition of lipid peroxidation (Heleno et al. 2012, Tseng et al. 2008). Saltarelli et al. (2009) stated that among different polysaccharides of *G. lucidum* extracted from mycelia, the low-molecular-weight polysaccharides had the highest antioxidative activity, based on the chelating activity on Fe^{2+}, lipoxygenase assay, and 1,1-diphenyl-dipicrylhydrazyl (DPPH) free radical scavenging, while intracellular polysaccharides were ineffective as antioxidants. Also, *in vitro* studies showed that the *G. lucidum* peptidoglucan could protect the mitochondria, endoplasmic reticulum, and microvilli of macrophages from chemically induced damage and malfunction (You and Lin 2002). In addition, methanolic extracts of *G. lucidum* and *G. tsugae* glucans and proteoglucans act as antioxidants by scavenging reactive oxygen species (ROS), which are linked both to oncogenesis and to lipid oxidation (Lakhanpal and Rana 2005). Another mechanism of antioxidant activity is the ability of some mushroom polysaccharides (e.g., those from *G. lucidum*) to limit the production of oxygen-free radicals and the activity of peripheral mononuclear cells in murine peritoneal macrophages, which are related to the respiratory burst and the ageing process (Xie et al. 2012, You and Lin 2002), or to enhance the activity of antioxidant enzymes in blood serum (XiaoPing et al. 2009). Methanolic extracts from *G. frondosa, M. esculenta,* and *Termitomyces albuminosus* mycelia have also exhibited antioxidant properties, but these were mainly associated with the presence of phenolic compounds in the extract (Mau et al. 2004). In submerged cultures of *H. erinaceum* with the addition of selenium sources (sodium selenite and Selol) in the fermentation medium, a selenium-containing exopolysaccharide was produced, which showed excellent antioxidant capacity, based on reducing power, inhibition of lipid peroxidation, and DPPH radical scavenging (Malinowska et al. 2009). Interestingly, Selol also induced a 2.5-fold increase in the formation of the exopolysaccharide. Other antioxidant mushroom polysaccharides include the polysaccharides from water-soluble extracts of *A. auricula* and *C. militaris* fruiting bodies, which showed free radical-scavenging, chelating, and reducing power properties, and an increase in the total antioxidant capacity (Chen et al. 2008, Luo et al. 2009, Wu et al. 2011).

8.4.3 Antimicrobial Properties

Mushroom polysaccharides are active against bacterial and viral infections *in vitro* or *in vivo,* as they can stimulate the phagocytosis of microbes by neutrophils and macrophages. Lentinan has shown antimicrobial activity against *Listeria monocytogenes, Staphylococcus aureus, Salmonella enteritis, Escherichia coli,* as well as tuberculosis (Giavasis 2013, Mattila et al. 2000, van Nevel et al. 2003). In addition, crude extracts from different *Agaricus* fruiting bodies restricted the growth of *S. aureus, Bacillus subtilis,* and *B. cereus,* although the antimicrobial effect might also be due to nonpolysaccharide components of these extracts (Barros et al. 2008). Several mushroom glucans are reported to have antiviral activity, which is believed to occur via the increased release of IFN-γ and enhanced proliferation of peripheral blood mononuclear cells (PBMC) (Lindequist et al. 2005, Markova et al. 2002, Sasidhara and Thirunalasundari 2012). Ganoderan has exhibited antiviral activity against the herpes virus, schizophyllan can enhance immune responses of hepatitis B patients, while lentinan has expressed significant antiviral activity against influenza virus and polio virus (Eo et al. 2000, Kakumu et al. 1991, Sasidhara and Thirunalasundari 2012). Notably, lentinan and an acidic *G. lucidum* proteoglucan have been applied successfully as adjunct therapy of HIV in combination with conventional anti-HIV drugs, as they could enhance host resistance to the HIV virus, and limit the toxicity of synthetic anti-HIV drugs. Similar anti-HIV activities were also reported for glucans from *G. frondosa* and *T. versicolor* (Giavasis and Biliaderis 2006, Lindequist et al. 2005, Markova et al. 2002, Sasidhara and Thirunalasundari 2012). Selegean et al. (2009) studied the antiviral activity of expolysaccharides of *P. ostreatus* against the infectious bursal disease virus in young broilers and noticed an enhanced antiviral activity, stimulation of maternal antibodies, and increased survival rate when the biopolymer was used (as part of the daily water intake) alone or in combination with conventional antiviral vaccines. As the antimicrobial activity of mushroom glucans seems to be indirect and related to immunomodulation (Giavasis and Biliaderi 2006), and to affect the intestinal microflora after oral administration (van Nevel et al. 2003), it seems feasible to formulate glucan-based nutraceuticals with prophylactic antimicrobial properties.

8.4.4 Hypolipidemic, Hypoglycemic, and Prebiotic Properties

Most of the bioactive mushroom polysaccharides can serve as dietary fiber, as they cannot be digested in the human intestine (Giavasis 2013). Fungal glucans from *L. edodes*, *G. lucidum*, *S. commune*, *P. ostreatus*, *G. frondosa*, *A. blazei*, *C. sinensis*, and *Cordiceps miltaris* are able to reduce blood sugar and serum cholesterol according to several animal and human studies (Chen et al. 2013, Lakhanpal and Rana 2005, Lindequist et al. 2005).

Hypoglycemic effects occur via the attachment of the indigestible polysaccharides to the intestinal epithelium, which decelerates glucose absorption, while hypolipidemic effects are due to the interruption of the enterohepatic circulation of bile acids, which favors their excretion in the feces (Giavasis 2013, Lakhanpal and Rana 2005).

Also, bioactive mushroom polysaccharides exert a hypoglycemic effect via the modulation of carbohydrate metabolism and insulin synthesis. For instance, glucans from *G. frondosa* exhibit antidiabetic and antiobesity properties (Lakhanpal and Rana 2005). An acidic xylomannan of *T. mesenterica* has been shown to regulate glycemic responses in normal and diabetic rats after ingestion, by decreasing serum concentration of fructosamines (Lo et al. 2006). The effectiveness of orally administered polysaccharides is important as they can be utilized as active components in functional foods for diabetic people.

According to Zhou et al. (2009), polysaccharide extracts of *C. sinensis* exhibit hypoglycemic, hypolipidemic, and antihypertensive effects, while alcohol extracts of this mushroom protect against myocardial injury (induced by adriamycin in rats), due to the mannitol, amino acids, and polysaccharides present in the extracts, which have a nourishing effect upon the myocardium and induce its anti-injury capacity.

Lentinan has been used as a hypocholesterolemic agent in humans, as it reduces the blood levels of lipoproteins [both high density lipoproteins (HDL) and low density lipoproteins (LDL)] (Lakhanpal and Rana 2005). In addition, glucan-rich water extracts from *P. ostreatus* are reported to decrease the formation of atherogenic plaques in animal studies (Bobek and Galbavy 1999). Notably, in the case of *P. ostreatus* extracts, other nonpolysaccharide molecules the mushroom contains may also contribute to the cholesterol-lowering effect, such as plovatin, lovastatin, or menivolin, which inhibit 3-hydroxy-3-methylglutaryl CoA reductase, the major rate-limiting enzyme in the cholesterol biosynthetic pathway (Gunde-Cimerman 1993, Gunde-Cimerman and Cimerman 1995, Lakhanpal and Rana 2005). In recognition of the dietary fiber effects of *Pleurotus* mushroom, the National Mushroom Development and Extension Centre in Bangladesh recommends a daily dosage in human diet, which ranges from 5 to 10 g of dried mushroom for healthy individuals to 20 g for patients with diabetes, hypertension, cardiovascular complications, or cancer (Asaduzzaman and Mousumi 2012).

Chen et al. (2008) studied the hypolipidemic effects of polysaccharides extracted from *A. auricula* in hypercholesterolemic mice after a daily oral administration of 120 mg/kg body weight. Their results pointed out that the polysaccharides significantly lowered the concentrations of serum total cholesterol and LDL-cholesterol, improved lipoprotein lipase activity, and reduced lipid peroxidation and atherosclerotic index, showing a prophylactic activity against hypercholesterolemia. Similar hypolipidemic effects were also obtained by Luo et al. (2009) after an oral administration of 300 mg/kg/day of *A. auricula* polysaccharide in hyperlipidemic mice. The antithrombotic activity of purified acidic glucans from extracts of *A. auricula* was found to be equivalent to that of aspirin and depended largely upon the glucuronic acid content of the biopolymer, which activated antithrombin (a thrombin inhibitor), causing an inhibition of platelet aggregation in rats orally fed with the polysaccharide (Yoon et al. 2003).

In other studies, the hypocholesterolemic effect of *T. fuciformis* on hyperlipidemic mice was described, which reduced total blood cholesterol and LDL-cholesterol, without affecting the levels of the HDL fraction. Furthermore, the crude preparations of *T. fuciformis* reduced triacylglycerol levels in the serum and total cholesterol levels in the liver (Cheng et al. 2002, Guillamón et al. 2010).

The prebiotic effects of edible mushroom polysaccharides have also been described by many researchers. As the human digestive enzyme is unable to hydrolyze β-glucosidic bonds, several mushroom polysaccharides are capable of acting as a source of prebiotics (Aida et al. 2009). Synytsya et al. (2009) tested the prebiotic effect of glucans isolated from fruiting bodies of *P. ostreatus* and *P. eryngii* on several *Lactobacillus*, *Bifidibacterium*, and *Enterococcus* probiotic strains. Both water-soluble branched β-1,3/β-1,6-glucans and alkali-soluble linear α-1,3-glucans of these mushrooms were found to stimulate the growth of probiotic bacteria, especially those from *P. eryngii*. In another study, β-glucans from the sclerotia of *P. tuber-regium* were evaluated for their bifidogenic effect on *Bifidobacterium infantis*, *Bifidobacterium longum*, and *Bifidobacterium adolescentis* in liquid cultures, using inulin as a control prebiotic (Zhao and Cheung 2011). It was shown that after a 24-h fermentation, the populations of bifidobacteria supplemented with mushroom glucan had a 3–4 log increase in their population, which was similar to the increase achieved by the addition of inulin (Zhao and Cheung 2011).

Recently, Chou et al. (2013) reported that polysaccharides from mushroom waste, namely, *L. edodes* stipe, *P. eryngii* base, and *F. velutipes* base, can increase the survival rate of *Lactobacillus acidophilus*, *Lactobacillus casei*, and *B. longum* in refrigerated yogurt. The authors observed synergistic effects of these polysaccharides with the peptides and amino acids from a yogurt culture, which maintained probiotics above 10^7 cfu/mL during cold storage. They also noticed that the mushroom polysaccharides had a significant protective effect (increased survival rate) on the probiotic bacteria in simulated gastric and bile juice.

8.5 Applications of Mushroom Bioactive Polysaccharides in Functional Foods and Nutraceuticals

Many of the above-mentioned bioactive polysaccharides have been used as purified molecules in pharmaceutical studies *in vitro* or *in vivo*, and some of them have formed the basis of novel drugs (especially anticancer drugs) but few of them have been commercialized worldwide as novel nutraceuticals. In Asia, however, such dietary and therapeutic food products have entered the market in the last few years, and their regular intake is believed (or claimed) to boost human health (Lakhanpal and Rana 2005). It is thought that some issues of production economics, quality standardization, and stable availability need to be resolved and that clinical studies on the therapeutic effects and the effective dosages of such functional foods need to be performed in order to allow a more global commercialization (Giavasis 2013, Wasser 2011).

In order to consolidate a health claim for nutraceuticals based on mushroom polysaccharides, apart from the pharmacological studies with pure polysaccharide solutions, one needs to consider the potential impact of food processing (heating, high-pressure, irradiation, acidification, etc.) and food physicochemical properties and composition (pH, moisture, presence of other biopolymers, enzymes, organic acids, and salts) on the bioactivity of the medicinal biopolymers. For example, ganoderan can be degraded by pectinases and dextranases, which may limit its bioactivity in a food matrix containing these enzymes (Xie et al. 2012). Moreover, when lentinan interacted with carrageenans, its antitumor capacity was reduced (Maeda and Chihara 1999). With regard to the effect of the heating and drying methods on the bioactivity of mushroom glucans, Fan et al. (2012) showed that freeze drying, in comparison to vacuum drying and heat drying, was the best method of drying G. lucidum polysaccharides in order to retain their antioxidant properties, measured as reducing powder and DPPH, hydroxyl radicals, and superoxide radical-scavenging ability. Heat drying was by far the least favorable method for retaining antioxidant activity (Fan et al. 2012). Apart from reducing antioxidant capacity, heating may also alter the composition of mushrooms. Indeed, after boiling several types of mushrooms (Agaricus bisporus, L. edodes, G. frondosa, and F. velutipes) for 10 min, it was observed that total dietary fiber content was increased while chitin and crude protein content was reduced. However, β-glucan concentration was largely unaffected by boiling (Dikeman et al. 2005).

There are several examples of novel nutraceuticals and functional foods that have recently been developed based on bioactive mushroom polysaccharides. Glucans from L. edodes have been successfully applied as a partial replacement of wheat flour in fiber-rich, low-calorie functional baked foods (with up to 2% glucan concentration), where they improved pasting parameters, batter viscosity, and elasticity, or in noodles where they conferred antioxidant and hypocholesterolemic effects and improved quality characteristics (Kim et al. 2009, 2011). Fan et al. (2006) produced a functional bread where wheat flour was partly substituted with A. auricula polysaccharides. In this study, an up to 9% substitution of flour with bioactive polysaccharides markedly increased the antioxidant capacity of bread (tested as DPPH free radical-scavenging ability), without altering the palatability and acceptance of the blended bread. The same mushroom was the main functional ingredient (along with Hawthorn fruit) in another experimental nutraceutical containing ethanolic extracts of A. auricula and Hawthorn, which exhibited antioxidant and hypolipidemic properties in vitro and in animal studies (Luo et al. 2009).

Interestingly, Okamura-Matsui et al. (2001) produced a functional cheese-like food containing live cultures of S. commune. In their novel approach, the fungus was added as a proteolytic, milk-clotting starter culture, which was also able to ferment lactose and produce up to 0.58% β-glucan in this novel "cheese," which had significant antithrombotic effects.

In other studies, the use of mushroom polysaccharides or mushroom powder has been proposed for the formulation of functional snack food. For instance, oyster mushroom powder has been added in an Indian papad snack to improve its fiber content while *Agaricus* extracts were utilized in snacks offering high antioxidant and free radical-scavenging properties (Parab et al. 2012, Singla et al. 2009). Similarly, snack foods where starch was partially replaced (by up to 15%) by powdered extracts of *Agrocybe aegerita* (chestnut mushroom) had a low glycemic response after consumption, due to the dietary fiber content (Brennan et al. 2012). *A. brasiliensis* polysaccharides have also been suggested as a functional ingredient in antiobesity and antidiabetic functional foods (Yamanaka et al. 2013).

With regard to sensory characteristics and consumer acceptance, a potential additional advantage of using mushroom polysaccharides in functional foods may be the fact that some mushroom crude extracts also contain monosodium glutamate-like components and an intense umami taste, which might improve the flavor of the final product (Tsai et al. 2006, Tseng et al. 2005).

In China, there are nowadays several commercial nutraceutical products that are based on medicinal mushroom extracts and mushrooms biopolymers. For instance, a tonic liquor made of extracts of *L. edodes, Poria cocos,* and *G. lucidum*, which is claimed to have anticarcinogenic, antiviral, and hypolipidemic effects, and a similar potable extract of *C. sinensis, G. lucidum,* and some medicinal herbs, which is marketed as an antiageing dietary supplement that improves cardiovascular function and reduces blood lipids (Xu 2001). Also, in a traditional Chinese medicine recipe, which could form the basis of a novel nutraceutical, a soup of *A. auricula* and *Tremella* mushrooms is recommended for the treatment of hypertension (Xu 2001). Other marketed mushroom-based nutraceuticals (found mostly in Asia) include "Reishi Plus" (50% *G. lucidum* and 50% *L. edodes* extract), which is a daily nutritional supplement for good health vitality, "Trimyco-Gene" (33% *C. sinensis*, 33% *G. lucidum*, 33% *L. edodes*), which is a good immunomodulant that is supposed to promote good health and longevity, "Mycoplex-7" (14% *C. sinensis*, 14% *T. fuciformis*, 14% *A. blazei*, 14% *C. versicolor*, 14% *P. cocos*, 14% *S. commune*, 14% *Hericium erinaceous*), which is believed to promote general health vitality, and the "Garden of Life" (RM-120), which contains 10 medicinal mushrooms, along with *Aloe vera* and *Uncaria tomentosa*, and is said to stimulate the immune system, offer antitumor, antiviral, and antibacterial protection, regulate blood cholesterol, and facilitate the treatment of cardiovascular diseases (Lakhanpal and Rana 2005).

8.6 Conclusions

Medicinal mushrooms are a very interesting and versatile source of bioactive polysaccharides (and other medicinal compounds), which exhibit numerous therapeutic properties and are or can be at the core of the development of novel functional foods and nutraceuticals. As most of the studied mushroom biopolymers derive from edible mushrooms and are nontoxic, and some of them are already used as pharmaceuticals in purified form, the idea of utilizing them as a general-purpose dietary and health-fortifying food, or as a specialized therapeutic edible supplement for groups of patients (e.g., suffering from cancer or cardiovascular diseases) becomes very attractive.

However, one has to bear in mind that the production of nutraceuticals and functional foods based on such biopolymers requires a thorough understanding of structure–function relationships, an economically viable and controllable production process and a stable polysaccharide quality. In addition, such products will require clinical studies to prove their therapeutic efficacy and the relative health claims, in order to be adopted in a global market. Although at a relatively early stage yet, the development of functional foods and nutraceuticals based on mushroom polysaccharides seems to have great potential and a bright future.

References

Aida, F. M. N. A., M. Shuhaimi, M. Yazid, and A. G. Maaruf. 2009. Mushroom as a potential source of prebiotics: A review. *Trends Food Sci Technol* 20:567–575.

Aleem, E. 2013. β-Glucans and their applications in cancer therapy: Focus on human studies. *Anti-Cancer Agent Med Chem* 13:709–719.

Asaduzzaman, K. and T. Mousoumi. 2012. Nutritional and medicinal importance of *Pleurotus* mushrooms: An overview. *Food Rev Int* 28:313–329.

Bao, X. F., X. S. Wang, Q. Dong, J. N. Fang, and X. Y. Li. 2002. Structural features of immunologically active polysaccharides from *Ganoderma lucidum*. *Phytochemistry* 59:175–181.

Barros, L., T. Cruz, P. Baptista, L. M. Estevinho, and I. C. F. R. Ferreira. 2008. Wild and commercial mushrooms as source of nutrients and nutraceuticals. *Food Chem Toxicol* 46:2742–2747.

Bergendiova, K., E. Tibenska, and J. Majtan. 2011. Pleuran (β-glucan from *Pleurotus ostreatus*) supplementation, cellular immune response and respiratory tract infections in athletes. *Eur J Appl Physiol* 111:2033–2040.

Bisen, P. S., R. K. Baghel, B. S. Sanodiya, G. S. Thakur, and G. B. K. S. Prasad. 2010. *Lentinus edodes*: A macrofungus with pharmacological activities. *Curr Med Chem* 17:2419–2430.

Bobek, P. and S. Galbavy. 1999. Hypocholesteremic and antiatherogenic effect of oyster mushroom (*Pleurotus ostreatus*) in rabbits. *Nahrung* 43:339–342.

Boh, B. and M. Berovic. 2007. *Grifola frondosa* (Diks.:Fr.) S. F. Gray: (Maitake mushroom): Medicinal properties, active compounds, and biotechnological cultivation. *Int J Med Mushrooms* 9:89–108.

Bohn, J. A. and J. N. BeMiller. 1995. (1 → 3)-β-D-glucans as biological response modifiers: A review of structure-functional activity relationships. *Carbohydr Polym* 28:3–14.

Borges, C. D., A. S. daMoreira, C. T. Vendruscolo, and M. A. Ayub. 2008. Influence of agitation and aeration in xanthan production by *Xanthomonas campestris* pv pruni strain 101. *Rev Argent Microbiol* 40:81–85.

Brennan, M. A., E. Derbyshire, B. K. Tiwari, and C. S. Brennan. 2012. Enrichment of extruded snack products with coproducts from chestnut mushroom (*Agrocybe aegerita*) production: Interactions between dietary fiber, physicochemical characteristics, and glycemic load. *J Agric Food Chem* 60:4396–4401.

Camelini, C. M., M. Maraschin, M. M. de Mendonca, C. Zucco, A. G. Ferreira, and L. A. Tavares. 2005. Structural characterization of β-glucans of *Agaricus brasiliensis* in different stages of fruiting body maturity and their use in nutraceutical products. *Biotech Lett* 27:1295–1299.

Chan, G. C. F., W. K. Chan, and D. M. U. Sze. 2009. The effects of β-glucan on human immune and cancer cells. *J Hematol Oncol* 2:25–36.

Chang, S. T. and S. P. Wasser 2012. The Role of culinary-medicinal mushrooms on human welfare with a pyramid model for human health. *Int J Med Mushr* 14:95–134.

Chang, S. T. 1993. Mushroom biology: The impact on mushroom production and mushroom products. In *Proceedings of the First International Conference on Mushroom Biology and Mushroom Products*, ed. S. T. Chang, S. W. Chiu, and J. A. Buswell, 3–20. Hong Kong: The Chinese University Press.

Chen, G., Y. C. Luo, B. P. Ji et al. 2008. Effect of polysaccharide from *Auricularia auricula* on blood lipid metabolism and lipoprotein lipase activity of ICR mice fed a cholesterol-enriched diet. *J Food Sci* 73:103–108.

Chen, P. X., S. Wang, S. Nie, and M. Marcone. 2013. Properties of *Cordyceps sinensis*: A review. *J Funct Food* 5:550–569.

Cheng, H. H., W. C. Hou, and M. L. Lu. 2002. Interactions of lipid metabolism and intestinal physiology with *Tremella fuciformis* Berk edible mushroom in rats fed a high-cholesterol diet with or without nebacitin. *Agric Food Chem* 50:7438–7443.

Cheng, K. C., A. Demirci, and J. M. Catchmark. 2011. Pullulan: Biosynthesis, production, and applications. *Appl Microbiol Biotechnol* 92:29–44.

Cho, S. M., J. S. Park, K. P. Kim, D. Y. Cha, H. M. Kim, and I. D. Yoo. 1999. Chemical features and purification of immunostimulating polysaccharides from the fruit bodies of *Agaricus blazei*. *Korean J Mycol* 27:170–174.

Chou, W. T., I. C. Sheih, and T. J. Fang. 2013. Various mushroom wastes as prebiotics in different systems. *J Food Sci* 78:M1041–M1048.

Cui, F. J., W. Y. Tao, Z. H. Xu et al. 2007. Structural analysis of anti-tumor heteropolysaccharide GFPS1b from the cultured mycelia of *Grifola frondosa* GF9801. *Biores Technol* 98:395–401.

De Baets, S. and E. J. Vandamme. 2001. Extracellular *Tremella* polysaccharides: Structure, properties and applications. *Biotechnol Lett* 23:1361–1366.

Deng, G., H. Lin, A. Seidman et al. 2009. A phase I/II trial of a polysaccharide extract from *Grifola frondosa* (Maitake mushroom) in breast cancer patients: Immunological effects. *J Cancer Res Clin Oncol* 135:1215–1221.

Dikeman, C. L., L. L. Bauer, E. A. Flickinger, and G. C. Jr. Fahey. 2005. Effects of stage of maturity and cooking on the chemical composition of select mushroom varieties. *J Agric Food Chem* 53:1130–1138.

Donot, F., A. Fontana, J. C. Baccou, and S. Schorr-Galindo. 2012. Microbial exopolysaccharides: Main examples of synthesis, excretion, genetics and extraction. *Carbohydr Polym* 87:951–962.

Duncan, C. J. G., N. Pugh, D. S. Pasco, and S. A. Ross. 2002. Isolation of a galactomannan that enhances macrophage activation from the edible fungus *Morchella esculenta*. *J Agric Food Chem* 50:5683–5685.

Elisashvili, V. 2012. Submerged cultivation of medicinal mushrooms: Bioprocesses and products (review). *Int J Med Mushr* 14:211–239.

Eo, S. K., Y. S. Kim, C. K. Lee, and S. S. Han. 2000. Possible mode of antiviral activity of acidic protein bound polysaccharide isolated from *Ganoderma lucidum* on herpes simplex viruses, *J Ethnopharm* 72:475–481.

Falch, B. H., T. Espevik, L. Ryan, and B. T. Stokke. 2000. The cytokine stimulating activity of $(1 \rightarrow 3)$-β-D-glucans is dependent on the triple helix conformation. *Carbohydr Res* 329:587–596.

Fan, L., J. Li, K. Deng, and L. Ai. 2012. Effects of drying methods on the antioxidant activities of polysaccharides extracted from *Ganoderma lucidum*. *Carbohydr Polym* 87:1849–1854.

Fan, L., S. Zhang, L. Yu, and L. Ma. 2006. Evaluation of antioxidant property and quality of breads containing *Auricularia auricula* polysaccharide flour. *Food Chem* 101:1158–1163.

Fan, L., A. T. Soccol, A. Pandey, and C. R. Soccol. 2007. Effect of nutritional and environmental conditions on the production of exo-polysaccharide of *Agaricus brasiliensis* by submerged fermentation and its antitumor activity. *LWT* 40:30–35.

FAO (Food and Agriculture Organization of the United Nations). 2011. FAOSTAT—FAO Statistics Division, Data for Worldwide Production of Crops. http://faostat. fao.org/site/567/DesktopDefault.aspx?PageID=567#ancor (accessed: September 6, 2013).

Firenzuoli, F., L. Gori, and G. Lombard. 2008. The medicinal mushroom *Agaricus blazei* Murrill: Review of literature and pharmaco-toxicological problems. *Evid Based Complement Altern Med* 5:3–15.

Fujimiya, Y., Y. Suzuki, K. Oshiman et al. 1998. Selective tumoricidal effect of soluble proteoglucan extracted from the basidiomycete *Agaricus blazei* Murill, mediated via the natural killer cell activation and apoptosis. *Cancer Immunol Immunother* 46:147–159.

Ganeshpurkar, A., G. Rai, and A. P. Jain. 2010. Medicinal mushrooms: Towards a new horizon. *Pharmacogn Rev* 4:127–135.

Giavasis, I. 2013. Production of microbial polysaccharides for use in food. In *Microbial Production of Food Ingredients, Enzymes and Nutraceuticals*, ed. B. McNeil, D. Archer, I. Giavasis, and L. M. Harvey, pp. 413–468. Cambridge: Woodhead Publishing.

Giavasis, I. and C. Biliaderis. 2006. Microbial polysaccharides. In *Functional Food Carbohydrates*, ed. C. Biliaderis, and M. Izydorczyk, pp. 167–214. Boca Raton: CRC Press.

Giavasis, I., L. M. Harvey, and B. McNeil. 2006. The effect of agitation and aeration on the synthesis and molecular weight of gellan in batch cultures of *Sphingomonas paucimobilis*. *Enzyme Microb Technol* 38:101–108.

Guillamón, E., A. García-Lafuente, M. Lozano et al. 2010. Edible mushrooms: Role in the prevention of cardiovascular diseases. *Fitoterap* 81:715–723.

Gunde-Cimerman, N. and A. Cimerman. 1995. *Pleurotus* fruiting bodies contain the inhibitor of 3-hydroxy-3-methylglutaryl-coenzyme A reductase-lovastatin. *Exp Mycol* 19:1–6.

Gunde-Cimerman, N., A. Plemenitag, and A. Cimerman. 1993. *Pleurotus* fungi produce mevinolin, an inhibitor of HMG CoA reductase. *FEMS Microbiol Lett*, 113:333–337.

Habijanic, J., M. Berovic, B. Wraber, D. Hodzar, and B. Boh. 2001. Immunostimulatory effects of fungal polysaccharides from *Ganoderma lucidum* submerged biomass cultivation. *Food Technol Biotechnol* 39:327–331.

Heleno, S. A., L. Barros, A. Martins, M. J. R. P. Queiroz, C. Santos-Buelga, and I. C. F. R. Ferreira. 2012. Fruiting body, spores and *in vitro* produced mycelium of *Ganoderma lucidum* from Northeast Portugal: A comparative study of the antioxidant potential of phenolic and polysaccharidic extracts. *Food Res Int* 46:135–140.

Hobbs, C. 2004. Medicinal value of Turkey Tail fungus *Trametes versicolor* (L.:Fr.) Pilát (*Aphyllophoromycetideae*). *Int J Med Mushrooms* 6:195–218.

Hsieh, C., H. L. Wang, C. C. Chena, T. H. Hsub, and M. H. Tseng. 2008. Effect of plant oil and surfactant on the production of mycelial biomass and polysaccharides in submerged culture of *Grifola frondosa*. *Biochem Eng J* 38:198–205.

Huang, H. C., C. I. Chen, C. N. Hung, and Y. C. Liu. 2009. Experimental analysis of the oil addition effect on mycelia and polysaccharide productions in *Ganoderma lucidum* submerged culture. *Bioproc Biosyst Eng* 32:217–224.

Ikekawa, T. 2001. Beneficial effects of edible and medicinal mushrooms in health care. *Int J Med Mushrooms* 3:291–298.

Jeong, S. C., B. K. Yang, K. S. Ra et al. 2004. Characteristics of anti-complementary biopolymer extracted from *Coriolus versicolor*. *Carbohydr Polym* 55:255–263.

Jeurink, P. V., C. L. Noguera, H. F. J. Savelkoul, and H. J. Wichers. 2008. Immunomodulatory capacity of fungal proteins on the cytokine production of human peripheral blood mononuclear cells. *Int Immunopharmacol* 8:1124–1133.

Kakumu, S., T. Ishikawa, T. Wakita, K. Yoshioka, Y. Ito, and T. Shinagawa. 1991. Effect of sizofiran, a polysaccharide, on interferon gamma, antibody production and lymphocyte proliferation specific for hepatitis-B virus antigen in patients with chronic hepatitis-B. *Int J Immunopharm* 13:969–975.

Khan, M. A., T. Mousumi, D. Z. Zhang, and H. C. Chen. 2010. *Cordyceps* mushroom: A potent anticancer nutraceutical. *Open Nutraceut J* 3:179–183.

Khondkar, P. 2009. Composition and partial structure characterization of *Tremella* polysaccharides. *Mycobiology* 37:286–294.

Kim, G., G. Choi, S. Lee, and Y. Park. 2004. Acidic polysaccharide isolated from *Phellinus linteus* enhances through the up-regulation of nitric oxide and tumor necrosis factor-alpha from peritoneal macrophages. *J Ethnopharmacol* 95:69–76.

Kim, J., S. Lee, I. Y. Bae, H. G. Park, H. G. Lee, and S. Lee. 2011. (1–3)(1–6)-β-Glucan-enriched materials from *Lentinus edodes* mushroom as a high-fibre and low-calorie flour substitute for baked foods. *J Sci Food Agric* 91:1915–1919.

Kim, S. W., H. J. Hwang, J. P. Park, Y. J. Cho, C. H. Song, and J. W. Yun. 2002. Mycelial growth and exo-biopolymer production by submerged culture of various edible mushrooms under different media. *Lett Appl Microbiol* 34:56–61.

Kim, S. Y., S. I. Chung, S. H. Nam, and M. Y. Kang. 2009. Cholesterol lowering action and antioxidant status improving efficacy of noodles made from unmarketable Oak Mushroom (*Lentinus edodes*) in high cholesterol fed rats. *J Korean Soc Appl Biol Chem* 52:207–212.

Kim, S. Y., H. J. Song, Y. Y. Lee, K. H. Cho, and Y. K. Roh. 2006. Biomedical issues of dietary fibre β-glucan. *J Korean Med Sci* 21:781–789.

Kobayashi, H., K. Matsunaga, and Y. Oguchi. 1995. Antimetastatic effects of PSK (Krestin), a protein-bound polysaccharide obtained from basidiomycetes: An overview. *Cancer Epidemiol Biomarkers Prev* 4:275–281.

Kozarski, M., A. Klaus, M. Niksic, D. Jakovljevic, J. P. F. G. Helsper, and L. J. L. D. van Griensven. 2011. Antioxidative and immunomodulating activities of polysaccharide extracts of the medicinal mushrooms *Agaricus bisporus, Agaricus brasiliensis, Ganoderma lucidum* and *Phellinus linteus. Food Chem* 129:1667–1675.

Kulicke, W. M., A. I. Lettau, and H. Thielking. 1997. Correlation between immunological activity, molar mass, and molecular structure of different (1 → 3)-β-D-glucans. *Carbohydr Res* 297:135–143.

Kumari, M., S. A. Survase, and R. S. Singhal. 2008. Production of schizophyllan using *Schizophyllum commune* NRCM. *Biores Technol* 99:1036–1043.

Lakhanpal, T. N. and M. Rana. 2005. Medicinal and nutraceutical genetic resources of mushrooms. *Plant Genet Resource* 3:288–303.

Largeteau, M. L., R. C. Llarena-Hernández, C. Regnault-Roger, and J. M. Savoie. 2011. The medicinal *Agaricus* mushroom cultivated in Brazil: Biology, cultivation and non-medicinal valorisation. *Appl Microbiol Biotechnol* 92:897–907.

Lee, B. C., J. T. Bae, H. B. Pyo et al. 2003. Biological activities of the polysaccharides produced from submerged culture of the edible Basidiomycete *Grifola frondosa. Enzyme Microb Technol* 32:574–581.

Lee, C., J. T. Bae, H. B. Pyo et al. 2004. Submerged culture conditions for the production of mycelial biomass and exopolysaccharides by the edible basidiomycete *Grifola frondosa. Enzyme Microb Technol* 35:369–376.

Li, S. P., K. J. Zhao, Z. N. Ji et al. 2003. A polysaccharide isolated from *Cordyceps sinensis*, a traditional Chinese medicine, protects PC12 cells against hydrogen peroxide-induced injury. *Life Sci* 73:2503–2513.

Li, S. P., G. H. Zhang, Q. Zeng et al. 2006. Hypoglycemic activity of polysaccharide, with antioxidation, isolated from cultured *Cordyceps* mycelia. *Phytomedicine* 13:428–433.

Lindequist, U., T. H. Niedermeyer, and W. D. Jülich. 2005. The pharmacological potential of mushrooms. *Evid Based Complement Altern Med* 2:285–299.

Liu, Y. J., J. Shen, Y. M. Xia, J. Zhang, and H. S. Park. 2012. The polysaccharides from *Ganoderma lucidum:* Are they always inhibitors on human hepatocarcinoma cells? *Carbohydr Polym* 90:1210–1215.

Lo, H. C., F. A. Tsai, S. P. Wasser, J. G. Yang, and B. M. Huang. 2006. Effects of ingested fruiting bodies, submerged culture biomass, and acidic polysaccharide glucuronoxylomannan of *Tremella mesenterica* Retz.:Fr. on glycemic responses in normal and diabetic rats. *Life Sci* 78:1957–1966.

Lo, T. C. T., F. M. Hsu, C. A. Chang, and J. C. H. Cheng. 2011. Branched α-(1,4) glucans from *Lentinula edodes* (L10) in combination with radiation enhance cytotoxic effect on human lung adenocarcinoma through the Toll-like receptor 4 mediated induction of THP-1 differentiation/activation. *J Agric Food Chem* 59:11997–12005.

Lu, H., Y. Yang, E. Gad et al. 2011. Polysaccharide Krestin is a novel TLR2 agonist that mediates inhibition of tumor growth via stimulation of CD8 T cells and NK cells. *Clin Cancer Res* 17:67–76.

Luo, Y., G. Chen, B. Li, B. Ji, Y. Guo, and F. Tian. 2009. Evaluation of antioxidative and hypolipidemic properties of a novel functional diet formulation of *Auricularia auricula* and Hawthorn. *Innov Food Sci Emerg Technol* 10:215–221.

Maeda, Y. Y. and G. Chihara. 1999. Lentinan and other antitumor polysaccharides. In *Immunomodulatory Agents from Plants*, ed. H. Wagner, pp. 203–221. Berlin: Birkhäuser.

Mahajna J., N. Dotan, B. Z. Zaidman, R. D. Petrova, and S. P. Wasser. 2009. Pharmacological values of medicinal mushrooms for prostate cancer therapy: The case of *Ganoderma lucidum. Nutr Cancer* 61:16–26.

Maji, P. K., K. I. Sen, K. S. P. Devi, T. K. Maiti, S. R. Sikdar, and S. S. Islam. 2013. Structural elucidation of a biologically active heteroglycan isolated from a hybrid mushroom of *Pleurotus florida* and *Lentinula edodes*. *Carbohydr Res* 368:22–28.

Malinowska, E., W. Krzyczkowski, F. Herolda et al. 2009. Biosynthesis of selenium-containing polysaccharides with antioxidant activity in liquid culture of *Hericium erinaceum*. *Enzyme Microb Technol* 44:334–343.

Manitchotpisit, P., C. D. Skory, T. D. Leathers et al. 2011. α-Amylase activity during pullulan production and α-amylase gene analyses of *Aureobasidium pullulans*. *J Ind Microbiol Biotechnol* 38:1211–1218.

Markova, N., V. Kussovski, T. Radoucheva, K. Dilova, and N. Georgieva. 2002. Effects of intraperitoneal and intranasal application of Lentinan on cellular response in rats, *Int Immunopharm* 2:1641–1645.

Mattila, P., K. Suonpaa, and V. Piironen. 2000. Functional properties of edible mushrooms. *Nutrition* 16:694–696.

Mau, J. L., C. N. Chang, S. J. Huang, and C. C. Chen. 2004. Antioxidant properties of methanolic extracts from *Grifola frondosa*, *Morchella esculenta* and *Termitomyces albuminosus* mycelia. *Food Chem* 87:111–118.

McNeil, B. and L. M. Harvey. 2006. Fungal biotechnology. In *Encyclopedia of Molecular Cell Biology and Molecular Medicine*, ed. R. Meyers. New York: Wiley-VCH.

Minato, K., M. Mizuno, H. Terai, and H. Tsuchida. 1999. Autolysis of lentinan, an anti-tumor polysaccharide, during storage of *Lentinus edodes*, Shiitake mushroom. *J Agric Food Chem* 47:1530–1532.

Mizuno, T. 1998. Bioactive substances in Yamabushitake, the *Hericium erinaceum* fungus, and its medicinal utilization. *Food Food Ingred Japan J* 167:69–81.

Mizuno, T. 2002. Medicinal properties and clinical effects of culinary-medicinal mushroom *Agaricus blazei Murill (Agaricomycetidae)*. *Int J Med Mushrooms* 4:299–312.

Mizuno, M. and Y. Nishitani. 2013. Immunomodulating compounds in basidiomycetes. *J Clin Biochem Nutr* 52:202–207.

Morin, A. 1998. Screening of polysaccharide-producing microorganisms, factors influencing the production, and recovery of microbial polysaccharides. In *Polysaccharides: Structural Diversity and Functional Versatility*, ed. S. Dumitriu, pp. 275–296. New York: Marcel Dekker Inc.

Nie, S., S. W. Cui, M. Xie, A. O. Phillips, and G. O. Phillips. 2013a. Bioactive polysaccharides from *Cordyceps sinensis*: Isolation, structure, features and bioactivities. *Bioact Carbohydr Diet Fiber* 1:38–52.

Nie, S., H. Zhang, W. Li, and M. Xie. 2013b. Current development of polysaccharides from *Ganoderma*: Isolation, structure and bioactivities. *Bioact Carbohydr Diet Fiber* 1:10–20.

Oba, K., M. Kobauashi, T. Matsui, Y. Kodera, and J. Sakamoto. 2009. Individual patient based meta-analysis of lentinan for unresectable/recurrent gastric cancer. *Anticancer Res* 29:2739–2746.

Okamura-Matsui, T., K. Takemura, M. Sera et al. 2001. Characteristics of a cheese-like food produced by fermentation of the mushroom *Schizophyllum commune*. *J Biosci Bioeng* 92:30–32.

Ooi, V. E. C. and F. Liu. 2000. Immunomodulation and anti-cancer activity of polysaccharide protein complexes. *Curr Med Chem* 7:715–729.

Parab, D. N., J. R. Dhalagade, A. K. Sahoo, and R. C. Ranvee. 2012. Effect of incorporation of mushroom (*Pleurotus sajor-caju*) powder on quality characteristics of Papad (Indian snack food). *Food Compos Anal* 63:866–870.

Paulik, S., Svrcec, J. Mojisova, A. Durove, Z. Benisek, and M. Huska. 1996. The immunomodulatory effect of the soluble fungal glucan (*Pleurotus ostreatus*) on the delayed hypersensitivity and phagocytic ability of blood leucocytes in mice. *J Vet Med* 43:129–135.

Peng, Y., L. Zhang, F. Zeng, and J. F. Kennedy. 2005. Structure and antitumor activities of the water-soluble polysaccharides from *Ganoderma tsugae* mycelium. *Carbohydr Polym* 59:385–392.

Rau, U., E. Gura, E. Olzewski, and F. Wagner. 1992. Enhanced glucan formation of filamentous fungi by effective mixing, oxygen limitation and fed-batch processing. *J Industr Microbiol* 9:19–26.

Rau, U., A. Kuenz, V. Wray, M. Nimtz, J. Wrenger, and H. Cicek. 2009. Production and structural analysis of the polysaccharide secreted by *Trametes (Coriolus) versicolor* ATCC 200801. *Appl Microbiol Biotechnol* 81:827–837.

Reshetnikov, S. V., S. P. Wasser, E. Nevo, I. Duckman, and K. Tsukor. 2000. Medicinal value of the genus *Tremella* Pers. (Heterobasidiomycetes). *Int J Med Mushr* 2:169–193.

Saltarelli, R. P. Ceccaroli, M. Iotti et al. 2009. Biochemical characterisation and antioxidant activity of mycelium of *Ganoderma lucidum* from Central Italy. *Food Chem* 116:143–151.

Sasidhara, R. and T. Thirunalasundari. 2012. Antimicrobial activity of mushrooms. *Biomedicine* 32:455–459.

Schmid, J., V. Meyer, and V. Sieber. 2011. Scleroglucan: Biosynthesis, production and application of a versatile hydrocolloid. *Appl Microbiol Biotechnol* 91:937–947.

Selegean, M., M. V. Putz, and T. Rugea. 2009. Effect of the polysaccharide extract from the edible mushroom *Pleurotus ostreatus* against infectious Bursal disease virus. *Int J Mol Sci* 10:3616–3634.

Shu, C. H., P. F. Chou, and I. C. Hsu. 2005. Effects of morphology and oxygen supply on schizophyllan formation by *Schizophyllum commune* using a pellet size controlling bioreactor. *J Chem Technol Biotechnol* 80:1383–1388.

Shu, C. H., K. J. Lin, and B. J. Wen. 2004. Effects of culture pH on the production of bioactive polysaccharides by *Agaricus blazei* in batch cultures. *J Chem Technol Biotechnol* 79:998–1002.

Singla, R., M. Ghosh, and A. Ganguli. 2009. Phenolics and antioxidant activity of a ready-to-eat snack food prepared from the edible mushroom (*Agaricus bisporous*). *Nutr Food Sci* 39:227–234.

Sletmoen, M. and B. T. Stokke. 2008. Higher order structure of (1,3)-β-ᴅ-glucans and its influence on their biological activities and complexation abilities. *Biopolymer* 89:310–321.

Stachowiak, B. and J. Reguła. 2012. Health-promoting potential of edible macromycetes under special consideration of polysaccharides: A review. *Eur Food Res Technol* 234:369–380.

Sullivan, R., J. E. Smith, and N. J. Rowan. 2006. Medicinal mushrooms and cancer therapy: Translating a traditional practice into Western medicine. *Perspect Biol Med* 49:159–170.

Sutherland, I. W. 1990. *Biotechnology of Microbial Exopolysaccharides*. I. W. Sutherland, Cambridge: Cambridge University Press.

Synytsya, A., K. Mickova, A. Synytsya et al. 2009. Glucans from fruit bodies of cultivated mushrooms *Pleurotus ostreatus* and *Pleurotus eryngii*: Structure and potential prebiotic activity. *Carbohydr Polym* 76:548–556.

Tang, Y. J. and J. J. Zhong. 2003. Role of oxygen in submerged fermentation of *Ganoderma lucidum* for production of *Ganoderma* polysaccharide and ganoderic acid. *Enzyme Microb Technol* 32:478–484.

Thakur, M. P. and H. K. Singh. 2013. Mushrooms, their bioactive compounds and medicinal uses: A review. *Med Plants* 5:1–20.

Torkelson, C. J., E. Sweet, M. R. Martzen et al. 2012. Phase 1 clinical trial of *Trametes versicolor* in women with breast cancer. *ISRN Oncol* 251632:1–7.

Tsai, S. Y., C. C. Wenga, S. J. Huang, C. C. Chen, and J. L. Mau. 2006. Nonvolatile taste components of *Grifola frondosa*, *Morchella esculenta* and *Termitomyces albuminosus* mycelia. *LWT/Food Sci Technol* 39:1066–1071.

Tseng, Y. G, Y. L. Lee, R. C. Li, and J. L. Mau. 2005. Non-volatile flavour components of *Ganoderma tsugae*. *Food Chem* 90:409–415.

Tseng, Y. H., J. H. Yang, and J. L. Mau. 2008. Antioxidant properties of polysaccharides from *Ganoderma tsugae*. *Food Chem* 107:732–738.

Tsuchida, H., M. Mizuno, Y. Taniguchi, H. Ito, M. Kawade, and K. Akasaka. 2001. Glucomannan separated from *Agaricus blazei* mushroom culture and antitumor agent containing as active ingredient. Japanese Patent 11-080206.

van Nevel, C. J., J. A. Decuypere, N. Dierick, and K. Molly. 2003. The influence of *Lentinus edodes* (Shiitake mushroom) preparations on bacteriological and morphological aspects of the small intestine in piglets. *Arch Anim Nutr* 57:399–412.

Vannucci, L., J. Krizan, P. Sima et al. 2013. Immunostimulatory properties and antitumor activities of glucans. *Int J Oncol* 43:357–364.

Vetter, J. 2004. Arsenic content of some edible mushroom species. *Eur Food Res Technol* 219:71–74.

Vinichuk, M., A. F. S. Taylor, K. Rosen, and K. J. Johanson. 2010. Accumulation of potassium, rubidium and caesium (^{133}Cs and ^{137}Cs) in various fractions of soil and fungi in a Swedish forest. *Sci Total Environ* 408:2543–2548.

Wagner, R., D. A. Mitchella, G. L. Sassakia, and M. A. L. D. A. Amazonas. 2004. Links between morphology and physiology of *Ganoderma lucidum* in submerged culture for the production of exopolysaccharide. *J Biotechnol* 114:153–164.

Wang, Z. M., Y. C. Cheung, P. H. Leung, and J. Y. Wu. 2010. Ultrasonic treatment for improved solution properties of a high-molecular weight exopolysaccharide produced by a medicinal fungus. *Biores Technol* 101:5517–5522.

Wasser, S. P. 2002. Medicinal mushrooms as a source of antitumor and immunomodulating polysaccharides. *Appl Microbiol Biotechnol* 60:258–274.

Wasser, S. P. 2011. Current findings, future trends, and unsolved problems in studies of medicinal mushrooms. *Appl Microbiol Biotechnol* 89:1323–1332.

Wenner, C. A., M. R. Martzen, L. U. Hailing, M. R. Verneris, H. Wang, and J. W. Slaton. 2012. Polysaccharide-K augments docetaxel-induced tumor suppression and antitumor immune response in an immunocompetent murine model of human prostate cancer. *Int J Oncol* 40:905–913.

Whitfield, C. and M. A. Valvano. 1993. Biosynthesis and expression of cell-surface polysaccharides. *Adv Microb Physiol* 35:135–246.

Wong, K. H., C. K. M. Lai, and P. C. K. Cheung. 2011. Immunomodulatory activities of mushroom sclerotial polysaccharides. *Food Hydrocoll* 25:150–158.

Wu, F., H. Yan, X. Ma et al. 2011. Structural characterization and antioxidant activity of purified polysaccharide from cultured *Cordyceps militaris*. *Afr J Microbiol Res* 5:2743–2751.

XiaoPing, C., C. Yan, L. ShuiBing, C. YouGuo, L. JianYun, and L. LanPing. 2009. Free radical scavenging of *Ganoderma lucidum* polysaccharides and its effect on antioxidant enzymes and immunity activities in cervical carcinoma rats. *Carbohydr Polym* 77:389–393.

Xie, J., J. Zhao, D. J. Hu, J. A. Duan, Y. P. Tang, and S. P. Li. 2012. Comparison of polysaccharides from two species of *Ganoderma*. *Molecules* 17:740–752.

Xu, Y. 2001. Perspectives on the 21st century development of functional foods: Bridging Chinese medicated diet and functional foods. *Int J Food Sci Technol* 36:229–242.

Yamanaka, D., Y. Liu, M. Motoi, and N. Ohno. 2013. Royal Sun medicinal mushroom, *Agaricus brasiliensis* Ka21 (Higher Basidiomycetes), as a functional food in humans. *Int J Med Mushr* 15:335–343.

Yang, F. C. and C. B. Liau. 1998. The influence of environmental conditions on polysaccharide formation by *Ganoderma lucidum* in submerged cultures. *Process Biochem* 33:547–553.

Yang, W., Y. Fang, J. Liang, and H. Qiuhui. 2011. Optimization of ultrasonic extraction of *Flammulina velutipes* polysaccharides and evaluation of its acetylcholinesterase inhibitory activity. *Food Res Int* 44:1269–1275.

Ye, L., J. Li, J. Zhang, and Y. Pan. 2010. NMR characterization for polysaccharide moiety of a glycopeptide. *Fitoterapia* 81:93–96.

Yin, H., Y. Wang, Y. Wang, T. Chen, H. Tang, and M. Wang. 2010. Purification, characterization and immuno-modulating properties of polysaccharides isolated from *Flammulina velutipes* mycelium. *Am J Chin Med* 38:191–204.

Yoon, S. J., M. A. Yu, Y. R. Pyun et al. 2003. The nontoxic mushroom *Auricularia auricula* contains a polysaccharide with anticoagulant activity mediated by antithrombin. *Thromb Res* 112:151–158.

You, Y. H. and Z. B. Lin. 2002. Protective effects of *Ganoderma lucidum* polysaccharides peptide on injury of macrophages induced by reactive oxygen species. *Acta Pharmacol Sinica* 23:789–791.

Yu, Z. Y. L., Q. Yang, and Y. Liu. 2009. Effect of *Lentinus edodes* polysaccharide on oxidative stress, immunity activity and oral ulceration of rats stimulated by phenol. *Carbohydr Polym* 75:115–118.

Yuen, J. W. M. and M. D. I. Gohel. 2005. Anticancer effects of *Ganoderma lucidum*: A review of scientific evidence. *Nutr Cancer* 53:11–17.

Zhang, M., P. C. K. Cheung, and L. Zhang. 2001. Evaluation of mushroom dietary fiber (nonstarch polysaccharides) from sclerotia of *Pleurotus tuber-regium* (Fries) Singer as a potential antitumor agent. *J Agric Food Chem* 49:5059–5062.

Zhang, M., S. W. Cui, P. C. K. Cheung, and Q. Wang. 2007. Antitumor polysaccharides from mushrooms: A review on their isolation process, structural characteristics and antitumor activity. *Trends Food Sci Technol* 18:4–19.

Zhang, Y., S. Li, X. Wang, L. Zhang, and P. C. K. Cheung. 2011. Advances in lentinan: Isolation, structure, chain conformation and bioactivities. *Food Hydrocoll* 25:196–206.

Zhao, J. and P. C. K. Cheung. 2011. Fermentation of β-glucans derived from different sources by bifidobacteria: Evaluation of their bifidogenic effect. *J Agric Food Chem* 59:5986–5992.

Zhong, S., H. Pan, L. Fan et al. 2009. Advances in research of polysaccharides in *Cordyceps* species. *Food Technol Biotechnol* 47:304–312.

Zhou, S., Y. Gao, and E. Chan. 2005. Clinical trials for medicinal mushrooms: Experience with *Ganoderma lucidum* (W. Curt.:Fr.) Lloyd (Lingzhi mushroom). *Int J Med Mushr* 7:111–117.

Zhou, X., Z. Gong, Y. Su, J. Lin, and K. Tang. 2009. *Cordyceps* fungi: Natural products, pharmacological functions and developmental products. *J Pharm Pharmacol* 61:279–291.

CHAPTER **9**

Nonstarch Polysaccharides from Food Grains

Their Structure and Health Implications

MURALIKRISHNA GUDIPATI and LYNED D. LASRADO

Contents

9.1	Introduction	208
9.2	Free Sugars and Undigestible Oligosaccharides	208
9.3	Starch	209
9.4	Nonstarch Polysaccharides	210
	9.4.1 Isolation	211
	9.4.2 Purification	211
	9.4.3 Purification Criteria	212
	9.4.4 Structural Analysis	212
	9.4.5 Health Benefits of NSP in Alleviation of Disease Symptoms	213
9.5	β-1,3/1,4-Glucans	214
9.6	Arabinoxylans	216
	9.6.1 Effect of Structure on Physicochemical Characteristics of AXs	219
	9.6.2 Nutraceutical Importance of Arabinoxylan	220
9.7	Arabinogalactan-Proteins	221
9.8	Pectins	223
9.9	Future Perspectives	224
	Acknowledgment	225
	References	225

9.1 Introduction

Plant carbohydrates can be broadly classified into mono-, di-, oligo-, and polysaccharides. Glucose, fructose, galactose, and ribose are the most preponderant monosaccharides in the plant kingdom. Sucrose, maltose, and melibiose are the important disaccharides present in several plants and they undergo hydrolysis into monosaccharides depending on the energy needs based on various metabolic activities (Tharanathan et al. 1987).

Carbohydrates present in animals, as well as plants, are one of the major biomolecules along with proteins and lipids. They provide energy in the form of free sugars, such as glucose, fructose, sucrose, lactose, maltotriose, and polymers in the form of starch and glycogen. In addition, they serve as structural compounds in plants such as cellulose, pectin, 1,3/1,4-β-D-glucans, and arabinogalacto-proteins. In animals, they exist as glyco-conjugates such as glycoproteins, proteoglycans, and glycolipids that are collectively called as glyco-calyx and modulate several biological functions (Aspinall 1982).

Nutritionally, the plant dietary fiber compounds play a pivotal role in alleviating several disease symptoms such as diabetes, atherosclerosis, and colon cancer. However, the exact mechanism in most of the cases is more speculative rather than based on experimental facts. Dietary fiber research got a face-lift in the 1960s and 1970s with respect to its beneficial effects in decreasing some adverse effects with respect to several nutritional disorders. The exact structure–function relationship of individual components of various dietary fiber components is still in the infancy stage although extensive structural details of the same are well documented (Dreher 2001).

Nutritionally, the plant polysaccharides can be demarcated as starch and nonstarch polysaccharides. Starch, in most cases, is easily digested by the human gut secretions/enzymes, which is not true in the case of dietary fiber components. Even, some of the starch is undigestible based on how it is processed, resulting in resistant starch that is not available for the amylolytic enzymes secreted by the salivary gland as well as pancreas. Dietary fiber is further divided into cellulose and noncellulosic polysaccharides such as 1,3/1,4-β-D-glucans, soluble arabinoxylans (AXs)/insoluble AXs, glucomannans, and proteoglycan moieties such as arabinogalactan proteins (Muralikrishna and Subba Rao 2007). In this chapter, emphasis is mostly laid on noncellulosic polysaccharides.

9.2 Free Sugars and Undigestible Oligosaccharides

Glucose, fructose, galactose, melibiose, sucrose, maltose, and maltotriose are the free sugars present in many cereals and pulses that are further metabolized in the human intestine to get energy in the form of acetyl CoA. However, some undigestible oligosaccharides such as raffinose, stachyose, verbascose, and ajugose are present to the extent of 1–3% in several pulses and are responsible for flatulence, a social discomfort caused due to the absence of the α-galactosidase enzyme in the small intestine. The above oligosaccharides are extensively fermented in the large intestine by various beneficial bacteria such as lactic acid bacteria to short-chain fatty acid such as acetic acid, propionic acid, and butyric acid. These oligosaccharides are also responsible for increase in the beneficial bacterial populations such as lactobacillus and bifidogenic species and can be bracketed under prebiotics.

9.3 Starch

Most of the carbohydrates present in plants exist as polysaccharides and polymers of high molecular weight (Mw). The most important storage polysaccharide in plants and nature is starch, which occurs as clusters or granules. Starch is heavily hydrated because it has several hydroxyl groups that can react with water. Starch consists of two polymers, amylose, and amylopectin. Amylose consists of long unbranched chains of D-glucose units connected by α-1 → 4 linkages. Such chains vary in Mw from 50,000 to 1 million daltons. Amylopectin is a branched polymer with α-1 → 6 linkages (5–10%) in addition to α-1 → 4 linkages (~90–95%) and has a very high Mw running into several million daltons (Figure 9.1). Starch is the main carbohydrate that gives energy since it is digested by the salivary and intestinal amylolytic enzymes (Muralikrishna

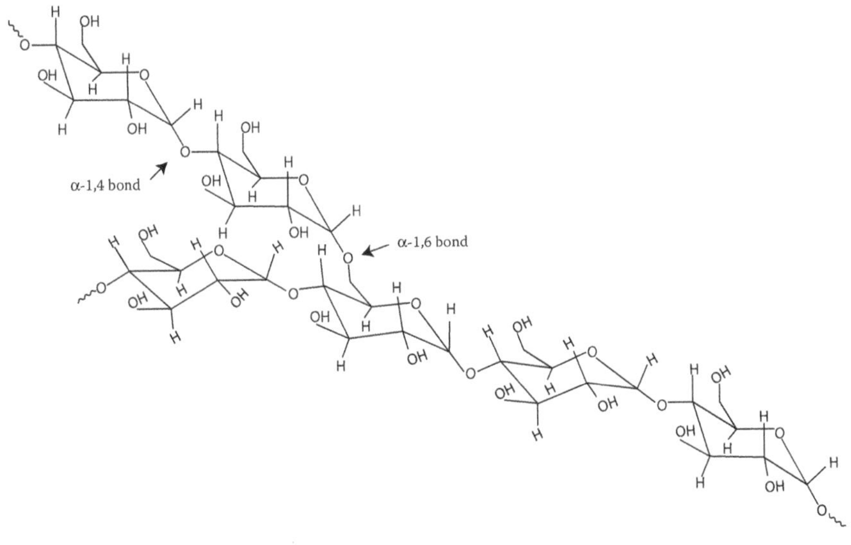

Figure 9.1 Starch structure. (Wikipedia. http://shikob.wikispaces.com/Biochemistry + Topics.)

Table 9.1 Resistant Starches: Nutritional Classification

Type of Resistant Starch (RS)	Nature	Example
RS1	Physically inaccessible	Partially milled grains and seeds
RS2	Resistant granules	Raw potato, green banana, some pulses, high amylose starch
RS3	Retrograded granules	Cooked and cooled potato, bread, cornflakes
RS4	Chemically modified	Etherized, esterified, cross linked starch

Source: Data from Brown, I. L., K. J. McNaught, and E. Moloney. 1995. *Food Aust* 47:272–275; Englyst, H. N., S. M. Kingman, and J. H. Cummings. 1992. *Eur J Clin Nutr* 46:S33–S50.

and Nirmala 2005). However, some amount of starch that escapes digestion is called as resistant starch. Resistant starch is classified into four classes based on its origin into RS1, RS2, RS3, and RS4 (Table 9.1). Among the various resistant starches, retrograded amylose formed by heating and cooling is the major one. This acts like dietary fiber with respect to its beneficial effects.

9.4 Nonstarch Polysaccharides

Cereals and pulses are rich sources of nonstarch polysaccharides that can be extracted with both aqueous and nonaqueous solutions, which are designated as water-extractable polysaccharides (WEPs) and water-unextractable polysaccharide (WUP) (Table 9.2). Nonstarch polysaccharides (NSPs) can be broadly divided into three classes, namely, cellulose, noncellulosic polymers, and pectic polysaccharides (Figure 9.2). Cellulose, a β-1,4-linked

Table 9.2 Nonstarch Polysaccharides in Cereals and Pulses

	WEP(%)	WUP(%)
Rice	1.16	8.19
Wheat	2.35	13.6
Maize	3.56	20.4
Ragi	0.60	20.3
Chickpea	3.3	7.4
Pea	2.5	32.2
Navy bean	5.7	1.7
Pinto bean	6.3	13.1
Rape seed	11.3	34.8

Source: Data from Rao, R. S. and G. Muralikrishna. 2004. *Food Chem* 84:527–531; Kumar, V. et al. 2012. *Crit Rev Food Sci Nutr* 52:899–935.

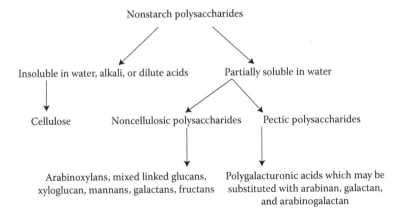

Figure 9.2 Classification of NSP.

polysaccharide, is completely insoluble in water due to its structural orientation and rigidity and is almost completely undigested and excreted without much change. Cellulose exists in the form of lignocelluloses where it forms a covalent linkage with lignin, a polyphenyl propionoid biomolecule. These lignocellulosic complexes are almost completely unfermented in the human gut with very little change. However, noncellulosic polysaccharides undergo fermentation to a different extent in the large intestine and exert various health benefits (Narasingha Rao 2002). In the following section, various aspects pertaining to the isolation, purification, and structural characterization of nonstarch polysaccharides are dealt with.

9.4.1 Isolation

NSP can be extracted with various extractants, such as (a) water for mixed linked 1,3/1,4-β-D-glucans and AXs, (b) chelating agents such as 0.5% ethylene diaminotetra acetic acid and ammonium oxalate for pectins, (c) 10% alkali for hemicelluloses and arabinogalacto-proteins, and (d) *N*-methyl morpholine–*N*-oxide (MMNO) for cellulose (Aspinall 1982).

9.4.2 Purification

Nonstarch polysaccharides are rarely homogeneous and require extensive fractionation and purification steps before proceeding to structural analysis. They differ in size, shape, and charge and can be fractionated by different methods such as fractional precipitation using solvents such as ethanol, acetone, or graded ammonium sulfate precipitation. Acidic polysaccharides can be separated from neutral polysaccharides by using quaternary salts such as cetyl trimethyl ammonium bromide (CTAB). Column chromatographic methods such as ion exchange and gel filtration will yield pure polysaccharides based on the separation with respect to charge as well as Mw (Rao and Muralikrishna 2010).

9.4.3 Purification Criteria

Polysaccharides are highly heterogeneous with respect to their Mw, physical properties, and chemical characteristics since their biosynthesis is indirectly controlled by several glycosyl transferase genes. These variations may be due to: (a) departure from absolute specificity of the transferases, (b) incomplete formation of segments (side chains), or (c) post polymerization changes. The separation into discrete molecular species is almost impossible if these variations are continuous with respect to parameters such as molecular size, proportions of sugar constituents, and linkage type and accordingly, the polysaccharide is called as polydisperse. Alternately, if the heterogeneity lies in their molecular size but not in their chemical composition, they are called polymolecular. Consequently, it would be very difficult to establish the purity of the polysaccharide beyond ambiguity. However, showing the absence of heterogeneity by as many independent criteria as possible is sufficient to go for further characterization, that is, determination of the structure. Many methods were developed to show the absence of heterogeneity in any given polysaccharide sample (Aspinall 1982). The most important of these methods are: (a) consistency in chemical composition and physical properties such as optical rotation and viscosity; (b) chromatographic methods (ion exchange, gel permeation, and affinity); (c) ultracentrifugation pattern; (d) electrophoretic methods (cellulose acetate and capillary electrophoresis); and (e) spectroscopic methods (nuclear magnetic resonance [NMR] and infrared [IR]) (Muralikrishna and Subba Rao 2007).

9.4.4 Structural Analysis

Nonstarch polysaccharides may contain hundreds to millions of sugar residues that are either arranged in a linear or branched manner. The sugar residues may be of the same type (homoglycans) or of different types (heteroglycans). The length of a polymer chain called the degree of polymerization is specified by the number of structural units it contains. The building units commonly have pyranose ring form, but sometimes, they may have the furanose ring too. The major problems in the determination of the molecular structure of polysaccharides are to establish: (a) the nature of constituent sugar residues including their ring size; (b) the positions and configurations of the inter glycosidic linkages; (c) the sequence of residues and linkages; and (d) the overall arrangement of polymeric chains. Several methods as reported in the literature can be used to elucidate the structural features of homogeneous polysaccharides that are: Methylation analysis (conversion of all the free hydroxyl groups into methoxyl groups) is the most extensively used technique to obtain information on the ring size and linkage positions, and also the extent and kind of branching. Out of several methylation procedures reported till date, the Hakomori methylation procedure and the use of gas chromatography–mass spectrometry (GC–MS) to examine the resulting sugar derivatives have radically altered the scope and depth of the studies on oligo-/polysaccharides. Partial fragmentation data obtained by employing several conditions (acidic and enzymatic) are extremely useful to deduce the monosaccharide sequences. Specific degradative methods such as periodate oxidation and Smith degradation, β-elimination of glycouronans, chromium trioxide oxidation, Barry degradation, and so on are also useful as supportive methods to the structural information as obtained by methylation analysis. Electrospray ionization-mass spectrometry (ESI-MS), fast atom bombardment-mass spectrometry (FAB-MS), and NMR have paved the way for understanding the intricate/complete structural details of oligo- and polysaccharides (Rao and Muralikrishna 2010). Positive functional attributes of water-soluble NSP from rice and ragi were documented with respect to foam-stabilizing activity and wheat-dough properties. The positive effect on dough characteristics was reflected on the baking studies wherein significant increase in the bread quality was attained by incorporating water-soluble NSP from rice and ragi (Rao and Muralikrishna 2007).

9.4.5 Health Benefits of NSP in Alleviation of Disease Symptoms

NSP plays an important role in protecting against degenerative diseases such as: (a) diabetes; (b) cardiovascular disease; and (c) cancer. NSP has a protective role against diabetes wherein it controls the postprandial blood glucose levels and in addition, it also inhibits the absorption of cholesterol by bile acids, thereby alleviating atherosclerosis symptoms. These NSP also help in preventing bowel cancer by binding carcinogens and toxins. The disease-preventing potential of the total NSP depends on (a) the proportion of the various fractions; (b) their actual content; (c) their viscosity; (d) hexose-to-pentose ratio; and (e) presence/absence of uronic acid, ester-linked groups of acetic acid, and ferulic acid. Various mechanisms have been proposed with respect to the beneficial preventive effects of NSP. One of the mechanisms is by exerting viscosity due to the swelling/solubility properties of polysaccharides that result in reducing the transit time in the small intestine as well as reducing the rate of release of glucose from dietary carbohydrates, thereby affecting their absorption. In addition, the NSP can also bind the bile acids and thereby prevents the absorption of cholesterol and promotes its excretion from the liver. The third mechanism is through binding of carcinogens and toxins by the charged moieties of uronic acids of pectins and glucuronoarabinoxylans of NSP that prevents or slows down the absorption of the carcinogens and toxins. In the fourth mechanism, NSP exerts beneficial effects on chronic diseases through their fermentation in the large intestine (colon). Soluble NSP is completely fermented in the large intestine whereas the insoluble fibers are partially fermented (Narasingha Rao 2002). As a consequence of this fermentation, bacterial cell mass increases several fold and this increased bulk reduces the transit time of undigested food material. Short-chain fatty acids such as butyrates, propionates, and acetates are produced as a result of colon fermentation of NSP. Butyrate helps in rejuvenation of colon mucosal cells by serving as a ready source of energy. Butyrate also promotes the differentiation and inhibition of cell proliferation in human carcinoma cells and facilitates deoxyribonucleic acid (DNA) repair, thereby reducing the risk of colon cancer as well as inflammatory bowel disease. The other short-chain fatty acids, namely, propionates and acetates, enter into blood circulation that are then transported to the liver wherein they exert a direct inhibitory effect on the release of glucose and synthesis of cholesterol. Thus, the NSP indirectly contributes to the hypoglycemic and hypocholesterolemic effects. NSP does not bind to minerals and vitamins and therefore, does not restrict their absorption, but rather, evidence exists that fermentable fiber sources improve absorption of minerals, especially calcium. Some plant foods can reduce the absorption of minerals and vitamins such as magnesium, calcium, zinc, and vitamin C but this is caused by the presence of phytate rather than fiber.

Among the various NSP, β-1,3/1,4-glucans, AXs, pectins, and arabinogalactan (AG) proteins were documented to have several health benefits that are highlighted in the following section.

9.5 β-1,3/1,4-Glucans

β-1,3/1,4-Glucans are enriched in barley, oat, and rye (Van-den et al. 2002, Ingelbrecht et al. 2002, Butt et al. 2008, Cui and Wang 2009). β-1,3/1,4-Glucans content varies from 2.5% to 17%, depending on the genetic background of the cereal varieties as well as environmental conditions under which they are grown. They are linear homopolysaccharides of β-D-glucopyranosyl residues alternately linked by (≈70%) (1 → 4) linkages interrupted by a single (1 → 3) glucose residue (≈30%) (Izydorczyk and Dexter 2008) (Figure 9.3). These components have different functional properties with their diverse structures that in turn will have a bearing on the product development and play a pivotal role in improving the health of the consumers (Urala and Lahteenmaki 2007). β-1,3/1,4-Glucans vary with respect to their localization in various cereals, that is, endosperm cell walls, pericarp, and aleurone layers (Izydorczyk and Dexter 2008). For example, 75% of starch endosperm cell walls of barley correspond to β-1,3/1,4-glucans

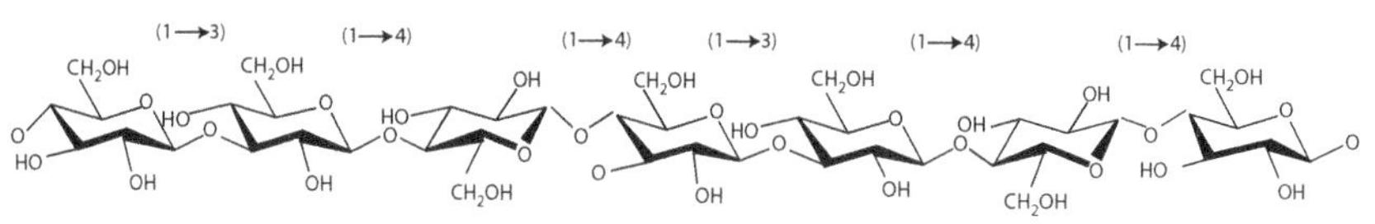

Figure 9.3 Structure of mixed linked glucan. (From Fincher, G. B. and B. A. Stone. 1986. In *Advances in Cereal Science and Technology*, pp. 207–295. American Association of Cereal Chemists, USA. With permission.)

while they constitute around 26% of aleurone walls (Fincher and Stone 1986). However, with respect to these polymers, distribution varies from cereal to cereal as observed in oats, rye, as well as wheat (Cui and Wang 2009).

Structural analysis of β-1,3/1,4-glucans indicated that the ratio of 1.3–1.4 is 9:1 (Cui and Wang 2009). The ratio of trisaccharides to tetrasaccharide forms a fingerprint of the particular grain and is unique to each cereal. It was reported to be the highest for wheat (3.7:4.8), followed by barley/rye (2.7:3.6) then oats (1.7:2.4) and the yield of β-1,3/1,4-glucans also depends on the method that is adopted (Wood 2010). The molar ratio of DP3/DP4 is the determining factor for the solubility of β-1,3/1,4-glucans (Cui et al. 2000). It is documented in the literature that long cellulose-like sequences of $(1 \rightarrow 4)$-linked β-D-glucose residues are one of the important factors responsible for the formation of strong internal or external aggregation that is through hydrogen bonding, resulting in its sparingly soluble property (Izydorczyk et al. 1998, Lazaridou and Biliaderis 2007).

Different Mws of β-1,3/1,4-glucans have been reported from various sources such as oats (0.65–31.0 × 10^5 g/mol), barley (0.31–27.0 × 105 g/mol), rye (0.21–11.0 × 105 g/mol), and wheat (2.1–4.9 × 105 g/mol) (Lazaridou and Biliaderis 2007). Environmental as well as varietal factors along with the method of extraction are determining factors with respect to the variation in Mw (Ajithkumar et al. 2005). In addition, improper inactivation of endogenous microbial β-glucanases as well as extraction in alkaline or acidic conditions at high temperatures (Lazaridou and Biliaderis 2007, Wood 2010) may also be responsible for variation in Mw.

β-1,3/1,4-Glucans are used as biological response modifier (BRM) to enhance the functioning of the immune system and also to lower blood cholesterol, triglycerides, and low-density lipoprotein (LDL) cholesterol. The activation of white blood cells such as macrophages and neutrophils is mediated by β-1,3/1,4-glucans by way of recognizing and subsequently killing abnormal cancerous cells (Pelley and Strickland 2000, Mayell 2001). This is one of the possible underlying mechanisms for tumor apoptosis.

Currently, β-1,3/1,4-glucans are widely available as a neutraceutical in the liquid form as well as in capsules and tablets. β-1,3/1,4-Glucans are well accepted as a food supplement but not as a medication. It cannot give energy to the body since it is not degraded in the human gastrointestinal tract; hence, the intact polysaccharide is absorbed and plays its useful role in cardiovascular and immune systems (Pelley and Strickland 2000, Mayell 2001).

It has been established that neutrophils (or polymorphonuclear leukocytes [PMNs]) recognize β-glucan (component of yeast cell wall) as a key molecular pattern in response to *Candida albicans* and produce antibodies specific to β-glucan to block this reaction (Lavigne et al. 2006). β-Glucan can stimulate phagocytic activity and also the synthesis and release of interleukins (IL-1, IL-2, IL-4, IL-6, IL-8, and IL-13) and α-tumor necrosis factor (Vetvicka et al. 2008). Cell surface receptors, namely, complement receptor 3 (CR3 and CD11b/CD18), lactosylceramide, selected scavenger receptors, and dectin-1 specifically interact with β-glucan and mediate macrophage, neutrophil, and natural killer (NK) cells activity (Akramiene et al. 2007, Chen and Seviour 2007, Harada and Ohno 2008). β-Glucan administration decreases the infectious complication rate in patients undergoing a major surgery (Babineau et al. 1994); also, the perioperative administration of β-glucan has been reported to reduce serious postoperative infections (Dellinger et al. 1999). β-Glucan oligosaccharides derived from oat bran were almost as effective as raffinose and slightly better than fructooligomers with respect to their prebiotic activity (Jaskari et al. 1998).

9.6 Arabinoxylans

AXs are the major noncellulosic polysaccharides, constituting 60–70% of endosperm cell walls in most of the cereal grains, with the exception of oats and barley (≈20%) and rice (40%) (Fincher and Stone 1986, Stone 2006). The backbone of the AX consists of (1 → 4)-linked β-D-xylopyranosyl residues, which may be either mono- or di substituted by α-L-arabinofuranosyl residue at O-2 or O-3 position or at both, respectively (Figure 9.4).

Barley AXs content vary with respect to endosperm (20–25%) (Balance and Manners 1978) and aleurone (85%) (McNeil et al. 1975). Structural studies of barley AXs indicated a (1 → 4)-β-D-xylan back bone, substituted to varying extents by arabinofuranose residues either at O-2 or O-3 or at both O-2 and O-3. They are made up of two types of structures: (a) isolated, substituted

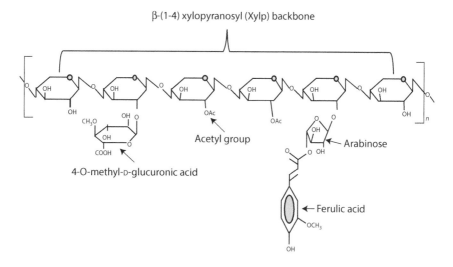

Figure 9.4 Structure of arabinoxylan.

xylose residues separated by one or two unsubstituted residues (region A); and (b) two or more unsubstituted xylose residues (region B) (Vietor et al. 1994, Han 2000).

Wheat water-unextractable arabinoxylan indicated two different regions, namely, regions A and B. Variations exist in region B depending on the composition as well as Ara/Xyl ratio whereas region A is constant. Region A is highly branched, consisting of unsubstituted and double arabinofuranosylated xylose residues (both O-2,3) of tetrameric repeating units. Region B is less branched and it includes contiguous unsubstituted xylose residues. However, the substituted xylose residues are either isolated or present in pairs (Gruppen et al. 1993).

Rice endosperm cell walls consist of highly branched arabinoxylan, in which the arabinofuranose residues are attached at the C3 position of the $(1 \rightarrow 4)$-β-D-xylan backbone (Shibuya 1984). Few O-2-linked arabinofuranosyl residues were also present in both the endosperm and the bran. Disubstituted (74–79%) $1 \rightarrow 4$-β-D-xylose residues are present in the acidic AXs. AXs derived from rice bran contain appreciable amounts of nonreducing end xylose and galactose and $(1 \rightarrow 2)$, $(1 \rightarrow 3)$, and $(1 \rightarrow 5)$-linked arabinose residues, indicating complex structural features of their side chains as compared with endosperm AXs, wherein most of the side chains are single arabinose residues. In glucuronoarabinoxylan of rice, the uronic acid is linked to xylose residues at the O-2 position as indicated by the presence of 2-O-(4-methyl-D-glucopyranosylurono)-D-xylose (Shibuya et al. 1983, Shibuya 1984, Shibuya and Iwasaki 1985).

Sorghum flour contains cell-wall material {5–6%; (w/w)} that consists of nonstarch polysaccharides and associated proteins (Verbruggen et al. 1993). Arabinoxylan is the major constituent of water-extractable NSP (Verbruggen et al. 1995), whereas the glucuronoarabinoxylan is the major constituent in the water-insoluble material (Woolard et al. 1976). Water-insoluble glucuronoarabinoxylans of sorghum were extracted with aqueous solutions of $Ba(OH)_2$ and KOH, resulting in nine fractions among which, BE-I was shown to be homogeneous with a high amount of substitution (45%) at O-3. In addition, it also contained a substantial amount of disubstituted O-2 and O-3 (17%) and unsubstituted (28%) xylose units. Most of the arabinose residues (88%) were present as nonreducing terminal units. The uronic acids were attached to the $(1 \rightarrow 4)$ xylan at the O-2 position of xylose (Verbruggen et al. 1995). Homogeneous glucuronoarabinoxylans were also isolated from the sorghum husk and structural analysis indicated the presence of arabinose residues at the O-2 and O-3 positions of the $1 \rightarrow 4$-linked xylan backbone. Uronic acid residues (glucuronic acid and 4-0-methylglucuronic acid) were attached to some of the O-2 positions of the xylose residues.

Maize bran contains very high amounts of {~40% (w/w)} heteroxylans. The sequential extraction of purified maize bran with 0.5 M NaOH followed by 1.5 M KOH yielded three fractions, namely, S1, S2, and R2 in different amounts (Chanliaud et al. 1995). Structural details obtained by methylation analysis of S1 and S2 indicated similar types of linkages with almost identity in the distributions of side chains. The xylan backbone was highly substituted with 77% oligomeric side chains containing xylose, arabinose, and galactose. Single arabinose residues substitutions were observed both at O-2 (22%) and O-3 (15%) along with unsubstituted (15%) and disubstituted (20%) xylose residues. Galactose residues (84%) were mainly present as the nonreducing terminals (Montgomery et al. 1957, Chanliaud et al. 1995).

Rye water-insoluble AXs have been divided into three classes, differing in extractability, solubility, and structure (Vinkx et al. 1995). Class I obtained by neutralization of the 1 M KOH alkaline extract had a low Ara/Xyl ratio (0.2). Class II has an intermediate Ara/Xyl ratio and remained in solution after neutralization of the saturated $Ba(OH)_2$ containing 1% $NaBH_4$; however, it precipitated upon saturation with ammonium sulfate. Classes I and II have some similarities in structure with mono-/di-/unsubstituted xylose residues along with nonreducing terminal arabinose residues. Class III was soluble both in water and ammonia solution and has a very high ratio of arabinose to xylose (1:1). Structural analysis of these AXs indicated the presence of substituted arabinoses (40% of the arabinose), terminal xyloses (26% of xyloses), and terminal galactose (Vinkx and Delcour 1996).

Finger millet also known as ragi is extensively used by the South Indian rural population both in native and germinated forms. It is rich in calcium (0.34%) and dietary fiber (17%) and used in infant and geriatric food preparations. Alkali-soluble (hemicellulose) AXs were isolated from both native and malted finger millet malt. Structural elucidation of purified AXs isolated from finger millet and its malt by performing methylation, gas liquid chromatography–mass spectrometry (GLC–MS), periodate oxidation, Smith degradation, NMR, IR, optical rotation, and oligosaccharide analysis indicated 1,4-β-D-xylan backbone with the majority of the residues substituted at C-3. The major oligosaccharide generated by endoxylanase treatment was homogeneous with an Mw of 1865 Da corresponding to 14 pentose residues as determined by matrix-assisted laser desorption–ionization-time-of-flight-mass spectrometry (MALDI-TOF-MS) and gel filtration on Biogel P-2. The structural analysis of this oligosaccharide showed that it contained eight xylose and six arabinose residues, substituted at C-3 (monosubstituted) and at both C-2 and C-3 (disubstituted). In addition, water-soluble feruloyl AXs (feraxans), isolated from native and malted (96 h) rice (*Oryza sativa*) and ragi (*Eleusine coracana*) grains, were purified and structural characterization of the purified polysaccharides by methylation, followed by GLC–MS, and also by ^{1}H NMR and ^{13}C NMR spectroscopy, indicated very high branching and the presence of high amounts of O-2-substituted xylans. The amount of O-2,3-disubstituted xylopyranosyl residues and the arabinose:xylose ratio was higher in malt feraxans. All feraxan samples consumed almost equal amounts of periodate (4.02–4.30 μmol/mg of polysaccharide). High amounts of xylose (40%), as identified by Smith degradation, further substantiated the high branching of feraxans (Rao and Muralikrishna 2007).

9.6.1 Effect of Structure on Physicochemical Characteristics of AXs

The degree and pattern of substitution by arabinose residues along the xylan backbone and the degree of polymerization of the xylan chain are important determinants of the structural heterogeneity and physicochemical properties of AX (Vinkx and Delcour 1996). For example, arabinoxylan with decreasing arabinose substituents tends to become less soluble, due to the tendency of unsubstituted xylan chains to associate and form stable and insoluble aggregates (Andrewartha et al. 1979). However, due to possibly stronger embedment in cell walls or interactions with other compounds, highly branched AXs in the plant matrix are difficult to extract (Cyran et al. 2003). The extent of branching has a bearing on the action of pentosanases and highly branched AX molecules are less prone to enzymatic degradation (Vinkx and Delcour 1996, Ordaz-Ortiz et al. 2005).

Water-extractable AX (WE-AX) structure is slightly different from that of water-unextractable AX solubilized by alkaline extraction (Gruppen et al. 1993). The alkali-extracted AX is believed to have higher Mw and slightly higher A/X ratio due to more arabinose branching (Fincher and Stone 1986, Gruppen et al. 1992). It has been reported that about 50% of the xylose residues are unsubstituted, 30% are monosubstituted, and 20% are disubstituted in rye alkali-extractable AXs (Cyran et al. 2004, Verwimp et al. 2007). The rheological properties of AX also strongly depend on its fine structure, apart from its solubility and Mw distribution (Bach Knudsen and Lærke 2010, Cyran and Ceglinska 2011). Both Mw and structure influence the hydrodynamic volume of the polymer that in turn influences viscosity (Courtin and Delcour 2002). Substitution of arabinose either as monosubstitutes or disubstitutes has an influence on the variation of the extract viscosity (of rye grains) (Bengtsson et al. 1992). This underscores the importance of AX structural features for its various functional properties. Huge variability in Mw of AX is reported in the literature, mainly because of different methods of extraction and analysis (Bach Knudsen and Lærke 2010). Girhammar and Nair (1992) reported weight average Mw of 7.70×105 g/mol in rye AX using gel permeation chromatography, while Andersson et al. (2009) reported 20.0×105 g/mol Mw using size-exclusion chromatography coupled with light-scattering and refractive index detection.

The structure–function relationship with respect to minor constituents of dietary fiber such as acetic acid and ferulic acid in conjunction with AXs is not deciphered. The role of acetyl and feruloyl groups has been documented with respect to foam stabilization, gelling, and bread-making characteristics for the first time (Madhavilatha and Muralikrishna 2009). Minor enzymes such as acetic acid and ferulic acid esterases have been characterized from ragi malt (Madhavilatha and Muralkrishna 2007, Madhavilatha et al. 2007). Hegde et al. (2009) reported a single-step method for the synthesis of the para-nitrophenyl ferulate, a substrate for spectrophotometric assay of ferulic acid esterase, one of the most sought-after enzyme in the food, cosmetic, and pharmaceutical industries. Methods have been developed with respect to the isolation of bound phenolic acid-rich dietary fibers, cell wall-degrading enzymes, and xylooligosaccharides, which have an impact on prebiotic and synbiotic preparations, used for various health benefits (Rao and Muralikrishna 2006b, Madhavilatha and Muralkrishna 2007, Chithra and Muralikrishna 2008).

9.6.2 Nutraceutical Importance of Arabinoxylan

In recent years, a lot of emphasis has been laid on the domain of nutrition with respect to beneficial effects of dietary fiber for the amelioration of various lifestyle-related diseases. Among the dietary fiber components, AXs occupy the prime place due to their structural variation in having various antioxidant phenolic acids such as ferulic acid, coumaric acid, and caffeic acid covalently linked to side chain arabinose residues (Slavin 2008, Cummings et al. 2009). Owing to the presence of these phenolic acid moieties, AXs do act like antioxidants, thereby exerting health benefits. In a seminal study, water-soluble feruloyl AXs were isolated from both native and malted rice and ragi and their antioxidant activities were determined by different methods; this study was the first of its kind with respect to the determination of the importance of bound phenolic acid, especially ferulic acid (Rao and Muralikrishna 2006a). Prior to this, it was documented that germination/malting of finger millet resulted in the increase of free phenolic acids that resulted in higher antioxidant activity as compared to the native finger millet (Subba Rao and Muralikrishna 2002). This is due to the induction of esterases, mainly, ferulic acid esterase that was purified and characterized from finger millet malt (Madhavilatha et al. 2007).

Various health benefits of AXs such as controlling diabetes mellitus, cardiovascular disorders, improving colon function, and improving the general body health were reported (Lu et al. 2000, Johnson 2005, Nino-Medina et al. 2009). The consumption of AX fiber is associated with significant reduction in: (a) blood glucose; (b) fructosamine; and (c) insulin concentrations (Garcia et al. 2007). The mechanism by which AX-rich fiber reduces blood glucose is yet to be deciphered (Lu et al. 2004); however, its high viscosity and soluble nature are ascribed as possible factors responsible for its hypoglycemic activity. It is assumed by many investigators that viscous substances slow the rate of gastric emptying and reduce small intestinal motility, thereby resulting in delayed glucose absorption (Lu et al. 2000, Johnson 2005). Lu et al. (2000) and Zunft et al. (2004) also supported this hypothesis of slow gastric emptying in reduced glucose absorption from intestines. Another additional advantage of arabinoxylan is related to its higher palatability and this property can be used in the preparation of AX-rich food products (Lu et al. 2004, Garcia et al. 2007).

In contrast, insoluble AXs affect the total fecal output at significantly lower rates, thus yielding very little influence on glycemic control. This is further substantiated that insoluble arabinoxylan has no tangible hypoglycemic effect (Crittenden et al. 2002). Hence, the consumption of soluble fiber such as arabinoxylan can possibly be used as a remedy against diabetes mellitus as it ameliorates its complications. The consumption of AX-rich fiber (practical range of 2–10 g/day) also has an influence on controlling the plasma lipid concentrations to some extent as revealed by the study carried out by Hunninghake et al. (2005). However, such effects are less pronounced in normal lipidemic subjects as compared to hypercholesterolemic subjects. Owing to their high viscosity, AXs exert significant influence on the digestion and the metabolic fate of nutrients (Fengler and Marquardt 1988) as they tend to increase fecal bulk (Lu et al. 2000).

AXs from cereal brans and husk pectins can be digested with xylanase to obtain xylooligosaccharides (Chithra and Muralikrishna 2010, Madhukumar and Muralikrishna 2010). The prebiotic activity of xylooligosaccharide has been documented using various probiotic cultures of lactobacillus and bifidogenic sps (Crittenden et al. 2002, Chithra and Muralikrishna 2012, Madhukumar and Muralikrishna 2012) and a β-D-xylosidase is purified and characterized from *Lactobacillus brevis* (Lasrado and Muralikrishna 2013). *In vitro* antioxidant activity of xylooligosaccharide derived from cereal and millet indicated that xylooligosaccharides derived from ragi bran showed maximum antioxidant activity (Veenashri and Muralikrishna 2011). Xylooligosaccharides from Bengal gram induced a nitric acid release from macrophages in a dose-dependent manner. However, these oligosaccharides did not exhibit mitogenic and comitogenic activities (Madhukumar et al. 2011).

9.7 Arabinogalactan-Proteins

AG proteins are proteoglycan type of polymers, and they are involved in plant development, especially root generation and seed germination (Rao et al. 2007). They are linked with peptides via covalent linkages and exist as AG peptides. Arabinose and galactose constitute the major part (84–93%) while the rest is hydroxyproline-rich peptide. The galactan backbone is linked to β-D-1,3 or β-D-1,6-linked arabinose that is in turn covalently linked to peptide moiety through 4-hydroxyproline residues (Figure 9.5). AG proteins are present in coffee beans, soybeans, broad beans, and cereals. They are usually water extractable; however, they can also be obtained with alkaline extracts.

They have several health implications since they act against cytokines, allergies, hay fever, asthma, autoimmune disease, cancer, arthritis, fibromyalgia,

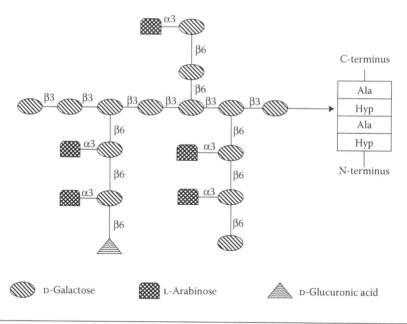

Figure 9.5 Structure of AG protein.

and viral and bacterial infections (Meuser and Suckow 1986, Labat et al. 2002). They can boost the immune responses by inhibiting tumor progression, viruses, and bacteria infiltration (Majewska-Sawka and Nothnagel 2000, Schultz et al. 2004, Garcia et al. 2007). They can also inhibit the adherence of toxic bacteria to the intestinal wall, thereby having anti-infectious potential (Girhammar and Nair 1992). In addition, AG is not amenable to human small intestinal enzymes (Loosveld and Delcour 2000) and hence, has the capacity to act as prebiotics for microorganisms residing in the large intestinal tract. These microorganisms break the AG proteins into short-chain fatty acids, which are important to mucosal health due to their role as an energy reservoir for cells forming a colon endothelial layer (Loosveld et al. 1998) as well as in overcoming inflammatory disorders and cancer (Suzuki et al. 2002). AG can have a beneficial role in decreasing ammonia levels in portal–systemic encephalopathy, a disease characterized by ammonia buildup in the liver (Showalter 2001). AG proteins also have a positive effect with respect to changes in bloating, flatulence, or stool consistency (Hunninghake et al. 2005). Contrary to arabinoxylan, AG at 30 g enhanced the blood glucose level significantly in subjects who had fasted (Toole et al. 2007, Revanappa et al. 2010). This is due to the effects that include the production of specific fermentation end products such as propionate that leads to enhancement of the process of gluconeogenesis in the liver (Van-den et al. 2002). Thus, AXs and AG are of prime importance in diabetes mellitus as well to boost immunity and fight against infection, respectively.

9.8 Pectins

Pectic substances present in the primary cell walls and middle lamellae play an important role as hydrating agents as well as cementing material for the cellulosic network (Muralikrishna and Tharanathan 1994). In the food industry in addition to their use as dietary fiber, they are used for thickening and gelling purpose (Rees 1969). Pectic substances are complex polysaccharides and are composed of (1 → 4)-linked α-D-galacturonopyranosyl residues either in free or methyl ester forms (Aspinall 1980). Arabinans, AGs, and galactan are attached at intervals to these homogalacturonan sequences at O-2-linked β-L-rhamnopyranosyl residues (Darvill et al. 1980) (Figure 9.6). The structural analysis of several pectic polysaccharides isolated from several fruit peels and also from the pulse endosperms was reported (Gordon and Christensen 1973, Tharanathan et al. 1987). Even though there are several reports available on the total pectins from various sources, the information on cereal and pulse pectins and the oligosaccharides derived from them are very limited (Salimath and Tharanathan 1982, Muralikrishna and Tharanathan 1994).

Several important biological functions of pectins were unraveled as suggested by the published literature (Willats et al. 2001, Yamada et al. 2003). Pectic polysaccharides from the roots of the medicinal herb of *Bupleurum falcatum* L. were tested for their B-cell proliferation activity (Sakurai et al. 1999). Bioactive polysaccharides from *Glinus oppositifolius* L. Aug. DC., a Malian medicinal plant, were extracted and partially characterized with

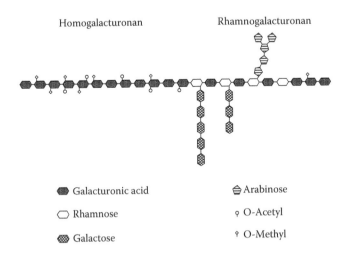

Figure 9.6 Schematic structure of pectin. Pectin consists of four different types of polysaccharides, and their structures are shown. Kdo, 3-deoxy-D-manno-2-octulosonic acid; DHA, 3-deoxy-D-lyxo-2-heptulosaric acid. HG and RGI are much more abundant than the other components. (From Harholt, J., A. Suttangkakul, and H. V. Scheller. 2010. *Plant Physiol* 153:384–395. With permission.)

respect to complement fixation activities and induced chemotaxis of macrophages, T cells, and NK cells (Inngjerdingen et al. 2005). It was reported that pectins and pectic oligosaccharides inhibit *Escherichia coli* O157:H7 shiga toxin as directed toward the human colonic cell line HT29 (Olano-Martin et al. 2003). *In vitro* evaluation of the prebiotic activity of pectic oligosaccharides derived from orange juice manufacturing by product stream as well as bergamot peel was carried out (Manderson et al. 2005, Mandalari et al. 2007).

9.9 Future Perspectives

Cereal and pulse noncellulosic polysaccharides are highly heterogeneous in their Mw, physical properties, and chemical characteristics, mainly because their biosynthesis is indirectly controlled by glycosyltransferase genes. The enzymes with individual specificities are responsible for the transfer of sugar residues from particular glycosyl donors. There are many parameters that influence the solution property of individual nonstarch polysaccharide that in turn determines its functionality and nutritional attribute. Parameters such as the overall structural integrity of the individual polysaccharide with respect to either linearity or branching; the hexose-to-pentose ratio; presence of uronic acid and its nature; Mw of the individual polysaccharide; the associated protein and its nature; esterified minor constituents such as acetic acid, phenolic acid (ferulic acid/caffeic acid/coumaric acid), diferulate bridges; hydrogen bonding; van der Waals forces; and hydrophobic interaction with other polymers such as proteins, lipids, and other nonstarch polysaccharides will have bearing on the complex behavior of the dietary fiber components. Even though the structure of most of the nonstarch polysaccharides is determined beyond ambiguity, the same is not true with respect to its nutritional implications. Another important factor is the effect of food processing on the nonstarch and noncellulosic polysaccharides that has to be studied in detail followed by functional and nutritional studies. How these dietary fiber polysaccharides affect the satiety, brain, and neurological behavior are yet to be addressed. The effect of individual polysaccharides in (a) alleviating the various disease symptoms of diabetes, atherosclerosis, colon cancer; (b) modulating functions of the liver and kidney; and (c) affecting the various beneficial/harmful bacterial populations in the large intestine is yet to be addressed in detail. Another approach is to study the dietary fiber effects on different populations with respect to diet–gene modulation. Since the cereals, millets, and pulses are the major staple foods for most of the population across the globe and the dietary fiber, being the major constituent of these grains, research on these components in untraversed paths with respect to nutrition, health, and genetics is very much warranted.

Acknowledgment

The authors thank Professor Ram Rajasekharan, director, CSIR-CFTRI for his encouragement and support.

References

Ajithkumar, A., R. Andersson, and P. Åman. 2005. Content and molecular weight of extractable β-glucan in American and Swedish oat samples. *J Agr Food Chem* 53:1205–1209.

Akramiene, D., A. Kondrotas, J. Didziapetriene, and E. Kevelaitis. 2007. Effects of beta-glucans on the immune system. *Medicina (Kaunas)* 43:597–606.

Andersson, R., G. Fransson, M. Tietjen, and P. Åman. 2009. Content and molecular-weight distribution of dietary fiber components in whole-grain rye flour and bread. *J Agric Food Chem* 57:2004–2008.

Andrewartha, K. A., D. R. Phillips, and B. A. Stone. 1979. Solution properties of wheat flour arabinoxylans and enzymatically modified arabinoxylans. *Carbohydr Res* 77:191–204.

Aspinall, G. O. 1980. Chemistry of cell wall polysaccharides. In *The Biochemistry of Plants*, ed. J. Preiss, pp. 473–500. Academic Press, New York.

Aspinall, G. O. 1982. Chemical characterization and structure determination of polysaccharides. In *The Polysaccharides* (Vol 1). ed. G. O. Aspinall, pp. 35–131. Academic Press, New York.

Babineau, T. J., A. Hackford, A.B. Kenler et al. 1994. A phase II multicenter double-blind randomized placebo-controlled study of three dosage of an immunomodulator (PGG-glucan) in high-risk surgical patients. *Arch Surg* 129:1204–1210.

Bach Knudsen, K. E. and H. N. Lærke. 2010. Rye arabinoxylans: Molecular structure, physicochemical properties and physiological effects in the gastrointestinal tract. *Cereal Chem* 87:353–362.

Balance, G. M. and D. J. Manners. 1978. Structural analysis and enzymic solubilisation of barley endosperm cell-walls. *Carbohydr Res* 61:107–118.

Bengtsson, S., R. Andersson, E. Westerlund, and P. Åman. 1992. Content, structure and viscosity of soluble arabinoxylans in rye grain from several countries. *J Sci Food Agr* 58:331–337.

Brown, I. L., K. J. McNaught, and E. Moloney. 1995. HI-MAIZE™: New directions in starch technology and nutrition. *Food Aust* 47:272–275.

Butt, M. S., M. Tahir-Nadeem, M. K. I. Khan, R. Shabir, and M. S. Butt. 2008. Oat: Unique among the cereals. *Eur J Nutr* 47:68–79.

Chanliaud, E., L. Saulnier, and J. F. Thibault. 1995. Alkaline extraction and characterisation of heteroxylans from maize bran. *J Cereal Sci* 21:195–203.

Chen, J. and R. Seviour. 2007. Medicinal importance of fungal beta-(1→3), (1→6)-glucans. *Mycol Res* 111:635–652.

Chithra, M. and G. Muralikrishna. 2012. Prebiotic activity of purified xylobiose obtained from ragi (*Eleusine coracana*, Indaf-15) bran. *Indian J Microbiol* 52: 251–257.

Chithra, M. and G. Muralkrishna. 2008. An improved process for obtaining xylanase from finger millet (*Eleusine coracana*, Indaf-15) malt. *J Food Sci Tech Mys* 45:166–169.

Chithra, M. and G. Muralikrishna. 2010. Bioactive xylo-oligosaccharides from wheat bran polysaccharides. *LWT-Food Sci Technol* 43:421–430.

Courtin, C. M. and J. A. Delcour. 2002. Arabinoxylans and endoxylanases in wheat flour breadmaking. *J Cereal Sci* 35:225–243.

Crittenden, R., S. Karpinnen, S. Ojanen et al. 2002. *In vitro* fermentation of cereal dietary fiber carbohydrates by probiotic and intestinal bacteria. *J Sci Food Agric* 82:781–789.

Cui, S. W. and Q. Wang. 2009. Cell wall polysaccharides in cereals: Chemical structures and functional properties. *Struct Chem* 20:291–297.

Cui, W., P. J. Wood, B. Blackwell, and J. Nikiforuk. 2000. Physicochemical properties and structural characterization by two-dimensional NMR spectroscopy of wheat β-D glucan—Comparison with other cereal β-D-glucans. *Carbohyd Polym* 41:249–258.

Cummings, J. H., J. I. Mann, C. Nishida, and H. H. Vorster. 2009. Dietary fibre: An agreed definition. *Lancet* 373:365–366.

Cyran, M. R. and A. Ceglinska. 2011. Genetic variation in the extract viscosity of rye (*Secale cereale* L.) bread made from endosperm and whole meal flour: Impact of high molecular-weight arabinoxylan, starch and protein. *J Sci Food Agr* 91:469–479.

Cyran, M., C. M. Courtin, and J. A. Delcour. 2003. Structural features of arabinoxylans extracted with water at different temperatures from two rye flours of diverse bread making quality. *J Agric Food Chem* 51:4404–4416.

Cyran, M., C. M. Courtin, and J. A. Delcour. 2004. Heterogeneity in the fine structure of alkali-extractable arabinoxylans isolated from two rye flours with high and low bread making quality and their coexistence with other cell wall components. *J Agric Food Chem* 52:2671–2680.

Darvill, J. E., M. McNeil, A. G. Darvill, and P. Albersheim. 1980. Structure of plant cell walls. XI. Glucuronoarabinoxylan, a second hemicellulose in primary cell walls of suspension cultured sycamore cells. *Plant Physiol* 66:1135–1139.

Dellinger, E. P., T. J. Babineau, P. Bleicher et al. 1999. Effect of PGG glucan on the rate of serious postoperative infection or death observed after high risk gastrointestinal operations. Beta fectin gastrointestinal study. *Arch Surg* 13:977–983.

Dreher, M. L. 2001. Dietary fibre overview. In *Handbook of Dietary Fibre*, eds., S. S. Cho and M. L. Dreher, pp. 1–16. Marcel Dekker, Inc, New York.

Englyst, H. N., S. M. Kingman, and J. H. Cummings. 1992. Classification and measurement of nutritionally important starch fraction. *Eur J Clin Nutr* 46:S33–S50.

Fengler, A. and R. R. Marquardt. 1988. Water-soluble pentosans from rye: I. Isolation, partial purification, and characterization. *Cereal Chem* 65: 291–297.

Fincher, G. B. and B. A. Stone. 1986. Cell walls and their components in cereal grain technology. In *Advances in Cereal Science and Technology*, ed. Y. Pomeranz, pp. 207–295. American Association of Cereal Chemists, USA.

Garcia, A., B. Otto, S. C. Reich et al. 2007. Arabinoxylan consumption decreases postprandial serum glucose, serum insulin and plasma total ghrelin response in subjects with impaired glucose tolerance. *Eur J Clin Nutr* 61: 334–341.

Girhammar, U. and B. M. Nair. 1992. Certain physical properties of water soluble non-starch polysaccharides from wheat, rye, triticale, barley and oats. *Food Hydrocolloid* 6:329–343.

Gordon, A. T. and O. Christensen. 1973. Pectin. In *Industrial Gums Polysaccharides and Their Derivatives.*, eds., R. L. Whistler and J. N. BeMiller, pp. 429–461. Academic Press, New York.

Gruppen, H., F. J. M. Kormelink, and A. G. J. Voragen. 1993. Water-unextractable cell wall material from wheat flour. 3. A structural model for arabinoxylans. *J Cereal Sci* 18:111–128.

Gruppen, H., R. A. Hoffmann, F. J. Kormelink, A. G. Voragen, J. P. Kamerling, and J. F. Vliegenthart. 1992. Characterisation by ^{1}H NMR spectroscopy of enzymically derived oligosaccharides from alkali-extractable wheat-flour arabinoxylan. *Carbohydr Res* 233:45–64.

Han, J. Y. 2000. Structural characteristics of arabinoxylan in barley, malt and beer. *Food Chem* 70:131–138.

Harada, T. and N. Ohno. 2008. Contribution of dectin-1 and granulocyte macrophage–colony stimulating factor (GMCSF) to immunomodulating actions of beta-glucan. *Int Immunopharmacol* 8:556–566.

Harholt, J., A. Suttangkakul, and H. V. Scheller. 2010. Biosynthesis of pectin. *Plant Physiol* 153:384–395.

Hegde, S., P. B. Srinivas, and G. Muralikrishna. 2009. Single step synthesis of 4-nitophenyl ferulate for spectrophotometric assay for feruloyl esterases. *Anal Biochem* 387:128–129.

Hunninghake, D. B., V. T. Miller, J. C. La Rosa et al. 2005. Hypercholesterolemic effect of dietary fiber supplement. *Am J Clin Nutr* 59:1050–1054.

Ingelbrecht, J. A., A. M. A. Loosveld, P. J. Grobet, H. Schols, E. Bakx, and J. A. Delcour. 2002. Characterization of the carbohydrate part of arabinogalactan peptides in *Triticum durum* Desf. Semolina. *Cereal Chem* 79:322–325.

Inngjerdingen, K. T., S. C. Debes, M. Inngjerdingen et al. 2005. Bioactive pectic polysaccharides from *Glinus oppositifolius* L. Aug. DC., a Malian medicinal plant, isolation and partial characterization. *J Ethnopharmacol* 101:204–214.

Izydorczyk, M. S. and J. E. Dexter. 2008. Barley β-glucans and arabinoxylans: Molecular structure, physicochemical properties, and uses in food products—A review. *Food Res Int* 41:850–868.

Izydorczyk, M. S., L. J. Macri, and A. W. MacGregor. 1998. Structure and physicochemical properties of barley non-starch polysaccharides—I. Water-extractable beta-glucans and arabinoxylans. *Carbohyd Polym* 35:249–258.

Jaskari, J., P. Konbula, A. Siitonen, H. Jousimes-Somen, T. Matilla-Sandholm, and K. Poutamen. 1998. Oat beta-glucan and xylan hydrolyzates as selective substrates for *Bifidobacterium* and *Lactobacillus* strains. *Appl Microbiol Biot* 49:175–181.

Johnson, I. T. 2005. Dietary fiber: Physiological effects on absorption. In *Encyclopedia of Human Nutrition*, 2nd edition, eds., B. Caballero, L. Allen, and A. Prentice. Elsevier, Oxford, UK.

Kumar, V., A. K. Sinha, H. P. S. Makkar, G. D. Boeck, and K. Becker. 2012. Dietary roles of non-starch polysaccharides in human nutrition: A review. *Crit Rev Food Sci Nutr* 52:899–935.

Labat, E., X. Rouau, and M.-H. Morel. 2002. Effect of flour water-extractable pentosans on molecular associations in gluten during mixing. *LWT Food Sci Technol* 35:185–189.

Lasrado, L. D. and G. Muralikrishna. 2013. Purification and characterization of β-D-xylosidase from *Lactobacillus brevis* grown on xylo-oligosaccharides. *Carbohyd Polym* 92:1978–1983.

Lavigne, L. M., J. E. Albina, and J. S. Reichner. 2006. Beta-glucan is a fungal determinant for adhesion-dependent human neutrophil functions. *J Immunol* 177:8667–8867.

Lazaridou, A. and C. G. Biliaderis. 2007. Molecular aspects of cereal β-glucan functionality: Physical properties, technological applications and physiological effects. *J Cereal Sci* 46:101–118.

Loosveld, A. M. A. and J. A. Delcour. 2000. The significance of arabinogalactan-peptide for wheat flour bread-making. *J Cereal Sci* 32:147–157.

Loosveld, A., C. Maes, W. H. M. Van-Casteren, H. A. Schols, P. F. Grobet, and J. A. Delcour. 1998. Structural variation and levels of water-extractable arabinogalactan-peptide in European wheat flours. *Cereal Chem* 75: 815–819.

Lu, Z. X., K. Z. Walker, J. G. Muir, and K. O'Dea. 2004. Arabinoxylan fiber improves metabolic control in people with type II diabetes. *Eur J Clin Nutr* 58:621–628.

Lu, Z. X., K. Z. Walker, J. G. Muir, T. Mascara, and K. O'Dea. 2000. Arabinoxylan fiber, a byproduct of wheat flour processing reduces the postprandial glucose response in normo glycemic subjects. *Am J Clin Nutr* 71:1123–1128.

Madhavilatha, G. and G. Muralikrishna. 2007. Isolation, purification and partial characterization of acetic acid esterase from malted ragi. *J Agr Food Chem* 55:895–902.

Madhavilatha, G. and G. Muralikrishna. 2009. Effect of finger millet malt esterases on the functional characteristics of non-starch polysaccharides. *Food Hydrocolloid* 23:1007–1014.

Madhavilatha, G., P. Srinivas, and G. Muralikrishna. 2007. Purification and characterization of ferulic acid esterase from malted finger millet (*Eleusine coracana*, Indaf-15). *J Agr Food Chem* 55:9704–9712.

Madhukumar, M. S. and G. Muralikrishna. 2010. Structural characterization and determination of prebiotic activity of purified xylo-oligosaccharides isolated from Bengal gram husk (*Cicer arietinum*) and wheat bran (*Triticum aestivum*). *Food Chem* 118:215–223.

Madhukumar, M. S. and G. Muralikrishna. 2012. Fermentation of xylo-oligosaccharides obtained from wheat bran and Bengal gram husk by lactic acid bacteria and bifidobacteria. *J Food Sci Tech* 49:745–752.

Madhukumar, M. S. P. M. Chandrashekar, Y. P. Venkatesh, and G. Muralikrishna. 2011. Immunomodulatory activity of xylo-oligosaccharides from Bengal gram (*Cicer arietinum* L.) husk. *Trends Carbohydr Res* 3:44–50.

Majewska-Sawka, A. and E. A. Nothnagel. 2000. The multiple roles of arabinogalactan proteins in plant development. *Plant Physiol* 122:3–10.

Mandalari, G., C. NuenoPalop, K. Tuohy et al. 2007. *In vitro* evaluation of the prebiotic activity of a pectic oligosaccharide-rich extract enzymatically derived from bergamot peel. *Appl Microbiol Biotechnol* 73:1173–1179.

Manderson, K., M. Pinart, K. M. Tuohy et al. 2005. *In vitro* determination of prebiotic properties of oligosaccharides derived from an orange juice manufacturing by-product stream. *Appl Environ Microb* 71:8383–8389.

Mayell, M. 2001. Maitake extracts and their therapeutic potential. *Altern Med Rev* 6:48–60.

McNeil, M., P. Albersheim, L. Taiz, and R. L. Jones. 1975. The structure of plant cell walls: VII. Barley aleurone cells. *Plant Physiol* 55:64–68.

Meuser, F. and P. Suckow. 1986. Non-starch polysaccharides. In *Chemistry and Physics of Baking*, eds., J. M. V. Blanshard, P. J. Frazier, and T. Gaillard, pp. 42–61. The Royal Society of Chemistry, London.

Montgomery, R., F. Smith, and H. C. Srivastava. 1957. Structure of corn hull hemicelluloses. Part IV. Partial hydrolysis and identification of 3-O-α-ᴅ-xylopyranosyl-ʟ-arabinose and 4-O-β-ᴅ-galactopyranosyl-β-ᴅ-xylose. *J Am Chem Soc* 79:698–700.

Muralikrishna, G. and M. Nirmala. 2005. Cereal α-amylases—An overview. *Carbohyd Poly* 60:163–175.

Muralikrishna, G. and M. V. S. S. T. Subba Rao. 2007. Non-cellulosic polysaccharides—Structure and function relationship—An overview. *CRC Cr Rev Food Sci* 47:599–610.

Muralikrishna, G. and R. N. Tharanathan. 1994. Characterization of pectic polysaccharides from pulse husks. *Food Chem* 50:87–89.

Narasingha Rao, B. S. 2002. Pulses and legumes as functional food. *NFI Bull* 23:1.

Nino-Medina, G., E. Carvajal-Millan, J. Lizardi et al. 2009. Maize processing waste water arabinoxylans: Gelling capability and crosslinking content. *Food Chem* 115:1286–1290.

Olano-Martin, E., M. R. Williams, G. R. Gibson, and R. A. Rastall. 2003. Pectins and pectic-oligosaccharides inhibit *Escherichia coli* O157:H7 Shiga toxin as directed towards the human colonic cell line HT29. *FEMS Microbiol Lett* 218:101–105.

Ordaz-Ortiz, J. J., M. F Devaux, and L. Saulnier. 2005. Classification of wheat varieties based on structural features of arabinoxylans as revealed by endoxylanase treatment of flour and grain. *J Agric Food Chem* 53:8349–8356.

Pelley, R. P. and F. M. Strickland. 2000. Plants, polysaccharides, and the treatment and prevention of neoplasia. *Crit Rev Oncog* 11:189–225.

Rao, R. S. and G. Muralikrishna. 2004. Non starch—Polysaccharides and phenolic acid complexes from native (N) and malted (M) cereals. *Food Chem* 84: 527–531.

Rao, R. S. and G. Muralikrishna. 2006a. Water soluble feruloyl arabinoxylans from rice and ragi: Changes upon malting and their consequence on antioxidant activity. *Phytochemistry* 67:91–99.

Rao, R. S. and G. Muralikrishna. 2006b. Efficient process of obtaining high content of bound phenolic acid rich dietary fibre by activity *in situ* amylases through stepwise increase in temperature. Patent—703 7537/2006.

Rao, R. S. and G. Muralikrishna. 2007. Structural characteristics of water-soluble feruloyl arabinoxylans from rice (*Oryza sativa*) and ragi (finger millet, *Eleusine coracana*): Variations upon malting. *Food Chem* 104:1160–1170.

Rao, R. S. and G. Muralikrishna. 2010. Dietary fibers—Purification, structure and their health benefits with particular reference to feruloyl arabinoxylans. In *Dietary Fibre, Fruit, and Vegetable Consumption and Health.*, eds., F. Klein and G. Moller, pp. 83–118. Nova Publications, USA.

Rao, R. S., R. Sai Manohar, and G. Muralikrishna. 2007. Functional properties of water soluble non-starch polysaccharides from rice and ragi, effect on dough characteristics and baking quality. *LWT-Food Sci Technol* 40:1678–1686.

Rees, D. A. 1969. Structure, conformation, and mechanism in the formation of polysaccharide gels and networks. *Adv Carbohyd Chem Biol* 24:267–332.

Revanappa, S. B., C. D. Nandini, and P. V. Salimath. 2010. Structural characterization of pentosans from hemicellulose B of wheat varieties with varying chapati-making quality. *Food Chem* 119:27–33.

Sakurai, M. H., T. Matsumoto, H. Kiyohara, and H. Yamada. 1999. B-cell proliferation activity of pectic polysaccharides from a medicinal herb, the roots of *Bupleurum falcatum* L. and its structural requirement. *Immunology* 97:540–547.

Salimath, P. V. and R. N. Tharanathan.1982. Structural features of two pectic fractions from field bean (*Dolichos lab lab*) husks. *Carbohydr Res* 106:251–257.

Schultz, C. J., K. L. Ferguson, J. Lahnstein, and A. Bacic. 2004. Post-translational modifications of arabinogalactan-peptides of *Arabidopsis thaliana*. Endoplasmic reticulum and glycosyl phosphatidyl inositol—Anchor signal cleavage sites and hydroxylation of proline. *J Biol Chem* 279:45503–45511.

Shibuya, N. 1984. Phenolic-acids and their carbohydrate esters in rice endosperm cell-walls. *Phytochemistry* 23:2233–2237.

Shibuya, N., A. Misaki, and T. Iwasaki. 1983. The structure of arabinoxylan and arabinoglucuroxylan isolated from rice endosperm cell walls. *Agric Biol Chem* 47:2223–2230.

Shibuya, N. and T. Iwasaki. 1985. Structural features of rice bran hemicellulose. *Phytochemistry* 24:285–289.

Showalter, A. M. 2001. Arabinogalactan: Structure, expression and function. *Cell Mol Life Sci* 58:1399–1417.

Slavin, J. L. 2008. Position of the American Dietetic Association: Health implications of dietary fiber. *J Am Diet Assoc* 108:1716–1731.

Stone, B. A. 2006. Cell walls of cereal grains. *Cereal Food World* 51:62–65.

Subba Rao, M. V. S. S. T. and G. Muralikrishna. 2002. Evaluation of the antioxidant properties of free and bound phenolic acids from native and malted finger millet (ragi, *Eleusine coracana* Indaf-15). *J Agric Food Chem* 50:889–892.

Suzuki, Y., M. Kitagawa, J. P. Knox, and I. Yamaguchi. 2002. A role of arabinogalactan proteins in gibberellin-induced α-amylase production in barley aleurone cells. *Plant J* 29:733–741.

Tharanathan, R. N., G. Muralikrishna, P. V. Salimath, and M. S. Raghavendra Rao. 1987. Plant carbohydrates—An overview. *Plant Indian Assoc—Plant Soc* 97: 81–155.

Toole, G. A., R. H. Wilson, M. L. Parker et al. 2007. The effect of environment on endosperm cell wall development in *Triticum aestivum* during grain filling: An infrared spectroscopy imaging study. *Planta* 225:1393–1403.

Urala, N. L. and L. Lahteenmaki. 2007. Consumers changing attitudes towards functional foods. *Food Qual Prefer* 18:1–12.

Van-den B. K., A. M. A. Loosveld, C. M. Courtin et al. 2002. Amino acid sequence of wheat flour arabinogalactan-peptide, identical to part of grain softness protein GSP-1, leads to improved structural model. *Cereal Chem* 79:329–331.

Veenashri, B. R. and G. Muralikrishna. 2011. *In vitro* anti-oxidant activity of xylo-oligosaccharides derived from cereal and millet brans—A comparative study. *Food Chem* 126:1475–1481.

Verbruggen, M. A., G. Beldman, A. G. J. Voragen, and M. Hollemans. 1993. Water-unextractable cell wall material from sorghum: Isolation and characterization. *J Cereal Sci* 17:71–82.

Verbruggen, M. A., G. Beldman, and A. G. J. Voragen. 1995. The selective extraction of glucuronoarabinoxylans from sorghum endosperm cell walls using barium and potassium hydroxide solutions. *J Cereal Sci* 21:271–282.

Verwimp, T., V. Van Craeyveld, C. M. Courtin, and J. A. Delcour. 2007. Variability in the structure of rye flour alkali-extractable arabinoxylans. *J Agric Food Chem* 55:1985–1992.

Vetvicka, V., A. Vashishta, S. Saraswat-Ohri, and J. Vetvickova. 2008. Immunological effects of yeast and mushroom derived beta-glucans. *J Med Food* 11:615–622.

Vietor, R. J., F. J. M. Kormelink, S. A. G. F. Angelino, and A. G. J. Voragen. 1994. Substitution patterns of water-unsoluble arabinogalactans from barley and malt. *Carbohydr Polym* 24:113–118.

Vinkx, C. J. A. and J. A. Delcour. 1996. Rye (*Secale cereale* L.) arabinoxylans: A critical review. *J Cereal Sci* 24:1–14.

Vinkx, C. J. A., J. A. Delcour, M. A.Verbruggen, and H. Gruppen. 1995. Rye water-soluble arabinoxylans also vary in their 2-monosubstituted xylose content. *Cereal Chem* 72:227–228.

Willats, W. G., L. McCartney, W. Mackie, and J. P. Knox. 2001. Pectin: Cell biology and prospects for functional analysis. *Plant Mol Biol* 47:9–27.

Wood, P. J. 2010. Oat and rye β-glucan: Properties and function. *Cereal Chem* 87: 315–330.

Woolard, G. R., L. Novellie, and S. J. Van der Walt. 1976. Note on the isolation of sorghum husk polysaccharides and fractionation of hemicellulose B. *Cereal Chem* 53:601–618.

Yamada, H., H. Kiyohara, and T. Matsumoto. 2003. Recent studies on possible functions of bioactive pectins and pectic polysaccharides from medicinal herbs. In *Advances in Pectin and Pectinase Research*, eds., F. Voragen, H. Schols, and R. Visser, pp. 481–490. Kluwer Academic Publishers, Dordrecht.

Zunft, H. J., W. Lueder, C. Koebnick, and D. Imhof. 2004. Reduction of postprandial glucose and insulin response in serum of healthy subjects by an arabinoxylan concentrate isolated from wheat starch plant process water. *Asia Pac J Clin Nutr* 13:147.

CHAPTER 10

Barley β-Glucan

*Natural Polysaccharide for Managing Diabetes and
Cardiovascular Diseases*

PARIYARATH SANGEETHA THONDRE

Contents

10.1 Introduction   233
10.2 Structure of β-Glucan   234
10.3 Physical Properties of β-Glucan   236
10.4 Food Products with Barley β-Glucan   237
10.5 Health Benefits of Barley β-Glucan   240
    10.5.1 Effect on Glycemic and Insulin Response   240
    10.5.2 Effect on Blood Lipids   248
10.6 Concluding Remarks   253
References   253

10.1 Introduction

Natural polysaccharides are mainly grouped under the name "dietary fiber," a term coined by Hipsley (1953) in the 1950s to refer to cellulose, hemicellulose, lignin, and so on, which form the outer walls of cereals and other plant products. This term was defined by Trowell (1972, p. 926) after almost two decades as *"the remnants of the plant cell wall that are not hydrolyzed by the alimentary enzymes of man."* The beneficial physiological effects of dietary fiber identified by Trowell (1972) were then used in the official definition of dietary fiber proposed by the American Association of Cereal Chemists (AACC) in 2001 as given below.

"Dietary fiber is the edible parts or analogous carbohydrates that are resistant to digestion and absorption in the small intestine with complete or partial fermentation in the large intestine. Dietary fiber includes polysaccharides, oligosaccharides, lignin, and associated plant substances. Dietary fibers promote beneficial physiological effects including laxation, and/or blood cholesterol attenuation, and/or blood glucose attenuation" (AACC 2001, p. 113).

Dietary fiber includes a variety of compounds such as nonstarch polysaccharides, resistant oligosaccharides, resistant starch, and lignin (EFSA 2007). β-Glucan comes under the classification of nonstarch polysaccharides that comprise cellulose, hemicelluloses, hydrocolloids, and pectins (Buttriss and Stokes 2008). Cereals such as barley and oats are rich sources of this hydrocolloid. β-Glucan from oats has received a lot of attention due to the popularity of oats as a food, but barley is not very widely used as food by humans in the developed countries. Although barley (*Hordeum vulgare* L.) was a popular staple in prehistoric days, the use of refined grains such as wheat and rice resulted in the depletion of barley from the diet of modern man. Even now, barley holds the fourth position among cereals in worldwide production after wheat, rice, and maize, and the Russian Federation, Canada, Germany, Ukraine, and France cultivate the majority of the barley produced worldwide (Mahdi et al. 2008). Only 15% of the world's barley production is used for food purposes and the rest is used in the production of malt for the brewing industry and also for animal feed. However, the diminished nutrient status of livestock fed with barley led to the identification of the role of β-glucan-soluble fiber in reducing nutrient release and absorption. This revelation later came to be utilized for preparing foods to prevent the development of chronic diseases such as obesity, type 2 diabetes, and cardiovascular diseases.

10.2 Structure of β-Glucan

β-Glucan is a long-chain polysaccharide of glucose primarily found in the endosperm cell walls of cereal grains such as oats and barley. The normal level of β-glucan in barley ranges from 3% to 7% and is comparable to oats, but there are specific breeds of barley with a high β-glucan content of around 17% with starch and total dietary fiber present in almost the same proportion. One such barley variety called Prowashonupana (Sustagrain)—abbreviated from **pro**tein rich, **wa**xy (amylopectin rich), **sho**rt awn, **nu**de (hulless), and Com**pana** (the parent variety)—bred in Canada (Eslick 1981) has 30% total dietary fiber compared to the native hulless barley with 13% total dietary fiber. Another high amylose barley called Himalaya 292 developed in Australia contains higher levels of β-glucan along with high resistant starch content as compared to native hulless barley (Bird et al. 2008). The amount of β-glucan in barley is influenced by genetic and environment factors such as drought, excessive precipitation, heat stress, and the use of nitrogen fertilizer. Other factors such as sowing period, use of fungicides, foliar disease, and so on ... were also shown to influence the yield of β-glucan from barley (Dickin

Table 10.1 β-Glucan Content in Different Varieties of Barley

Variety	Starch (%)	Protein (%)	Total Fiber (%)	β-Glucan (%)
Hulless barley	60	13	13	5
Himalaya 292	30	15	27	8
Prowashonupana	21	20	30	15

et al. 2011). Table 10.1 shows the nutrient content of three barley varieties varying in β-glucan content.

Chemically, β-glucan is a polysaccharide of glucose with (1 → 4) and (1 → 3) linkages between β-D-glucopyranose residues. But, it is different from other common glucose polysaccharides such as starch and cellulose due to some differences in the linkages between the glucose units. While starch is a polymer of α-D-glucopyranose residues with (1 → 4) linkages that makes it water soluble and easily digestible by the digestive enzymes, cellulose is a polymer of β-D-glucopyranose units with (1 → 4) linkages that makes it a nondigestible fiber (El Khoury et al. 2012). The presence of β-linkages makes β-glucan nondigestible while the intermittent (1 → 3) linkages are the characteristic features of β-glucan that make it water soluble (El Khoury et al. 2012). Figure 10.1 illustrates the representation of a barley grain showing the presence of cellulose, starch, and β-glucan with differences in the linkages associated with each polysaccharide.

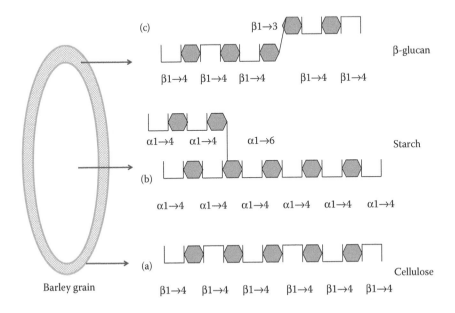

Figure 10.1 Barley grain showing the structure of barley β-glucan in comparison with cellulose and glucose. R represents glucose.

10.3 Physical Properties of β-Glucan

Water solubility is the property that allows β-glucan to form a very thick and viscous solution in the human stomach and intestines (Table 10.2). Subsequent effects of delayed gastric emptying and restricted access of the digestive enzymes to the food bolus are all proposed as the underlying mechanisms for the reduction in glycemic and insulin response to β-glucan-rich foods. The presence of the thick unstirred viscous layer generated by β-glucan in the small intestine reduces the absorption of nutrients into the circulation, thereby maintaining a slow and steady supply of energy (Jenkins et al. 2004).

Another important property responsible for the metabolic effects of β-glucan is its high molecular weight (MW). Many studies have linked the MW of β-glucan with the viscosity developed in solution (Wood 2007). The MW of β-glucan that might influence its physiological effects also depends on the methods of processing and extraction of β-glucan. While cooking increases the extractability of β-glucan, baking causes depolymerization of β-glucan and decreases its MW (Andersson et al. 2004). Efforts have been made to isolate and purify β-glucan from barley to be used in various food products. However, this result in β-glucan concentrates with a variety of MW and purity may have different effects on glycemic responses and cholesterol levels. Barley β-glucan forms aggregates in solutions *via* a very fast process that depends on diffusion mechanism and the MW of the glucans. This means that the higher the MW, the lower the rate of diffusion and the subsequent aggregate formation (Li et al. 2011), which will be different in the concentrates prepared by various methods.

β-Glucan physically binds to the cholesterol and bile acids and facilitates their excretion from the body (Chen and Huang 2009). The excretion of bile acids from the body facilitates the conversion of existing cholesterol stores into bile acids to promote fat digestion. This is the most important property that enables the lowering and maintenance of cholesterol levels in the body, following a β-glucan-rich diet. Fermentation is another property of β-glucan that produces short-chain fatty acids in the colon, which inhibits the enzyme HMG CoA reductase involved in cholesterol synthesis.

Table 10.2 Physical Properties of Barley β-Glucan

Solubility and water retention
Viscosity
Gel formation
Elasticity
Binding with fat and bile acids
Foam- and emulsion-stabilizing property
Fermentation

10.4 Food Products with Barley β-Glucan

β-Glucan is consumed as part of a normal diet by incorporating barley or oats in the diet. However, the dose suggested to deliver health benefits such as cholesterol lowering may not be achieved by using barley and oats in our diet. Hence, there has been a lot of interest in either breeding high β-glucan barley varieties or developing β-glucan-rich barley flour concentrates to use in food products (Table 10.3). β-Glucan-rich barley flour is prepared by different methods. Bourdon et al. (1999) described a repeated milling method and sifting through a 325 mesh sieve to get rid of the barley starch, resulting in a β-glucan-rich flour fraction called Waxbar flour.

The physical properties associated with β-glucan allow its use in various food products to improve their textural and nutritional characteristics. However, food manufacturers endeavoring to produce food products enriched with β-glucan face many challenges, including increasing the nutritional quality without deteriorating the consumer acceptability and product palatability. Tiwari and Cummins (2012) recently highlighted the development of a human exposure assessment model that predicted an uptake of 0.77 g per portion of β-glucan from bread baked with 70% substitution of wheat flour with barley flour. Substitution of wheat flour at 30% and 50% by barley flour was able to meet the demand of β-glucan at only 50% and 70% levels, respectively, based on the recommendations by Food and Drug Administration (FDA). Bread baking may also influence the MW of β-glucan as reported by Cleary et al. (2007). The dough became stiff with the incorporation of β-glucan, resulting in loaves of low volume and height. The high MW of β-glucan underwent degradation following baking, whereas the low MW of β-glucan was left unaffected by the baking process. *In vitro* digestion methods showed a reduction in the reducing sugar release in both breads containing high and low MW of β-glucan and thus, the authors suggested that it may be beneficial to use the low MW of β-glucan for better properties of bread and for beneficial effects on blood glucose. A 5% supplementation with the low MW of β-glucan, glucagel reduced the release of reducing sugars from the bread following *in vitro* digestion (Brennan and Cleary 2007).

Symons and Brennan (2004) reported the effect of 2.5% and 5% addition of a β-glucan-rich fraction from barley in bread, resulting in an increase in the dough elasticity at a 5% level but having a negative effect on loaf volume and height. But, the breads with 5% β-glucan-rich extract did result in lowering the reducing sugars released by *in vitro* digestion methods. The same β-glucan-rich barley was also used for the preparation of pasta, leading to the attenuation of reducing sugar release following *in vitro* digestion (Cleary and Brennan 2006). The incorporation of β-glucan at 2.5%, 5%, 7.5%, and 10% affected the cooking quality of pasta resulting in the loss of hardness, adhesiveness, and increased cooking loss mainly in the form of starch and protein. In a double-layered flat bread, the addition of 20% barley fiber-rich fraction

Table 10.3 Summary of Studies Using Barley β-Glucan in Various Food Products

Product	β-Glucan	Characteristics	Reference
Low-fat yogurt	Glucagel (0.5%, 1.0%, and 1.5%)	Decreased syneresis, increased viscosity, and improved sensory attributes	Brennan and Tudorica (2008)
Synbiotic yogurt	60% barley β-glucan (0.1–1% level)	Improved viability and stability of the probiotic bacterium and increased organic acid production	Vasiljevic et al. (2007)
Bread	5.77% β-glucan and hulled waxy feed barley variety (2.5% and 5%)	Improved elasticity, decreased loaf height, and volume	Symons and Brennan (2004)
Two-layered flat bread	Barley fiber-rich fraction with 8.9% β-glucan	Increased water absorption of the dough	Izydorczyk et al. (2008)
Pasta	5.77% β-glucan and hulled waxy feed barley variety (2.5%, 5%, 7.5%, and 10%)	Greater cooking loss, reduced hardness, and adhesiveness	Cleary and Brennan (2006)
Spaghetti	75% and 25% β-glucan at 2%, 4%, 6%, 8%, and 10% concentration	Increased cooking loss and adhesiveness with increasing β-glucan concentration	Chillo et al. (2011b)
Reduced fat sausages	0.3% and 0.8% β-glucan	Comparable to high and reduced fat controls in terms of textural and sensory attributes	Morin et al. (2002)
Frying batter	Prowash steam jet cooked flour with 15.6% β-glucan (2.5% and 5%)	Increased moisture retention and reduced oil uptake of fried batters	Lee and Inglett (2006)
Soup	34.5% β-glucan (0.5%, 1%, and 2%)	Feasible thickening agents with no adverse effect on sensory qualities	Lyly et al. (2004)
Potato and leek soup (instant)	75% and 25% β-glucan at 4 g per serving	Increased viscosity with 25% β-glucan of high MW	Thondre et al. (2013)

to wheat flour increased the water absorption and compared well with a control flat bread without the barley fraction (Izydorczyk et al. 2008). With flat breads prepared using high and low MW of β-glucan, the apparent reduction in the reducing sugars was evident only with the inclusion of high MW of β-glucan and not the low MW of β-glucan (Thondre et al. 2010, Thondre and Henry 2011). High and low MW of β-glucan incorporated into spaghetti also showed similar results with respect to the release of reducing sugars following *in vitro* digestion (Chillo et al. 2011a). Although most researchers have highlighted the undesirable characteristics of barley bread, Kinner et al. (2011) recently modified the amount of water, malt flour, and margarine to develop barley-based bread with sufficient β-glucan to fulfill the EFSA requirements in the recommended portion size. This bread could provide 0.81 g per serving of 50 g, thus contributing to the daily recommended dose of β-glucan to lower the cholesterol level from four servings a day.

Barley β-glucan is very useful as a fat replacer. In comparison to some other carbohydrate-based fat replacers such as guar gum and inulin, Brennan and Tudorica (2008) found that barley β-glucan was an excellent substitute, improving the rheological, textural, and sensory quality of yogurt. The amount of β-glucan required was only 0.5% compared to 2% required for inulin and guar gum to achieve reduced syneresis comparable to full-fat yogurt. At 1% addition, barley β-glucan improved the textural characteristics such as viscosity, product firmness, and consistency along with the sensory characteristics such as creaminess, mouthfeel, and smoothness without affecting the color and appearance of the yogurts. The prebiotic properties of β-glucan could be improved by incorporating it in a yogurt with a specific probiotic microorganism of *Bifidobacterium* species (Vasiljevic et al. 2007). The resultant symbiotic product showed an effect similar to the commonly used prebiotic inulin and produced more organic acids during the 4-week storage. The viability and stability of the probiotic bacterium was also improved with the incorporation of barley β-glucan with 60% purity at levels from 0.1% to 1%.

The high viscosity, water-binding ability and foam, and emulsion-stabilizing properties of β-glucan promoted its use as a fat replacer in sausages (Morin et al. 2002). Reduced fat sausages with 0.3% and 0.8% β-glucan were comparable to their high fat and reduced fat controls in both sensory attributes and textural characteristics and there was no loss of β-glucan after cooking.

The β-glucan-rich natural variety of barley Prowashonupana or Sustagrain barley has also been used in various food matrices to increase the soluble fiber in our diet. This specific variety has shown reduction in the oil absorption when used in frying batters (Lee and Inglett 2006). This steam jet-cooked flour added to the batter increased the water absorption, prevented moisture loss from the fried batter, and reduced the oil retention following frying, which could reduce the intake of fat and increase the intake of fiber. Although different food-processing techniques have been used for the development of food products with β-glucan, roasting may be one process to avoid because it seemed to reduce the β-glucan levels in flours without affecting its extractability (Sharma et al. 2011).

It was desirable to use β-glucan in solid foods due to its rheological and textural characteristics; however, some liquid foods were also formulated using low doses of β-glucan. An orange-flavored beverage with 0.5% β-glucan was added with whey protein isolate at different concentrations ranging from 0% to 1.5% to improve the overall acceptability and shelf life stability for this functional product (Temelli et al. 2004). While the addition of whey protein isolate decreased the intensity of the sourness and flavor of the beverage, it also resulted in the increased viscosity and cloudiness of the β-glucan beverage. Owing to the viscous properties associated with β-glucan, it can be used as a thickener in soups with no effect on freezing and thawing (Lyly et al. 2004). The addition of 0.5%, 1.0%, and 2.0% β-glucan in soups influenced the sensory perception of soups depending on the MW and concentration of β-glucan. β-Glucan of lower MW <200 kDa is best suitable to include the required amounts in a portion of the soup, but it is important to consider the additional beneficial effects associated with high MW of β-glucan. The use of β-glucan in an instant potato and leek soup showed differences in viscosity, depending on the MW of the β-glucan (Thondre et al. 2013). The soup with high MW of β-glucan had higher viscosity as compared to the soup with low MW of β-glucan and the control soup with no β-glucan. Table 10.4 summarizes the studies in which food products were developed using barley β-glucan of different purity and physical properties. The effects of physical properties of β-glucan observed in the *in vitro* studies were supported by the *in vivo* studies, highlighting the importance of maintaining the MW of β-glucan during purification and food preparation for beneficial physiological effects (Thondre and Henry 2009, 2011).

10.5 Health Benefits of Barley β-Glucan

10.5.1 *Effect on Glycemic and Insulin Response*

Diabetes mellitus has emerged as a worldwide public health problem in the past 20 years, especially with the increased prevalence of obesity. Previous research has shown that lifestyle and pharmacological interventions can prevent or delay the progression of impaired glucose intolerance (IGT) to type 2 diabetes. The use of barley β-glucan in foods with a high glycemic index could result in lowering the glycemic response and maintaining healthy blood glucose levels in people with IGT. Glycemic and insulin response to β-glucan-rich foods depended on the physical properties mentioned above and also on the form of the test meals used as described in this section (Table 10.5).

Table 10.4 Summary of the Randomized Controlled Trials and Long-Term Studies Carried Out to Test the Effect of Barley β-Glucan on Glycemic and Insulin Responses

Study	β-Glucan	Subjects	Results
Ostman et al. (2002)	Barley bread (80% barley flour and 20% wheat flour) with 81 g lactic acid	Healthy subjects	23% reduction in glycemic response and 21% reduction in insulin response
Ostman et al. (2006)	Bread baked by substituting 50% and 75% Prowashonupana barley flour	Healthy men	Reduction in the GI and II of bread
Biorklund et al. (2005)	Beverage with 5 or 10 g barley β-glucan	Hypercholester-olemic subjects for 8 weeks	No effect on glucose or insulin
Li et al. (2003)	Barley and rice 30:70 for 4 weeks	Normal healthy women	No effect on glucose tolerance
Bourdon et al. (1999)	Pasta with 40% substitution of wheat flour with β-glucan-enriched barley flour or naturally β-glucan-rich barley flour	Healthy men	Reduced insulin response
Liljeberg et al. (1996)	Porridge (17.5%) and flat bread with β-glucan-rich barley flour (11.1% and 14.9%)	Healthy subjects	Low GR, IR, and GI and II
Bays et al. (2011)	Beverages with low viscosity β-glucan; 6 g/day	Healthy subjects with baseline hyperglycemia, but no diabetes	Improved insulin sensitivity in 12 weeks
Keogh et al. (2003)	75% purity glucagel, cooked into various foods; 10 g/day	Mildly hyperlipidemic, overweight men	No effect on blood glucose profile
Poppitt et al. (2007)	Solid and liquid high-carbohydrate foods; Cerogen; 6.3 g per serving	Healthy men	Only solid food reduced glycemic response
Cavallero et al. (2002)	Bread baked with β-glucan-enriched water-extracted barley flour. 5.7%	Healthy subjects	28% reduction in GI

continued

Table 10.4 (continued) Summary of the Randomized Controlled Trials and Long-Term Studies Carried Out to Test the Effect of Barley β-Glucan on Glycemic and Insulin Responses

Study	β-Glucan	Subjects	Results
Thondre and Henry (2009)	25% purity, MW, chapatis with 4 and 8 g per serving	Healthy subjects	43% reduction in GI and 47% reduction in GI
Yokoyama et al. (1997)	Durum wheat pasta with β-glucan (12 g)	Healthy subjects	Reduced glycemic response
Behall et al. (2006)	Muffins with 0.1, 3, and 6 g β-glucan with 0.1, 6, and 12 g resistant starch	Overweight, mildly insulin resistant, and healthy subjects	Reduction in GR and IR
Casiraghi et al. (2006)	Barley cookies and crackers; 38% β-glucan; 3.5–3.6 g per 40 g of available CHO serving	Healthy subjects	50% reduction in GI and II
Alminger and Eklund-Jonsson (2008)	Tempe-fermented barley (4.6% β-glucan)	Healthy subjects	Reduced GI to 30
Rendell et al. (2005)	Prowashonupana barley cereal compared to a liquid meal replacer	Nondiabetic and diabetic subjects	Reduced glycemic response to 1/4th in nondiabetic and 1/2 in diabetic and insulin response 1/10th in nondiabetic and 1/3rd in diabetic
Hinata et al. (2007)	Mugimeshi, a mixture of rice and barley in 7:2 ratio	Type 2 diabetes	Reduction in HbA1c and fasting plasma glucose over 2 years
Kim et al. (2009)	Breakfast cereal with 10 g β-glucan	Overweight women with risk of insulin resistance	Reduced GR and IR

Healthy men fed with high carbohydrate solid and liquid meals with β-glucan showed reduced postprandial glycemic response only to the solid food (Poppitt et al. 2007). The liquid food consumption showed no effect probably due to inadequate time available for the development of viscosity in the case of the beverages and also due to quick gastric emptying and absorption of sugars due to the absence of starch in liquid foods. Cavallero et al. (2002) tested the glycemic index (GI) to bread with barley flour and sieved, water-extracted fractions of β-glucan-enriched barley flour in healthy people.

Table 10.5 Summary of Studies That Tested the Effect of β-Glucan on Blood Lipids

Study	β- Glucan	Subjects	Results
Rondanelli et al. (2011)	Foods with 6 g/day β-glucan (BB)	Mildly hypercholester-olemic men	5% reduction in total cholesterol and 8.6% reduction in LDL cholesterol
Behall and Hallfrisch (2006)	Foods containing 3 and 6 g barley β-glucan	Moderately hypercholester-olemic men	17% and 20% reduction in total cholesterol
		Mildly hypercholester-olemic men and women	9% and 10% reduction in total cholesterol
Biorklund et al. (2005)	Beverage with 5 or 10 g barley β-glucan	Hypercholester-olemic subjects for 8 weeks	No effect on serum lipids
Lia et al. (1995)	Bread with barley β-glucan (13 g /day) for 2 days	Ileostomy patients	Increased cholesterol excretion
Aman (2006)	Aktivated barley with 5% β-glucan	Mildly hypercholester-olemic subjects	Reduced LDL cholesterol by 5% in 4 weeks
Hallfrisch et al. (2003)	Whole-grain barley with 6 g β-glucan	Moderately hypercholester-olemic subjects	Reduced systolic blood pressure
Keenan et al. (2007)	High and low MW of β-glucan at 3 and 5 g/day in the form of breakfast cereal or low-calorie fruit juice	Hypercholester-olemic subjects	9% reduction in LDL cholesterol with 3 g dose, 13% reduction in LDL cholesterol using 5 g LMW β-glucan, and 15% reduction in LDL cholesterol using 5 g HMW β-glucan
Li et al. (2003)	Barley and rice 30:70 for 4 weeks	Normal healthy women	Reduced total and LDL cholesterol
Keogh et al. (2003)	75% purity glucagel, cooked into various foods; 10 g/day	Mildly hyperlipidemic, overweight men	No effect on lipid profile
Behall et al. (2004)	β-glucan at 3 and 6 g/day for 5 weeks	Mildly hypercholester-olemic subjects	Lowered total and LDL cholesterol Altered LDL particle size

continued

Table 10.5 (continued) Summary of Studies That Tested the Effect of β-Glucan on Blood Lipids

Study	β-Glucan	Subjects	Results
Shimizu et al. (2008)	Barley with 3.5 g β-glucan mixed with rice (50% each)	Hypercholestr-olemic Japanese men	Lowered total and LDL cholesterol and visceral fat
Sundberg (2008)	Barley flakes with 3% β-glucan	Subjects with moderately elevated cholesterol	Total and LDL cholesterol lowered
Smith et al. (2008)	Low and high MW β- glucan in powder form; 6 g/day for 6 weeks	Hypercholestr-olemic men and women	No difference in cholesterol levels. Only body weight reduced more by high MW β-glucan
Ikegami et al. (1996)	Barley and rice 50:50; 2 times a day for 4 weeks	Hyperlipidemic men and hypercholester-olemic women	Reduction in total and LDL cholesterol and triglycerides
Liljeberg et al. (1996)	Porridge (17.5%) and flat bread with β-glucan-rich barley flour (11.1% and 14.9%)	Healthy subjects	Low GR, IR, and GI and II

The proportion of substitution was 50% for the barley flour and the sieved fraction and 20% for the water-extracted fraction, resulting in the β-glucan content of 2%, 2.8%, and 5.7%, respectively compared to 0.1% in the control wheat flour bread. A 28% reduction in GI was obtained for the bread with the water-extracted fraction of barley flour rich in β-glucan. However, a similar concentration of β-glucan in the bread made with high β-glucan Prowashonupana barley flour did not show a significant reduction in GI (Ostman et al. 2006). The common barley flour was used to substitute for 50% of wheat flour, whereas, with Prowashonupana barley flour, three substitutions at 35%, 50%, and 75% were used to bake bread with barley β-glucan. The bread prepared using common barley flour had 2.6% β-glucan while the β-glucans in the bread prepared using Prowashonupana barley flour were 5.75%, 7.95%, and 12.24% for the 35%, 50%, and 75% substitution, respectively. A significant reduction in the GI and insulinemic index (II) of the bread was observed only with the 50% and 75% substitution of Prowashonupana barley flour. The mechanisms proposed for this effect include reduced motility of the intestinal contents and high viscosity generated by the thick layer that remains unstirred, thereby slowing down the absorption of nutrients from the intestinal lumen into the blood stream.

Additional ingredients such as lactic acid in barley bread have shown an impact on the blood glucose and insulin response to a second meal of high GI (Ostman et al. 2002). A significant lowering of glycemic and insulin response in healthy subjects was observed after a high GI lunch following the breakfast of barley bread with lactic acid. This reduction in starch digestion may have been due to a prolonged starch digestion caused by lactic acid rather than the delayed gastric emptying exhibited by other acids such as acetic and propionic acids in some other studies (Ostman et al. 2005). The effect of high amylose barley bread with 30% Prowashonupana barley flakes was also used to identify the second meal effect to a high GI lunch (Liljeberg et al. 1999). Unlike the previous study, this trial tested the glycemic and insulin response after the second meal lunch following breakfast with predetermined glycemic and insulin indices. The high amylose bread with barley flakes had a low GI and resulted in a significant reduction in the second meal glycemic response, whereas another low GI breakfast of white wheat bread with vinegar did not result in the lowering of the glycemic response after the second meal. This reiterated the superior effect of β-glucan on a day-long glucose tolerance over other hypoglycemic agents such as acids.

In healthy subjects, the high-molecular-weight barley β-glucan in unleavened flat breads lowered the GI by 43% at a dose of 4 g per serving of 50 g available carbohydrate (CHO) and also, a reduction of 47% was observed at a dose of 8 g per serving (Thondre and Henry 2009). Similar results were observed for durum wheat pasta containing 12 g β-glucan that reduced the glycemic response in healthy subjects (Yokoyama et al. 1997). Behall et al. (2006) prepared muffins with β-glucan using various barley sources such as spent malt barley and standard barley flour with added β-glucan. The muffins with low (0.1 g), medium (3.1 g), and high (5.8 g) β-glucan were also supplemented with 0.1, 6.1, or 11.6 g resistant starch, respectively, per 75 g of available CHO. These muffins were effective in lowering the glucose and insulin responses in overweight men with mild insulin resistance and the result was attributed to β-glucan and not to resistant starch. A coarse barley flour fraction with 38% β-glucan was used by Casiraghi et al. (2006) to prepare cookies and crackers to compare with wheat bran-based control products. The dose of β-glucan was 3.5–3.6 g in a 40 g available carbohydrate portion. The GI and II of both barley-based cookies and crackers were 50% lower than the wheat-based control samples when tested in healthy subjects. Of the two barley-based products, cookies were better than crackers probably due to a processing effect resulting in lower moisture content, water activity, and starch gelatinization. The authors did not test the MW of the β-glucan used and hence, no conclusion may be drawn.

Another method used for preparing β-glucan-based products is fermentation. Alminger and Eklund-Jonsson (2008) evaluated the effect of fermented high amylose barley with 4.6% β-glucan on healthy volunteers. The glycemic response was lowered by the tempe-fermented barley with a

GI of 30. In overweight women with normoglycemic status, barley-based cereal meals with 0, 2.5, 5, 7.5, and 10 g were tested (Kim et al. 2009). The 10 g dose showed an acute reduction in insulin response that was more pronounced than the reduction in glycemic response. This could be attributed to the reduction in gastric inhibitory peptide (GIP) or glucagon-like peptide (GLP-1) hormones.

In healthy women subjected to a 4-week diet with either rice or 30% barley and 70% rice, there was no effect on glucose tolerance at the end of the intervention period, suggesting that the duration was not enough to induce a significant difference on glucose tolerance (Li et al. 2003). However, a recent study investigated the effect of a low-viscosity barley β-glucan on insulin resistance in healthy subjects (Bays et al. 2011). The subjects were administered a placebo drink or a test drink containing either a low or high dose of low-viscosity barley β-glucan daily for 12 weeks. The outcome of the study was measured by oral glucose tolerance test (OGTT) at the end of the intervention to identify the effect on fasting and postprandial glucose and insulin responses. While the low dose of β-glucan treatment was effective in lowering the glucose area under the curve, the high-dose treatment successfully reduced the insulin response and improved insulin sensitivity in the subjects measured by homeostasis model assessment-estimated insulin resistance (HOMA IR). Despite the advice to the subjects to follow a weight-maintenance diet, there were no changes in the weight after intervention and this supports the hypothesis that the beneficial effect on insulin sensitivity was not just due to low-calorie intake and weight loss. This suggests that barley β-glucan may have an effect on glucose homeostasis beyond weight loss. The consumption of a rice meal mixed with barley (7:2 ratio) has also shown a significant improvement in the long-term management of blood glucose in Japanese prisoners (Hinata et al. 2007). During a 2-year follow-up, the prisoners showed a significant reduction in HbA1c and fasting plasma glucose levels with some subjects being able to discontinue the use of insulin or oral hypoglycemic agents.

Bourdon et al. (1999) compared the effect of wheat pasta with barley pasta prepared by substituting 40% of wheat flour with barley flour naturally rich in β-glucan or enriched barley flour by processing to increase the high β-glucan. The high-fiber version had 15.7 g fiber, whereas the low-fiber version had only 5 g fiber. Postprandial measures of glucose, insulin, and the satiety hormone cholecystokinin (CCK) were recorded to identify the benefits of consuming this barley flour pasta. The control pasta had only 0.3 g β-glucan, whereas the pasta naturally rich in β-glucan (Prowash) and the pasta made of β-glucan-enriched barley flour had 5 g of β-glucan per serving. Although both glucose and insulin increased postprandial in the plasma, the insulin increase was more blunted with the β-glucan-rich pasta meals. The satiety hormone CCK was increased after the barley pasta, suggesting the influence of barley β-glucan in slowing carbohydrate digestion and absorption.

Porridges made with commercial whole-meal barley or oats flour and a mixture of β-glucan-rich barley and common barley in equal proportions were compared with flat breads made by mixing the β-glucan-rich barley (Prowashonupana) and commercial barley mixed in equal ratios or in an 80:20 ratio (Liljeberg et al. 1996). The glucose and insulin response to the commercial barley and oat flours were similar to that of a reference food of white wheat bread, whereas the β-glucan-rich barley flour used in the test meals reduced the postprandial glucose and insulin response significantly, leading to a low GI value. The main difference in the test meals was the low β-glucan content in the oats and common barley porridges (4 and 4.7 g per 100 g, respectively) in comparison with the higher β-glucan content in the bread prepared with a 50:50 ratio of Prowash flour and common barley flour (11.1/100 g), bread baked with an 80:20 ratio of Prowash flour and common barley flour (14.9/100 g) and high-fiber barley porridge (17.5/100 g).

In a study carried out to test the effect of 5 or 10 g of β-glucan from oats or barley in beverages against a control beverage administered for 8 weeks to hypercholesterolemic subjects, a significant difference in glucose and insulin was observed using only 5 g of oat β-glucans and not the higher dose of oat β-glucan or both the doses of barley β-glucans. The barley used in this study was milled and treated with enzymes to remove the insoluble fiber and the remaining fraction was freeze dried to obtain flour with 36% β-glucan content. The MW for the β-glucan in this preparation was only 40,000 Da. The authors believed that this low MW must have affected the viscosity development resulting from β-glucan and might have been responsible for no effect on glycemic and insulin response (Biorklund et al. 2005).

The high β-glucan barley named Prowashonupana barley has shown a significant reduction in the glycemic and insulin responses in both nondiabetic and diabetic subjects as compared with oat meal and a low-energy meal replacement reference meal (Rendell et al. 2005). The barley cereal had 10 g soluble fiber and lower starch content compared to the oat meal with 3 g soluble fiber and double the starch present in the barley meal. The glycemic response to the liquid meal replacer reference was 4 times more than the barley cereal in nondiabetic subjects and double in diabetic subjects. The insulin response to barley meal was reduced by 10 times in the nondiabetic subjects and 3 times in the diabetic subjects in comparison with the liquid meal replacer. The mechanisms behind the beneficial effects of Prowashonupana barley were tested by growing it with normal barley in the presence of $^{13}CO_2$. Both the varieties were then consumed by healthy subjects to test the rate of digestion and fermentation of the two barley cultivars varying in β-glucan content. Breath samples collected from the subjects for 450 min after consumption of the cereals showed a reduction in the oxidation of ^{13}C and increase in expulsion of hydrogen, indicating delayed absorption and increased colonic fermentation of β-glucan-rich barley (Lifschitz et al. 2002). Different types of meals varying in particle size prepared using the high β-glucan barley produced similar results in terms of the glycemic response in overweight and obese subjects. Both the barley flour and flakes reduced the postprandial glycemic and insulin response significantly as compared to a reference glucose, highlighting the predominant effect of soluble fiber β-glucan over the difference in particle size of the food (Behall et al. 2005).

A recently published study established a relation between the MW of β-glucan and gastric emptying (Thondre et al. 2013). Using a soup test meal with high and low MW of β-glucan, the authors demonstrated that the glycemic response and gastric emptying of the test soups depended on the MW of β-glucan. This effect could be attributed to the differences in viscosity generated in the soup following the addition of β-glucan.

10.5.2 Effect on Blood Lipids

The mechanisms behind the cholesterol-lowering effect of β-glucan are varied mainly due to its effects on bile acids and cholesterol. β-Glucan increases the excretion of cholesterol and bile acids and thereby reduces their reabsorption in the intestine and promotes the hepatic production of bile acids from existing cholesterol stores in the body. Another mechanism relates to the fermentation of β-glucan in the colon and the resultant production of short-chain fatty acids such as acetate, propionate, and butyrate. Propionate is known to inhibit the enzyme HMG CoA reductase that is involved in cholesterol biosynthesis (Pins and Kaur 2006).

β-Glucan has an important role in reducing cholesterol levels in human subjects as discussed in many reviews (AbuMweis et al. 2010, Aman 2006, El Khoury et al. 2012, Tiwari and Cummins 2011). However, physical properties have been shown to have variable effects on the efficacy of β-glucan in cholesterol lowering (Wolever et al. 2010). Among the factors that may influence the efficacy of β-glucan are MW, viscosity, solubility, mode of delivery, and processing methods used to prepare test foods with β-glucan (AbuMweis et al. 2010). While some researchers have reported the MW of β-glucan in the studies, others have not always attempted to discuss the MW of the β-glucan used in the human studies, making it harder to arrive at a conclusion based on changes in physical properties associated with β-glucan.

Changes in physical properties of β-glucan can happen during domestic cooking or industrial processing. When mildly hyperlipidemic men were on a diet of a variety of snacks and meals cooked with β-glucan-enriched barley powder (75% purity) for 4 weeks, there were no changes in their triglycerides, total, low-density lipoprotein (LDL), or high-density lipoprotein (HDL) cholesterol levels. Neither was any change noted in their fasting or postprandial blood glucose levels after the intervention period (Keogh et al. 2003). This was despite the higher-than-normal recommended daily dose of 10 g/day and the authors thought that the unfavorable results may have been due to the structural changes undergone by β-glucan during processing for commercialization. Such changes have been known to reduce the MW and the resultant viscosity, which are very important properties that improve the efficacy of β-glucan (Wood 2007).

The effect of MW on cardiovascular disease markers has been investigated but the range of MW has varied widely between studies. In a randomized parallel design, 90 hypercholesterolemic subjects were allocated to consume 6 g of low or high MW of β-glucan per day for 6 weeks (Smith et al. 2008). The MW was 62,000 Da in the low MW variant and had 75% purity, whereas the high MW version had a MW of 139,000 Da with 85% purity. The β-glucan was supplied as a supplement in powder form and the subjects were instructed to consume it mixed with a beverage. After 6 weeks of intervention, a reduction from baseline was noticed only in the LDL cholesterol, C-reactive protein (CRP), and cholesterol/HDL ratio in the low MW group. The cholesterol/HDL ratio was slightly increased in the high molecular weight (HMW) group. However, there were no significant differences between the two groups in blood glucose, insulin, or blood pressure. Against the hypothesis of the authors, the high MW of β-glucan did not result in a better cholesterol profile due to its increased viscosity effect and the authors concluded that the MW is not just the effective parameter (Smith et al. 2008). The effect on hypertension may be due to the influence of β-glucan on insulin sensitivity. Other potential mechanisms are those mediated by improvement in body weight and blood cholesterol levels. In another study comparing β-glucan of different MWs, Keenan et al. (2007) investigated the effect of concentrated barley β-glucan (Barliv) in two doses (3 and 5 g/day) and in the form of a ready-to-eat breakfast cereal and a reduced calorie fruit juice beverage on lipid levels in hypercholesterolemic subjects. After 6 weeks of intervention, there was a 15% reduction in the LDL cholesterol in 5 g of high MW of β-glucan group. The beneficial effects were also noticed in 5 g of low MW of β-glucan group with a 13% reduction in LDL cholesterol closely followed by a 9% reduction in LDL cholesterol in the 3 g dose of high and low MW barley β-glucan groups. Similar results were obtained for total cholesterol also, but the HDL cholesterol did not show any change after the treatment. One limitation of this study was the failure to specify the exact MW of the β-glucan used.

Not many studies have investigated the effects of barley β-glucan on both serum lipids and glucose and insulin concentration in one trial. Interestingly, some studies that followed such a design compared oats and barley β-glucan and reported that barley β-glucan is not as effective as oat β-glucan in lowering cholesterol (Biorklund et al. 2005). The effect of 5 or 10 g of β-glucan from oats or barley was tested in beverages against a control beverage administered for 8 weeks to hypercholesterolemic subjects. A significant difference in serum lipids was observed using only 5 g of oat β-glucans and not the higher dose of oat β-glucan or both the doses of barley β-glucans. The barley used in this study was milled and treated with enzymes to remove the insoluble fiber and the remaining fraction was freeze dried to obtain flour with 36% β-glucan content. The MW for the β-glucan in this preparation was only 40,000 Da.

The authors believed that this low MW affected the viscosity development and might have been responsible for no effect on the cholesterol levels.

Instead of using concentrated or purified β-glucan, some trials have compared barley alone or mixed with other grains. One such study compared normolipidemic, hyperlipidemic, and hypercholesterolemic subjects and showed the lowering of cholesterol by a 50:50 mixture of rice and barley in only the hyperlipidemic men and women. The test foods were administered 2 times a day for 4 weeks. There was no effect on the normolipidemic subjects, which suggests that the benefits will be more obvious in hyperlipidemic subjects (Ikegami et al. 1996). In hypercholesterolemic Japanese subjects, barley was used to replace rice to test the effect of β-glucan on body fat levels. The barley used had a high β-glucan content to provide 7 g/day when mixed with rice and was consumed against a placebo rice meal for 12 weeks. The test diet had 50% rice and 50% barley, providing a β-glucan dose of 3.5 g per portion. The consumption of barley with rice significantly lowered both the total and LDL cholesterol and there was a time-dependent effect on the total cholesterol. A significant difference was also noticed in the visceral fat of the test and placebo groups with the test group showing a significant reduction from baseline in visceral fat at the end of 12 weeks (Shimizu et al. 2008). The effects may have been due to the soluble fiber effect that decreases gastric emptying, digestion, and absorption. The reduction in glucose and insulin may have resulted in lowering fatty acid synthesis, whereas the β-glucan may also have excreted cholesterol by its binding effects on cholesterol and bile acids. The authors were not clear about the effect of barley on visceral fat, but believed that it may be due to the low GI effect or due to compounds other than β-glucan present in barley. Whole-grain foods containing 0, 3, or 6 g β-glucan from barley were also tested in mildly hypercholesterolemic subjects for 5 weeks (Behall et al. 2004). There was a significant reduction in total cholesterol after the 3 and 6 g dose of β-glucan, especially in men and postmenopausal women. Although there were no effects on the HDL cholesterol or triacyl glycerol concentrations, there was a significant lowering of large LDL and small very-low-density lipoprotein (VLDL) fractions and mean LDL particle size after the incorporation of β-glucan in the diets. This indicated a possible mechanism to reduce the risk of cardiovascular disease (CVD) caused by the increased prevalence of small LDL particles (Behall et al. 2004).

When healthy women were subjected to a 4-week diet with either rice or 30% barley and 70% rice, a significant improvement was noticed in their total and LDL cholesterol and triglyceride levels. The total cholesterol was reduced by 14.5%, whereas triacyl glycerol was reduced by 13.9% (Li et al. 2003). Lia et al. (1995) explained the mechanism of cholesterol lowering using β-glucan-rich barley fraction in ileostomy patients. Breads prepared using barley containing 13 g β-glucan per day were served for two consecutive days and compared with wheat flour bread and oat bran bread. Analysis revealed an increased excretion of cholesterol and a decreased excretion of bile acids after barley bread (Lia et al. 1995). In moderately hypercholesterolemic men, the use of whole-grain barley reduced the systolic blood pressure compared to those who used the wheat and brown rice diet or a mixture of the whole-grain barley and brown rice/wheat diet with equivalent dietary fiber content. The authors did not relate this effect to any proposed mechanisms on blood pressure lowering such as loss of electrolytes in urine, changes in gastric emptying, or fecal losses of minerals due to lack of data on gastric emptying. However, they found differences in the excretion of potassium in the urine samples collected from the subjects after consumption of the whole-grain barley. But the results were inconclusive because there was no significant difference in the blood pressure following the three whole-grain diets (Hallfrisch et al. 2003).

A comparison of barley flakes with 3% β-glucan against wheat flakes for 4 weeks in individuals with moderately elevated cholesterol levels showed a significant reduction in total and LDL cholesterol in the barley flake group compared to the placebo that had identical nutrient content (Sundberg 2008). Bourdon et al. (1999) compared the effect of wheat pasta with barley pasta prepared by substituting 40% of wheat flour with barley flour naturally rich in β-glucan or enriched and processed barley flour high in β-glucan. The high-fiber version had 15.7 g fiber, whereas the low-fiber version had only 5 g fiber. Postprandial measures of lipids were recorded to identify the benefits of consuming this barley flour pasta. The control pasta had only 0.3 g β-glucan, whereas the pasta naturally rich in β-glucan (Prowashonupana) and the pasta made of β-glucan-enriched barley flour had 5 g β-glucan per serving. The cholesterol levels dropped below fasting and remained significantly lower than the control meals after 4 h of the pasta meals, suggesting the influence of barley β-glucan in slowing lipid digestion and absorption. Lowering of cholesterol may have also resulted from the reverse transport of cholesterol that lowers cholesterol in the plasma. Hyperlipidemic subjects who consumed 8 g/day of fiber from barley combined with psyllium fiber showed significant improvements in their cholesterol and apolipoprotein levels that might reduce the risk of cardiovascular diseases (Jenkins et al. 2002). A new barley product called Aktivated barley containing 5% β-glucan produced by boiling, flaking, and milling of barley showed a reduction in total and LDL cholesterol in mildly hypercholesterolemic human subjects after 4 weeks of consumption (Aman 2006). However, it may be noted that another highly purified β-glucan called glucagel did not elicit a similar reduction in blood cholesterol.

While most trials have used the same food with different doses or MW of β-glucan, others have compared different types of foods. Behall et al. (2006) conducted two studies in subjects with varied degrees of hypercholesterolemia evaluating barley β-glucan at doses of 0, 3, or 6 g/day in different foods prepared using barley flour, flakes, and pearled barley. In the first study with moderately hypercholesterolemic men, the total cholesterol concentrations were lowered by 14%, 17%, and 20% with the three doses after 5 weeks. In mildly hypercholesterolemic men and women, the total cholesterol marginally decreased by 4%, 9%, and 10% at the three doses of β-glucan. The authors speculated the role of β-glucan in the micelle formation of fats and bile acids. In another study using barley foods in hypercholesterolemic men for 4 weeks, there was a reduction in the total cholesterol (6%) observed with the barley diet as compared to a control wheat diet. While LDL cholesterol also showed a reduction by 7%, there was no change to the HDL levels of the subjects. The amount of β-glucan consumed from the mixed diet was around 8 g/day (Mcintosh et al. 1991). In a recent 14-week trial in mildly hypercholesterolemic men randomized to consume either barley β-glucan or rice bran for 4 weeks, a significant lowering of total and LDL cholesterol was observed for the β-glucan group as compared to the rice bran group (Rondanelli et al. 2011). β-Glucan and rice bran were incorporated into various foods such as pasta, tomato sauce, vegetable soup, rice cakes, and bread to provide 6 g of β-glucan per day, whereas the rice bran diet provided no soluble dietary fiber. The β-glucan used was of high MW but of low purity with 30% concentration. The reduction in LDL cholesterol (8.6%) was more following the β-glucan intervention compared to 1.1% after the rice bran consumption. While the total cholesterol reduced by 5% in the β-glucan group, there was an increase in total cholesterol in the rice bran group by 1.3%. This confirmed the results from the previous studies where β-glucan mimics the effect of statins that are HMG CoA reductase inhibitors causing a reduction in cholesterol levels.

A recent meta-analysis and systematic review has reported lowering of total blood cholesterol, LDL cholesterol, and triglycerides in people consuming barley in various forms containing 3–10 g of β-glucan (Talati et al. 2009). This finding was important because the results were independent of whether the participants were consuming a normal or low-fat diet, which suggests that the effect on cholesterol is due to the consumption of β-glucan and not just by a change in the normal diet followed by the participants. There was no effect on improving the HDL cholesterol levels in the subjects. The cholesterol-lowering effects of barley β-glucan may depend on various factors such as MW, solubility, dose, food matrix, and the subject's baseline characteristics (AbuMweis et al. 2010). A recent meta-analysis of randomized controlled trials showed that both barley and β-glucan from barley are efficient in reducing the total and LDL cholesterol levels, but the authors did not see a dose-dependent effect or any influence of subject characteristics or food matrix responsible for the effect. The lack of a dose response effect may be attributed to the variations in the MW of the β-glucan used in the studies. Another factor to be considered is the solubility of β-glucan, which might also affect the response to cholesterol levels. Low MW and low solubility properties reduce the efficacy of β-glucan in lowering cholesterol levels. Like many soluble fibers, barley β-glucan also did not show an increase in HDL cholesterol levels in the studies where it reduced the LDL cholesterol levels. Not all studies report the MW and solubility of β-glucan that makes it difficult to derive any conclusion based on their effect on cholesterol lowering. At higher doses above 5 g/day, the effect plateaus do not show a dose-dependent increase in the effect. This makes complete sense as the required dose for cholesterol lowering is 3 g/day. Another issue with the effect of β-glucan is the change it undergoes during processing in terms of solubility and MW such that sometimes the effect on cholesterol lowering is not observed if the food matrix incorporating β-glucan is highly processed. Some studies have also speculated that the presence of β-glucanase enzymes in wheat flour that get activated following processing methods may depolymerize β-glucan chains and thereby reduce their hypocholesterolemic effect. Another more recent meta-analysis compared the role of oat and barley β-glucan in cholesterol lowering and glycemic response (Tiwari and Cummins 2011). Unlike the earlier meta-analysis, this report showed a dose response effect of oat and barley β-glucan on both cholesterol and glucose levels and also an increase in HDL cholesterol levels. However, separate analysis did not show the beneficial effect on HDL cholesterol following barley β-glucan consumption.

10.6 Concluding Remarks

The effect of barley β-glucan on lowering glucose and cholesterol levels has been illustrated in many studies although there is still some discrepancy in deciding the precise MW and viscosity required for demonstrating the beneficial health effects. Nevertheless, the European Food Safety Authority (EFSA) has approved the cholesterol-lowering health claim for barley β-glucan ranging from 100 to 2000 kDa in MW (EFSA 2011). Including barley in the daily diet is thus a viable strategy to control and manage some of the chronic diseases prevalent worldwide.

References

AbuMweis, S. S., S. Jew, and N. P. Ames. 2010. β-glucan from barley and its lipid-lowering capacity: A meta-analysis of randomized, controlled trials. *Eur J Clin Nutr* 64:1472–1480.

Alminger, M. and C. Eklund-Jonsson. 2008. Whole-grain cereal products based on a high fiber barley or oat genotype lower post-prandial glucose and insulin responses in healthy humans. *Eur J Nutr* 47:294–300.

Aman, P. 2006. Cholesterol-lowering effects of barley dietary fiber in humans: Scientific support for a generic health claim. *Scand J Food Nutr* 50:173–176.

American Association of Cereal Chemists. 2001. The definition of dietary fiber. Report of the Dietary Fiber Definition Committee to the Board of Directors of the American Association of Cereal Chemists. *Cereal Foods World* 46:112–126. http://www.scisoc.org/aacc/DietaryFiber/report.html (accessed: 26 June 2013).

Andersson, A. A. M., E. Armo, E. Grangeon, H. Fredriksson, R. Andersson, and P. Aman. 2004. Molecular weight and structure units of (1–3, 1–4)-β-glucans in dough and bread made from hull-less barley milling fractions. *J Cereal Sci* 40:195–204.

Bays, H., J. L. Frestedt, M. Bell et al. 2011. Reduced viscosity barley β-glucan versus placebo: A randomized controlled trial of the effects on insulin sensitivity for individuals at risk for diabetes mellitus. *Nutr Metabol* 8:58.

Behall, K. M. and J. G. Hallfrisch. 2006. Effects of barley consumption on CVD risk factors. *Cereal Foods World* 51:12–15.

Behall, K. M., D. J. Scholfield, and J. Hallfrisch. 2004. Diets containing barley significantly reduce lipids in mildly hypercholesterolemic men and women. *Am J Clin Nutr* 80:1185–1193.

Behall, K. M., D. J. Scholfield, and J. Hallfrisch. 2005. Comparison of hormone and glucose responses of overweight women to barley and oats. *J Am Coll Nutr* 24:182–188.

Behall, K. M., D. J. Scholfield, and J. G. Hallfrisch. 2006. Barley β-glucan reduces plasma glucose and insulin responses compared with resistant starch in men. *Nutr Res* 26:644–650.

Biorklund, M., A. van-Rees, R. P. Mensink, and G. Onning. 2005. Changes in serum lipids and postprandial glucose and insulin concentrations after consumption of beverages with β-glucans from oats or barley: A randomized dose-controlled trial. *Eur J Clin Nutr* 59:1272–1281.

Bird, A. R., M. S. Vuaran, R. A. King et al. 2008. Wholegrain foods made from a novel high-amylose barley variety (Himalaya 292) improve indices of bowel health in human subjects. *Brit J Nutr* 99:1032–1040.

Bourdon, I., W. Yokoyama, P. Davis et al. 1999. Postprandial lipid, glucose, insulin and cholecystokinin responses in men fed barley pasta enriched with beta glucan. *Am J Clin Nutr* 69:55–63.

Brennan, C. S. and L. J. Cleary. 2007. Utilisation glucagel in the β-glucan enrichment of breads: A physicochemical and nutritional evaluation. *Food Res Intl* 40:291–296.

Brennan, C. S. and C. M. Tudorica. 2008. Carbohydrate-based fat replacers in the modification of the rheological, textural and sensory quality of yogurt: Comparative study of the utilisation of barley beta-glucan, guar gum and inulin. *Intl J Food Sci Technol* 43:824–833.

Buttriss, J. L. and C. S. Stokes. 2008. Dietary fibre and health: An overview. *Nutr Bull* 33:186–200.

Casiraghi, M. C., M. Garsetti, G. Testolin, and F. Brighenti. 2006. Post-prandial responses to cereal products enriched with barley β-glucan. *J Am Coll Nutr* 25:4313–4320.

Cavallero, A., S. Empilli, F. Brighenti, and A. M. Stanca. 2002. High $(1 \rightarrow 3, 1 \rightarrow 4)$-b-glucan barley fractions in bread making and their effects on human glycemic response. *J Cer Sci* 36:59–66.

Chen, J. and X. Huang. 2009. The effects of diets enriched in beta-glucans on blood lipoprotein concentrations. *J Clin Lipidol* 3:154–158.

Chillo, S., D. V. Ranawana, and C. J. K. Henry. 2011a. Effect of two barley β-glucan concentrates on *in vitro* glycaemic impact and cooking quality of spaghetti. *LWT-Food Sci Technol* 44:940–948.

Chillo, S., D. V. Ranawana, M. Pratt, and C. J. K. Henry. 2011b. Glycemic response and glycemic index of semolina spaghetti enriched with barley β-glucan. *Nutrition* 27:653–658.

Cleary, L. and C. Brennan. 2006. The influence of a $(1 \rightarrow 3)(1 \rightarrow 4)$-β-D-glucan rich fraction from barley on the physico-chemical properties and *in vitro* reducing sugars release of durum wheat pasta. *Intl J Food Sci Technol* 41:910–918.

Cleary, L. J., R. Andersson, and C. S. Brennan. 2007. The behaviour and susceptibility to degradation of high and low molecular weight barley b-glucan in wheat bread during baking and *in vitro* digestion. *Food Chem* 102:889–897.

Dickin, E., K. Steele, G. Frost, G. Edwards-Jones, and D. Wright. 2011. Effect of genotype, environment and agronomic management on β-glucan concentration of naked barley grain intended for health food use. *J Cereal Sci* 54:44–52.

EFSA. 2007. Statement of the scientific panel on dietetic products, nutrition and allergies on a request from the commission related to dietary fibre. Available at: http://www.icc.or.at/news/EFSA_Panel_Statement_on_Dietary_Fibre.pdf (accessed: 20 May 2008).

EFSA. 2011. Scientific opinion on the substantiation of a health claim related to barley beta-glucans and lowering of blood cholesterol and reduced risk of (coronary) heart disease pursuant to Article 14 of Regulation (EC) No. 1924/2006. Available at: http://www.efsa.europa.eu/en/efsajournal/pub/2470.htm (accessed: 26 July 2013).

El Khoury, D., C. Cuda, B. L. Luhovyy, and G. H. Anderson. 2012. Beta glucan: Health benefits in obesity and metabolic syndrome. *J Nutr Metabol* Article ID 851362, 28, http://dx.doi.org/10.1155/2012/851362.

Eslick, R. F. 1981. Mutation and characterization of unusual genes associated with the seed. In *Barley Genetics IV, Proceedings of the IV International Barley Genetics Symposium.* ed. R. N. H. Whitehouse, pp. 864–867. Edinburgh: Edinburgh University Press.

Hallfrisch, J., D. J. Scholfield, and K. M. Behall. 2003. Blood pressure reduced by whole grain diet containing barley or whole wheat and brown rice in moderately hypercholesterolemic men. *Nutr Res* 23:1631–1642.

Hinata, M., M. Ono, S. Midorikawa, and K. Nakanishi. 2007. Metabolic improvement of male prisoners with type 2 diabetes in Fukushima Prison, Japan. *Diabetes Res Clin Prac* 77:327–332.

Hipsley, E. H. 1953. Dietary "fibre" and pregnancy toxaemia. *Brit Med J* 2: 420–422.

Ikegami, S., M. Tomita, S. Honda et al. 1996. Effect of boiled barley–rice feeding in hypercholesterolemic and normolipidemic subjects. *Plant Food Hum Nutr* 49:317–328.

Izydorczyk, M. S., T. L. Chornick, F. G. Paulley, N. M. Edwards, and J. E. Dexter. 2008. Physicochemical properties of hull-less barley fibre-rich fractions varying in particle size and their potential as functional ingredients in two-layer flat bread. *Food Chem* 108:561–570.

Jenkins, D. J. A., C. W. C. Kendall, V. Vuksan et al. 2002. Soluble fiber intake at a dose approved by the US Food and Drug Administration for a claim of health benefits: Serum lipid risk factors for cardiovascular disease assessed in a randomized controlled crossover trial. *Am J Clin Nutr* 75:834–839.

Jenkins, D. J. A., A. Marchie, L. S. A. Augustin, E. Ros, and C. W. C. Kendall. 2004. Viscous dietary fibre and metabolic effects. *Clin Nutr Supp* 1:39–49.

Keenan, J. M., M. Goulson, T. Shamliyan, N. Knutson, L. Kolberg, and L. Curry. 2007. The effects of concentrated barley beta glucan on blood lipids in a population of hypercholesterolemic men and women. *Brit J Nutr* 97:1162–1168.

Keogh, G. F., G. J. S. Cooper, T. B. Mulvey et al. 2003. Randomized controlled crossover study of the effect of a highly beta-glucan-enriched barley on cardiovascular disease risk factors in mildly hypercholesterolemic men. *Am J Clin Nutr* 78:711–718.

Kim, H., K. S. Stote, K. M. Behall, K. Spears, B. Vinyard, and J. M. Conway. 2009. Glucose and insulin responses to whole grain breakfasts varying in soluble fiber, β-glucan. *Eur J Nutr* 48:170–175.

Kinner, M., S. Nitschko, J. Sommeregger et al. 2011. Naked barley optimized recipe for pure barley bread with sufficient beta-glucan according to the EFSA health claims. *J Cereal Sci* 53:225–230.

Lee, S. and G. E. Inglett. 2006. Functional characterization of steam jet-cooked β-glucan-rich barley flour as an oil barrier in frying batters. *J Food Sci* 71: E308–E313.

Li, J., T. Kaneko, L. Qin, J. Wang, and Y. Wang. 2003. Effects of barley intake on glucose tolerance, lipid metabolism, and bowel function in women. *Nutrition* 19:926–929.

Li, W., S. W. Cui, Q. Wang, and R. Y. Yada. 2011. Studies of aggregation behaviors of cereal β-glucans in dilute aqueous solutions by light scattering: Part I. Structure effects. *Food Hydrocoll* 25:189–195.

Lia, A., G. Hallmans, A. S. Sundberg, P. Aman, and H. Andersson. 1995. Oat beta glucan increases bile acid excretion and a fibre rich barley fraction increases cholesterol excretion in ileostomy subjects. *Am J Clin Nutr* 62:1245–1251.

Lifschitz, C. H., M. A. Grusak, and N. F. Butte. 2002. Carbohydrate digestion in humans from a beta-glucan-enriched barley is reduced. *J Nutr* 132: 2593–2596.

Liljeberg, H. G. M., A. K. E. Akerberg, and I. M. E. Bjorck. 1999. Effect of the glycemic index and content of indigestible carbohydrates of cereal-based breakfast meals on glucose tolerance at lunch in healthy subjects. *Am J Clin Nutr* 69:647–655.

Liljeberg, H. G. M., Y. E. Granfeldt, and I. M. E. Bjorck. 1996. Products based on a high fibre barley genotype, but not on common barley or oats, lower postprandial glucose and insulin responses in healthy humans. *J Nutr* 126:458–466.

Lyly, M., M. Salmenkallio-Marttila, T. Suortti, K. Autio, K. Poutanen, and L. Lahteenmaki. 2004. The sensory characteristics and rheological properties of soups containing oat and barley β-glucan before and after freezing. *LWT-Food Sci Technol* 37:749–761.

Mahdi, G. S., M. Abdal, B. C. Behera, N. Verma, A. Sonone, and U. Makhija. 2008. Barley is a healthful food: A review. *Elec J Environ, Agric Food Chem* 7:2686–2694.

Mcintosh, G. H., J. Whyte, R. McArthur, and P. J. Nestel. 1991. Barley and wheat foods: Influence on plasma cholesterol concentrations in hypercholesterolemic men. *Am J Clin Nutr* 53:1205–1209.

Morin, L. A., F. Temelli, and L. McMullen. 2002. Physical and sensory characteristics of reduced-fat breakfast sausages formulated with barley β-glucan. *J Food Sci* 67:2391–2396.

Ostman, E. M., H. M. L. Elmstahl, and I. M. E. Bjorck. 2002. Barley bread containing lactic acid improves glucose tolerance at a subsequent meal in healthy men and women. *J Nutr* 132:1173–1175.

Ostman, E., E. Rossi, H. Larssen, F. Brighenti, and I. Bjorck. 2006. Glucose and insulin responses in healthy men to barley bread with different levels of (1/3;1/4)-β-glucans; predictions using fluidity measurements of *in vitro* enzyme digests. *J Cereal Sci* 43:230–235.

Ostman, E., Y. Granfeldt, L. Persson, and I. Björck. 2005. Vinegar supplementation lowers glucose and insulin responses and increases satiety after a bread meal in healthy subjects. *Eur J Clin Nutr* 59:983–988.

Pins, J. J. and H. Kaur. 2006. A review of the effects of barley β- glucan on cardiovascular and diabetic risk. *Cereal Foods World* 51:8–11.

Poppitt, S. D., J. D. E. van Drunen, A. McGill, T. B. Mulvey, and F. E. Leahy. 2007. Supplementation of a high-carbohydrate breakfast with barley β-glucan improves postprandial glycaemic response for meals but not beverages. *Asia Pac J Clin Nutr* 16:16–24.

Rendell, M., J. Vandehoof, M. Venn et al. 2005. Effect of a barley breakfast cereal on blood glucose and insulin response in normal and diabetic patients. *Plant Food Hum Nutr* 60:63–67.

Rondanelli, M., A. Opizzi, F. Monteferrario, C. Klersy, R. Cazzola, and B. Cestaro. 2011. Beta-glucan- or rice bran-enriched foods: A comparative crossover clinical trial on lipidic pattern in mildly hypercholesterolemic men. *Eur J Clin Nutr* 65:864–871.

Sharma, P., H. S. Gujral, and C. M. Rosell. 2011. Effects of roasting on barley b-glucan, thermal, textural and pasting properties. *J Cereal Sci* 53:25–30.

Shimizu, C., M. Kihara, S. Aoe et al. 2008. Effect of high β-glucan barley on serum cholesterol concentrations and visceral fat area in Japanese men—A randomized, double-blinded, placebo-controlled trial. *Plant Food Hum Nutr* 63:21–25.

Smith, K. N., K. M. Queenan, W. Thomas, G. Fulcher, and J. L. Slavin. 2008. Physiological effects of concentrated barley beta glucan in mildly hypercholesterolemic adults. *J Am Coll Nutr* 27:434–440.

Sundberg, B. 2008. Cholesterol lowering effects of a barley fibre flake product. *Agro Food Ind Hi-Tech* 19:14–17.

Symons, L. J. and C. S. Brennan. 2004. The influence of $(1 \to 3)$ $(1 \to 4)$-β-D-glucan-rich fractions from barley on the physicochemical properties and *in vitro* reducing sugar release of white wheat breads. *J Food Sci* 69:C463–C467.

Talati, R., W. L. Baker, M. S. Pabilonia, C. M. White, and C. I. Coleman. 2009. The effect of barley-derived soluble fibre on serum lipids. *Ann Fam Med* 7:157–163.

Temelli, F., C. Banesma, and K. Stobbe. 2004. Development of an orange-flavored barley β-glucan beverage with added whey protein isolate. *J Food Sci* 69:S237–S242.

Thondre, P. S. and C. J. K. Henry. 2009. High-molecular-weight barley β-glucan in chapatis (unleavened Indian flatbread) lowers glycemic index. *Nutr Res* 29:480–486.

Thondre, P. S. and C. J. K. Henry. 2011. Effect of a low molecular weight, high-purity β-glucan on *in vitro* digestion and glycemic response. *Intl J Food Sci Nutr* 62:678–684.

Thondre, P. S., J. A. Monro, S. Mishra, and C. J. K. Henry. 2010. High molecular weight barley beta-glucan decreases particle breakdown in chapatis (Indian flat breads) during *in vitro* digestion. *Food Res Intl* 43:1476–1481.

Thondre, P. S., A. Shafat, and M. E. Clegg. 2013. Molecular weight of barley β-glucan influences energy expenditure, gastric emptying and glycaemic response in human subjects. *Brit J Nutr* 110:2173–2179.

Tiwari, U. and E. Cummins. 2011. Meta-analysis of the effect of β-glucan intake on blood cholesterol and glucose levels. *Nutrition* 27:1008–1016.

Tiwari, U. and E. Cummins. 2012. Dietary exposure assessment of beta glucan in a barley and oat-based bread. *LWT-Food Sci Technol* 47:413–420.

Trowell, H. 1972. Ischemic heart disease and dietary fiber. *Am J Clin Nutr* 25: 926–932.

Vasiljevic, T., T. Kealy, and V. K. Mishra. 2007. Effects of β-glucan addition to a probiotic containing yogurt. *J Food Sci* 72:C405–C411.

Wolever, T. M. S., S. M. Tosh, A. L. Gibbs et al. 2010. Physicochemical properties of oat b-glucan influence its ability to reduce serum LDL cholesterol in humans: A randomized clinical trial. *Am J Clin Nutr* 92:723–732.

Wood, P. J. 2007. Cereal beta glucans in diet and health. *J Cereal Sci* 46:230–238.

Yokoyama, W. H., C. A. Hudson, B. E. Knuckles et al. 1997. Effect of barley beta-glucan in durum wheat pasta on human glycemic response. *Cereal Chem* 74:293–296.

CHAPTER 11

Chicory Fructans in Nutrition and the Formulation of Foods Dedicated to Blood Glucose Disorder Management

CATHY SIGNORET and HEIDI JACOBS

Contents

11.1 Introducing Chicory Fructans   260
11.2 Glucose Metabolism Disorders   261
    11.2.1 Glucose Disposal in the Body   261
    11.2.2 Regulation of Postprandial Blood Glucose Levels   262
    11.2.3 Type 2 Diabetes   263
    11.2.4 Impaired Fasting Glucose and Impaired Glucose Tolerance   264
    11.2.5 Insulin Resistance   264
    11.2.6 Metabolic Syndrome   265
11.3 Nutritional Interest of Chicory Fructans for People Suffering from Glucose Metabolism Disorders   265
    11.3.1 Dietary Fiber and Diabetes   265
    11.3.2 Impact of Chicory Fructans on Postprandial Blood Glucose Response   266
    11.3.3 Impact of Chronic Chicory Fructans Intake on Serum Glucose Concentrations   272
    11.3.4 Potential Role of Gut Microbiota in Glucose-Associated Metabolic Disorders   276
    11.3.5 Chicory Fructans and Gut Microbiota Modulation in the Context of Metabolic Disorders   282
11.4 Formulation of Foods Dedicated to People Suffering from Glucose Metabolism Disorders   288
    11.4.1 Chicory Fructans Are Low-Calorie Ingredients   289

11.4.2 Sugar Substitution by Chicory Fructans 290
11.4.3 Glycemic Index Reduction by Chicory Fructans 290
11.5 Overall Conclusion 290
References 291

11.1 Introducing Chicory Fructans

Fructans were first described in 1804 by Rose, a German scientist, who found a "peculiar" substance of plant origin in a boiling water extract from *Inula helenium*. Chemically, fructans are defined as any compound in which one or more fructosyl–fructose linkages constitute a majority of the linkages. The material included in this definition may or may not contain attached glucose (Lewis 1993).

Fructans are widely distributed in the plant kingdom, and they can also be found in some bacterial species. Up to 200 fructose units can be linked in a single fructan molecule in plants. Bacterial fructans are often even much larger and can achieve a degree of polymerization (DP) of 100,000 or more fructose units.

There are several types of fructans present in nature. They can be classified into three main groups based on the glycosidic linkages by which the fructose residues are linked to each other:

- The inulin group consists of linear fructans where the fructose units are mostly linked via a $\beta(2\text{-}1)$ bond.
- Levans (phlein group) are fructans where the fructose units are mostly linked via a $\beta(2\text{-}6)$ bond.
- The branched group, also referred to as the gramminan type, has both $\beta(2\text{-}1)$ and $\beta(2\text{-}6)$ fructosyl–fructose linkage in significant amounts.

Inulin, one of the most well-known fructans, belongs to the linear fructans group. It is the energy reserve in various flowering plants such as dahlia, agave, and so on. Inulin is a very widespread carbohydrate and is one of the

Table 11.1 Inulin in Nature

Food	Inulin (g/100 g Fresh Matter)
Banana	1
Onion	1–7.5
Globe artichoke	2–6.8
Asparagus	2–3
Leek	3–10
Garlic	16
Jerusalem artichoke	16–20
Chicory root	15–20

most common subjects of fructan research. Inulin is present in noticeable amounts that are suitable for industrial extraction in chicory (*Cichorium intybus*) and Jerusalem artichoke (*Helianthus tuberosus*). Other food sources of inulin-type fructans are, for instance, salsify, asparagus, wheat, and onions as shown in Table 11.1 (Roberfroid 2005).

Chicory inulin has had a long safe history of consumption. Old Egyptian (the Ebers Papyrus, 4000 BC), Greek (Aristophane, 450 BC; Threophaste, 371 BC), and Roman (Horatius, Ovidius) sources indicate chicory as a vegetable that was commonly consumed raw, cooked, or roasted. Based on archaeological data, a publication even suggests that Paleolithic men may have consumed inulin in significant amounts (Leach et al. 2006). Closer to us in time, it was reported that the first "industrial" production of torrified chicory was conducted in the Netherlands in the 1650s. Moreover, since the end of the eighteenth century, roasted chicory, used as a coffee substitute, has been prepared on a vast industrial scale (Van Loo et al. 1995).

Consumption of naturally occurring inulin (through fruits and vegetables) has been evaluated by Van Loo et al. in 1995. They found that the European population was consuming between 3.2 and 11.3 g/day and the North American population between 1 and 4 g/day (Van Loo et al. 1995).

Chicory inulin is industrially obtained from chicory roots by hot water extraction, a process very close to the one of sugar beet-extracted sucrose. Chicory roots are one of the local agricultural resources of the area from the north of France to the Netherlands including Belgium. Chemically, chicory inulin is a mixture of linear fructans with different chain lengths, which have mostly the $\beta(2\text{-}1)$ fructosyl–fructose linkage with glucose as the end group. The DP of chicory inulin naturally varies from 3 to 60 units. Molecules with a DP lower than 20 are the most abundant in chicory. Moreover, the chain length distribution is influenced by the harvesting as well as by the processing conditions. Usually, native chicory inulin is produced with an average DP of about 10. Particular processing enables the reduction of this average chain length or the production of fractions with a different one. For example, when partial hydrolysis is applied to native chicory inulin in order to obtain shorter chains, the ingredient obtained is usually called oligofructose or sometimes fructo-oligosaccharide. The selection of long chains by physical means leads to the production of long-chain inulin.

11.2 Glucose Metabolism Disorders

11.2.1 Glucose Disposal in the Body

Glucose is an essential substrate for the body, notably for the proper functioning of the brain. The brain is the main glucose consumer in the fasting or postabsorptive phase, accounting for around 50% of the body's glucose use (DeFronzo 2004). Next, 25% of glucose use occurs in the splanchnic area (liver and gastrointestinal tissues) and the remaining 25% in insulin-dependent tissues (primarily in muscle but also in adipose tissue).

Basal glucose use is matched by the rate of endogenous glucose production. Eighty-five percent of the endogenous glucose is derived from the liver by the breakdown of endogenous glycogen stores (glycogenolysis) and by gluconeo-genesis (glucose formation from noncarbohydrate carbon sources such as pyru-vate). The remaining endogenous glucose is produced in the kidneys (Bryant et al. 2002). Endogenous stores of glucose are replenished by dietary glucose.

Dietary glucose disposal following digestion and absorption is under the con-trol of several hormones and in particular of insulin. Following the consump-tion of a digestible carbohydrate-containing meal, the resulting increase in blood glucose concentration triggers insulin release at the pancreatic level that will, in return, stimulate splanchnic and peripheral (primarily muscles) glucose uptake and suppress endogenous (primarily hepatic) glucose production (Triplitt 2012).

When considering the disposal of a theoretical meal containing 100 g of glucose, it is usually admitted that about 30% of the ingested glucose is initially extracted by splanchnic tissues with the most important part being incorporated into glycogen in the liver. Of the remaining 70% that enters the systemic circulation, 25–30 g is taken up by skeletal muscle, initially to be oxidized in place of free fatty acids (FFA) and later to be stored as glycogen. About 15 g is taken up by the brain in place of the endogenously produced glucose. Another 15 g is extracted from the systemic circulation by the liver for glycogen formation. Finally, the kidneys may take up as much as 8 g, and 5–10 g of the ingested glucose entering the systemic circulation remains for adipose and other tissue uses (Shrayyef and Gerich 2010).

11.2.2 Regulation of Postprandial Blood Glucose Levels

In healthy adults, blood glucose levels are tightly regulated within a range of 70–99 mg/dL by targeted hormones such as insulin and glucagon that are both produced in the pancreas by the islets of Langerhans (Triplitt 2012). As mentioned previously, insulin reduces blood glucose levels following a meal ingestion by stimulating glucose transport into insulin-sensitive cells and facilitating its conversion into storage compounds via glycogenesis (conver-sion of glucose into glycogen) and lipogenesis (fat formation). Insulin is also a potent antilipolytic hormone (inhibitor of fat breakdown); its release leads to a decline in the FFA plasma level that in turn increases muscle glucose uptake, playing an important role in the maintenance of normal glucose homeostasis. The main regulator of insulin secretion is the plasma glucose concentration.

On the contrary, glucagon, which is the major counterpart of insulin, is released when blood glucose levels are low in order to stimulate glycoge-nolysis and gluconeogenesis. Following glucose-containing meal ingestion, glucagon secretion is inhibited by hyperinsulinemia, contributing, by the resulting hypoglucagonemia, to the suppression of hepatic glucose produc-tion (DeFronzo 2004). Another hormone, amylin, contributes to a reduction in postprandial glucagon and has been implicated in progressive β-cell fail-ure in type 2 diabetes mellitus.

Incretins released from intestinal tissue cells, such as glucagon-like peptide 1 (GLP-1) and glucose-dependent insulinotropic polypeptide (GIP), are also involved in blood glucose regulation as they have a stimulating effect on the release of insulin following oral glucose administration. Notably, GLP-1, which is considered to be one of the more significant incretins, stimulates insulin secretion in response to the presence of carbohydrates in the gut in a glucose-dependent manner (DeFronzo 2004).

Other molecules, such as catecholamines, growth hormone, and cortisol, are also impacting on glucose homeostasis, underlying the complexity of this process.

11.2.3 Type 2 Diabetes

Type 2 diabetes mellitus is a metabolic disease characterized by hyperglycemia resulting from defects in insulin secretion, insulin action, or both (American Diabetes Association 2013). Type 2 diabetes develops from the chronic and progressive loss of insulin secretion with a background of chronic and often progressive insulin resistance. It accounts for 90–95% of the total cases of diagnosed diabetes (the remainder being type 1 diabetes, resulting from a cellular-mediated autoimmune destruction of the β-cells of the pancreas usually leading to absolute insulin deficiency).

Type 2 diabetes is one of the leading causes of morbidity and mortality worldwide and has become a major health issue not only in developed countries but also in developing countries (Kumanyika et al. 2002, Yang et al. 2010). According to the latest figures from the World Health Organization (WHO), 347 million people worldwide have diabetes with more than 80% of them living in low- and middle-income countries. Diabetes is associated with an increase in the risk of stroke occurrence and is a leading cause of renal failure, visual impairment, and blindness. The risk of tuberculosis is also three times higher among people with diabetes (WHO 2011).

The risk factors of type 2 diabetes are closely related to lifestyle and include being overweight and obesity, sedentarity, and diet composition (Parillo and Riccardi 2004). This explains why type 2 diabetes belongs to the category of the so-called civilization diseases and is often associated with the "westernization" of populations of developing countries in particular with regard to diet composition. The risk of developing type 2 diabetes is closely linked to the presence and duration of being overweight and obesity, with 90% of type 2 diabetic patients being either overweight or obese (Kumanyika et al. 2002). In particular, waist adiposity is acknowledged as a strong predictor of type 2 diabetes risk (Wang et al. 2005). Results obtained from the EPIC-InterAct case-cohort study pointed out that obese men with a high waist circumference are 22 times more likely to develop diabetes than men with a low normal weight and a low waist circumference. This figure was close to 32 times in obese women (The InterAct Consortium 2012). Conversely, a reduction in body weight has a positive effect on the incidence of diabetes. For example, in the long-term prospective Swedish Obese Subjects (SOS) study, a large amount of weight loss in obese volunteers *via* gastric surgery had a dramatic effect on the incidence of diabetes after 8 years (Sjostrom et al. 2000).

As the importance given to lifestyle habits is key in the occurrence and management of this disease, strategies involving lifestyle modifications, notably dietary changes toward weight loss or regular practice of physical activity, have been promoted for years. The Diabetes Prevention Program (DPP), a U.S. multicenter randomized clinical trial, is a good example of how individual lifestyle intervention, achieved by at least 7% weight loss and at least 150 min of physical activity per week, can reduce the incidence of diabetes by 58% in nondiabetic but high-risk individuals with elevated fasting and postload plasma glucose concentrations (Knowler et al. 2002).

11.2.4 Impaired Fasting Glucose and Impaired Glucose Tolerance

The early metabolic abnormalities that precede diabetes are impaired fasting glucose (IFG) and impaired glucose tolerance (IGT). IFG is defined by an elevated fasting plasma glucose concentration (≥ 100 and <126 mg/dL), whereas IGT is defined by an elevated 2-h plasma glucose concentration (≥ 140 and <200 mg/dL) after a 75 g glucose load on the oral glucose tolerance test (OGTT) in the presence of an elevated fasting plasma concentration over 126 mg/dL (Nathan et al. 2007). Both isolated IFG and IGT are insulin-resistant states, which differ by their site of insulin resistance: only hepatic in the case of IFG and mostly muscular and slightly hepatic in the case of IGT. IFG and IGT are often associated with obesity.

11.2.5 Insulin Resistance

The impaired ability of muscle, liver, and adipocytes to respond to insulin by decreasing hepatic glucose output and increasing glucose uptake and utilization is called insulin resistance. As a consequence of insulin resistance, inefficient glucose utilization is eventually replaced by the cellular utilization of fats and proteins for energy. The real origin of insulin resistance is still unclear as genetics are involved but environmental factors such as obesity and visceral adiposity are connected to its appearance (Triplitt 2012).

One common hypothesis is that fat accumulation in the adipose tissue, following a sustained overnutrition frequently observed in developed countries, may trigger inflammation that leads to insulin resistance. Adipose tissue is not only composed of adipocytes, which are the fat storage elements, but also of numerous immune cells, including macrophages (Shoelson et al. 2007). Both cell types (adipocytes and immune cells) secrete substances that help regulate metabolic homeostasis. Several data point out that, in obesity, the infiltration of the adipose tissue by macrophages initiates a proinflammatory response and blocks adipocyte insulin action (Harford et al. 2011). Insulin-resistant adipocytes are characterized by low liposynthetic and high lipolytic capacities, leading to an increased release of FFA that may activate toll-like receptors 4 (TLR-4) located at the surface of the macrophages, contributing to the amplification of the inflammatory response in the adipose tissue (Lionetti et al. 2009). The significant role of the tumor necrosis factor-α (TNF-α), a macrophage-derived factor involved in adipose tissue inflammation, is also clearly established in insulin resistance through its ability to decrease the tyrosine kinase activity of the insulin receptor (IR), which is an absolute requirement for the biological activities of insulin (Hotamisligil et al. 1996). Moreover, it is now well established that high-fat feeding not only increases fat storage in the adipose tissue and FFA release but also augments circulating levels of lipopolysaccharide (LPS), an important constituent of the outer membranes of Gram-negative bacteria that contributes to inflammation and insulin resistance (Greiner and Backhed 2011).

11.2.6 Metabolic Syndrome

Metabolic syndrome refers to a cluster of abnormalities, which are inter-related risk factors for cardiovascular diseases and diabetes (Delzenne and Cani 2005). For example, the metabolic syndrome confers a fivefold increase in risk for type 2 diabetes mellitus. First described in the 1920s, this syndrome has seen its prevalence increasing worldwide not only in adult or older populations but also in children and young people and is now both a public health and a clinical problem (Galisteo et al. 2008).

A recent joint statement of the International Diabetes Federation Task Force on Epidemiology and Prevention, the National Heart, Lung and Blood Institute, the American Heart Associations, the World Heart Federation, the International Atherosclerosis Society, and the International Association for the Study of Obesity has proposed common criteria for the clinical diagnosis of the metabolic syndrome that includes elevated waist circumference, elevated triglycerides, reduced high-density lipoprotein (HDL)-cholesterol, elevated blood pressure, and elevated fasting glucose (Alberti et al. 2009). Despite the fact that it is not listed in these criteria, insulin resistance is believed to play a central role in the pathogenesis of metabolic syndrome (Eckel et al. 2005). Moreover, the homeostatic model assessment for insulin resistance ($HOMA_{IR}$) test, which generates indices of pancreatic cell function and tissue insulin sensitivity, is seen as a good index of metabolic syndrome (Russo et al. 2010).

11.3 Nutritional Interest of Chicory Fructans for People Suffering from Glucose Metabolism Disorders

11.3.1 Dietary Fiber and Diabetes

Dietary fibers are highly complex substances that can be described as any nondigestible carbohydrates and lignins not degraded in the upper gut (Weickert and Pfeiffer 2008). Two subclasses are usually used to categorize dietary fiber. Although some differences exist with regard to physiological effects, this classification is commonly based on their solubility in water. The insoluble dietary fiber (which is insoluble in an aqueous enzyme solution) category is the predominant class. The main components are cellulose and its derivatives, hemicellulose, lignin, and resistant starch. Soluble dietary fiber is soluble in an aqueous enzyme solution but can be precipitated with ethanol. This category includes, among others, chicory fructans, pectin, gums, and β-glucans. The major effects of dietary fiber occur in the colon. Those effects strongly correlate to the fermentability of the fiber. Roughly, soluble fiber is fermented (either rapidly or either slowly) by the resident gut microbiota whereas insoluble fiber is hardly fermented (FAO/WHO 1998).

The consumption of insoluble dietary fibers from cereals is significantly associated with reduced diabetes risk in prospective cohort studies but the mechanism associated with this effect, to date, remains unclear. On the contrary, despite the fact that the properties of some soluble dietary fiber (such as gel-forming and increased viscosity) are associated with reduced postprandial glucose responses, the effect on reduced diabetes risk is not confirmed by meta-analysis (Weickert and Pfeiffer 2008). Nevertheless, the interest of the consumption of soluble fiber, as nondigestible carbohydrates, in the context of the management of type 2 diabetes, remains indisputable.

11.3.2 Impact of Chicory Fructans on Postprandial Blood Glucose Response

The nondigestibility of dietary fibers in the upper intestinal system and in consequence their limited effect on the increase of blood glucose levels following a meal remains an important property in the context of diabetes management. Chicory fructans (inulin, oligofructose) are not degraded (and therefore not absorbed) in the upper part of the gastrointestinal tract, reaching the colon intact, where they undergo bacterial fermentation. Studies conducted on ileostomic volunteers have shown that the recovery of fructans from various sources (chicory and Jerusalem artichoke) in the ileostomy effluent is nearly 90% of the ingested dose (BachKnudsen and Hessov 1995, Ellegard et al. 1997, Rumessen et al. 1990), demonstrating its resistance to digestion in the upper intestinal system.

There are only a limited number of studies regarding the acute effect of chicory fructans on postprandial glucose and insulin responses, which are summarized in Table 11.2.

In the study by Grysman and coworkers, inulin was used as a nondigestible carbohydrate to partially replace high-fructose corn syrup (HFCS) in a beverage used as a control in the study of the effect of sucromalt on postprandial glucose and insulin responses. The beverage, containing either 80 g HFCS or 80 g sucromalt or a mixture of 35 g fructose, 21 g glucose, and 24 g inulin, was consumed by 10 healthy volunteers on three separate occasions after an overnight fast. Blood samples were drawn before the beverage consumption and at 15, 30, 45, 60, 90, 120, 180, 240, 270, 300, 330, and 360 min after. The beverage containing inulin elicited a significantly lower level of blood glucose than the two other beverages at 60 min and less than the sucromalt-containing beverage at 90 and 120 min ($p < 0.05$). The mean 0–2 h glucose

Table 11.2 Summary of the Human Studies Regarding the Acute Effect of Chicory Fructans on Postprandial Blood Glucose and Insulin

Reference	Ingredient	Dose	Endpoint(s)	Duration	Design	Volunteers	Outcome(s)
Chicory Fructan Used in *Substitution* to Digestible Carbohydrates							
Grysman et al. (2008)	Inulin	One test drink (360 mL containing 24 g inulin, 35 g fructose, and 21 g glucose)	Postprandial glucose and insulin	One-day test on three separate occasions	RCT, CO	10 healthy volunteers	Significantly lower glucose level at 60 min compared to HFCS and at 60, 90, and 120 min compared to sucromalt ($p < 0.05$) AUC for glucose 32% lower compared to HFCS (NS). Similar finding for insulin levels
Tarini and Wolever (2010)	Inulin	One test drink (400 mL containing 24 g inulin and 56 g HFCS)	Postprandial glucose and insulin	One-day test on three separate occasions separated by 1 week washout	RCT, CO single-blind	12 young and healthy	Trend for lower AUC for glucose Significantly lower AUC for insulin compared to HFCS80 beverage ($p < 0.05$)
Chicory Fructan Used in *Addition* to Digestible Carbohydrates							
Granfeldt and Björck (2004)	Inulin, OF, LC-inulin	10 g of the chicory fructan dissolved in 150 mL of water	Postprandial glucose and insulin	One-day test on four separate occasions	RCT, CO	15 healthy volunteers	No impact of none of the fructans tested on the glycemic and insulinemic responses

continued

Table 11.2 (Continued) Summary of the Human Studies Regarding the Acute Effect of Chicory Fructans on Postprandial Blood Glucose and Insulin

Reference	Ingredient	Dose	Endpoint(s)	Duration	Design	Volunteers	Outcome(s)
Meyer (2007)	Inulin, OF, LC-inulin	One test drink (250 mL) containing 25 g of chicory fructan	Postprandial glycemic response	One-day test	RCT	10 healthy volunteers	Glycemic response expressed in percentage of one of glucose (reference): LC-inulin: 5 ± 2%, inulin: 14 ± 3%, oligofructoses: 20 ± 5%, and 48 ± 6%

Abbreviations: OF: oligofructose, LC-inulin: long-chain inulin, RCT: randomized controlled trial, CO: crossover, AUC: area under the curve.

area under the curve (AUC) after inulin was 32% less than that after HFCS ($p = 0.064$, NS). Similarly, insulin levels were significantly lower in the inulin beverage at 60 and 90 min compared to the HFCS beverage and at 90 and 120 min ($p < 0.05$) compared to the sucromalt beverage. Finally, mean 0–2 h and 0–4 h AUC after inulin were 47% and 42%, respectively, less than after HFCS (both $p < 0.05$) (Grysman et al. 2008).

In another study conducted by the same team on 12 young healthy volunteers, a beverage containing 80 g of HFCS (HFCS80) was compared to a beverage combining 24 g inulin and 56 g HFCS and another one containing only 56 g HFCS (HFCS56) on three separate occasions with a washout of 1 week between each. Blood samples were drawn before the beverage consumption and at 0.5, 1, 1.5, 2, 3, and 4 h after, when a standardized lunch was served to the volunteers. Further blood samples were drawn at 4.5, 5, 5.5, and 6 h. The AUCs with the inulin and the HFCS56 beverages tended to be lower for glucose and were significantly lower for insulin ($p < 0.05$) as compared to the HFCS80 beverage (Tarini and Wolever 2010). These results indicate that, when used to substitute for digestible carbohydrates, chicory fructans significantly impact postprandial blood glucose and insulin responses.

The effect of the addition of various chicory fructans (long-chain inulin, native inulin, and oligofructose) to a bread reference meal on the immediate postprandial glucose and insulin responses has been evaluated in another human study (Granfeldt and Björck 2004). The reference and test breakfast meals were served randomized after an overnight fast to the same 15 healthy adult volunteers (6 men and 9 women) on four separate occasions with a minimum of 1 week of washout. The compositions of the breakfast meals are presented in Table 11.3. The test meals consisted of white wheat bread (50 g

Table 11.3 Composition of Test Breakfasts

Meals	Ingredients	Water (mL)	Available Starch (g)	Chicory Fructans (g)	Sugar (g)
Reference meal	126 g white wheat bread	300	50	–	–
Test meal Long-chain inulin	10.6 g Fibruline® XL 126 g white wheat bread	300	50	10	0.09
Test meal Oligofructose	10.7 g Fibrulose® F97 126 g white wheat bread	300	50	10	0.10
Test meal Native inulin	11.5 g Fibruline® Instant 126 g white wheat bread	300	50	10	0.94

available starch) and a glass of water (150 mL) in which one of the three chicory fructans (10 g pure chicory fructan) was dissolved according to data presented in Table 11.3. In the case of the reference test, the glass of water was free from chicory fructans. Another glass of water (150 mL) and tea (150 mL) were also included in the breakfast that was eaten over 10 min. Capillary blood was taken from the fingertips prior to the breakfast meal for the determination of the fasting value for blood glucose and insulin. Blood samples were also drawn at 15, 30, 45, 60, 90, and 120 min after the start of the breakfast for the analysis of glucose and insulin levels (except at 60 min). The blood glucose was analyzed the same day with a glucose oxidase peroxidase reagent while serum was frozen. After finishing the study, the serum insulin was analyzed in all samples with an ELISA method (Biorad, Coda Automated EIA Analyzer). Approval of the study was given by the Ethic Committee in Lund, Sweden.

For each volunteer, glucose and insulin curves were printed and the area under each curve (above the fasting value) was calculated from 0 to 120 min after the reference and test breakfasts, respectively. At all measuring points, a mean value was calculated to receive mean glucose and insulin curves. Glycemic index (GI) and insulinemic index (II) were calculated for each volunteer and product from the area (0–120 min after breakfast) under glucose and insulin curves, respectively, divided by the corresponding area after the reference bread. Mean values for glucose and insulin areas, together with GI and II values, were calculated. Significant differences were calculated by statistical ANOVA models, each volunteer being his/her own control. The results are presented in Table 11.4.

Table 11.4 Fasting Values and Postprandial Responses of Blood Glucose and Insulin in Healthy Humans after White Wheat Bread Consumed with and without Chicory Fructans

	Blood Glucose			Serum Insulin		
	Fasting Concentration (nmol/L)	AUC 0–120 h (nmol/L min)	GI	Fasting Concentration (mmol/L)	AUC0–120h (nmol/L min)	II
Reference Test meal	4.6 ± 0.1	168 ± 13	100	0.06 ± 0.01	20 ± 4	100
Long-chain inulin	4.5 ± 0.1	174 ± 18	105 ± 8	0.06 ± 0.01	20 ± 4	117 ± 15
Test meal Oligofructose	4.6 ± 0.1	163 ± 21	99 ± 13	0.06 ± 0.01	$23 \pm 5^*$	121 ± 11
Test meal Native inulin	4.5 ± 0.1	145 ± 19	90 ± 13	0.05 ± 0.01	$17 \pm 3^*$	98 ± 12

Mean values ± SEM, $n = 14$. $^*p = 0.0505$.

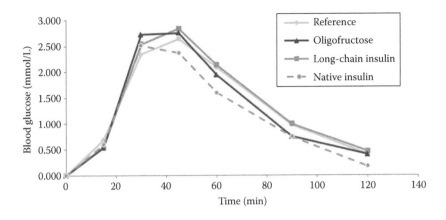

Figure 11.1 Mean incremental blood glucose after ingestion of bread together with different chicory fructans.

Blood glucose graphs after ingestion of the different breakfast meals with or without the addition of various chicory fructans are presented in Figure 11.1. There were no significant differences between the mean glucose values, the glucose areas under the curve, and the GI values after the different breakfast meals. Insulin responses after different breakfast meals are shown in Figure 11.2. At 45 min, the insulin level after the breakfast with native inulin was significantly lower than the one with oligofructose ($p = 0.0505$). Besides that, there were no significant differences either in insulin response at different time points or in insulin areas after different breakfast meals. However, the AUC after the breakfast with native inulin was nearly significantly

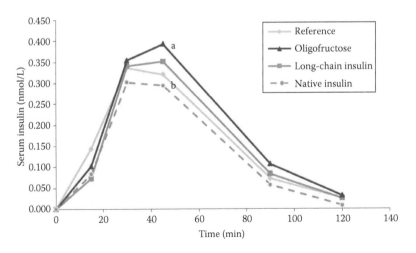

Figure 11.2 Mean incremental serum insulin after ingestion of bread together with different chicory fructans.

($p = 0.0505$) lower than after oligofructose. From the observed results, it was concluded that the consumption of 10 g of chicory fructans in addition to the test breakfast, whatever their chain length, did not influence either the acute glycemic or insulinemic responses.

In another study, the glycemic response of 25 g of various chicory fructans (two types of oligofructoses, native inulin, and long-chain inulin) compared to that of glucose was measured in 10 healthy adults after an overnight fast. The glycemic response of the tested products was closely related to their residual free sugar content, indicating that pure chicory fructans themselves have a negligible glycemic effect (Meyer 2007).

Taken altogether, these data lead to the conclusion that, owing to their nondigestibility, chicory fructans do not impact on the postprandial blood glucose and insulin responses and that they can be used to substitute for digestible carbohydrates.

11.3.3 Impact of Chronic Chicory Fructans Intake on Serum Glucose Concentrations

Besides the fact that chicory fructans do not impact the postprandial glycemic and inulinemic responses in the acute phase, the potential benefits on blood glucose concentrations following chronic consumption have also been investigated. Studies conducted in humans have shown mixed results whereas animal studies consistently report positive effects. For a summary of the human studies regarding the effect of chicory fructans on blood glucose, see Table 11.5.

According to a recently published review of some of the available data regarding those effects, also including data coming from studies conducted with short-chain fructo-oligosaccharides (sc-FOS) obtained from sucrose polymerization, it does not appear that fructan consumption has a significant serum glucose-lowering effect. The authors acknowledged however that the limited available studies may account for such a result and that further research, especially targeting at-risk populations, such as those with diabetes, is required (Bonsu et al. 2011).

In most of the human studies, a chronic intake of chicory fructans did not lead to a change in fasting blood glucose concentrations in various populations, healthy, diabetic, or overweight/obese (Alles et al. 1999, Bonsu and Johnson 2012, Cani, Lecourt, et al. 2009, Causey et al. 2000, Daubioul et al. 2005, Jackson et al. 1999, Letexier et al. 2003, van Dokkum et al. 1999). However, other parameters related to glucose metabolism have been positively impacted by chicory fructans in some of them.

Despite the fact that it had no effect on fasting blood glucose concentrations, the daily chronic supplementation of 10 g long-chain inulin for 8 weeks in healthy, middle-aged men and women with moderately raised blood lipids was able to significantly reduce fasting insulin concentrations ($p < 0.01$) (Jackson et al. 1999).

Table 11.5 Summary of Human Studies Regarding the Chronic Effect of Chicory Fructans on Blood Glucose

Reference	Ingredient	Dose	Endpoint(s)	Duration	Design	Volunteers	Outcome(s)
				Type 2 Diabetes Volunteers			
Alles et al. (1999)	OF	15 g/day (7.5 g twice a day) Dose gradually increased during the first 3 days by 5 g/day	Fasting blood glucose	6 weeks (2*20 days treatments and 2 weeks washout)	RCT, single-blind,CO	20 volunteers with type 2 diabetes	No effect on fasting blood glucose (capillary)
Bonsu and Johnson (2012)	Inulin	10 g/day (one sachet at breakfast with a beverage)	Fasting blood glucose	12 weeks	RCT, parallel, DB	36 volunteers with type 2 diabetes	No effect on fasting blood glucose
				Healthy Volunteers			
Cani, Lecourt, et al. (2009)	OF-INU	16 g/day (8 g twice daily)	Plasma glucose and insulin (fasting and postprandial)	14 days	RCT, parallel, DB	10 healthy volunteers	No effect on fasting blood glucose and insulin. Lower postprandial AUC for glucose in the OF-INU group ($p < 0.05$)
Jackson et al. (1999)	LC-inulin	10 g/day (5 g twice daily). One sachet added to a beverage	Fasting blood glucose and insulin	8 weeks	RCT, parallel, DB	54 healthy volunteers with moderately raised blood lipids	Decreased fasting insulin in the LC-inulin group after 4 weeks ($p < 0.01$). No effect on fasting blood glucose

continued

Table 11.5 (Continued) Summary of Human Studies Regarding the Chronic Effect of Chicory Fructans on Blood Glucose

Reference	Ingredient	Dose	Endpoint(s)	Duration	Design	Volunteers	Outcome(s)
Letexier et al. (2003)	LC-inulin	10 g/day (5 g twice daily at breakfast and at the evening meal)	Fasting blood glucose, insulin, and glucagon	2*6 weeks (plus a washout period of minimum 4 months)	RCT, CO, DB	8 healthy volunteers	No changes in fasting blood glucose, insulin, and glucagon levels
Russo et al. (2010)	LC-inulin	100 g/day of pasta formulated with 11% of inulin instead of durum semolina corresponding to ~11 g/day inulin	Fasting blood glucose and insulin resistance	18 weeks (2*5 weeks of pasta consumption plus 8 weeks washout)	RCT, CO, DB	22 healthy males enrolled (15 completed)	Significant reduction in insulin resistance. Significantly lower fasting blood glucose, serum fructosamine, HbA1c, and HOMA ($p < 0.05$) compared to baseline
van Dokkum et al. (1999)	Inulin, OF	15 g/day	Fasting and postprandial blood glucose and insulin	4*3 weeks (one period with inulin, one with OF, one with GOS, and one without any fiber)	RCT, parallel, DB	12 healthy males	No differences on fasting or postprandial blood glucose and insulin between the four test periods
				Other Populations			
Causey et al. (2000)	LC-inulin	20 g/day (consumed as low-fat vanilla ice-cream)	Postprandial plasma glucose and insulin (oral glucose test = 75 g)	2*3 weeks	RCT, CO, diet controlled, DB	12 adult males with mild-HP	No differences in postprandial blood glucose levels. Trend for an increased insulin level 1 h post-glucose load ($p = 0.07$)

Daubioul et al. (2005)	OF	8 g/day (4 g twice daily)	Fasting blood glucose and insulin	2*8 weeks plus a washout of minimum 5 weeks	RCT, CO, DB	7 volunteers with NASH	No changes in fasting blood glucose or insulin
Parnell and Reimer (2009)	OF	21 g/day (3*7 g daily) to be added in 250 mL drinks before meals with an adaptation period of 2 weeks (doses increase)	Plasma glucose and insulin (fasting and postprandial)	12 weeks	RCT, parallel, DB	48 overweight or obese volunteers	Lower postprandial blood glucose and insulin with OF at the final test compared to the initial test ($p < 0.05$). Trend for reduced AUC for glucose (-5%) and insulin (-10%) at the final test compared to the initial test ($p = 0.16$ and 0.19 respectively).

Abbreviations: GOS: galactooligosaccharides, OF: oligofructose, OF-INU: oligofructose-enriched inulin, LC-inulin: long-chain inulin, RCT: randomized controlled trial, DB: double blind, HP: hypercholesterolemia, AUC: area under the curve, NASH: non-alcoholic steatohepatitis.

The consumption of long-chain inulin-enriched pasta (around 11 g of inulin daily) for 8 weeks induced an improved metabolic control as compared to baseline in 15 young healthy males. In this study, fasting glucose, serum fructosamine, and glycosylated hemoglobin (HbA1c) were significantly lower ($p < 0.05$) in the inulin-treated group as compared to the baseline. Serum fructosamine reflects glycemic control during a short period (2–3 weeks) and HbA1c is a measurement of the mean blood glucose level during the life span of red blood cells, which is commonly used as a parameter of chronic glycemic control in patients with diabetes. Moreover, insulin resistance, measured by the HOMA test, was significantly reduced as compared to the control group (Russo et al. 2010).

In normoglycemic overweight and obese adults, the daily intake of 21 g of oligofructose for 12 weeks led to a significant decrease of glucose as well as of insulin between initial and final meal tolerance test ($p < 0.05$). The opposite was observed in the placebo group. Interestingly, the authors suggested, among other hypothesis, that the weight loss observed in the oligofructose group (-1.03 ± 0.43 kg) after 12 weeks of intake may have played a role in the improvement of glucoregulation in this population (Parnell and Reimer 2009).

Also, in the study from Cani and coworkers, conducted with healthy adult volunteers, the AUC for plasma glucose concentration was significantly lower ($p < 0.05$) after the daily consumption of 16 g of oligofructose-enriched inulin for 2 weeks (Cani, Lecourt, et al. 2009). Interestingly, the glucose response was inversely correlated with a gut microbial fermentation activity marker (breath-hydrogen excretion).

Increased fermentation following chicory fructans intake, reflecting an increased activity of the colonic microbiota, is a common pattern of those ingredients. There is room to suggest that potential benefits of chicory fructans for people suffering from metabolic disorders such as metabolic syndrome or type 2 diabetes should then be considered at a wider level, and not only be limited to the impact on glycemia. Indeed, the role of intestinal microbiota on the genesis of such disorders has recently come into focus. The following section aims at presenting the scientific data supporting this hypothesis.

11.3.4 Potential Role of Gut Microbiota in Glucose-Associated Metabolic Disorders

11.3.4.1 Microbiota Profile in Populations Suffering from Glucose-Associated Metabolic Disorders Larsen and coworkers have shown that the intestinal microbiota in humans with type 2 diabetes is different from that of nondiabetic persons. In their study conducted with 36 male adults who were diagnosed with type 2 diabetes, the proportion of Firmicutes was significantly higher in healthy individuals as compared to their type 2 diabetic counterparts, whereas the class Betaproteobacteria was highly enriched in diabetic volunteers (Larsen et al. 2010). Furthermore, ratios of Bacteroidetes to Firmicutes and of Bacteroides–Prevotella group to *Clostridium coccoides–Eubacteria rectale* group correlated positively and significantly with the values of plasma glucose. The authors suggested that the Bacteroidetes and Proteobacteria groups may affect the risk of acquiring diabetes *via* an endotoxin-induced inflammatory response as both are Gram-negative bacteria with LPS being the main component of their outer membrane.

Additionally, in severe obese subjects (including some type 2 diabetic patients), Bacteroides–Prevotella group was lower (versus lean control subjects) and increased post bariatric surgery. Also, levels of *Faecalibacterium prausnitzii*, a species from the Firmicutes phyla, were negatively correlated with inflammatory markers (Furet et al. 2010).

Wu and coworkers have also shown that the *Bifidobacterium* genus is poorly represented in the fecal samples of diabetic patients compared with healthy individuals (Wu et al. 2010). The authors further suggested that the gut microbiota of type 2 diabetes patients may have some changes associated with occurrence and diabetes development. The modulation of the gut microbiota would even now been considered as having therapeutic potential in obesity and type 2 diabetes (Kootte et al. 2012).

As an illustration of this concept, the gut levels of both aerobic and anaerobic bacteria were decreased in obese mice after 2 weeks of antibiotic treatment (norfloxacin and ampicillin), resulting in an improved glucose tolerance in antibiotic-treated mice (Membrez et al. 2008).

Recent science, notably due to the tremendous development of culture-independent approaches based on 16S ribosomal RNA analysis, suggests that the intestinal microbiota could be a potential contributor to the development of obesity and type 2 diabetes. As the human gut harbors 10^{14} bacteria, the gut microbiome (microbial genome) therefore represents 150-fold more genes than the human genome, leading to a tremendous metabolic potential of the gut microbiota (Delzenne et al. 2011). Gut microbiota may act on obesity and type 2 diabetes development via several mechanisms, including energy harvesting in the gut, the regulation of fat storage, metabolic endotoxemia inflammation, and the modulation of gut-derived peptide secretion (Snedeker and Hay 2012).

11.3.4.2 Energy Harvesting A now common hypothesis is that the composition of the gut microbiota affects the amount of energy extracted from the diet (DiBaise et al. 2008). Studies have shown that the gut microbiota of obese mice is more effective at releasing calories from food during digestion than the one of their lean siblings, resulting in greater adiposity (Turnbaugh et al. 2006). The role of the gut microbiota in nutrient harvest regulation has also been suggested in humans with an increased energy harvest associated with changes in microbiota toward higher counts of Firmicutes and lower counts of Bacteroidetes (Jumpertz et al. 2011). According to Eckburg et al. (2005), Bacteroidetes and Firmicutes account for more than 90% of all phylotypes of bacteria in the colon.

The Firmicutes phyla includes genera such as *Clostridium, Enterococcus,* and *Lactobacillus,* whereas Bacteroidetes is composed of *Bacteroides* and *Prevotella* genera (DiBaise et al. 2008). In addition, studies show that the relative proportion of Bacteroidetes is decreased in obese people in comparison to lean people and that this proportion increases with weight loss with the ratio of Bacteroides to Firmicutes approaching a lean-type profile after 52 weeks of weight loss in obese volunteers (Ley et al. 2005, 2006). However, those findings may be subject to controversy as they were not confirmed in other studies conducted with obese volunteers (Duncan et al. 2008, Zhang et al. 2009).

More recently, three robust clusters referred to as "enterotypes" have been identified from sequenced fecal metagenomes of individuals from four countries (Arumugam et al. 2011). Those enterotypes, identified by variations at the level of one of the following genera: *Bacteroides, Prevotella,* and *Ruminococcus,* cannot be explained by body mass index (BMI), age, or gender. However, marker genes or functional modules can be identified for each of these host properties. Notably, three functional modules correlate with BMI, supporting the link between microbiota, energy harvest, and obesity development in the host. Despite the fact that a clear causal relationship remains to be established, the potential role of the gut microbiota in the development of obesity and other metabolic disorders (including type 2 diabetes) henceforth deserves particular attention (Harris et al. 2012).

11.3.4.3 Regulation of Fat Storage   Lipoprotein lipase (LPL) activity leads to an increased cellular uptake of fatty acids and adipocyte triglycerides accumulation. The colonization of adult, germ-free mice with a microbiota harvested from the cecum of conventionally raised mice (a process known as conventionalization) produces a 60% increase in body fat content and insulin resistance within 2 weeks despite reduced food intake (Backhed et al. 2004). The authors found that the microbiota promoted the storage of fat in white adipose tissue through the suppression of the intestinal expression of a circulating LPL inhibitor: the fasting-induced adipose factor (Fiaf). Fiaf is selectively suppressed in the intestinal epithelium of normal mice by conventionalization (thus by microbial colonization). The central role of Fiaf suppression in the promotion of adiposity was confirmed in another study where germ-free Fiaf-deficient mice, compared to the germ-free wild-type mice, gain more weight when put on a Western high-fat diet (Backhed et al. 2007). In the same publication, the authors proposed that increased adiposity was not only resulting from Fiaf suppression but also from the suppression by the gut microbiota of AMP-activated protein kinase (AMPK) activity, leading to lower fatty acid oxidation.

11.3.4.4 Metabolic Endotoxemia Inflammation   Obesity is one of the most important risk factors for the increased occurrence of type 2 diabetes. It is also well established that an increase in visceral adiposity confers higher metabolic risk, associated with low-grade chronic inflammation (Creely et al. 2007). Low-grade inflammation is found in the metabolic syndrome and is a common comorbidity of type 2 diabetes. Its cause is still unclear but there is evidence to suggest that a factor from microbial origin would trigger and maintain a low-tone continuous inflammatory state.

This proposed factor is the LPS originating from Gram-negative bacteria in the gut that induces low-grade inflammation and insulin resistance (Wellen and Hotamisligil 2005). LPS has a major role in both acute and chronic infections. It is located at the outer membrane of the bacteria, whereas, in the circulation system, it is mostly bound to lipoproteins (Pussinen et al. 2011). LPS is believed to enter into the circulation by two primary routes. In paracellular transport, also known as "leaky gut," compromised intestinal tight junctions enhance the possibility of bacteria translocation. In transcellular transport, LPS is taken up in circulation by chylomicrons (Harris et al. 2012). LPS activates both innate and adaptive immune systems characterized by a release of antibodies, cytokines, and other inflammatory mediators, which may promote hepatic insulin resistance (Pussinen et al. 2011). Notably, LPS has been shown to signal through TLR-4, an important toll-like receptor in the response to common bacterial infections, and to induce interleukin, and notably interleukin-6 (IL-6), and cytokine, particularly tumor TNF-α, secretion (Creely et al. 2007). For example, TNF-α has been shown to cause insulin resistance by increasing serine phosphorylation on insulin receptor substrate-1 (IRS-1) leading to its inactivation (Hotamisligil et al. 1996).

However, TLR-4 alone is not able to recognize LPS. By using CD14 (LPS-receptor deleted) mutant mice, Cani and coworkers found that the occurrence of insulin resistance, obesity, and diabetes was delayed in response to high-fat feeding, suggesting a critical role for the LPS:CD14 system in the onset of those metabolic disorders. CD14 is a glycoprotein, strongly expressed on the surface of monocytes, macrophages, and neutrophils, which binds with LPS present at the surface of Gram-negative bacteria and allows it to be recognized by other receptors such as TLR-4. LPS was also shown to increase TLR-2 expression.

High-fat feeding in mice induces a sufficient level of LPS in the blood to increase body weight, fasted glycemia, and inflammation. This increase in plasma LPS concentration induced by high-fat feeding is defined as "metabolic endotoxemia" (Cani, Amar, et al. 2007). Mice that were fed a high-energy diet (either high-fat or high-carbohydrate) showed a significant increase in plasma LPS with fat having the strongest effect (Amar et al. 2008). Low-dose chronic subcutaneous LPS administration to mice for 1 month caused weight gain and insulin resistance (Cani, Amar, et al. 2007).

Creely and coworkers found that circulating serum LPS is twofold higher in type 2 diabetic patients than in BMI-, sex-, and age-matched lean healthy subjects (Creely et al. 2007). In apparently healthy humans, increased endotoxemia was found to be associated with energy intake (Amar et al. 2008). In a large population-based cohort followed up for 10 years, an increased risk for clinically incident diabetes was found to be associated with endotoxemia (Pussinen et al. 2011). Therefore, endotoxemia has been suggested to be a key player in the pathogenesis of diabetes by initiating or promoting obesity, insulin resistance, metabolic syndrome, and finally diabetes.

A potential link between microbiota changes and endotoxemia has been suggested several times. Metabolic endotoxemia was associated with reduced numbers of *Bifidobacterium* species in the cecal contents of mice fed a high-fat diet (Cani, Amar, et al. 2007). In another animal study, the negative correlation between *Bifidobacterium* spp. counts and endotoxemia was confirmed (Cani, Neyrinck, et al. 2007). Moreover, *Bifidobacterium* spp. have been shown to reduce intestinal endotoxin levels in rodents and to improve mucosal barrier function (Cani and Delzenne 2009).

In high-fat diet-fed mice, the modulation of the gut microbiota is associated with an increased intestinal permeability, which precedes the development of metabolic endotoxemia, inflammation, and associated disorders (Cani et al. 2008). Notably, fat feeding participates in the disruption of the gut barrier by mechanisms, including tight-junction proteins such as zonula occludens-1 (ZO-1) and occludin, strongly associated with gut microbiota modulation. The involvement of the glucagon-like peptide-2 (GLP-2)-mediated pathway on gut barrier function has also been recently underlined (Cani, Possemiers, et al. 2009). GLP-2 is a proglucagon-derived peptide, cosecreted with GLP-1 in the gut, which enhances intestinal epithelial proliferation and reduces gut permeability. In the study from Cani and coworkers, selective gut microbiota modulation, driven by the consumption of prebiotic fibers, controlled and increased endogenous production of GLP-2 and consequently improved gut barrier function.

Another interesting mechanism regarding the gut barrier function is related to the endocannabinoid system (eCB) and in particular one of its receptors: the cannabinoid receptor 1 (CB$_1$). Recently discovered, eCB is involved in the regulation of the energy balance at the level of food intake and peripheral control of metabolism (Matias et al. 2008). Greater eCB tone (altered expression of CB$_1$, higher plasma eCB levels, or increased adipose tissue eCB content) was found to be associated with obesity. Moreover, LPS is a potent stimulator of eCB synthesis. Muccioli and cowokers found that not only does the eCB system control gut permeability via a CB$_1$-dependent mechanism but also that microbiota selectively modulates colonic CB$_1$ mRNA expression in normal and obese mice underlying again its critical role in gut barrier function (Muccioli et al. 2010).

11.3.4.5 Gut-Derived Peptides　In the gut, the resident microbiota uses various substrates and more particularly complex plants oligosaccharides to produce monosaccharides and short-chain fatty acids (SCFA), mainly acetate, propionate, and butyrate. These SCFA are an important energy source for *de novo* lipogenesis in hepatocytes and adipocytes. Propionate, acetate, and, to a lesser extent, butyrate are also specific ligands for G-protein-coupled receptors 41 and 43 (GPR41 and GPR43), which are largely expressed in the distal small intestine, colon, and adipocytes. In adipocytes, SCFA, via GPR41, stimulate the expression of leptin and PYY, two gut-derived peptides involved in appetite regulation (Samuel et al. 2008, Xiong et al. 2004). PYY normally inhibits gut motility and slows intestinal transit thereby enhancing nutrient absorption. Leptin can also contribute to energy harvest. SCFA (again acetate and propionate) also stimulate adipogenesis via GPR43 with upregulation of peroxisome proliferator-activated receptor γ 2 (PPARγ2) (Hong et al. 2005).

Another gut-derived peptide, GLP-1, deserves particular attention. GLP-1 is cleaved from proglucagon (which is expressed in the gut, pancreas, and brain) by L cells in the distal small intestine and colon. Its secretion is stimulated by some nutrients, especially fats and carbohydrates. GLP-1 delays gastric emptying contributing to the ileal break, which is a feedback phenomenon whereby ingested food activates distal-intestinal signals that inhibit proximal gastrointestinal motility and gastric emptying (Pironi et al. 1993). As already mentioned in a previous part of this chapter, GLP-1 is considered to be a key peptide in the control of glucose tolerance and insulin secretion by pancreatic β-cells (Drucker 2002, Meier and Nauck 2005). GLP-1 also participates in pancreatic β-cell proliferation and neogenesis (Cani et al. 2005). In humans, intravenous administration of GLP-1 decreases food intake in both lean and obese individuals in a dose-dependent manner (Verdich et al. 2001). Obese subjects, given subcutaneous GLP-1 prior to each meal, reduce their calorie intake by 15% and lose 0.5 kg in weight over 5 days (Naslund et al. 2004). Animal data show that SCFA, either directly infused or produced by microbial fermentation of dietary fiber, increase intestinal proglucagon expression as well as GLP-1 secretion in rats (Reimer and McBurney 1996, Reimer et al. 1997).

11.3.4.6 Diet as a Target for Microbiota Modulation   It is well acknowledged that diet modulates the composition of the gut microbiota. Indeed, gut microbiota is able to adapt to the available nutrients provided by the diet in order to maximize their extractable energy. For example, in mice, the Western diet, high in fat and low in fiber, is known to increase the relative abundance of Firmicutes at the expense of the Bacteroidetes (Musso et al. 2010). On the contrary, the microbiota of children in a rural African village, consuming a fiber-rich diet, exhibits a significant enrichment in Bacteroidetes and a depletion in Firmicutes ($p < 0.001$) with a unique abundance of bacteria from the genus *Prevotella* and *Xylanibacter* that possess the adequate enzymatic equipment to degrade such substrate (De Filippo et al. 2010). Interestingly, the microbiota may adapt to dietary changes but this would not occur on the short term (Wu et al. 2011).

It has been suggested that diet is also a strong factor of the composition of the gut microbiota in animals suffering from metabolic disorders. In a study conducted with Apoa-I knockout mice with IGT and increased body fat and their wild-type counterparts, both fed a high-fat diet aiming at inducing metabolic syndrome, it was found that the diet explained 57% of the bacterial variation in the gut whereas genetic background only accounted for 12% (Zhang et al. 2010). Most notably, gut barrier-protecting *Bifidobacterium* spp. were nearly absent in all animals on high-fat diet, regardless of genotype. If diet can play such a significant role, the optimization of microbiota composition through the choice of particular nutrients, and notably prebiotic substances, should then be considered as a valuable part of the dietary strategy in the management of metabolic disorders associated with obesity and diabetes.

11.3.5 Chicory Fructans and Gut Microbiota Modulation in the Context of Metabolic Disorders

11.3.5.1 Back to Basics: Chicory Fructans Are Prebiotic Ingredients   Chicory fructans belong to the category of the so-called prebiotic ingredients. The concept of a prebiotic was first defined in 1995 by Gibson and Roberfroid as "nondigestible food ingredients that beneficially affect the host by selectively stimulating the growth and/or activity of one or a limited number of bacterial species already resident in the colon, and thus attempt to improve host health" (Gibson and Roberfroid 1995). This definition was updated twice to take into account the improved knowledge of the gut microbiota composition and properties, as summarized in the recent publication from Roberfroid and coworkers, to reach the following: "a dietary prebiotic is a selectively fermented ingredient that results in specific changes, in the composition and/or activity in the gastrointestinal microbiota, thus conferring benefit(s) upon host health" (Roberfroid et al. 2010).

Chicory fructans are resistant to digestion in the upper intestinal system as mentioned in the previous section. What makes their specificity is that they are totally fermented in the large intestine with no fructan residue being found in feces (Alles et al. 1996). Notably, they are specifically utilized by bifidobacteria (mostly) and lactobacilli residing in the large intestine. They are not or much less used by potentially harmful bacteria, such as *Clostridium perfringens, Escherichia coli*, and *Streptococcus faecalis* (Boeckner et al. 2001). In some cases, even a repressive effect of the chicory fructans on the potential pathogen microflora (clostridia, coliforms, *Escherichia coli*) can be observed (Fooks and Gibson 2002, Gibson and Wang 1994, van de Wiele et al. 2007, Wang and Gibson 1993). The selectivity toward bifidobacteria is probably due to the specific β(2-1) bonds between the fructose units in the fructan chain and to the fact that bifidobacteria are able to produce the enzymes able to cut such bonds (Wang and Gibson 1993).

A beneficial effect on the modulation of the microbiota, and more specifically an increase of bifidobacteria following chicory fructans intake, has been constantly observed in human studies (for a nonexhaustive summary of some of those studies, see Table 11.6). Other changes following chicory fructans intake, such as the increase of *Faecalibacterium prausnitzii*, have also been observed (Ramirez-Farias et al. 2009).

Table 11.6 Summary of Human Studies Regarding the Effects of Chicory Fructans on the Microbiota Modulation in Various Populations (Nonexhaustive)

Reference	Ingredient	Age	Daily Dose; Duration	Volunteers	Results
				Infants and Young Children	
Kapiki et al. (2007)	OF	0–2 weeks	4 g/L of product ready to use; 2 week	56	Higher numbers of bifidobacteria ($p = 0.032$) Higher counts of bacteroides ($p = 0.029$) Reduced counts of *Escherichia coli* and enterococci ($p = 0.029$ and $p = 0.025$, respectively) in the stools of OF-fed babies compared to placebo
Kim et al. (2007)	Inulin	± 3 months	1.5 g (3×0.5) (0.25 g inulin/kg body weight); 3 weeks	14 before weaning	Significant increase in bifidobacteria and lactobacilli ($p < 0.05$)
Yap et al. (2008)	Inulin	Average 7.7 months	0.75, 1, and 1.25 g/day; 35 days	36	Significant ($p < 0.05$) reduction of potential pathogenic microorganisms such as clostridia at all levels of inulin intake Significant ($p < 0.05$) increase of *Bifidobacterium* spp. as well as a significant ($p < 0.05$) decline in Gram-positive cocci and coliform bacteria with 1.25 g/day of inulin
				Adults	
Bouhnik et al. (2007)	Inulin	20–58 years	5 g/day, 8 weeks	20 healthy	Significant 12-fold bifidobacteria increase ($p < 0.0001$)
Harmsen (2002)	LC-inulin	28–54 years	9 g/day, 2 weeks	10 healthy	Significant 2.3-fold increase in bifidobacteria and 1.4-fold decrease of the *Eubacteria rectale–Clostridium coccoides* group ($p < 0.05$)

continued

Table 11.6 (Continued) Summary of Human Studies Regarding the Effects of Chicory Fructans on the Microbiota Modulation in Various Populations (Nonexhaustive)

Reference	Ingredient	Age	Daily Dose; Duration	Volunteers	Results
Kleessen et al. (2007)	Inulin	21–26 years	7.7 g/day for 1 week and 15.4 g/day for 2 weeks (in a snack bar)	45 healthy	Significant 1.2 log increase in bifidobacteria ($p<0.05$) Significant decrease in *Bacteroides/Prevotella* numbers and in *Clostridium histolyticum/C. lituseburense* group in frequency ($p < 0.05$)
Menne et al. (2000)	OF	20–50 years	8 g/day, 5 weeks	8 healthy	Significant increase in bifidobacteria, from $10^{8.6}$ to $10^{9.6}$ ($p < 0.01$) Trend for increased lactobacilli Trend for decreased coliforms and *Clostridium perfringens*
Ramirez-Farias et al. (2009)	Inulin	35–41 years	10 g/day, 21 days	12 healthy	Strongest response to inulin of *Bifidobacterium adolescentis* (from 0.89% to 3.9% of the total microbiota) ($p = 0.001$) *Bifidobacterium bifidum* increased from 0.22% to 0.63% ($p < 0.001$) Significant increase of *Faecalibacterium prausnitzii* (10.3% for control period *vs.* 14.5% during inulin intake, $p = 0.019$)
Rao (2001)	OF	24–48 years	5 g/day, 3 weeks	8 healthy	Close to 1 $\log_{10}$ cycle increase in bifidobacteria ($p < 0.001$)
Kleessen et al. (1997)	Inulin	68–89 years	20 g/day for 8 days, then 40 g/day for 11 days	**Elderly** 10 elderly constipated women	Significant increase in bifidobacteria, from 7.9 to 8.8 and 9.2 $\log_{10}$/g feces ($p < 0.05$) at 20 and 40 g/day, respectively. Decrease in enterococci ($p < 0.01$) and enterobacteria at 40 g/day
Marteau et al. (2011)	Inulin	51–62 years	15 g/day, 4 weeks	50 elderly constipated volunteers	Significant 0.6 log increase in bifidobacteria ($p < 0.01$)

Abbreviations: OF: oligofructose, OF-INU: oligofructose-enriched inulin, LC-inulin: long-chain inulin.

Microbiota modulation is not the only beneficial effect that can be ascribed to prebiotic ingredients. The bacterial fermentation of chicory fructans in the large intestine also promotes the release of SCFA, namely, acetate, propionate, and butyrate. SCFA may enhance ileal motility and increase intestinal cell proliferation. They also stimulate water and salt absorption, preventing diarrhea. Some may also be absorbed through the colonic epithelial cells into the blood, thus becoming a source for host energy and regulators of several metabolic processes. SCFA production also leads to a decrease in the intestinal pH.

Propionate has been demonstrated to lower cholesterol synthesis, both *in vitro* (Demigne et al. 1995) and *in vivo* in rats and in humans (Wolever et al. 1995). Conversely, acetate stimulates gluconeogenesis and is a well-known precursor of cholesterol. However, more recent data suggest that acetate may be used as a substrate by certain bacterial species of the clostridial cluster such as *Roseburia intestinalis* or *Fusobacterium prausnitzii* in order to produce butyrate in the colon (Duncan et al. 2004). Other data suggest that acetate is also able to support intestinal mucoprotection by increasing intestinal mucin expression and secretion (Scholtens et al. 2006). Butyrate is the preferred energy substrate for the colonocytes. Butyrate, and to a lesser extent propionate, may have a role in preventing certain types of colitis and may inhibit the proliferation of colon cancer cells (Scheppach 1998). Butyrate also has important effects on the development of the gene expression in intestinal cells (Falony et al. 2006).

Prebiotics can easily double the pool of SCFA in the GI tract. The capacity of chicory fructans to increase SCFA production has been demonstrated in several *in vitro* (Gibson and Wang 1994, Langlands et al. 2004, Sauer et al. 2007, van de Wiele et al. 2007) or animal studies (Juskiewicz et al. 2005). Usually the molar ratio between the different SCFA is altered by the fermentation of chicory fructans (Djouzi and Andrieux 1997, Femia et al. 2002). A higher level of propionate and butyrate produced compared to the control group or even to other substrates is reported (Licht et al. 2006). It is interesting to underline that despite the fact that bifidobacteria, which are the primary users of chicory fructans in the gut, are not butyrate producers themselves, butyrate secretion is strongly increased by chicory fructan fermentation. According to Duncan and coworkers, butyrate is believed to be produced by other bacterial species such as *Roseburia intestinalis* or *Faecalibacterium prausnitzii* (Duncan et al. 2004). A hypothesis would then be that microorganisms use the substrates by a cross-feeding metabolism. Indeed, butyrate production by *Roseburia intestinalis* from the fermentation of chicory oligofructose is achieved by its use of acetate released by oligofructose fermentation as this bacteria is not able to degrade oligofructose directly (Falony et al. 2006). Such interactions may play a significant role in the colon ecosystem.

Nevertheless, as potent modulators of the microbiota, notably toward higher counts of bifidobacteria, and of the release of SCFA and in particular butyrate, chicory fructans may be promising avenues to play a role on the management of metabolic disorders.

11.3.5.2 Effects of Chicory Fructans on Gut Barrier Function It has been suggested that as bifidobacteria have been reported to reduce intestinal endotoxin levels and to improve mucosal barrier function, the increase of gut bifidobacteria contents by a prebiotic ingredient such as a chicory fructan may modulate metabolic endotoxemia, the inflammatory tone, and the development of diabetes. Indeed, in chicory oligofructose-treated mice fed a high-fat diet, the levels of *Bifidobacterium* significantly and positively correlate with improved glucose tolerance and normalized inflammatory tone (Cani, Neyrinck, et al. 2007).

The selective modulation of the microbiota by a prebiotic ingredient and its effect on the intestinal permeability and endotoxemia has been further explored in other animal studies. Obese mice treated with chicory oligofructose exhibited lower plasma LPS and cytokines levels as well as a better tight-junction integrity, associated with significantly increased GLP-2 production, as compared to obese control under a nonprebiotic diet (Cani, Possemiers, et al. 2009). In addition, the cecal content of *Bifidobacterium* spp. and the portal plasma levels of LPS showed a negative correlation. In obese mice, chicory oligofructose treatment normalized the eCB tone in both the gut and adipose tissue and led to significantly ($p < 0.05$) lower plasma LPS levels (Muccioli et al. 2010). Taken together, these data demonstrate that supplementing the diet with chicory fructans counteracts the increased plasma LPS levels observed in obese mice by affecting both GLP-2 and endocannabinoid signalings, which independently regulate gut permeability.

Similarly, chicory oligofructose enrichment of the diet of genetic or diet-induced obese and diabetic mice significantly lowered fasting glycemia and improved glucose tolerance ($p < 0.05$). In addition, prebiotic treatment improved gut barrier function with better jejunum ZO-1 and occludin distribution. Plasma LPS levels were twofold lower in the prebiotic group. Also, significant changes in the microbiota profile and not only in bifidobacteria were observed under oligofructose treatment. In particular, prebiotic feeding decreased Firmicutes and increased Bacteroidetes phyla and changed more than 100 taxa of bacteria (Everard et al. 2011).

11.3.5.3 Chicory Fructans and Fat Storage (Insulin Resistance) G-protein coupled receptor 43 (GPR43), highly expressed in adipocytes, is involved in both lipolysis regulation and adipocyte differentiation leading to an increased adiposity. A high-fat diet increases GPR43 mRNA expression. Moreover, the role of SCFA in adiposity increase via GPR43 has already been described previously.

Surprisingly, under chicory oligofructose supplementation in high-fat diet-fed mice, the resulting increased fermentation led to a decrease in the expression of the genes responding to the SCFA such as GPR43 mRNA. Selective changes in the cecal microbiota composition, notably a 100-fold increase in bifidobacteria and a drop in *Roseburia* spp. and in *Eubacterium rectal–Clostridium coccoides*, were observed in the chicory fructan-supplemented group. Also, the chicory fructan supplementation normalized mean adipocyte size, restored the release of FFA in the medium, and counteracted the increase in insulin resistance (Dewulf et al. 2011).

11.3.5.4 Chicory Fructans and Gut-Derived Peptides
11.3.5.4.1 GLP-2 The impact of chicory fructans on GLP-2 secretion involved in gut barrier function has already been described in a previous section about the gut barrier function.

11.3.5.4.2 Leptin In diet-induced leptin-resistant mice, chicory oligofructose supplementation improved leptin sensitivity in association with changes in gut microbiota, notably with increased counts of bifidobacteria. Adiposity index as well as plasma glucose levels were also significantly reduced in the prebiotic-supplemented group (Everard et al. 2011).

11.3.5.4.3 PYY In humans, the daily consumption of 16 g of chicory oligofructose significantly increased plasma PYY concentration (Cani, Lecourt, et al. 2009). The effects of 12 weeks of 21 g chicory oligofructose daily supplementation on weight loss, energy intake, plasma satiety hormone and glucose concentrations, and subjective appetite rating have been assessed in 48 over weight/obese adults in a parallel double-blind randomized design (Parnell and Reimer 2009). After 12 weeks of intake, a 13% plasma PYY levels increase after a meal was observed in the oligofructose group (compared to baseline). Unfortunately, in none of those studies, an effect on blood glucose metabolism was investigated.

11.3.5.4.4 GLP-1 The colonic fermentation of chicory fructans by the resident microbiota led to considerable enlargement of the cecal wall and to the production of SCFA (Gibson and Wang 1994, Langlands et al. 2004, Sauer et al. 2007, van de Wiele et al. 2007). Butyrate is metabolized by colonocytes, whereas acetate and propionate reach the liver through the portal vein. Repeatedly, the consumption of prebiotic fibers such as chicory fructans has demonstrated an effect on the release of GLP-1 in the gut (Cani et al. 2005, Cani, Lecourt, et al. 2009, Delmée et al. 2006).

In streptozotocin (STZ)-treated rats (a classical animal model for diabetes), oligofructose supplementation (10% in the diet) reduced all symptoms associated with diabetic stage (postprandial hyperglycemia, hyperphagia, polydypsia, weight loss) normally observed in such animals. It also increased portal and colonic GLP-1 levels and doubled colonic proglucagon (Cani et al. 2005).

In diabetic mice, 10% of oligofructose added to the diet, increased by 66% portal GLP-1 concentration and by 100% GLP-1 concentration in the proximal colon as compared to the control group. Proglucagon mRNA was also increased by 80% in the proximal colon and a linear correlation between proglucagon mRNA and the concentration of GLP-1 has been underlined (Delmée et al. 2006). In a second part of this study, diabetic mice were put under two differents high-fat (HF) diets. In HF-1, high-fat diet was given alone or with oligofructose supplementation during 4 weeks, whereas in HF-2, high-fat diet was first given for 8 weeks before the introduction of the oligofructose. Oligofructose treatment significantly increased proglucagon mRNA in the proximal colon by about 50% in HF-1 diet but not in HF-2 diet. It has been suggested by the authors that an enrichment of the diet with oligofructose is less effective in more advanced states of metabolic disturbances due to a longer period of high-fat treatment. In another animal study, Cani et al. (2006) have demonstrated that the antidiabetic effect of oligofructose requires a functional GLP-1 receptor.

Further to the data on animals, some publications have focused on the release of GLP-1, following chicory fructans consumption in humans. In patients with gastroesophageal reflux disease, oligofructose feeding at 20 g/day for 1 week significantly increased plasma GLP-1 after a mixed meal (Piche et al. 2003). In healthy adult volunteers, the AUC for plasma glucose concentration was significantly lower after the daily consumption of 16 g of oligofructose-enriched inulin for 2 weeks (Cani, Lecourt, et al. 2009). The glucose response was inversely correlated with a gut microbial fermentation activity marker (breath-hydrogen excretion). In addition to this effect, a significant increase in plasma GLP-1, also inversely correlated with breath-hydrogen excretion (reflecting colonic microbial fermentation) after the meal, was observed.

GLP-1 is produced from proglucagon by L cells in the distal small intestine and colon. All the research conducted on inulin-type fructans shows an increase in the concentration of proglucagon mRNA and GLP-1 in the proximal and, to a lesser extent, in the medial colon (Delzenne et al. 2005, 2007). The number of GLP-1-expressing cells is doubled in the proximal colon of oligofructose-treated rats, a phenomenon correlated with the increase in proglucagon mRNA and peptide content in this tissue (Cani, Hoste, et al. 2007).

Altogether, the data presented above show that, through their impact on gut activity, prebiotics such as chicory fructans can be interesting contributors to the improvement of the conditions associated with metabolic disorders such as metabolic syndrome, diabetes type 2, and obesity.

11.4 Formulation of Foods Dedicated to People Suffering from Glucose Metabolism Disorders

Chicory fructans have been used as food ingredients for decades, notably because of their low calorie value and their ability to substitute for sugar and/or fat in food formulations. Moreover, owing to their nondigestibility, inulin and oligofructose are suitable for consumption by diabetics.

11.4.1 Chicory Fructans Are Low-Calorie Ingredients

The caloric value of chicory fructans in human subjects has been estimated using different methodologies.

Oligofructose was fed to volunteers, followed by measurement of the amounts excreted in urine and feces, as well as the amount exiting the small intestine by using intestinal aspiration (Molis et al. 1996). The authors determined the amount of oligofructose absorbed and metabolized from the small intestine and the amount fermented in the colon as 11% and 89%, respectively. Caloric value was then calculated by multiplying small intestine utilization by 4 kcal/g (which is the accepted energy value for digested carbohydrates) and by assuming that the amount fermented in the large bowel yields 50% of the energy for a digestible carbohydrate. The analysis resulted in a 2.3 kcal/g caloric value.

However, in 1993, Roberfroid et al. (1993) demonstrated that the energy generated from the fermentation of oligofructose as being only 38% of digestible carbohydrate and not the 50% used in the study by Molis et al. By studying the biochemical balance charts for carbon atoms, metabolic pathways, and energy yield to the host, Roberfroid et al. have shown that the caloric value of inulin is likely to be close to 1 kcal/g. Furthermore, it has been shown that the technique of small intestinal aspiration overestimates the amount of material absorbed in the small intestine (Livesey et al. 1993), leading to the conclusion that the amount fermented in the small intestine is minimal; therefore, the factor used in the Molis study for the small intestine may be as low as zero (Flamm et al. 2001). Reevaluation of the caloric value using these factors provides a caloric value for oligofructose of 1.5–1.8 kcal/g (assuming an 11% intestinal absorption in the small intestine).

In another publication on the caloric value of chicory fructans, Roberfroid (1999) applied the factorial method, which had been used before by a FASEB/LSRO (1994) expert group on evaluating caloric values of polyols. Using this formula, the calculated caloric value of chicory fructans is estimated to be 1.5–1.7 kcal/g or 6.3–7.3 kJ/g.

Another additional energy balance experiment using whole-body indirect calorimetry methods was performed, with reported caloric values for inulin ranging from 2.1 to 2.8 kcal/g (Castiglia-Delavaud et al. 1998). However, Livesey (1993) showed a certain amount of variability in employing this methodology, based on the ability to estimate within only 0.5 kcal/g precision (Livesey et al. 1993). The different study results reported by Castiglia, which employ the same number of subjects and methodology, seem to support Livesey's conclusion. In conclusion, based on these findings, it is evident that only 40–50% of the energy of digestible carbohydrates is the energy in chicory fructans, making the energy value for inulin and oligofructose 1.5–2.0 kcal/g (Flamm et al. 2001).

11.4.2 Sugar Substitution by Chicory Fructans

Chicory fructans are commonly used for sugar reduction and/or substitution in various food applications. This is because, first, their caloric value is lower as compared to that of digestible carbohydrates such as sucrose or starch, as explained in the previous section, but also because their physical and chemical characteristics closely match those of sucrose in a wide range of food applications. Chicory fructans are soluble, tasteless, heat stable, and combine easily with polyols and intensive sweeteners, particularly with *Stevia*, making them a perfect ingredient for sugar reduction and/or substitution (Franck 2002). For example, sucrose-free chocolate formulated with inulin is well accepted in terms of sensory attributes as well as physicochemical properties (Shah et al. 2010). Cookies, where sugars were partially replaced by oligofructose (up to 60%), were preferred over the control cookies because of improved color, texture, and appearance (Handa et al. 2012). Similar results were observed for partial sugar substitution by inulin in "kaya," a popular Malaysian jam-like food composed of egg, sugar, and coconut milk, and commonly consumed at breakfast. In this study, 10% and 30% sugar substitutions were found to be comparable to the commercial "kaya" sample (Phang and Chan 2009). All these examples demonstrate the versatility of chicory fructans that are easily used in many different food applications.

11.4.3 Glycemic Index Reduction by Chicory Fructans

Obviously, as chicory fructans do not impact on postprandial blood glucose levels (Granfeldt and Björck 2004, Meyer 2007), they are particularly attractive ingredients for the formulation of low or reduced GI foods. They may also present some interest not only in substitution but also in addition to digestible carbohydrates.

In a study from Brennan and coworkers, wheat durum pasta were enriched by various levels of inulin (0%, 2.5%, 5%, 7.5%, and 10% in g/100 g of flour) (Brennan et al. 2004). *In vitro* digestion of the pasta was performed using a multienzymatic method described by Brighenti and coworkers (Brighenti et al. 1995), which monitored the amount of reducing sugars (indicative of the rate of starch degradation) released over a 5 h period, allowing for the calculation of a predictive GI. Although the calculated values for the predictive GI of inulin-containing pasta were not significantly different from the control, a general trend was observed with a reduction of GI proportional to the amount of inulin used in the formulation. For example, the pasta with 10% of inulin addition decreased their predictive GI by 15% as compared to the control pasta.

11.5 Overall Conclusion

Despite the limited effect of chicory fructans on blood glucose levels in the long term, its interest on sugar replacement, thanks to its very limited impact on postprandial glucose and insulin levels, is well acknowledged. Moreover, recent practical recommendations for clinicians in diabetes care propose the inclusion of products containing fructans into the eating plans (Maziarz 2013).

Besides the interest of chicory fructans on food formulations targeting more specifically people with disturbed glucose metabolism, such as low GI or sugar-reduced, the potential of those ingredients on the management of such disorders may be considered at a wider level, notably toward their particular feature, which is their prebiotic effect. With a greater focus on the human gut microbiota's potential role on several metabolic disorders, including obesity and type 2 diabetes, and taking into account the latest scientific advances on microbiota identification and functions, the door is open to further explore the impact of the consumption of prebiotic chicory fructans on the management of those disorders. Existing data seem promising, but more research is needed to enhance the understanding of the exact mechanisms involved in the mediation of such effects.

References

Alberti, K. G., R. H. Eckel, S. M. Grundy et al. 2009. Harmonizing the metabolic syndrome: A joint interim statement of the International Diabetes Federation Task Force on Epidemiology and Prevention; National Heart, Lung, and Blood Institute; American Heart Association; World Heart Federation; International Atherosclerosis Society; and International Association for the Study of Obesity. *Circulation* 120:1640–5.

Alles, M. S., N. M. de Roos, J. C. Bakx et al. 1999. Consumption of fructooligosaccharides does not favorably affect blood glucose and serum lipid concentrations in patients with type 2 diabetes. *Am J Clin Nutr* 69:64–9.

Alles, M. S., J. G. Hautvast, F. M. Nagengast et al. 1996. Fate of fructo-oligosaccharides in the human intestine. *Br J Nutr* 76:211–21.

Amar, J., R. Burcelin, J. B. Ruidavets et al. 2008. Energy intake is associated with endotoxemia in apparently healthy men. *Am J Clin Nutr* 87:1219–23.

American Diabetes Association. 2013. Diagnosis and classification of diabetes mellitus. *Diabetes Care* 36(Suppl. 1):S67–74.

Arumugam, M., J. Raes, E. Pelletier et al. 2011. Enterotypes of the human gut microbiome. *Nature* 473:174–80.

Bach Knudsen, K. E., and I. Hessov. 1995. Recovery of inulin from Jerusalem artichoke (*Helianthus tuberosus* L.) in the small intestine of man. *Br J Nutr* 74:101–13.

Backhed, F., H. Ding, T. Wang et al. 2004. The gut microbiota as an environmental factor that regulates fat storage. *Proc Natl Acad Sci USA* 101:15718–23.

Backhed, F., J. K. Manchester, C. F. Semenkovich, and J. I. Gordon. 2007. Mechanisms underlying the resistance to diet-induced obesity in germ-free mice. *Proc Natl Acad Sci USA* 104:979–84.

Boeckner, L. S., M. I. Schnepf, and B. C. Tungland. 2001. Inulin: A review of nutritional and health implications. *Adv Food Nutr Res* 43:1–63.

Bonsu, N. K., C. S. Johnson, and K. M. McLeod. 2011. Can dietary fructans lower serum glucose? *J Diabetes* 3:58–66.

Bonsu, N. K., and S. Johnson. 2012. Effects of inulin fibre supplementation on serum glucose and lipid concentration in patients with type 2 diabetes. *Int J Diabetes Metab* 21:80–6.

Bouhnik, Y., L. Achour, D. Paineau et al. 2007. Four-week short chain fructo-oligo-saccharides ingestion leads to an increase in fecal bifidobacteria and cholesterol excretion in healthy elderly volunteers. *Nutr J* 6:42.

Brennan, C. S., V. Kuri, and C. M. Tudorica. 2004. Inulin-enriched pasta: Effects on textural properties and starch degradation. *Food Chem* 86:189–93.

Brighenti, F., N. Pellegrini, M. C. Casiraghi, and G. Testolin. 1995. *In vitro* studies to predict physiological effects of dietary fibre. *Eur J Clin Nutr* 49(Suppl. 3):S81–8.

Bryant, N. J., R. Govers, and D. E. James. 2002. Regulated transport of the glucose transporter GLUT4. *Nat Rev Mol Cell Biol* 3:267–77.

Cani, P. D., J. Amar, M. A. Iglesias et al. 2007. Metabolic endotoxemia initiates obesity and insulin resistance. *Diabetes* 56:1761–72.

Cani, P. D., R. Bibiloni, C. Knauf et al. 2008. Changes in gut microbiota control meta-bolic endotoxemia-induced inflammation in high-fat diet-induced obesity and diabetes in mice. *Diabetes* 57:1470–81.

Cani, P. D., C. A. Daubioul, B. Reusens et al. 2005. Involvement of endogenous gluca-gon-like peptide-1(7–36) amide on glycaemia-lowering effect of oligofructose in streptozotocin-treated rats. *J Endocrinol* 185:457–65.

Cani, P. D., and N. M. Delzenne. 2009. The role of the gut microbiota in energy metab-olism and metabolic disease. *Curr Pharm Des* 15:1546–58.

Cani, P. D., S. Hoste, Y. Guiot, and N. M. Delzenne. 2007. Dietary non-digestible carbohy-drates promote L-cell differentiation in the proximal colon of rats. *Br J Nutr* 98:32–7.

Cani, P. D., C. Knauf, M. A. Iglesias et al. 2006. Improvement of glucose tolerance and hepatic insulin sensitivity by oligofructose requires a functional glucagon-like peptide 1 receptor. *Diabetes* 55:1484–90.

Cani, P. D., E. Lecourt, E. M. Dewulf et al. 2009. Gut microbiota fermentation of pre-biotics increases satietogenic and incretin gut peptide production with conse-quences for appetite sensation and glucose response after a meal. *Am J Clin Nutr* 90:1236–43.

Cani, P. D., A. M. Neyrinck, F. Fava et al. 2007. Selective increases of bifidobacteria in gut microflora improve high-fat-diet-induced diabetes in mice through a mecha-nism associated with endotoxaemia. *Diabetologia* 50:2374–83.

Cani, P. D., S. Possemiers, T. Van de Wiele et al. 2009. Changes in gut microbiota con-trol inflammation in obese mice through a mechanism involving GLP-2-driven improvement of gut permeability. *Gut* 58:1091–103.

Castiglia-Delavaud, C., E. Verdier, J. M. Besle et al. 1998. Net energy value of non-starch polysaccharide isolates (sugarbeet fibre and commercial inulin) and their impact on nutrient digestive utilization in healthy human subjects. *Br J Nutr* 80:343–52.

Causey, J. L., J. M. Feirtag, D. D. Gallaher, B. C. Tungland, and J. L. Slavin. 2000. Effects of dietary inulin on serum lipids, blood glucose and the gastrointestinal environ-ment in hypercholestertolemic men. *Nutr Res* 20:191–201.

Creely, S. J., P. G. McTernan, C. M. Kusminski et al. 2007. Lipopolysaccharide activates an innate immune system response in human adipose tissue in obesity and type 2 diabetes. *Am J Physiol Endocrinol Metab* 292:E740–7.

Daubioul, C. A., Y. Horsmans, P. Lambert, E. Danse, and N. M. Delzenne. 2005. Effects of oligofructose on glucose and lipid metabolism in patients with nonalcoholic steatohepatitis: Results of a pilot study. *Eur J Clin Nutr* 59:723–6.

De Filippo, C., D. Cavalieri, M. Di Paola et al. 2010. Impact of diet in shaping gut microbiota revealed by a comparative study in children from Europe and rural Africa. *Proc Natl Acad Sci USA* 107:14691–6.

DeFronzo, R. A. 2004. Pathogenesis of type 2 diabetes mellitus. *Med Clin North Am* 88:787–835.

Delmée, E., P. D. Cani, G. Gual et al. 2006. Relation between colonic proglucagon expression and metabolic response to oligofructose in high fat diet-fed mice. *Life Sci* 79:1007–13.

Delzenne, N. M., and P. D. Cani. 2005. A place for dietary fibre in the management of the metabolic syndrome. *Curr Opin Clin Nutr Metab Care* 8:636–40.

Delzenne, N. M., P. D. Cani, C. Daubioul, and A. M. Neyrinck. 2005. Impact of inulin and oligofructose on gastrointestinal peptides. *Br J Nutr* 93(Suppl. 1):S157–61.

Delzenne, N. M., P. D. Cani, and A. M. Neyrinck. 2007. Modulation of glucagon-like peptide 1 and energy metabolism by inulin and oligofructose: Experimental data. *J Nutr* 137:2547S–51S.

Delzenne, N. M., A. M. Neyrinck, and P. D. Cani. 2011. Modulation of the gut microbiota by nutrients with prebiotic properties: Consequences for host health in the context of obesity and metabolic syndrome. *Microb Cell Fact* 10(Suppl. 1):S10.

Demigne, C., M. A. Levrat, H. Younes, and C. Remesy. 1995. Interactions between large intestine fermentation and dietary calcium. *Eur J Clin Nutr* 49(Suppl. 3):S235–8.

Dewulf, E. M., P. D. Cani, A. M. Neyrinck et al. 2011. Inulin-type fructans with prebiotic properties counteract GPR43 overexpression and PPARgamma-related adipogenesis in the white adipose tissue of high-fat diet-fed mice. *J Nutr Biochem* 22:712–22.

DiBaise, J. K., H. Zhang, M. D. Crowell et al. 2008. Gut microbiota and its possible relationship with obesity. *Mayo Clin Proc* 83:460–9.

Djouzi, Z., and C. Andrieux. 1997. Compared effects of three oligosaccharides on metabolism of intestinal microflora in rats inoculated with a human faecal flora. *Br J Nutr* 78:313–24.

Drucker, D. J. 2002. Biological actions and therapeutic potential of the glucagon-like peptides. *Gastroenterology* 122:531–44.

Duncan, S. H., G. Holtrop, G. E. Lobley et al. 2004. Contribution of acetate to butyrate formation by human faecal bacteria. *Br J Nutr* 91:915–23.

Duncan, S. H., G. E. Lobley, G. Holtrop et al. 2008. Human colonic microbiota associated with diet, obesity and weight loss. *Int J Obes (Lond)* 32:1720–4.

Eckburg, P. B., E. M. Bik, C. N. Bernstein et al. 2005. Diversity of the human intestinal microbial flora. *Science* 308:1635–8.

Eckel, R. H., S. M. Grundy, and P. Z. Zimmet. 2005. The metabolic syndrome. *Lancet* 365:1415–28.

Ellegard, L., H. Andersson, and I. Bosaeus. 1997. Inulin and oligofructose do not influence the absorption of cholesterol, or the excretion of cholesterol, Ca, Mg, Zn, Fe, or bile acids but increases energy excretion in ileostomy subjects. *Eur J Clin Nutr* 51:1–5.

Everard, A., V. Lazarevic, M. Derrien et al. 2011. Responses of gut microbiota and glucose and lipid metabolism to prebiotics in genetic obese and diet-induced leptin-resistant mice. *Diabetes* 60:2775–86.

Falony, G., A. Vlachou, K. Verbrugghe, and L. De Vuyst. 2006. Cross-feeding between *Bifidobacterium longum* BB536 and acetate-converting, butyrate-producing colon bacteria during growth on oligofructose. *Appl Environ Microbiol* 72:7835–41.

FAO/WHO. 1998. Carbohydrates in human nutrition. Report of a Joint FAO/WHO Expert Consultation. *FAO Food Nutr Pap* 66.

Femia, A. P., C. Luceri, P. Dolara et al. 2002. Antitumorigenic activity of the prebiotic inulin enriched with oligofructose in combination with the probiotics *Lactobacillus rhamnosus* and *Bifidobacterium lactis* on azoxymethane-induced colon carcinogenesis in rats. *Carcinogenesis* 23:1953–60.

Flamm, G., W. Glinsmann, D. Kritchevsky, L. Prosky, and M. Roberfroid. 2001. Inulin and oligofructose as dietary fiber: A review of the evidence. *Crit Rev Food Sci Nutr* 41:353–62.

Fooks, L. J., and G. Gibson. 2002. *In vitro* investigations of the effect of probiotics and prebiotics on selected human intestinal pathogens. *FEMS Microbiol Ecol* 39:67–75.

Franck, A. 2002. Technological functionality of inulin and oligofructose. *Br J Nutr* 87(Suppl. 2):S287–91.

Furet, J. P., L. C. Kong, J. Tap et al. 2010. Differential adaptation of human gut microbiota to bariatric surgery-induced weight loss: Links with metabolic and low-grade inflammation markers. *Diabetes* 59:3049–57.

Galisteo, M., J. Duarte, and A. Zarzuelo. 2008. Effects of dietary fibers on disturbances clustered in the metabolic syndrome. *J Nutr Biochem* 19:71–84.

Gibson, G. R., and M. B. Roberfroid. 1995. Dietary modulation of the human colonic microbiota: Introducing the concept of prebiotics. *J Nutr* 125:1401–12.

Gibson, G. R., and X. Wang. 1994. Enrichment of bifidobacteria from human gut contents by oligofructose using continuous culture. *FEMS Microbiol Lett* 118:121–7.

Granfeldt, Y., and I. Björck. 2004. Evaluation of the effects of the addition of chicory fructans to a meal on postprandial glucose and insulin responses. Confidential Report.

Greiner, T., and F. Backhed. 2011. Effects of the gut microbiota on obesity and glucose homeostasis. *Trends Endocrinol Metab* 22:117–23.

Grysman, A., T. Carlson, and T. M. Wolever. 2008. Effects of sucromalt on postprandial responses in human subjects. *Eur J Clin Nutr* 62:1364–71.

Handa, C., S. Goomer, and A. Siddhu. 2012. Physicochemical properties and sensory evaluation of fructoligosaccharide enriched cookies. *J Food Sci Technol* 49:192–9.

Harford, K. A., C. M. Reynolds, F. C. McGillicuddy, and H. M. Roche. 2011. Fats, inflammation and insulin resistance: Insights to the role of macrophage and T-cell accumulation in adipose tissue. *Proc Nutr Soc* 70:408–17.

Harmsen, H. J. 2002. The effect of the prebiotic inulin and the probiotic *Bifidobacterium longum* on the fecal microflora of healthy volunteers measured by FISH and DGGE. *Microbial Ecol Health Dis* 14:212–20.

Harris, K., A. Kassis, G. Major, and C. J. Chou. 2012. Is the gut microbiota a new factor contributing to obesity and its metabolic disorders? *J Obes* 2012:879151, doi: 10.1155/2012/879151.

Hong, Y. H., Y. Nishimura, D. Hishikawa et al. 2005. Acetate and propionate short chain fatty acids stimulate adipogenesis via GPCR43. *Endocrinology* 146:5092–9.

Hotamisligil, G. S., P. Peraldi, A. Budavari et al. 1996. IRS-1-mediated inhibition of insulin receptor tyrosine kinase activity in TNF-alpha- and obesity-induced insulin resistance. *Science* 271:665–8.

Jackson, K. G., G. R. Taylor, A. M. Clohessy, and C. M. Williams. 1999. The effect of the daily intake of inulin on fasting lipid, insulin and glucose concentrations in middle-aged men and women. *Br J Nutr* 82:23–30.

Jumpertz, R., D. S. Le, P. J. Turnbaugh et al. 2011. Energy-balance studies reveal associations between gut microbes, caloric load, and nutrient absorption in humans. *Am J Clin Nutr* 94:58–65.

Juskiewicz, J., Z. Zdunczyk, and M. Wroblewska. 2005. The effect of the administration of cellulose and fructans with different degree of polymerization to rats on caecal fermentation and biochemical indicators in the serum. *Czech J Anim Sci* 50:273–80.

Kapiki, A., C. Costalos, C. Oikonomidou et al. 2007. The effect of a fructo-oligosaccharide supplemented formula on gut flora of preterm infants. *Early Hum Dev* 83:335–9.

Kim, S. H., H. Lee da, and D. Meyer. 2007. Supplementation of baby formula with native inulin has a prebiotic effect in formula-fed babies. *Asia Pac J Clin Nutr* 16:172–7

Kleessen, B., S. Schwarz, A. Boehm et al. 2007. Jerusalem artichoke and chicory inulin in bakery products affect faecal microbiota of healthy volunteers. *Br J Nutr* 98:540–9.

Kleessen, B., B. Sykura, H. J. Zunft, and M. Blaut. 1997. Effects of inulin and lactose on fecal microflora, microbial activity, and bowel habit in elderly constipated persons. *Am J Clin Nutr* 65:1397–402.

Knowler, W. C., E. Barrett-Connor, S. E. Fowler et al. 2002. Reduction in the incidence of type 2 diabetes with lifestyle intervention or metformin. *N Engl J Med* 346:393–403.

Kootte, R. S., A. Vrieze, F. Holleman et al. 2012. The therapeutic potential of manipulating gut microbiota in obesity and type 2 diabetes mellitus. *Diabetes Obes Metab* 14:112–20.

Kumanyika, S., R. W. Jeffery, A. Morabia et al. 2002. Obesity prevention: The case for action. *Int J Obes Relat Metab Disord* 26:425–36.

Langlands, S. J., M. J. Hopkins, N. Coleman, and J. H. Cummings. 2004. Prebiotic carbohydrates modify the mucosa associated microflora of the human large bowel. *Gut* 53:1610–6.

Larsen, N., F. K. Vogensen, F. W. van den Berg et al. 2010. Gut microbiota in human adults with type 2 diabetes differs from non-diabetic adults. *PLoS One* 5:e9085.

Leach, J. D., G. R. Gibson, and J. Van Loo. 2006. Human evolution, nutritional ecology and prebiotics in ancient diet. *Biosci Microflora* 25:1–8.

Letexier, D., F. Diraison, and M. Beylot. 2003. Addition of inulin to a moderately high-carbohydrate diet reduces hepatic lipogenesis and plasma triacylglycerol concentrations in humans. *Am J Clin Nutr* 77:559–64.

Lewis, D. H. 1993. Nomenclature and diagrammatic representation of oligomeric fructans-a paper for discussion. *New Phytol* 124:583–94.

Ley, R. E., F. Backhed, P. Turnbaugh et al. 2005. Obesity alters gut microbial ecology. *Proc Natl Acad Sci USA* 102:11070–5.

Ley, R. E., P. J. Turnbaugh, S. Klein, and J. I. Gordon. 2006. Microbial ecology: Human gut microbes associated with obesity. *Nature* 444:1022–3.

Licht, T. R., M. Hansen, M. Poulsen, and L. O. Dragsted. 2006. Dietary carbohydrate source influences molecular fingerprints of the rat faecal microbiota. *BMC Microbiol* 6:98, doi:10.1186/1471-2180-6-98.

Lionetti, L., M. P. Mollica, A. Lombardi et al. 2009. From chronic overnutrition to insulin resistance: The role of fat-storing capacity and inflammation. *Nutr Metab Cardiovasc Dis* 19:146–52.

Livesey, G., I. T. Johnson, J. M. Gee et al. 1993. Determination of sugar alcohol and polydextrose absorption in humans by the breath hydrogen (H_2) technique: The stoichiometry of hydrogen production and the interaction between carbohydrates assessed *in vivo* and *in vitro*. *Eur J Clin Nutr* 47:419–30.

Marteau, P., H. Jacobs, M. Cazaubiel et al. 2011. Effects of chicory inulin in constipated elderly people: A double-blind controlled trial. *Int J Food Sci Nutr* 62:164–70.

Matias, I., S. Petrosino, A. Racioppi et al. 2008. Dysregulation of peripheral endocannabinoid levels in hyperglycemia and obesity: Effect of high fat diets. *Mol Cell Endocrinol* 286:S66–78.

Maziarz, M. 2013. Role of fructans and resistant starch in diabetes care. *Diabetes Spectrum* 26:35–39.

Meier, J. J., and M. A. Nauck. 2005. Glucagon-like peptide 1(GLP-1) in biology and pathology. *Diabetes Metab Res Rev* 21:91–117.

Membrez, M., F. Blancher, M. Jaquet et al. 2008. Gut microbiota modulation with norfloxacin and ampicillin enhances glucose tolerance in mice. *FASEB J* 22:2416–26.

Menne, E., N. Guggenbuhl, and M. Roberfroid. 2000. Fn-type chicory inulin hydrolysate has a prebiotic effect in humans. *J Nutr* 130:1197–9.

Meyer, D. 2007. Inulin for product development of low GI products to support weight management. In *Dietary Fibre: Components and Functions*, eds. H. Salovaraa, F. Gates, and M. Tenkanen, 257–270. The Netherlands: Wageningen Academic Publishers.

Molis, C., B. Flourie, F. Ouarne et al. 1996. Digestion, excretion, and energy value of fructooligosaccharides in healthy humans. *Am J Clin Nutr* 64:324–8.

Muccioli, G. G., D. Naslain, F. Backhed et al. 2010. The endocannabinoid system links gut microbiota to adipogenesis. *Mol Syst Biol* 6:392

Musso, G., R. Gambino, and M. Cassader. 2010. Obesity, diabetes, and gut microbiota: The hygiene hypothesis expanded? *Diabetes Care* 33:2277–84.

Naslund, E., N. King, S. Mansten et al. 2004. Prandial subcutaneous injections of glucagon-like peptide-1 cause weight loss in obese human subjects. *Br J Nutr* 91:439–46.

Nathan, D. M., M. B. Davidson, R. A. DeFronzo et al. 2007. Impaired fasting glucose and impaired glucose tolerance: Implications for care. *Diabetes Care* 30:753–9.

Parillo, M., and G. Riccardi. 2004. Diet composition and the risk of type 2 diabetes: Epidemiological and clinical evidence. *Br J Nutr* 92:7–19.

Parnell, J. A., and R. A. Reimer. 2009. Weight loss during oligofructose supplementation is associated with decreased ghrelin and increased peptide YY in overweight and obese adults. *Am J Clin Nutr* 89:1751–9.

Phang, Y. L., and H. K. Chan. 2009. Sensory descriptive analysis and consumer acceptability of original "kaya" and "kaya" partially substituted with inulin. *Int Food Res J* 16:483–92.

Piche, T., S. B. des Varannes, S. Sacher-Huvelin et al. 2003. Colonic fermentation influences lower esophageal sphincter function in gastroesophageal reflux disease. *Gastroenterology* 124:894–902.

Pironi, L., V. Stanghellini, M. Miglioli et al. 1993. Fat-induced ileal brake in humans: A dose-dependent phenomenon correlated to the plasma levels of peptide YY. *Gastroenterology* 105:733–9.

Pussinen, P. J., A. S. Havulinna, M. Lehto, J. Sundvall, and V. Salomaa. 2011. Endotoxemia is associated with an increased risk of incident diabetes. *Diabetes Care* 34:392–7.

Ramirez-Farias, C., K. Slezak, Z. Fuller et al. 2009. Effect of inulin on the human gut microbiota: Stimulation of *Bifidobacterium adolescentis* and *Faecalibacterium prausnitzii*. *Br J Nutr* 101:541–50.

Rao, V. A. 2001. The prebiotic properties of oligofructose at low intake levels. *Nutr Res* 21:843–8.

Reimer, R. A., and M. I. McBurney. 1996. Dietary fiber modulates intestinal proglucagon messenger ribonucleic acid and postprandial secretion of glucagon-like peptide-1 and insulin in rats. *Endocrinology* 137:3948–56.

Reimer, R. A., A. B. Thomson, R. V. Rajotte et al. 1997. A physiological level of rhubarb fiber increases proglucagon gene expression and modulates intestinal glucose uptake in rats. *J Nutr* 127:1923–8.

Roberfroid, M., G. R. Gibson, and N. Delzenne. 1993. The biochemistry of oligofructose, a nondigestible fiber: An approach to calculate its caloric value. *Nutr Rev* 51:137–46.

Roberfroid, M., G. R. Gibson, L. Hoyles et al. 2010. Prebiotic effects: Metabolic and health benefits. *Br J Nutr* 104(Suppl. 2):S1–63.

Roberfroid, M. B. 1999. Caloric value of inulin and oligofructose. *J Nutr* 129:1436S–7S.

Roberfroid, M. B. 2005. *Inulin-Type Fructans: Functional Food Ingredients*. CRC Series in Modern Nutrition. Boca Raton, FL: CRC Press.

Rumessen, J. J., S. Bode, O. Hamberg, and E. Gudmand-Hoyer. 1990. Fructans of Jerusalem artichokes: Intestinal transport, absorption, fermentation, and influence on blood glucose, insulin, and C-peptide responses in healthy subjects. *Am J Clin Nutr* 52:675–81.

Russo, F., G. Riezzo, M. Chiloiro et al. 2010. Metabolic effects of a diet with inulin-enriched pasta in healthy young volunteers. *Curr Pharm Des* 16:825–31.

Samuel, B. S., A. Shaito, T. Motoike et al. 2008. Effects of the gut microbiota on host adiposity are modulated by the short-chain fatty-acid binding G protein-coupled receptor, Gpr41. *Proc Natl Acad Sci USA* 105:16767–72.

Sauer, J., K. K. Richter, and B. L. Pool-Zobel. 2007. Products formed during fermentation of the prebiotic inulin with human gut flora enhance expression of biotransformation genes in human primarycolon cells. *Br J Nutr* 97:928–37.

Scheppach, W. 1998. Butyrate and the epithelium of the large intestine. In *Proceedings of Profibre Conference. Functional Properties of Non-Digestible Carbohydrates*. 3–6 March, Lisbon, Portugal.

Scholtens, P. A., M. S. Alles, L. E. Willemsen et al. 2006. Dietary fructo-oligosaccharides in healthy adults do not negatively affect faecal cytotoxicity: A randomised, double-blind, placebo-controlled crossover trial. *Br J Nutr* 95:1143–9.

Shah, A. B., G. P. Jones, and T. Vasiljevic. 2010. Sucrose-free chocolate sweetened with *Stevia rebaudiana* extract and containing different bulking agents—Effects on physicochemical and sensory properties. *Int J Food Sci Technol* 45:1426–35.

Shoelson, S. E., L. Herrero, and A. Naaz. 2007. Obesity, inflammation, and insulin resistance. *Gastroenterology* 132:2169–80.

Shrayyef, M. Z., and J. Gerich. 2010. Normal glucose homeostasis. In *Principles of Diabetes Mellitus*, ed. L. Poretsky, 19–36. Berlin: Springer.

Sjostrom, C. D., M. Peltonen, H. Wedel, and L. Sjostrom. 2000. Differentiated long-term effects of intentional weight loss on diabetes and hypertension. *Hypertension* 36:20–5.

Snedeker, S. M., and A. G. Hay. 2012. Do interactions between gut ecology and environmental chemicals contribute to obesity and diabetes? *Environ Health Perspect* 120:332–9.

Tarini, J., and T. M. Wolever. 2010. The fermentable fibre inulin increases postprandial serum short-chain fatty acids and reduces free-fatty acids and ghrelin in healthy subjects. *Appl Physiol Nutr Metab* 35:9–16.

The InterAct Consortium. 2012. Long-term risk of incident type 2 diabetes and measures of overall and regional obesity: The EPIC-InterAct case-cohort study. *PLoS Med* 9:e1001230.

Triplitt, C. L. 2012. Examining the mechanisms of glucose regulation. *Am J Manag Care* 18:S4–10.

Turnbaugh, P. J., R. E. Ley, M. A. Mahowald et al. 2006. An obesity-associated gut microbiome with increased capacity for energy harvest. *Nature* 444:1027–31.

van de Wiele, T., N. Boon, S. Possemiers, H. Jacobs, and W. Verstraete. 2007. Inulin-type fructans of longer degree of polymerization exert more pronounced *in vitro* prebiotic effects. *J Appl Microbiol* 102:452–60.

van Dokkum, W., B. Wezendonk, T. S. Srikumar, and E. G. van den Heuvel. 1999. Effect of nondigestible oligosaccharides on large-bowel functions, blood lipid concentrations and glucose absorption in young healthy male subjects. *Eur J Clin Nutr* 53:1–7.

Van Loo, J., P. Coussement, L. de Leenheer, H. Hoebregs, and G. Smits. 1995. On the presence of inulin and oligofructose as natural ingredients in the western diet. *Crit Rev Food Sci Nutr* 35:525–52.

Verdich, C., A. Flint, J. P. Gutzwiller et al. 2001. A meta-analysis of the effect of glucagon-like peptide-1 (7–36) amide on ad libitum energy intake in humans. *J Clin Endocrinol Metab* 86:4382–9.

Wang, X., and G. R. Gibson. 1993. Effects of the *in vitro* fermentation of oligofructose and inulin by bacteria growing in the human large intestine. *J Appl Bacteriol* 75:373–80.

Wang, Y., E. B. Rimm, M. J. Stampfer, W. C. Willett, and F. B. Hu. 2005. Comparison of abdominal adiposity and overall obesity in predicting risk of type 2 diabetes among men. *Am J Clin Nutr* 81:555–63.

Weickert, M. O., and A. F. Pfeiffer. 2008. Metabolic effects of dietary fiber consumption and prevention of diabetes. *J Nutr* 138:439–42.

Wellen, K. E., and G. S. Hotamisligil. 2005. Inflammation, stress, and diabetes. *J Clin Invest* 115:1111–9.

WHO. 2011. Global status report on noncommunicable diseases 2010: Description of the global burden of NCDs, their risk factors and determinants. Chapter 1: Burden: Mortality, morbidity and risk factors. Geneva: World Health Organization.

Wolever, T. M., P. J. Spadafora, S. C. Cunnane, and P. B. Pencharz. 1995. Propionate inhibits incorporation of colonic [1,2–13C]acetate into plasma lipids in humans. *Am J Clin Nutr* 61:1241–7.

Wu, G. D., J. Chen, C. Hoffmann et al. 2011. Linking long-term dietary patterns with gut microbial enterotypes. *Science* 334:105–8.

Wu, X., C. Ma, L. Han et al. 2010. Molecular characterisation of the faecal microbiota in patients with type II diabetes. *Curr Microbiol* 61:69–78.

Xiong, Y., N. Miyamoto, K. Shibata et al. 2004. Short-chain fatty acids stimulate leptin production in adipocytes through the G protein-coupled receptor GPR41. *Proc Natl Acad Sci USA* 101:1045–50.

Yang, W., J. Lu, J. Weng et al. 2010. Prevalence of diabetes among men and women in China. *N Engl J Med* 362:1090–101.

Yap, W. K. W., S. Mohamed, H. J. Mohamed, D. Meyer, and A. Y. Manap. 2008. Changes in infants faecal characteristics and microbiota by inulin supplementation. *J Clin Biochem Nutr* 43:159–66.

Zhang, C., M. Zhang, S. Wang et al. 2010. Interactions between gut microbiota, host genetics and diet relevant to development of metabolic syndromes in mice. *ISME J* 4:232–41.

Zhang, H., J. K. DiBaise, A. Zuccolo et al. 2009. Human gut microbiota in obesity and after gastric bypass. *Proc Natl Acad Sci USA* 106:2365–70.

CHAPTER 12

Dietary Fibers in Gastroenterology
From Prevention to Recommendations to Patients

MARTINE CHAMP

Contents

12.1 Introduction 302
12.2 Recommendations for the General Population 302
12.3 Epidemiological and Other Clinical Studies: DF Consumption
     and Prevention of Gastroenterological Diseases 303
     12.3.1 DF and Colonic Function in Healthy Subjects 303
     12.3.2 DF and Prevention of Diverticular Disease 305
     12.3.3 DF and Prevention of Colorectal Cancer and
            Other Digestive Tract Cancers 305
12.4 Epidemiological and Other Clinical Studies: DF in Therapy
     of Gastroenterological Diseases 309
     12.4.1 DF and Constipation 309
     12.4.2 DF and Hemorrhoids Complications 310
     12.4.3 DF and Irritable Bowel Syndrome 311
     12.4.4 DF and Diverticular Disease 312
     12.4.5 Prebiotics and Acute Pancreatitis 313
     12.4.6 DF in Enteral Formula as Means to Normalize
            Bowel Function 314
12.5 Prebiotic OS in Human Milk and Formula: What Benefits
     for the Infant? 314
12.6 What Mechanisms May Explain the Impact of DF
     on Gastrointestinal Diseases Prevention and/or Treatment? 316
12.7 Conclusions 318
References 321

12.1 Introduction

Dietary fibers (DFs) have to be part of a balanced diet and most recommendations are to consume 25–30 g DF per day. This figure (which is pretty high and larger than what is consumed in most Western countries) is based on epidemiological studies that associate a lack of DF to an increased risk of colon cancer as well as several gastrointestinal diseases such as constipation or diverticulosis. The recommendation is often associated with more concrete advices such as "eat five portions of fruits and vegetable a day" and "eat more whole meal cereal products and grain legumes." These foods contain diverse types of DF that are soluble or insoluble, small or high degree of polymerization, and have different physicochemical properties and, consequently, diverse physiological impacts.

Insoluble fibers such as wheat bran (WB) appear as the most efficient on transit time, whereas soluble fibers, especially when viscous, are known to have metabolic effects. Fermentability and fermentation profiles are more and more considered, as this property is linked to a proliferation of the microbiota and the production of short-chain fatty acids (SCFAs), including butyric acid, which are important metabolites for the colonic health.

This chapter will first consider the recommendations for the general population then to patients not only on a quantitative but also on a qualitative point of view. The scientific and medical literature will be reviewed to examine the basis of the recommendations and/or possibly to reconsider some of them.

12.2 Recommendations for the General Population

Most countries recommend, to the general population, a consumption of 25 g or 25–30 g of total fiber per day. Nordic Nutrition Recommendations (NNRs) are that the intake of DF should be at least 25–35 g/day, that is, approximately 3 g/MJ (>25 g for women and >35 g for men) (Øverby et al. 2013). Other countries do not propose a precise level of DF consumption to be reached but recommend an increased consumption of vegetables, fruits, nuts, whole cereals, and grain legumes.

The recommendations for children also vary between the countries. The recommendations of Øverby et al. (2013) are 2–3 g/MJ for children from 1 to 17 years of age.

Finally, precise recommendations for infants (<1 an) are very rare and most national and international countries indicate that there are no functional criteria for DF in infants; human milk is often being considered not to contain any DF (Australia/New Zealand (NHMRC 2006)). Human milk contains nondigestible oligosaccharides (OS) at a concentration from 12 to 23 g/L (12–15 g/L in mature milk and 20–23 g/L in colostrum) (Petherick 2010). Assuming that a newborn will drink from 150 to 200 mL of formula or human milk per kilogram of his body weight (BW) per day, the intake of OS from human milk would be around 2.4 g/kg of BW (i.e., 11.8 g/day when BW = 5 kg); it would be 4 g/L (galacto-oligosaccharides:inulin (9:1)) or an average of 0.7 g OS per kilogram of BW if he/she is fed with a formula containing prebiotics. Except in lactose-intolerant infants, lactose is supposed to be digested as the activity of lactase is optimal in newborns.

12.3 Epidemiological and Other Clinical Studies: DF Consumption and Prevention of Gastroenterological Diseases

12.3.1 DF and Colonic Function in Healthy Subjects

The impact of different fibers and/or high-fiber diets on colonic functions has been explored in healthy subjects. Low-fiber intake seems to be partly responsible for gastrointestinal symptoms such as constipation (IoM 2005). Constipation occurs in 5–18% of adults in different countries (average 12.3%) with a greater percentage of women and the elderly who are affected (Wald et al. 2008). Odds ratios (ORs) for constipation among women and elderly were 2.43 (95% CI: 2.18–2.71) and 1.5 (95% CI: 1.25–1.73) vs. men and young subjects.

It was thought that certain insoluble fibers such as WB were the most efficient to increase fecal bulk. The most recent data tend to prove that the efficiency of fiber source is not related to the criteria of solubility and fiber sources such as psyllium would be at least as efficient and may be more efficient than WB.

The meta-analysis published by Müller-Lissner, in 1988, mentioned nine papers reporting on the effect of WB on large bowel function. Bran increased the stool weight and decreased the transit time in each study in the healthy controls (Figure 12.1).

While considering the efficiency of insoluble fiber on transit time and stool weight, particle size seems to be a determinant factor. Indeed, for instance, WB with high particle size appears to be more efficient than WB with low particle size (Brodribb and Groves 1978, Heller et al. 1980, Wrick et al. 1983). However, more recently, Jenkins et al. (1999) observed that very fine particle size WB was an effective fecal bulking agent that might be explained by its fermentative pattern: substantial butyrate production as shown by butyrate concentration in stools.

Jenkins et al. (2000) described an increase of mean fecal outputs in healthy subjects with cocoa-bran cereals (25.0 g/d of total dietary fiber [TDF]) as compared to low-fiber cereals (5.6 g/d of TDF). A novel source of wheat fiber (product of the amylolytic digestion of milled wheat kernel) ingested as wheat flakes or a WB supplement (21 g TDF/d), compared to a negative control supplement providing 1.7 g TDF/d, had similar effects on fecal bulking (239.5 ± 19, 216.7 ± 19, and 165.6 ± 16 g/d, respectively) (Vuksan et al. 1999).

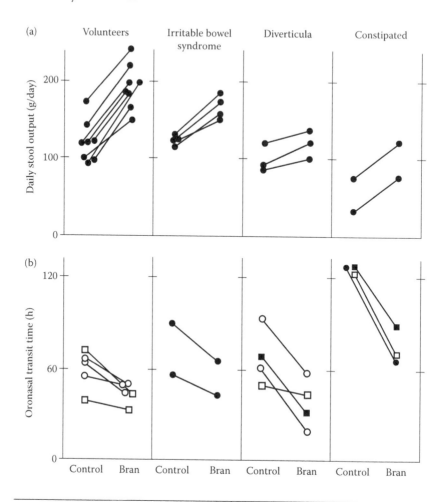

FIGURE 12.1 (a) Daily stool output in volunteers and patients with and without (controls) bran supplement. Each pair of dots represents the means from one of the analyzed papers. (b) Oro-anal transit times output in volunteers and patients with and without (controls) bran supplement. Each pair of dots represents the means from one of the analyzed papers. (From Müller-Lissner, S. A. 1988. Effect of wheat bran on weight of stool and gastrointestinal transit time: A meta analysis. *Brit Med J* (*Clin Res Ed*) 296:615–7. With permission.)

Resistant starches (RS2 and RS3) have also been shown to increase fecal bulk but are less efficient than WB; fecal bulks were respectively 22 ± 8 and 96 ± 14 g/d for RSs (mean for both RSs) and WB, respectively (30 g TDF of each fiber source) (Jenkins et al. 1998).

Jenkins et al. (2001) have observed that, compared to starch-based cereals and legumes (early agricultural diet) and low-fat (contemporary therapeutic diet for CVD) diets, a high-fiber vegetable (vegetable, fruit, and nut) diet (55 g TDF/1000 kcal) resulted in the greatest fecal bulk (906 ± 130 g/d, $P < 0.001$)

and also the greatest fecal bile acid output (1.13 ± 0.30 g/d, $P = 0.002$), and fecal SCFA outputs (78 ± 13 mmol/d, $P < 0.001$).

More recently, the same group (Vuksan et al. 2008) compared different fiber sources presented as breakfast cereals (2.5 servings/d) to healthy subjects. They received 25.0–28.7 g fiber/d as all-bran (AB), bran buds with corn (BBC), bran buds with psyllium (BBP), BBC, and viscous fiber blend (VFB), for 5 weeks. All the cereals under study induced significant ($P < 0.05$) increases in fecal bulk compared to the control diet, decreases in transit time, and increases in bowel movement frequency ($P < 0.05$). BBP was more effective than other fiber-containing cereals in terms of increasing fecal wet weight ($P < 0.05$) (247 ± 87 g/d), whereas AB was the less efficient (128 ± 38 g/d). Sources of water-insoluble fibers (AB and BBC) and their mixture with soluble fibers (BBP and VFB) had a good level of tolerance.

12.3.2 DF and Prevention of Diverticular Disease

The consumption of DF is commonly recommended for the prevention of diverticular disease (i.e., World Gastroenterology Organization 2007, European Association for Endoscopic Surgery (Köhler et al. 1999)); however, there are very few studies demonstrating the beneficial effects of high consumption of fiber. Among these, the prospective study of British vegetarians within European Prospective Investigation into Cancer and Nutrition (EPIC) (Crowe et al. 2011) showed that a risk of admission to the hospital or death from diverticular disease was 40% lower among patients with a high (>25 g/day) as compared with a low (<14 g/day) intake of DF after taking into account factors such as smoking and body mass index. However, the authors mentioned several reasons for caution. Among these, residual confounding or confounding by unmeasured variables might partially explain the results, although given the risk reductions of 40%, any effect of confounding would have to be substantial.

In a recent review, Tarleton and DiBaise (2011) mainly examined the evidence-supporting eviction of DF in the diet or recommendation of fiber-containing diet. They also reported the evidence that fiber intake may be beneficial in the prevention of diverticular disease.

12.3.3 DF and Prevention of Colorectal Cancer and Other Digestive Tract Cancers

A first meta-analysis was based on 16 of the 23 case-control studies published before 1990 (Trock et al. 1990). The authors concluded that the majority of studies gave support for a protective effect associated with fiber-rich diets. An estimated combined OR of 0.57 (95% CI: 0.50–0.64) was obtained when the highest and lowest quantiles of intake were compared. Risk estimates based on vegetable consumption (OR = 0.48) were only slightly more convincing than those based on an estimated fiber intake (OR = 0.58). However, the overall data were considered not to permit discrimination between effects due to fiber and nonfiber effects due to vegetables.

The Harvard pooled project also analyzed the original data for 13 prospective cohort studies (Park et al. 2005). More than 700 thousands of participants were followed up for 6–20 years with 8081 colorectal cases. A significant inverse association between fiber intake and risk of colorectal cancer was observed in the age-adjusted model while the association was no longer significant after adjusting for other risk factors.

The World Cancer Research Fund (WCRF) and the American Institute for Cancer Research (AICR) reported in 2007 that 16 cohort studies and 91 case-control studies investigated DF and *colorectal cancer*. An association was apparent from many, though not all, cohort studies. Ten of the studies showed decreased risk when comparing high and low intake groups but only one decreased risk was statistically significant (Bingham et al. 2003) (Figure 12.2a). Two studies reported nonsignificant increased risk (Giovannucci et al. 1994, Willett et al. 1990). Meta-analysis was considered as possible on eight studies, giving a summary effect estimate of a 0.90 (95% CI: 0.84–0.97) per 10 g fiber/day increment with moderate heterogeneity (Figure 12.2b).

In their report of 2007, the WCRF and the AICR considered the strength of evidence for "Foods containing dietary fibre" to decrease the risk of colorectal cancer to be "probable" whereas "non-starchy vegetable" and "fruits" would have "limited–suggestive" evidence and "cereals (grains)" would have "limited–no conclusion."

The report on the updated evidence for colorectal cancer was published by WCRF in 2010 and 2011. The evidence that food containing DF protect against colorectal cancer was upgraded from probable to convincing by the Expert Panel. The updated meta-analyses (per 10 g/d) showed a 10% decreased risk for colorectal cancer. These analyses included 15 studies compared with eight for the Second Expert Report and showed more consistent results. It is mentioned that both plant foods naturally containing DF and foods that have DF added have the potential to decrease the risk of colon cancer.

Another recent meta-analysis, investigating the association between the intake of DF and whole grains and the risk of colorectal cancer, has been published in 2011 (Aune et al. 2011). Twenty-five prospective studies were included in the analysis. The summary relative risk of developing colorectal cancer for 10 g daily of total DF (16 studies) was 0.90 (95% CI: 0.86–0.94, $I(2) = 0\%$) (Figure 12.3). It was 0.93 (0.82–1.05, $I(2) = 23\%$) for fruit fiber ($n = 9$), 0.98 (0.91–1.06, $I(2) = 0\%$) for vegetable fiber ($n = 9$), 0.62 (0.27–1.42, $I(2) = 58\%$) for legume fiber ($n = 4$), and 0.90 (0.83–0.97, $I(2) = 0\%$) for cereal fiber ($n = 8$). The summary relative risk for an increment of three servings daily of whole grains ($n = 6$) was 0.83 (0.78–0.89, $I(2) = 18\%$).

A recent study (Tantamango et al. 2011) on the protective effects of foods and food groups against colorectal polyps concluded to a protective association with higher frequency of cooked green vegetables (or 1 time/d vs. <5 times/wk = 0.76, 95% CI: 0.59–0.97) and dried fruits (OR 3+ times/wk vs. <1 time/wk = 0.76, 95% CI: 0.58–0.99). The consumption of legumes at least

(a) Dietary fiber and colorectal cancer:
cohort studies

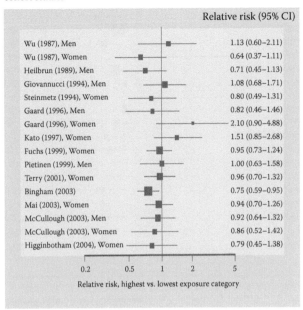

	Relative risk (95% CI)
Wu (1987), Men	1.13 (0.60–2.11)
Wu (1987), Women	0.64 (0.37–1.11)
Heilbrun (1989), Men	0.71 (0.45–1.13)
Giovannucci (1994), Men	1.08 (0.68–1.71)
Steinmetz (1994), Women	0.80 (0.49–1.31)
Gaard (1996), Men	0.82 (0.46–1.46)
Gaard (1996), Women	2.10 (0.90–4.88)
Kato (1997), Women	1.51 (0.85–2.68)
Fuchs (1999), Women	0.95 (0.73–1.24)
Pietinen (1999), Men	1.00 (0.63–1.58)
Terry (2001), Women	0.96 (0.70–1.32)
Bingham (2003)	0.75 (0.59–0.95)
Mai (2003), Women	0.94 (0.70–1.26)
McCullough (2003), Men	0.92 (0.64–1.32)
McCullough (2003), Women	0.86 (0.52–1.42)
Higginbotham (2004), Women	0.79 (0.45–1.38)

Relative risk, highest vs. lowest exposure category

(b) Dietary fiber and colorectal cancer:
cohort studies

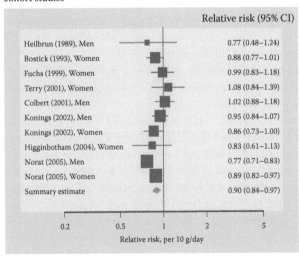

	Relative risk (95% CI)
Heilbrun (1989), Men	0.77 (0.48–1.24)
Bostick (1993), Women	0.88 (0.77–1.01)
Fuchs (1999), Women	0.99 (0.83–1.18)
Terry (2001), Women	1.08 (0.84–1.39)
Colbert (2001), Men	1.02 (0.88–1.18)
Konings (2002), Men	0.95 (0.84–1.07)
Konings (2002), Women	0.86 (0.73–1.00)
Higginbotham (2004), Women	0.83 (0.61–1.13)
Norat (2005), Men	0.77 (0.71–0.83)
Norat (2005), Women	0.89 (0.82–0.97)
Summary estimate	0.90 (0.84–0.97)

Relative risk, per 10 g/day

FIGURE 12.2 DF and colorectal cancer: cohort studies. (From WCRF (World Cancer Research Fund). 2011. *Colorectal Cancer.* http://www.wcrf.org/cancer_research/cup/key_findings/colorectal_cancer.php (accessed July 27th 2013).)

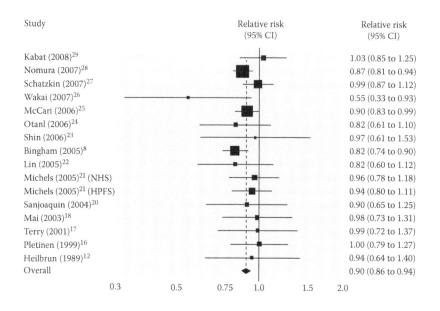

Study	Relative risk (95% CI)	Relative risk (95% CI)
Kabat (2008)[29]		1.03 (0.85 to 1.25)
Nomura (2007)[28]		0.87 (0.81 to 0.94)
Schatzkin (2007)[27]		0.99 (0.87 to 1.12)
Wakai (2007)[26]		0.55 (0.33 to 0.93)
McCari (2006)[25]		0.90 (0.83 to 0.99)
Otanl (2006)[24]		0.82 (0.61 to 1.10)
Shin (2006)[23]		0.97 (0.61 to 1.53)
Bingham (2005)[8]		0.82 (0.74 to 0.90)
Lin (2005)[22]		0.82 (0.60 to 1.12)
Michels (2005)[21] (NHS)		0.96 (0.78 to 1.18)
Michels (2005)[21] (HPFS)		0.94 (0.80 to 1.11)
Sanjoaquin (2004)[20]		0.90 (0.65 to 1.25)
Mai (2003)[18]		0.98 (0.73 to 1.31)
Terry (2001)[17]		0.99 (0.72 to 1.37)
Pletinen (1999)[16]		1.00 (0.79 to 1.27)
Heilbrun (1989)[12]		0.94 (0.64 to 1.40)
Overall		0.90 (0.86 to 0.94)

FIGURE 12.3 Summary relative risk of developing colorectal cancer for 10 g daily of total DF (16 studies). (From Aune, D., D. S. Chan, R. Lau et al. 2011. Dietary fibre, whole grains, and risk of colorectal cancer: Systematic review and dose-response meta-analysis of prospective studies. *Brit Med J* 343:d6617. With permission.)

3 times per week reduced the risk by 33% after adjusting for meat intake. Consumption of brown rice at least 1 time/wk reduced the risk by 40%. These associations showed a dose–response effect.

Zhang et al. (2013) recently published a meta-analysis on the impact of DF consumption and *gastric cancer risk*. They analyzed 21 articles that included 580,064 subjects. The summary ORs of gastric cancer for the highest (compared with the lowest) DF intake was 0.58 (95% CI: 0.49–0.67) with significant heterogeneity among studies ($P < 0.001$, I(2) = 62.2%). Dose–response analysis associated a 10 g/day increment in fiber with a significant (44%) reduction in gastric cancer risk. The authors concluded that DF intake is inversely associated with gastric cancer risk, the effect probably being independent of conventional risk factors.

Among studies investigating DF and *esophagus cancer*, one single cohort study has been published in 2002 (Kasum et al. 2002). It indicated a relative risk of 0.5 (without assessment of statistical significance) when high-fiber diets were compared to low-fiber diets. From nine case-control studies producing 13 independent effect estimates, 11 estimates were of decreased risk with eight being statistically significant. The most consistent data were observed for adenocarcinomas with five out of six reporting significantly decreased risk. There is no evidence of a plausible biological mechanism of an effect of DF on the esophagus and it cannot be excluded that the observed effects would be linked to components associated to fiber in fruits and vegetables.

12.4 Epidemiological and Other Clinical Studies: DF in Therapy of Gastroenterological Diseases

12.4.1 DF and Constipation

Constipation refers to bowel movements that are infrequent and hard to pass (Chatoor and Emmnauel 2009). Constipation is a symptom that may have multiple origins such as obstructed defecation and colonic slow transit and/or hypomotility. It can be caused or exacerbated by a low-fiber diet.

Functional constipation, known as chronic idiopathic constipation (CIC), is constipation that does not have a physical (anatomical) nor metabolic cause but may have a neurological, psychological, or psychosomatic cause. CIC is similar to constipation-predominant irritable bowel syndrome (IBS-C); however, people with CIC do not have other symptoms of IBS, such as abdominal pain. Patients with acute as well as chronic constipation are often told to increase DF intake.

Müller-Lissner (1988) performed a meta-analysis of studies reporting the effect of bran on large bowel function of patients with the IBS, with diverticula, and with chronic constipation (Figure 12.1). They concluded from these data that bran can be expected to be effective in restoring normal stool weight and transit time in patients who are constipated. However, these patients responded less well to bran treatment than healthy subjects.

Later on, Suares and Ford (2011) conducted a systematic review of the efficacy of soluble and insoluble fiber supplementation in the management of CIC. Six randomized controlled trials (RCTs) were eligible according to the criteria selected by the authors; four used soluble fibers and two used insoluble fibers. Formal meta-analysis was not undertaken due to the concern about methodological quality of identified studies. Compared with placebo, soluble fiber led to improvements in global symptoms (psyllium; 86.5% vs. 47.4%) (Fenn et al. 1986), straining (inulin vs. maltodextrin; 35.7% vs. 78.6%) (López Román et al. 2008), pain on defecation, and stool consistency, an increase in mean stool frequency per week (psyllium; 0.9 after therapy compared with 0.2 without therapy) (Ashraf et al. 1995). Evidence for any benefit of insoluble fiber was considered as less convincing. Adverse events data were limited, with no RCT reporting total numbers. The authors concluded that soluble fiber may be of benefit in CIC, but data for insoluble fiber are conflicting.

In 2012, the effect of DF intake on constipation was investigated by a new meta-analysis of five (out of 19) RCTs (Yang et al. 2012). Results showed either a trend or a significant difference in favor of the treatment group (bran (20 g, 12.5 g DF, in adults), glucomannan (100–200 mg/kg or 2.52 g, in children), cocoa husks (5.2 g, 52.3% fiber, in children)), and an increased number of stools per week in the treatment group as compared to the placebo group (OR = 1.19; 95% CI: 0.58–1.80, $P < 0.05$), with no significant heterogeneity among the studies (Figure 12.4). However, there was no significant difference

Study of subgroup	Experimental Mean	SD	Total	Control Mean	SD	Total	Weight	Mean difference IV, random, 95% CI	Mean difference IV, random, 95% CI
Badiali (1995)	6.4	3	24	5.1	2.7	24	14.3%	1.30 (−0.31, 2.91)	
Loening-Baucke (2004)	4.5	2.3	31	3.8	2.2	31	29.6%	0.70 (−0.42, 1.82)	
Castillejo (2006)	6.16	3.35	24	5.08	2.1	24	14.9%	1.08 (−0.50, 2.66)	
Chmielewska (2011)	6	3.7	36	4	3.15	36	14.8%	2.00 (0.41, 3.59)	
Staiano (2000)	4	1.3	10	2.7	1.4	10	26.5%	1.30 (0.12, 2.48)	
Total (95% CI)			125			125	100.0%	1.19 (0.58, 1.80)	

Heterogeneity: $\tau^2 = 0.00$; $\chi^2 = 1.80$, df = 4 ($P = 0.77$); $I^2 = 0\%$
Test for overall effect: $z = 3.83$ ($P = 0.0001$)

−10 −5 0 5 10
Favors experimental   Favors control

FIGURE 12.4 Meta-analysis of RCTs on the effect of DF on stool frequency. Pooled estimate of OR and 95% CI. (From Yang, J., H. P. L. Wang, and C. F. Xu. 2012. Effect of dietary fiber on constipation: A meta analysis. *World J Gastroenterol* 18:7378–83. With permission.)

in stool consistency, treatment success, laxative use, and painful defecation between the two groups.

12.4.2 DF and Hemorrhoids Complications

The impact of fibers as laxatives has been evaluated on a wide range of symptoms in patients with symptomatic hemorrhoids, through a systematic review and meta-analysis (Alonso-Coello et al. 2006). Seven trials randomized 378 patients to fiber or a nonfiber control. Studies were of moderate quality for most outcomes. Meta-analyses using random effects models suggested that fiber (i.e., ispaghula husk) has an apparent beneficial effect (Figure 12.5). The risk of not improving/persisting symptoms decreased by 47% in the fiber group (RR = 0.53, 95% CI: 0.38–0.73) and the risk of bleeding decreased

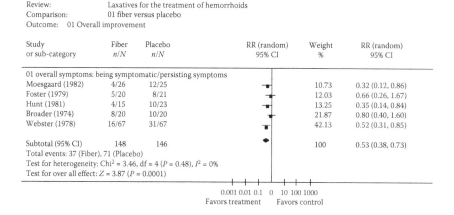

FIGURE 12.5 Meta-analysis of RCTs on the impact of DF for the treatment of hemorrhoid complications. Relative risk of being symptomatic/persisting symptoms for overall improvement. (From Alonso-Coello, P., E. Mills, D. Heels-Ansdell et al. 2006. Fiber for the treatment of hemorrhoids complications: A systematic review and meta-analysis. *Am J Gastroenterol* 101:181–8. With permission from Nature Publishing.)

by 50% (RR = 0.50, 95% CI: 0.28–0.89). Studies with multiple follow-ups, usually at 6 weeks and at 3 months, showed consistent results over time. Results are also compatible with large treatment effects in prolapse, pain, and itching, but even in the pooled analyses, confidence intervals were wide and compatible with no effect (RR = 0.79, 95% CI: 0.37–1.67; RR = 0.33, 95% CI: 0.07–1.65; and RR = 0.71, 95% CI: 0.24–2.10, respectively). One study suggested a decrease in recurrence. Results showed a nonsignificant trend toward increases in mild adverse events in the fiber group (RR = 6.0, 95% CI: 0.57–64.8). The authors concluded that trials with fiber as laxatives show a consistent beneficial for symptoms and bleeding in the treatment of symptomatic hemorrhoids.

12.4.3 DF and Irritable Bowel Syndrome

IBS is a chronic disease of cyclic nature characterized by recurrent symptoms (Evangelista 2012) (Table 12.1). The main symptoms, such as pain, bloating, and change in stool form, would be present in about 20% of the days (Hahn et al. 1998). The population prevalence is between 5% and 20% according to community surveys (Ford et al. 2008).

Traditional recommendations to patients with IBS were to increase their daily intake of DF, because of its potentially beneficial effects on intestinal transit time, in the case of both constipation and diarrhea (Harvey et al. 1973). Later on, the exclusion of fiber as well as unrefined carbohydrate and dairy products (for lactose) were the most common recommendations by physicians. However, in patients with constipation-dominant IBS, the traditional recommendation remained to adopt a high-fiber diet. However, WB therapy had to be kept when constipation was the major feature, due to the common increase of symptoms of abdominal pain and bloating (Gunn et al. 2003). The British Society of Gastroenterology guidelines for the management of IBS (Jones et al. 2000) proposed that patients with IBS and constipation must be given a trial

Table 12.1 Criteria for Diagnosis of IBS

Manning Criteria	Revised Rome II Criteria
1. Abdominal pain	Twelve weeks or more in the last 12 months of abdominal discomfort or pain that has two of the following three features:
2. Loose stools with onset of pain	
3. More frequent stools with onset of pain	1. Relieved by defecation
4. Abdominal distension	2. Associated with a change in frequency of stool
5. Passage of mucus in stools	3. Associated with a change in consistency of stool
6. Sensation of incomplete evacuation	

Source: Data from Gunn, M. C., A. A. Cavin, and J. C. Mansfield. 2003. Management of irritable bowel syndrome. *Postgrad Med J* 79:154–8.

of an increased intake of DF. When failing to respond to this first dietary recommendation or when intolerant to increased DF intake, a fiber supplement could be tried. In that case, ispaghula husk should be preferred to WB that may increase some of the symptoms. Most recent recommendations indicate that IBS patients should receive, as an initial therapeutic approach, a short course of treatment (i.e., antispamodics, 5HT-3 or four agonists, guanylate cyclase-C agonist, or prostaglandin E1 derivative). If effective, it has the additional value of confirming the diagnosis. Long-term treatment should then be reserved to diagnosed IBS patients with recurrent symptoms (Evangelista 2012).

A systematic review and meta-analysis of RCTs on the effects of fiber in the treatment of an irritable syndrome has been published in 2009 (Ford et al. 2008). Twelve studies compared fiber with placebo or no treatment in 591 patients with a relative risk of persistent symptoms of 0.87 (95% CI: 0.76–1.00). A positive effect was limited to ispaghula husks (six studies; RR: 0.78; 95% CI: 0.63–0.96) (doses: from 2 to 3 sachets per day or 30 g), whereas WB (five studies; 10–20 g/day) had no effect on the global symptoms of IBS or abdominal pain.

Qualitative changes of the microbiota have been associated with IBS without clear evolution of the microbial profile. However, it is suggested that quantitative changes in the colonic microbiota may lead to the proliferation and development of specific species that produce more SCFAs and gases (carbon dioxide, hydrogen, and methane), potentially resulting in abdominal bloating and distension. An increase in the concentration of SCFAs leads to acidification of the colon and deconjugation of bile salts. This in turn may cause significant changes in water and electrolyte transport in the colon that results in diarrhea. Malabsorption of carbohydrates may cause increased production of hydrogen, which is mainly associated with diarrhea-predominant IBS while excess methane production is associated with constipation-predominant IBS (Ghoshal et al. 2012). Targeting the gut microbiota using probiotics, antibiotics, or prebiotics has emerged as a potentially effective approach to the treatment (Ghoshal et al. 2012).

In 2011, Whelan reviewed the most recent and emerging evidence for the use of prebiotics (and probiotics) in the management of IBS. He came to the conclusion that there were no recent clinical trials of prebiotics in IBS, although the previous studies indicate the potential benefit at a low dose. More recently, Silk et al. (2009) concluded from a parallel crossover-controlled clinical trial of 12 weeks that galacto-oligosaccharide is effective in alleviating the symptoms of IBS when given at a low dose (3.5 g/d being apparently more efficient than 7 g/d for most symptoms).

12.4.4 DF and Diverticular Disease

Ünlü et al. (2012) recently published a review of high-fiber dietary therapy in diverticular disease. No studies concerning the prevention of recurrent diverticulitis, after a primary episode, with a high-fiber diet met the inclusion criteria of the authors. Three RCTs, considered by the authors of the review as moderate-quality studies, and one case-control study, were considered. One of the RCTs showed no difference in the primary endpoints (Brodribb 1977). A second RCT (Ornstein et al. 1981) and the case-control study (Leahy et al. 1985) found a significant difference in favor of a high-fiber diet in the treatment of symptomatic diverticular disease. The study of Ornstein and colleagues (1981) described improvement of the symptoms of constipation with the bran crisp bread and ispaghula husk, compared to the initial score. The third RCT (Hodgson 1977) found a significant difference in favor of methylcellulose (fiber supplement). This study also showed a placebo effect. The authors of the review concluded that high-quality evidence for a high-fiber diet in the treatment of diverticular disease is lacking. Most recommendations are based on inconsistent level-2 and mostly level-3 evidence. Nevertheless, a high-fiber diet is recommended in most guidelines as the hypothesis that a low-fiber diet that will prevent symptoms or complications of diverticular disease is still widely accepted (i.e., World Gastroenterology Organization 2007, European Association for Endoscopic Surgery (Köhler et al. 1999)).

12.4.5 Prebiotics and Acute Pancreatitis

There are apparently very few studies that consider the benefits of DF and/ or prebiotics on acute pancreatitis. Karakan et al. (2007) compared the beneficial effects of early enteral nutrition with prebiotic fiber supplementation (PFS) or without PFS (control) in patients with severe acute pancreatitis (15 patients per arm). The median duration of a hospital stay had been shorter in the PFS group 10 ± 4 (8–14) days vs. 15 ± 6 (7–26) days ($P < 0.05$); however, the median values of days in the intensive care unit (ICU) as well as the median duration of enteral nutrition were similar in both groups. The mean duration of APACHE II normalization (APACHE II score <8) was shorter in the PFS group than in the control group (4 ± 2 d vs. 6.5 ± 3 d, $P < 0.05$). Finally, the mean duration of C-reactive protein (CRP) normalization was also shorter in the PFS group than in the control group (7 ± 2 d vs. 10 ± 3 d, $P < 0.05$).

More recently, Plaudis et al. (2012) evaluated the benefits of prebiotic- or synbiotic-supplemented enteral formula to a standard, whole-protein feeding formula (control). Oral administration of synbiotic/prebiotic supplements was associated with a lower infection rate (pancreatic and peripancreatic necrosis) as compared to the control ($p = 0.03$, $p = 0.001$), lower rate of surgical interventions, $p = 0.005$, and shorter ICU ($p = 0.05$) and hospital stay ($p = 0.03$). Synbiotic but not prebiotic-supplemented enteral stimulation in the gut resulted in a reduced mortality rate compared to the control ($p = 0.02$).

If there are few studies examining the benefits of prebiotics in acute pancreatitis, more studies have been performed using pro- and synbiotics. Indeed, in 2010, Zhang and colleagues published a meta-analysis on the use of pre-, pro-, and synbiotics in patients with acute pancreatitis. Among the seven randomized studies (with 559 patients) that were included in the meta-analysis, 1, 3, and 4 were respectively evaluating pre-, pro-, and synbiotic as a supplement. On this single basis, synbiotics seems to be more efficient than prebiotics only on infectious morbidity but more studies of good quality would be necessary to conclude.

12.4.6 DF in Enteral Formula as Means to Normalize Bowel Function

A first meta-analysis on the application of DF in clinical enteral nutrition was published in 2005 by Yang and colleagues. The authors concluded, from seven RCTs with 400 patients included, that there was no evidence of a benefit of DF in the diarrhea of patients under enteral nutrition. Athough the length of hospital stay was shortened by the use of DF, there was no evidence available in preventing infection by DF.

In a more recent systematic review and meta-analysis on the effects of fiber supplementation of enteral feeds in healthy volunteers and patients from hospital and community settings, Elia and colleagues (2008) concluded to an important physiological effect and clinical benefits of the supplementation. Fifty-one studies (including 43 RCTs), enrolling 1762 subjects (1591 patients and 171 healthy volunteers) met the inclusion criteria of the authors. Fiber supplementation was usually well tolerated. In the hospital setting, the incidence of diarrhea was reduced as a result of fiber administration (OR 0.68, 95% CI: 0.48–0.96; 13 RCT) (Figure 12.6). Metaregression showed a more pronounced effect when the baseline incidence of diarrhea was high. In patients as well as in healthy subjects, fiber significantly reduced bowel frequency when the baseline frequency was high and increased it when it was low, confirming a significant moderating effect of fiber.

12.5 Prebiotic OS in Human Milk and Formula: What Benefits for the Infant?

OS (more than 115 different compounds) are present in the human milk. There is evidence suggesting that human milk oligosaccharides (HMOs) are absorbed unchanged by the small intestine of breast-fed infants but a fraction is excreted in the stools. It has been shown that only HMO that contains $Fuc(\alpha1–2)Gal(\beta1–4)$ GlcNac unit is able to inhibit the attachment of *Campylobacter jejuni* to colonic epithelial cells. These OS also appear to act as immune modulators within the systemic circulation. According to recent studies, the data suggest that type I HMOs (containing lacto-N-biose ([gal(b1-3)GlcNac]) structure) are utilized more predominantly than type II HMOs (containing N-acetyllactosamine ([gal(b1-4)GlcNac]) structure) by the colonic bacteria present in breast-fed infants. In addition, it has been found that the predominance of type I OS in milk and colostrum is a feature that is specific to humans, not found in other mammals, including other primates (Urashima et al. 2011).

Some of the infant milk contains prebiotics that are mostly OS not digested by the endogenous enzymes of the digestive tract. Prebiotics are defined as nondigestible food ingredients that beneficially affect the host by selectively

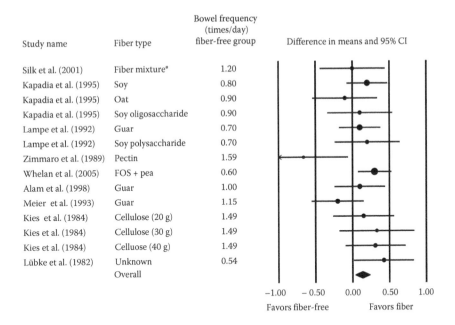

| | | Bowel frequency (times/day) | |
Study name	Fiber type	fiber-free group	Difference in means and 95% CI
Silk et al. (2001)	Fiber mixture*	1.20	
Kapadia et al. (1995)	Soy	0.80	
Kapadia et al. (1995)	Oat	0.90	
Kapadia et al. (1995)	Soy oligosaccharide	0.90	
Lampe et al. (1992)	Guar	0.70	
Lampe et al. (1992)	Soy polysaccharide	0.70	
Zimmaro et al. (1989)	Pectin	1.59	
Whelan et al. (2005)	FOS + pea	0.60	
Alam et al. (1998)	Guar	1.00	
Meier et al. (1993)	Guar	1.15	
Kies et al. (1984)	Cellulose (20 g)	1.49	
Kies et al. (1984)	Cellulose (30 g)	1.49	
Kies et al. (1984)	Celluose (40 g)	1.49	
Lübke et al. (1982)	Unknown	0.54	
	Overall		

−1.00   − 0.50   0.00   0.50   1.00

Favors fiber-free   Favors fiber

Figure 12.6 Meta-analysis (fixed effect model) of the incidence of diarrhea in tube-fed hospitalized patients participating in RCTs. OR <1.0 (favoring fiber) indicates that administration of a fiber-containing feed reduces the incidence of diarrhea. (Elia, M., M. B. Engfer, C. J. Green, and D. B. Silk. 2008. Systematic review and meta-analysis: The clinical and physiological effects of fibre-containing enteral formulae. *Aliment Pharmacol Ther* 2008. 27:120–45, Copyright Wiley-VCH Verlag GmbH & Co. KGaA. Reproduced with permission.)

stimulating the growth and/or activity of one or a limited number of bacterial species already resident in the colon, and thus attempt to improve host health. The intake of prebiotics can significantly modulate the colonic microbiota by increasing the number of specific bacteria and thus changing the composition of the microbiota (Gibson and Roberfroid 1995).

It is not clear from the literature which is the fraction of OS from human milk or galacto-oligosaccharides and inulin (90/10) from infant formula that is fermented or excreted in the stool of infants. On the one hand, it is likely that, at least, part of these OS are fermented by the infant microbiota as its profile is affected by the presence of this undigestible carbohydrate in the colon (Salvini et al. 2011, Veereman-Wauters et al. 2011, Holscher et al. 2012, Xia et al. 2012, Closa-Monasterolo et al. 2013). On the other hand, OS can be quantified in the feces from breast- and formula-fed babies. HMOS are mostly related to blood group characteristic OS (GalNAc-[fuc]-Gal-Glc and GalNAc-[fuc]-Gal-GlcNAc-Gal-Glc), at 2 months of age (Albrecht et al. 2010, 2011a,b). According to the same author (Albrecht et al. 2011b), galacto-oligosaccharides (GOS) supplemented to the formula was not recovered in baby feces, whereas HMOs as well as advanced degradation and bioconversion of HMOs were observed in the stools of breast-fed babies. However, GOS and fructo-oligosaccharides (FOS) were recovered in the feces of babies who received, during 28 days, a formula supplemented with a 0.8 g/dL GOS:FOS (9:1) (Moro et al. 2005).

As mentioned by S. Albrecht in her PhD thesis (2011) "so far, little is known about the implication of oligosaccharides structures on their gastrointestinal fate." However, several health-beneficial characteristics of breast milk are mainly connected to the complex HMO structures.

HMOs are proposed to be involved in the development of the immune system of infants (Klein et al. 2000, Bode et al. 2004, Newburg 2005). A double-blind randomized placebo controlled on 84 infants (41 infants receiving the prebiotic) from van Hoffen et al. (2009) showed that GOS/FOS supplementation induced a beneficial antibody profile in infants (6 months of age) at risk for allergies.

Direct pathogen inhibition and bifidogenicity of HMOs have been demonstrated recently. Indeed, HMOs can act as receptor analogs for preventing the adhesion of pathogenic bacteria to the mucosal surface. This ligand–receptor mechanism is based on the structural characteristics of HMOs, which are complementary to the structures of the carbohydrate epitopes in the mucosa (cited by Albrecht 2011). Enterogenic *Escherichia coli*, influenza A virus, campylobacter, and norovirus appear as microbes that would be inhibited by specific HMOs not present in all human milk (from Albrecht 2011). As an example, $(\alpha 1,2)$-fucosylated HMOs would be responsible of the inhibition of campylobacter, norovirus, and toxin-producing *E. coli in vitro* and a lower incidence of diarrhea in breast-fed babies (Newburg 2009, Albrecht 2011).

12.6 What Mechanisms May Explain the Impact of DF on Gastrointestinal Diseases Prevention and/or Treatment?

DF can be partly or totally fermented in the colon. When this fermentation is incomplete, DF can be excreted in the stools contributing to the fecal bulk. Before being fermented, insoluble fiber is able to directly interact with the digestive tract with impact on motility and transit time (Tomlin and Read 1988). When fermented, bacterial digestion and fermentation produces SCFAs (acetate, propionate, butyrate, and iso-acids), other organic acids (i.e., lactate), alcohols, and gases (carbon dioxide, hydrogen, and methane) (Cummings 1997). Several of these compounds are susceptible to take part in the physiological effect of DF in the colon and other segments of the digestive tract. Indeed, they can interact with

- Various exogenous and endogenous compounds and particles (including microbes) present in the colonic lumen;
- Digestive epithelium and also enteric nervous system and, when absorbed, with various organs.

Finally, when fermented, DF can influence microbiota composition.

Several hypotheses have been proposed to explain the protective role of DF on colon cancer (Cummings 1981, Jenkins et al. 2001):

- Fiber dilutes fecal contents, including potential carcinogenic compounds.
- Fiber decreases transit time, decreasing the time of contact of potential carcinogenic compounds with the colonic mucosa.
- Fiber increases stool weight, preventing constipation, probably, a risk factor for colon cancer. The increase of stool weight can be linked to:
  1. an excretion of DF residues (i.e., WB, sweet corn, or pulse husks);
  2. a high water-holding capacity of the fiber (i.e., ispaghula husk);
  3. an increased proliferation of bacteria.
- Fiber is fermented by the colonic microbiota producing SCFAs. Among these, butyrate has an important role as the preferred metabolic fuel and regulator of colonocyte proliferation, differentiation, and apoptosis. The production of butyrate is thus considered as a determinant factor to explain the protective effect of some DFs against colon cancer as shown mostly in animal models (rats or mice) (Le Leu et al. 2007).

Several of these mechanisms can also explain the beneficial effect of DF consumption on other gastrointestinal diseases (prevention and/or treatment).

DF can have a beneficial impact on gastrointestinal transit time and stool weight with a positive impact on constipation and some cases on diarrhea.

The following properties of DF might be involved:

- Particle size for insoluble fiber: Indeed, it has been shown by several authors that coarse WB is more efficient than finely ground bran (Wrick et al. 1983, Heller et al. 1980). Moreover, inert indigestible plastic particles can have a similar effect than WB (Tomlin and Read 1988).
- Water-holding capacity of the fiber matrix (Nakamura et al. 2001).
- Fermentability: On the one hand, a poor fermentability will favor the presence of undigested material in the stool and, on the other, a high fermentability will contribute to increase the biomass and thus the volume of the stools (Fischer et al. 2012).
- The production of SCFAs and mainly butyrate and also gases (Cherbut et al. 1998, Tazoe et al. 2008, Soret et al. 2010).

Among SCFA, butyrate regulates colonic mucosa homeostasis and can modulate excitability. This SCFA increased histone H3 acetylation in enteric neurons of rats, whereas effects of butyrate were prevented by inhibitors of the Src-signaling pathways (Soret et al. 2010). Butyrate also increased the cholinergic-mediated colonic circular muscle contractile response *ex vivo* (Soret et al. 2010). Among the DF, WB, RS, and soy fiber, most prebiotics have been shown to ferment with a high butyrate production, as compared to most DFs (Vitali et al. 2012, Damen et al. 2012 , Fung et al. 2012, Fredstrom et al. 1994, Titgemeyer et al. 1991, Walton et al. 2012).

Some OS, including some of the HMOs, have been shown to inhibit the adhesion of pathogenic bacteria and other microbes (Rhoades et al. 2008, Shoaf-Sweeney and Hutkins 2009, Coppa et al. 2006).

Indeed, a ligand–receptor mechanism based on the structural characteristics of OS (i.e., HMOs) that are complementary to the structures of the carbohydrate epitopes in the mucosa (Urashima et al. 2011).

For instance, pectic oligosaccharides (POS) have also been shown to inhibit the adhesion of verotoxigenic and enteropathogenic strains of *E. coli* to human intestinal epithelial cell cultures (HT29). Similar effect was observed on the adhesion of *Lactobacillus gasseri,* whereas the adhesion of *Lactobacillus acidophilus* was not significantly affected. POS also had a protective effect against *E. coli* verocytotoxins VT1 and VT2 at low concentrations (0.01 and 1 μgmL^{-1}, respectively) (Rhoades et al. 2008).

12.7 Conclusions

The role of DF in bowel function was considered, by EFSA (2010), the most suitable criterion for establishing an adequate intake (AI). On the basis of the available evidence on bowel function, EFSA considered a DF intake of 25 g/day to be adequate for normal laxation in adults. There is still limited evidence to set an AI for children. Consequently, EFSA considered that the AI for DF for children should be based on that for adults with appropriate adjustment for energy intake. A fiber intake of 2 g/MJ was considered adequate for normal laxation in children from the age of 1 year. Most recommendations also mention a diet rich in vegetable, fruits, whole cereals and legumes, and, sometimes, nuts.

There is no specific qualitative recommendation regarding the type of DF that should be preferred to prevent gastrointestinal disorders. From the literature (Table 12.2), it appears that a relative consensus on WB (coarse), psyllium, and a high-fiber diet (mixed fiber sources) as DF sources is able to prevent constipation and other diseases that are often partly associated with constipation (i.e., hemorrhoids and diverticulosis). Finally, the last WCRF report (2010) mentions that the scientific and clinical evidence that foods containing DF protect against colorectal cancer is now convincing (whereas it was only "probable" in the previous report of 2007).

Regarding the recommendation to patients with gastrointestinal diseases, conflicting results and thus recommendations are observed. However, WB and several other soluble or insoluble DFs seem to improve the symptoms linked to constipation in part of the patients. Several DF including soy polysaccharides, fiber mixes, and guar gum would be able to normalize bowel function in patients with enteral nutrition.

Table 12.2 Conclusions Regarding the Interest of DF Consumption for Prevention and Treatment of Main Gastroenterology Disorders

Dietary Fiber	Characteristics	Main Mechanisms	Degree of Evidence of the Benefit or Adverse Effect
Constipation			
Prevention			
WB (15–30 g)	Mostly insoluble fiber (coarse and finely ground)	Mechanical stimulation of the transit	++
Psyllium (25–30 g)	Mostly soluble fiber	Fermentation pattern (butyrate production)	+
High-fiber diet (25–35 g)	Various sources (fruits, vegetable, grain legumes, nuts, and whole cereals)	Mixed mechanisms	++
Treatment			
WB, glucomannan, and cocoa husks	Various characteristics	Mixed mechanisms	+
Enteral nutrition			
Normalization of bowel function			
Soy polysaccharides, multifiber mix, guar gum (hydrolyzed), and various other fibers	Various characteristics	Regulation of both small and large intestine transit time	++
Hemorrhoids			
Treatment (and avoidance of complications)			
Ispaghula husk	Mostly insoluble and high hydration capacity	Stools become softer	+
Irritable bowel syndrome			
Treatment of constipation-dominant IBS			
1. Trial of increased intake of DF (various sources)	Various characteristics	Mixed mechanisms	+
2. Trial with a fiber supplement (ispaghula husk) Avoid WB supplement	Mostly insoluble and high hydration capacity	Bulking effect	+

continued

Table 12.2 (continued) Conclusions Regarding the Interest of DF Consumption for Prevention and Treatment of Main Gastroenterology Disorders

Dietary Fiber	Characteristics	Main Mechanisms	Degree of Evidence of the Benefit or Adverse Effect
Prebiotic (galacto-oligosaccharides) (3.5 g/d)	Highly fermentable	Modification of the microbiota, production of butyrate	+
Diverticulosis			
Prevention			
High-fiber diet (>25 g)	Various sources (fruits, vegetable, grain legumes, nuts, and whole cereals)		+
Treatment			
Various DF (ispaghula, WB, and mixed fiber sources)	Various characteristics		+
Acute Pancreatitis			
Treatment			
Prebiotics	Highly fermentable—promotes specific microbiota	Decrease the level of infection	+
Colon Cancer			
Prevention			
High-fiber diet (>25 g)	Various sources (fruits, vegetable, grain legumes, nuts, and whole cereals)		+++
Gastric Cancer			
Prevention			
High-fiber diet (>25 g)	Various sources (fruits, vegetable, grain legumes, nuts, and whole cereals)		+

+++ Very high (convincing).
++ High (probable).
+ Poor (limited evidence).

IBS has multiple symptoms with predominant ones being constipation or diarrhea. Treatment of constipation-dominant IBS should include successive trials with: (1) increasing intake of DF-containing foods, avoiding during the first step presumably irritating DF such as WB and/or whole-meal flours and (2) if not successful in reducing the symptoms, a specific fiber supplement should be tried: DF with high hydration capacity might be the most efficient and/or a prebiotic (low doses to avoid gases accumulation in the colon) can be an appropriate alternative.

References

Albrecht, S. 2011. Gastrointestinal-active oligosaccharides from human milk in functional foods. Thesis, Wageningen University.

Albrecht, S., H. A. Schols, E. G. H. van den Heuvel, A. G. Voragen, and H. Gruppen. 2010. CE-LIF-MS n profiling of oligosaccharides in human milk and feces of breast-fed babies. *Electrophoresis* 31:1264–73.

Albrecht, S., H. A. Schols, E. G. van den Heuvel, A. G. Voragen, and H. Gruppen. 2011a. Occurrence of oligosaccharides in feces of breast-fed babies in their first six months of life and the corresponding breast milk. *Carbohydr Res* 346:2540–50.

Albrecht, S., H. A. Schols, D. van Zoeren et al. 2011b. Oligosaccharides in feces of breast- and formula-fed babies. *Carbohydr Res* 346:2173–81.

Alonso-Coello, P., E. Mills, D. Heels-Ansdell et al. 2006. Fiber for the treatment of hemorrhoids complications: A systematic review and meta-analysis. *Am J Gastroenterol* 101:181–8.

Ashraf, W., F. Park, J. Lof, and E. M. Quigley. 1995. Effects of psyllium therapy on stool characteristics, colon transit and anorectal function in chronic idiopathic constipation. *Aliment Pharmacol Ther* 9:639–47.

Aune, D., D. S. Chan, R. Lau et al. 2011. Dietary fibre, whole grains, and risk of colorectal cancer: Systematic review and dose-response meta-analysis of prospective studies. *Brit Med J* 343:d6617.

Bingham, S. A., N. E. Day, R. Luben et al. 2003. Dietary fibre in food and protection against colorectal cancer in the European Prospective Investigation into Cancer and Nutrition (EPIC): An observational study. *Lancet* 361:1496–501.

Bode, L., S. Rudloff, C. Kunz, S. Strobel, and N. Klein. 2004. Human milk oligosaccharides reduce platelet–neutrophil complex formation leading to a decrease in neutrophil beta 2 integrin expression. *J Leukoc Biol* 76:820–6.

Brodribb, A. J. 1977. Treatment of symptomatic diverticular disease with a high-fibre diet. *Lancet* 1:664–6.

Brodribb, A. J., and C. Groves. 1978. Effect of bran particle size on stool weight. *Gut* 19:60–3.

Chatoor, D., and A. Emmnauel. 2009. Constipation and evacuation disorders. *Best Pract Res Clin Gastroenterol* 23:517–30.

Cherbut, C., L. Ferrier, C. Roze et al. 1998. Short-chain fatty acids modify colonic motility through nerves and polypeptide YY release in the rat. *Am J Physiol* 275:G1415–22.

Closa-Monasterolo, R., M. Gispert-Llaurado, V. Luque, N. Ferre, C. Rubio-Torrents, M. Zaragoza-Jordana, and J. Escribano, 2013. Safety and efficacy of inulin and oligofructose supplementation in infant formula: Results from a randomized clinical trial. *Clin Nutr* 32:918–27.

Coppa, G. V., L. Zampini, T. Galeazzi et al. 2006. Human milk oligosaccharides inhibit the adhesion to Caco-2 cells of diarrheal pathogens: *Escherichia coli, Vibrio cholerae, and Salmonella fyris. Pediatr Res* 59:377–82.

Crowe, F. L., P. N. Appleby, N. E. Allen, and T. J. Key. 2011. Diet and risk of diverticular disease in Oxford cohort of European Prospective Investigation into Cancer and Nutrition (EPIC): Prospective study of British vegetarians and non-vegetarians. *BMJ* 343:d4131.

Cummings, J. H. 1981. Dietary fibre and large bowel cancer. *Proc Nutr Soc* 40:7–14.

Cummings, J. H. 1997. The large intestine in nutrition and disease. In: *Danone Chair Monograph*. Bruxelles, Belgium: Institut Danone.

Damen, B., L. Cloetens, W. F. Broekaert, et al. 2012. Consumption of breads containing in situ-produced arabinoxylan oligosaccharides alters gastrointestinal effects in healthy volunteers. *J Nutr* 142(3):470–7.

EFSA Panel on Dietetic Products, Nutrition, and Allergies (NDA). 2010. Scientific opinion on dietary reference values for carbohydrates and dieatry fibre. *EFSA J* 8:1462–538.

Elia, M., M. B. Engfer, C. J. Green, and D. B. Silk. 2008. Systematic review and meta-analysis: The clinical and physiological effects of fibre-containing enteral formulae. *Aliment Pharmacol Ther* 27:120–45.

Evangelista, S. 2012. Benefits from long-term treatment in irritable bowel syndrome. *Gastroenterol Res Pract* 2012:1–5.

Fenn, G. C., P. D. Wilkinson, C. E. Lee, and F. A. Akbar. 1986. A general practice study of the efficacy of Regulan in functional constipation. *Brit J Clin Pract* 40:192–7.

Fischer, M. M., A. M. Kessler, L. R. de Sá et al. 2012. Fiber fermentability effects on energy and macronutrient digestibility, fecal traits, postprandial metabolite responses, and colon histology of overweight cats. *J Anim Sci* 90:2233–45.

Ford, A. C., N. J. Talley, B. M. Spiegel et al. 2008. Effect of fibre, antispasmodics, and peppermint oil in the treatment of irritable bowel syndrome: Systematic review and meta-analysis. *BMJ* 337:a2313.

Fredstrom, S. B., J. W. Lampe, H. J. Jung, and J. L. Slavin. 1994. Apparent fiber digestibility and fecal short-chain fatty acid concentrations with ingestion of two types of dietary fiber. *JPEN J Parenter Enteral Nutr* 18:14–9.

Fung, K. Y., L. Cosgrove, T. Locket, R. Head, and D. L. Topping. 2012. A review of the potential mechanisms for the lowering of colorectal oncogenesis by butyrate. *Brit J Nutr* 108:820–31.

Ghoshal, U. C., R. Shukla, U. Ghoshal et al. 2012. The gut microbiota and irritable bowel syndrome: Friend or foe? *Int J Inflam* 2012:151085.

Gibson, G. R., and M. B. Roberfroid. 1995. Dietary modulation of the human colonic microbiota: Introducing the concept of prebiotics. *J Nutr* 125:1401–12.

Giovannucci, E., E. B. Rimm, M. J. Stampfer et al. 1994. Intake of fat, meat, and fiber in relation to risk of colon cancer in men. *Cancer Res* 54:2390–7.

Gunn, M. C., A. A. Cavin, and J. C. Mansfield. 2003. Management of irritable bowel syndrome. *Postgrad Med J* 79:154–8.

Hahn, B., M. Watson, S. Yan, D. Gunput, and J. Heuijerjans. 1998. Irritable bowel syndrome symptom patterns: Frequency, duration, and severity. *Dig Dis Sci* 43:2715–8.

Harvey, R. F., E. W. Pomare, and K. W. Heaton. 1973. Effects of increased dietary fibre on intestinal transit. *Lancet* 1:1278–80.

Heller, S. N., L. R. Hackler, J. M. Rivers et al. 1980. Dietary fiber: The effect of particle size of wheat bran on colonic function in young adult men. *Am J Clin Nutr* 33:1734–44.

Hodgson, W. J. 1977. The placebo effect. Is it important in diverticular disease? *Am J Gastroenterol* 67:157–62.

Holscher, H. D., K. L. Faust, L. A. Czerkies et al. 2012. Effects of prebiotic-containing infant formula on gastrointestinal tolerance and fecal microbiota in a randomized controlled trial. *JPEN J Parenter Enteral Nutr* 36:95–105S.

Institute of Medicine. 2005. *Dietary Reference Intakes for Energy, Carbohydrate, Fiber, Fat, Fatty Acids, Cholesterol, Protein, and Amino Acids.* Washington, DC: The National Academies Press.

Jenkins, D. J., C. W. Kendall, D. G. Popovich et al. 2001. Effect of a very-high-fiber vegetable, fruit, and nut diet on serum lipids and colonic function. *Metabolism* 50:494–503.

Jenkins, D. J., C. W. Kendall, V. Vuksan et al. 1999. The effect of wheat bran particle size on laxation and colonic fermentation. *J Am Coll Nutr* 18:339–45.

Jenkins, D. J., C. W. Kendall, V. Vuksan et al. 2000. Effect of cocoa bran on low-density lipoprotein oxidation and fecal bulking. *Arch Intern Med* 160:2374–9.

Jenkins, D. J., V. Vuksan, C. W. Kendall et al. 1998. Physiological effects of resistant starches on fecal bulk, short chain fatty acids, blood lipids and glycemic index. *J Am Coll Nutr* 17:609–16.

Jones, J., J. Boorman, P. Cann et al. 2000. British Society of Gastroenterology guidelines for the management of the irritable bowel syndrome. *Gut* 47:1–19.

Karakan, T., M. Ergun, I. Dogan et al. 2007. Comparison of early enteral nutrition in severe acute pancreatitis with prebiotic fiber supplementation versus standard enteral solution: A prospective randomized double-blind study. *World J Gastroenterol* 13:2733–7.

Kasum, C. M., D. R. Jacobs Jr., K. Nicodemus, and A. R. Folsom. 2002. Dietary risk factors for upper aerodigestive tract cancers. *Int J Cancer* 99:267–72.

Klein, N., A. Schwertmann, M. Peters, C. Kunz, and S. Strobel. 2000. Immunomodulatory effects of breast milk oligosaccharides. *Adv Exp Med Biol* 478:251–9.

Köhler, L., S. Sauerland, and E. Neugebauer. 1999. Diagnosis and treatment of diverticular disease: Results of a consensus development conference. The Scientific Committee of the European Association for Endoscopic Surgery. *Surg Endosc* 13:430–6.

Le Leu, R. K., I. L. Brown, Y. Hu, A. Esterman, and G. P. Young. 2007. Suppression of azoxymethane-induced colon cancer development in rats by dietary resistant starch. *Cancer Biol Ther* 6:1621–6.

Leahy, A. L., R. M. Ellis, D. S. Quill, and A. L. Peel. 1985. High fibre diet in symptomatic diverticular disease of the colon. *Ann R Coll Surg Engl* 67:173–4.

López Román, J., A. B. Martinez Gonzálvez, A. Luque et al. 2008. The effect of a fibre enriched dietary milk product in chronic primary idiopathic constipation. *Nutr Hosp* 23:12–9.

Moro, G. E., B. Stahl, S. Fanaro, J. Jelinek, G. Boehm, and G. V. Coppa. 2005. Dietary prebiotic oligosaccharides are detectable in the faeces of formula-fed infants. *Acta Paediatr Suppl* 94:27–30.

Müller-Lissner, S. A. 1988. Effect of wheat bran on weight of stool and gastrointestinal transit time: A meta analysis. *Brit Med J (Clin Res Ed)* 296:615–7.

Nakamura, T., K. Agata, M. Mizutani, and H. Lino. 2001. Effects of brewer's yeast cell wall on constipation and defecation in experimentally constipated rats. *Biosci Biotechnol Biochem* 65:774–80.

Newburg, D. S. 2005. Innate immunity and human milk. *J Nutr* 135:1308–12.

Newburg, D. S. 2009. Neonatal protection by an innate immune system of human milk consisting of oligosaccharides and glycans. *J Anim Sci* 87:26–34.

NHMRC (National Health and Medical Research Council). 2006. *Dietary Fibre*. http://www.nrv.gov.au/resources/_files/n35-dietaryfibre.pdf (accessed August 6th 2013).

Ornstein, M. H., E. R. Littlewood, I. M. Baird et al. 1981. Are fibre supplements really necessary in diverticular disease of the colon? A controlled clinical trial. *Brit Med J (Clin Res Ed)* 282:1353–6.

Øverby, N. C., E. Sonestedt, D. E. Laaksonen, and B. E. Birgisdottir. 2013. Dietary fiber and the glycemic index: A background paper for the Nordic Nutrition Recommendations 2012. *Food Nutr Res*. 57:20709.

Park, Y., D. J. Hunter, D. Spiegelman et al. 2005. Dietary fiber intake and risk of colorectal cancer: A pooled analysis of prospective cohort studies. *JAMA* 294:2849–57.

Petherick, A. 2010. Development: Mother's milk: A rich opportunity. *Nature* 468:S5–7.

Plaudis, H., G. Pupelis, K. Zeiza, and V. Boka. 2012. Early low volume oral synbiotic/prebiotic supplemented enteral stimulation of the gut in patients with severe acute pancreatitis: A prospective feasibility study. *Acta Chir Belg* 112:131–8.

Rhoades, J., K. Manderson, A. Wells et al. 2008. Oligosaccharide-mediated inhibition of the adhesion of pathogenic *Escherichia coli* strains to human gut epithelial cells *in vitro*. *J Food Prot* 71:2272–7.

Salvini, F., E. Riva, E. Salvatici et al. 2011. A specific prebiotic mixture added to starting infant formula has long-lasting bifidogenic effects. *J Nutr* 141:1335–9.

Shoaf-Sweeney, K. D., and R. W. Hutkins. 2009. Adherence, anti-adherence, and oligosaccharides preventing pathogens from sticking to the host. *Adv Food Nutr Res* 55:101–61.

Silk, D. B., A. Davis, J. Vulevic, G. Tzortzis, and G. R. Gibson. 2009. Clinical trial: The effects of a trans-galactooligosaccharide prebiotic on faecal microbiota and symptoms in irritable bowel syndrome. *Aliment Pharmacol Ther* 29:508–18.

Soret, R., J. Chevalier, P. de Coppet et al. 2010. Short-chain fatty acids regulate the enteric neurons and control gastrointestinal motility in rats. *Gastroenterology* 138:1772–82.

Suares, N. C., and A. C. Ford. 2011. Systematic review: The effects of fibre in the management of chronic idiopathic constipation. *Aliment Pharmacol Ther* 33:895–901.

Tantamango, Y. M., S. F. Knutsen, W. L. Beeson, G. Fraser, and J. Sabate. 2011. Foods and food groups associated with the incidence of colorectal polyps: The Adventist Health Study. *Nutr Cancer* 63:565–72.

Tarleton, S., and J. K. DiBaise. 2011. Low-residue diet in diverticular disease: Putting an end to a myth. *Nutr Clin Pract* 26(2):137–42.

Tazoe, H., Y. Otomo, I. Kaji, R. Tanaka, S. I. Karaki, and A. Kuwahara. 2008. Roles of short-chain fatty acids receptors, GPR41 and GPR43 on colonic functions. *J Physiol Pharmacol* 59:251–62.

Titgemeyer, E. C., L. D. Bourquin, G. C. Fahey Jr., and K. A. Garleb. 1991. Fermentability of various fiber sources by human fecal bacteria *in vitro*. *Am J Clin Nutr* 53:1418–24.

Tomlin, J., and N. W. Read. 1988. Laxative properties of indigestible plastic particles. *BMJ* 297:1175–6.

Trock, B., E. Lanza, and P. Greenwald. 1990. Dietary fiber, vegetables, and colon cancer: Critical review and meta-analyses of the epidemiologic evidence. *J Natl Cancer Inst* 82(8):650–61.

Ünlü, C., L. Daniels, B. C. Vrouenraet, and M. A. Boermeester. 2012. A systematic review of high-fibre dietary therapy in diverticular disease. *Int J Colorectal Dis* 27:419–27.

Urashima, T., K. Fukuda, M. Kitaoka, M. Ohnishi, T. Terabayashi, and A. Kobata. 2011. Milk oligosaccharides. In: *Nutrition and Diet Research Progress*. Ed. Nova Biomedical Books. New York: Nova Science Publishers.

van Hoffen, E., B. Ruiter, J. Faber, L. M'Rabet, E.F. Knol, B. Stahl, S. Arslanoglu, G. Moro, G. Boehm, J. Garssen, 2009. A specific mixture of short-chain galacto-oligosaccharides and long-chain fructo-oligosaccharides induces a beneficial immunoglobulin profile in infants at high risk for allergy. *Allergy* 64:484–7.

Veereman-Wauters, G., S. Staelens, H. Van de Broek et al. 2011. Physiological and bifidogenic effects of prebiotic supplements in infant formulae. *J Pediatr Gastroenterol Nutr* 52:763–71.

Vitali, B., M. Ndagijimana, S. Maccaferri et al. 2012. An *in vitro* evaluation of the effect of probiotics and prebiotics on the metabolic profile of human microbiota. *Anaerobe* 18:386–91.

Vuksan, V., A. L. Jenkins, D. J. Jenkins, A. L. Rogovik, J. L. Sievenpiper, and E. Jovanovski. 2008. Using cereal to increase dietary fiber intake to the recommended level and the effect of fiber on bowel function in healthy persons consuming North American diets. *Am J Clin Nutr* 88:1256–62.

Vuksan, V., D. J. Jenkins, E. Vidgen et al. 1999. A novel source of wheat fiber and protein: Effects on fecal bulk and serum lipids. *Am J Clin Nutr* 69:226–30.

Wald, A., C. Scarpignato, S. Mueller-Lissner et al. 2008. A multinational survey of prevalence and patterns of laxative use among adults with self-defined constipation. *Aliment Pharmacol Ther* 28:917–30.

Walton, G. E., E. G. van den Heuvel, M. H. Kosters, R. A. Rastall, K. M. Tuohy, and G. R. Gibson. 2012. A randomised crossover study investigating the effects of galacto-oligosaccharides on the faecal microbiota in men and women over 50 years of age. *Brit J Nutr* 107:1466–75.

WCRF (World Cancer Research Fund). 2011. *Colorectal Cancer*. http://www.wcrf.org/cancer_research/cup/key_findings/colorectal_cancer.php (accessed July 27th 2013).

WGO (World Gastroenterology Organization). 2007. http://www.worldgastroenterology.org/assets/downloads/en/pdf/guidelines/07_diverticular_disease.pdf (accessed July 15th 2013).

Whelan, K. 2011. Probiotics and prebiotics in the management of irritable bowel syndrome: A review of recent clinical trials and systematic reviews. *Curr Opin Clin Nutr Metab Care* 14:581–7.

Willett, W. C., M. J. Stampfer, G. A. Colditz, B. A. Rosner, and F. E. Speizer. 1990. Relation of meat, fat, and fiber intake to the risk of colon cancer in a prospective study among women. *N Engl J Med* 323:1664–72.

World Cancer Research Fund/American Institute for Cancer Research Food. 2007. *Nutrition, Physical Activity, and the Prevention of Cancer: A Global Perspective*. Washington, DC: American Institute for Cancer Research.

World Cancer Research Fund/American Institute for Cancer Research. 2010. WCRF/AICR systematic literature review—Continuous update project report. American Institute for Cancer Research.

Wrick, K. L., J. B. Robertson, P. J. Van Soest et al. 1983. The influence of dietary fiber source on human intestinal transit and stool output. *J Nutr* 113:1464–79.

Xia, Q., T. Williams, D. Hustead, P. Price, M. Morrison, and Z. Yu. 2012. Quantitative analysis of intestinal bacterial populations from term infants fed formula supplemented with fructo-oligosaccharides. *J Pediatr Gastroenterol Nutr* 55:314–20.

Yang, G., X. T. Wu, Y. Zhou, and Y. L. Wang. 2005. Application of dietary fiber in clinical enteral nutrition: A meta-analysis of randomized controlled trials. *World J Gastroenterol* 11:3935–8.

Yang, J., H. P. L. Wang, and C. F. Xu. 2012. Effect of dietary fiber on constipation: A meta analysis. *World J Gastroenterol* 18:7378–83.

Zhang, M. M., J. Q. Cheng, Y. R. Lu, Z. H. Yi, P. Yang, and X. T. Wu. 2010. Use of pre-, pro- and synbiotics in patients with acute pancreatitis: A meta-analysis. *World J Gastroenterol* 16:3970–8.

Zhang, Z., G. Xu, M. Ma, J. Yang, and X. Liu. 2013. Dietary fiber intake reduces risk for gastric cancer: A meta-analysis. *Gastroenterology* 145:113–20 e3.

CHAPTER **13**

Soluble Dietary Plant Nonstarch Polysaccharides May Improve Health by Inhibiting Adhesion, Invasion, and Translocation of Enteric Gut Pathogens

HANNAH L. SIMPSON and BARRY J. CAMPBELL

Contents

13.1 Introduction 328
13.2 Dietary Fiber 328
    13.2.1 Insoluble versus Soluble Fiber 329
    13.2.2 Dietary Fiber and Intestinal Health Benefits 329
13.3 Bacterial Adherence to the Intestinal Epithelium Is Mediated by Lectin (Adhesin)–Host Carbohydrate Interactions 331
    13.3.1 Bacterial Adhesins 331
    13.3.2 Bacterial Toxins with Lectin Activity 332
13.4 Use of Dietary Oligosaccharides to Block Bacterial Gut Infections 332
    13.4.1 Soluble Dietary Plant Nonstarch Polysaccharides Inhibit *E. coli*–Intestinal Epithelium Interactions 333
    13.4.2 Source and Composition of Plantain NSP 334
    13.4.3 Soluble Plantain NSP Blocks Adhesion and Translocation of Major Diarrheagenic Pathogens 336
13.5 Conclusions 339
Acknowledgments 341
Funding 341
Disclosures 342
References 342

13.1 Introduction

There is considerable evidence to suggest that dietary fiber is beneficial to man and that a high fiber intake promotes intestinal health. Mechanisms suggested have included accelerated transit time through the colon related to the bulking effects of fiber, the production of short-chain fatty acids (SCFAs) such as butyrate that act as a carbon and energy source for the colonic epithelium and the promotion of "probiotic" bacteria, such as Bifidobacteria. Although there is a growing interest in the beneficial effects of dietary components on the intestinal microbiota, this has focused largely on prebiotic effects that encourage the growth of "probiotic" bacteria. One potential beneficial effect of nondigested food components that has been largely overlooked is their ability to interfere with potentially harmful interactions between bacteria and the intestinal epithelium. Since adherence is often mediated by lectin–carbohydrate interactions, it is probable that bacterial–epithelial interactions in the intestine could be inhibited by nondigested food components that might include complex oligosaccharides. Bacterial adherence to epithelial cells can often be blocked by the presence of oligosaccharides or more complex glycans and glycoconjugates, such as milk oligosaccharides, mucins, or soluble plant polysaccharides. Our own recent studies have explored the possibility that soluble dietary plant nonstarch polysaccharide (NSP) preparations may improve health by inhibiting the adhesion, invasion, and translocation of pathogenic bacteria, something we have termed a "contrabiotic" effect. NSP from plantain bananas (*Musa* spp.) was particularly beneficial, potently inhibiting gut epithelial adhesion and translocation of intestinal pathogens (including *Escherichia coli* and *Salmonella* spp.), and at concentrations readily achievable *in vivo*. Our own studies have shown that soluble dietary fiber from other plant sources such as broccoli may also block bacteria–epithelial adherence, although other NSP preparations, including leek, oat, and apple, did not have this effect. This raises the possibility that dietary supplementation with specific soluble plant NSP preparations could be beneficial for the maintenance of intestinal health and the prevention of diarrheal episodes. These effects are likely relevant to man and to farm animals. Although different organisms and different receptors will often be relevant in different hosts, soluble plant fibers contain a wide range of oligosaccharide structures and might have the ability to inhibit a wide range of bacteria–epithelial interactions.

13.2 Dietary Fiber

Dietary fiber is defined as "the edible parts of plants or analogous carbohydrates that are resistant to digestion and absorption in the human small intestine with complete or partial fermentation in the large intestine" (AACC 2001). The primary source of dietary fiber is the plant cell wall, which forms a continuous extracellular matrix extending through the whole structure of the plant. Cellulose microfibrils form the basic structural framework into which diverse matrix polysaccharides are deposited, and are common to all classes of plant, ~30% of wall polymers. Key matrix components include NSPs, oligosaccharides, lignin (a cross-linked complex polymer of phenylpropane subunits), and associated plant substances (Asp 1987, Ha et al. 2000, Anderson et al. 2009). NSPs include cellulose, hemicelluloses, pectins, and arabinoxylans (Blackwood et al. 2000). The definition of dietary fiber was expanded in the mid-1970s by Trowel and colleagues to include nondigestible polysaccharides, such as mucilages and gums (Anderson et al. 2009). Although these nondigestible polysaccharides have been found to have physiological actions attributed to dietary fiber, their origins within the cell wall remain elusive (Buttriss and Stokes 2008, DeVries 2003).

13.2.1 Insoluble versus Soluble Fiber

Dietary fiber can be subdivided into insoluble and soluble components, classified according to their chemical, physical, and functional properties (Lattimer and Haub 2010, Raninen et al. 2011). There is a fine interplay between these properties, in that even a slight variance in the chemical and physical properties of dietary fiber can influence its physiological effect. Insoluble fiber refers to cellulose, lignin, and some hemicelluloses (Lattimer and Haub 2010), which by definition are not soluble in aqueous medium. They have low viscosity and are only fermented to a very limited extent in the colon (Kaczmarczyk et al. 2012). Common food sources of insoluble fiber include cereal brans and fruits with edible skins and seeds. Soluble fiber, that is, water-soluble NSPs, include pectins—the acid polysaccharides present in soluble fiber, gums, and some hemicelluloses (Lattimer and Haub 2010), which are capable of forming gels with a high viscosity. NSPs pass relatively intact through the digestive processes encountered in the human stomach and small intestine. They are, however, subject to fermentation by the resident fecal microbiota within the colorectal lumen (Kaczmarczyk et al. 2012, Kumar et al. 2012). Different types of soluble fiber may be derived from common foods such as fruits, especially apples and citrus species such as oranges, vegetables, cereal oats, bran and barley, and legumes. Different food sources will contain varying amounts of polysaccharides, such as hemicelluloses or pectins, which also vary in response to factors such as cultivar, ripeness, and geographical origin.

13.2.2 Dietary Fiber and Intestinal Health Benefits

There is considerable evidence to suggest that a diet rich in fiber has health benefit for the gut. Intestinal health benefits can be divided into two categories of action, "nonfermentative" and "fermentative" (Rose et al. 2007). The former describes effects that are due to the "physical" properties of the fiber itself. For example, soluble fiber can rapidly form gels when combined with water, while insoluble fiber acts more like a sponge to absorb water (James et al. 2003). High dietary fiber intake supports increase in fecal bulking and viscosity (Anderson et al. 2009, Kaczmarczyk et al. 2012). The studies of Burkitt highlighted the low rates of bowel cancer and diverticular disease in Africans and proposed this might be due to a rapid colonic transit time related to the bulking effects of dietary fiber (Burkitt et al. 1972). A plausible mechanism is that dietary fiber, through binding/interaction with ingested carcinogens, may decrease the availability and contact time of these cancer-promoting agents with the gut epithelium (Rose et al. 2007, Lattimer and Haub 2010). Furthermore, a diet rich in dietary fiber may also bind excess primary bile salts, facilitating their excretion and limiting their conversion by the fecal microbiota into potential procarcinogenic secondary bile acids (Hull 2008).

Subsequent studies showing that not all fiber sources provided equivalent defense against colon cancer implied more complex protective mechanisms (Potter 1996). Dietary fiber components are partially or completely degraded by resident gut microbiota in the colon, resulting in their conversion to SCFAs, primarily acetate, propionate, and butyrate, that act as a carbon and energy source for the colonic epithelium (Buttriss and Stokes 2008, Hamer et al. 2008). High concentrations of SCFAs lower the colonic luminal pH, thereby inhibiting the growth of pathogenic organisms such as Enterobactericiae, which is particularly sensitive to a low pH (Buttriss and Stokes 2008, Scott et al. 2008). Furthermore, butyrate has been reported to have a protective effect against inflammation (Inan et al. 2000, Havenaar 2011, Vinolo et al. 2011) and carcinogenesis (Sengupta et al. 2006, Scott et al. 2008).

Several epidemiological studies support the case that dietary fiber may have a protective effect against the development of colorectal cancer (Howe et al. 1992, Cassidy et al. 1994, Kim 2000, Park et al. 2005, Aune et al. 2011). The European Prospective Investigation on Cancer (EPIC) study reported a 40% reduction in colorectal cancer risk between patients with the highest quintiles of fiber intake, 35 g/day, compared to those with the lowest quintile, 15 g/day (Bingham et al. 2003).

More recently, the NSP component of dietary fiber has also attracted considerable attention as it has been shown to convey intestinal health benefit, and decrease the risk of colorectal cancer through a "prebiotic" effect (Lim et al. 2005, Davis and Milner 2009,)—that is, an effect that is mediated by the promotion of commensal beneficial gut bacteria, such as Lactobacilli and Bifidobacteria (Macfarlane et al. 2006, Brownawell et al. 2012). Beneficial resident bacteria of the gut microbiota (and probiotic bacteria) have been shown to suppress the growth of pathogenic bacteria through the release of bacteriocins (Corr et al. 2007, Fukuda et al. 2011) and to block their translocation across the gut epithelium via the improvement of tight junctions between intestinal epithelial cells (Ulluwishewa et al. 2011), thereby promoting intestinal health. So far though, the beneficial effects of dietary components on the composition of intestinal gut microbiome have mainly focused on these potential prebiotic effects. One potential beneficial effect of nondigested food components that has been largely overlooked is their ability to interfere with the potentially harmful adhesion, invasion, and translocation of pathogenic interaction of bacteria to the intestinal epithelium, that is, a "contrabiotic" effect.

13.3 Bacterial Adherence to the Intestinal Epithelium Is Mediated by Lectin (Adhesin)–Host Carbohydrate Interactions

To effectively colonize a host animal, many bacterial pathogens have evolved a means for attachment or adhesion to host epithelial cells and tissues. Bacterial adhesion is of paramount importance in that it allows the targeting of a given bacterium to a specific surface, such as a particular epithelial surface in a mammalian host (Klemm et al. 2010), as well as enabling the bacteria to withstand the natural defenses of the host (Sharon 2006, Klemm et al. 2010). The adhesion of pathogenic bacteria to the gut epithelium prevents the removal of the bacteria by the flow of mucous secretions (Tiralongo and Moran 2010). The adhesion of pathogenic bacteria to host tissues represents an early but critical step in the pathogenesis of virtually all infections (Lehmann et al. 2006). In fact, attachment to the intestinal epithelium facilitates bacterial access to sources of nutrition, promotes the delivery of toxic agents into host tissues, and also allows bacterial translocation to occur (Sharon 2006).

13.3.1 Bacterial Adhesins

Bacterial surface components that mediate adherence are collectively known as adhesins, many of which can be single proteins located directly on the bacterial surface. Examples include autotransporter adhesins of *E. coli* such as TibA and AIDA. However, most bacterial adhesins are associated with more complex thread-like protein structures known as fimbriae or pili (Tiralongo and Moran 2010). Fimbriae are heteropolymers with lengths of approximately 1 μm, where the bulk of the "organelle" is composed of a structural protein that serves as a scaffold to support the presentation of the functional adhesin commonly located at the tip, for example, FimH on type 1 pili of Enterobacteriaceae (Jones et al. 1995). Adhesins display a lectin-like activity, in that they recognize and bind to complementary carbohydrates present on the surface of the host epithelial cells (Sharon 2006).

Well-documented examples exist whereby gut pathogen adherence to the intestinal epithelium is mediated by lectin–carbohydrate interactions. Thus far, all fimbrial adhesins characterized from the gastrointestinal pathogen *Salmonella enterica* exhibit lectin activity. Adhesins StdA and PefA bind to $\alpha(1\text{-}2)$fucosylated receptors and the Lewis X blood group antigen, respectively, while FimH is highly specific for glycoforms rich in mannose (Wagner and Hensel 2011). Enterotoxigenic *E. coli* (ETEC) K99 also demonstrates carbohydrate-binding specificity, and binds to surface glycolipids containing *N*-glycolylneuraminic acid (NeuGc) in the form of NeuGc($\alpha2\text{-}3$)Galβ4Glc

(Sharon 2006). *Helicobacter pylori* that colonizes the gastric epithelium also expresses a range of surface adhesins, all of which exhibit complex lectin activity (Aspholm et al. 2006). For example, *H. pylori* adhesin BabA binds to the carbohydrate moiety of the fucosylated Lewis b (Le[b]) ABO blood group antigen on the surface of gastric epithelial cells (Delahay and Rugge 2012) and sialic acid (*N*-acetylneuraminic acid; NeuAc)-binding adhesin SabA recognizes all sialylated glycan structures expressing terminal α2,3-linked NeuAc (Roche et al. 2004, Delahay and Rugge 2012).

13.3.2 Bacterial Toxins with Lectin Activity

Some gut pathogens also express enterotoxins that display lectin activity and interact with host epithelial cell surface receptors through the recognition of specific carbohydrate moieties. These toxins have the ability to catalytically modify macromolecules that are required for essential cellular functions, such as cytoskeleton assembly or signaling, essential to their pathogenesis during infection. Many enterotoxins, particularly those that belong to the AB_5 family, show a high specificity for sialylated glycoconjugates. In this family, the A(or α)-subunit constitutes the toxin catalytic domain, while the B(or β)-subunit is responsible for binding to the glycosylated receptor on the epithelial cell surface (Lehmann et al. 2006). One of the classic examples is cholera toxin, produced by *Vibrio cholera* with the B(or β)-subunit exhibiting specificity for the monosialoganglioside GM1 (Lencer et al. 1999). Diarrheagenic *Clostridium difficile* also releases toxins TcdA and TcdB, which are involved in the monoglucosylation of Rho-GTPases, resulting in the subsequent dysregulation of host colonocyte actin cytoskeleton and loosening of intracellular tight junctions (Just et al. 1995, Ananthakrishnan 2011). The close proximity of *C. difficile* to the host epithelium is almost certainly necessary to produce toxic effects (Borriello et al. 1988). The toxins exhibit lectin activity and the direct binding of *C. difficile* TcdA to structures containing the disaccharide Galβ1–4GlcNac has been described (Just and Gerhard 2004, Voth and Ballard 2005). Preventing these interactions should therefore be of therapeutic benefit (Kelly and Younson 2000) and great commercial interest. Antiadhesion strategies could provide the much-needed alternative to, or be used in combination with, conventional antibiotic approaches that kill pathogens but often result in antibiotic resistance due to an increased selective pressure (Pieters 2007).

13.4 Use of Dietary Oligosaccharides to Block Bacterial Gut Infections

Bacterial adherence to epithelial cells can often be blocked by the presence of monosaccharides and oligosaccharides typically present in dietary food sources (Ofek et al. 2002) or more complex mixtures, such as milk oligosaccharides (deAraujo and Giugliano 2000), mucins, or soluble plant NSP preparations (Martin et al. 2004). Oligosaccharides present in human milk have been known for some time to prevent certain bacterial infections. Human milk-derived fucosylated oligosaccharides have been shown to inhibit adherence of gut pathogens, such as *Campylobacter jejuni*, to intestinal epithelial cells *in vitro*, as well as *in vivo* (Newburg 2000, Ruiz-Palacios et al. 2003). Similarly, a fucosylated oligosaccharide fraction isolated from milk was effective in reducing mortality in mice infected with ETEC heat-stable enterotoxin (Newburg et al. 1990, Cleary et al. 1983). Other oligosaccharide preparations from human milk have also been shown to inhibit the adherence of diarrhea-causing diffusely adherent *E. coli* (DAEC) and enteroaggregative *E. coli* (EAEC) (deAraujo and Giugliano 2000). Moreover, high-molecular-weight mucus glycoproteins (mucins) present in human milk are also effective in inhibiting a range of enteric bacteria, examples including the blockade of S-fimbriated *E. coli* to buccal epithelial cells (Schroten et al. 1992), as well as the epithelial invasion of *Salmonella enterica* serovar Typhimurium *in vitro* (Liu et al. 2012).

Plant-derived cell wall constituents have been shown to possess antiadhesive activity against pathogenic bacteria (Potter and Steinmetz 1996). This includes pectins, acidic polysaccharides rich in alpha-D-galacturonic acid (GalA), abundant in the primary cell wall of all land plants except grasses and their allies (Dumville and Fry 2000, Caffall and Mohnen 2009). Pectic oligosaccharides have been shown to inhibit *C. jejuni*'s adhesion to and invasion of, intestinal epithelial cells (Ganan et al. 2010), and to block the action of *E. coli* Shiga toxin (Olano-Martin et al. 2003).

13.4.1 Soluble Dietary Plant Nonstarch Polysaccharides Inhibit E. coli– Intestinal Epithelium Interactions

During studies in our own laboratory where we were examining bacteria recruitment to an inflamed and cancerous intestine, via lectin (adhesin) interactions to aberrant epithelial glycosylation observed in these condition (Campbell et al. 2001), it seemed to us highly plausible that nondigested polysaccharides may have a beneficial impact on intestinal health by their ability to inhibit potentially harmful interactions between bacteria and the human intestinal epithelium. We therefore investigated a range of complex oligosaccharides and soluble plant NSP for their ability to block the attachment of adherent, invasive *E. coli*, which we had observed to be increased in abundance within the colonic mucosae of both Crohn's disease and colon cancer patients to intestinal epithelial cells *in vitro* (Martin et al. 2004). As part of this study, we showed particular potency for soluble NSP extracted from boiled plantain fruit (Martin et al. 2004) (see Figure 13.1).

We established that the likely portal of entry for Crohn's mucosa-associated *E. coli* was via interaction with Peyer's patches in the ileum and lymphoid follicles in the colon, where early lesions in Crohn's disease occur, entering via the specialized microfold (M) cells (Roberts et al. 2010, Chassaing et al. 2011). M-cells of the "dome" or follicle-associated epithelium (FAE) overlying

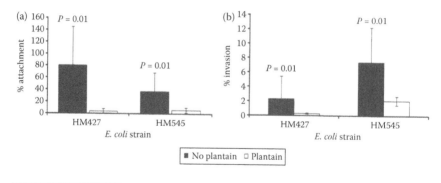

Figure 13.1 Inhibition of (a) attachment to and (b) invasion of I407 intestinal cells by two strains of *E. coli* (HM427 and HM545—colonic mucosa-associated isolates from patients with Crohn's disease and colon cancer, respectively) in the presence of soluble plantain fiber extracted by boiling 50 mg/mL starch-free fiber in water. $N = 4$; P values following analysis by Mann–Whitney U test. (From Martin, H. M., B. J. Campbell, C. A. Hart et al. 2004. Enhanced *Escherichia coli* adherence and invasion in Crohn's disease and colon cancer. *Gastroenterology* 127:80–93. With permission.)

Peyer's patches are the major antigenic sampling sites for microorganisms and the main portal of entry for various enteric gut pathogens, including *Salmonella* and *Shigella* (Sansonetti and Phalipon 1999). We found that soluble plantain fiber could block the translocation of a wide range Crohn's *E. coli* isolates across a validated *in vitro* M-cell model (Roberts et al. 2010). Furthermore, soluble dietary fibers from other plant sources, such as broccoli, were also shown to block bacterial–epithelial adherence. Other NSP preparations including leek, apple, and oat (data not shown) did not have this effect (Roberts et al. 2010) (see Figure 13.2).

13.4.2 Source and Composition of Plantain NSP

Plantain banana (*Musa* spp.) is traditionally cooked as a vegetable, and forms an important part of the staple diet in some parts of the world such as Africa, India, and Central America (Imam and Akter 2011), where the incidence of inflammatory bowel diseases and colorectal cancer is lower than that seen in the major developed nations. Our preferred source of soluble NSP has been from green plantain flour rather than that of ripe plantain fruits (see Table 13.1). The use of green plantain ensures that water-soluble components of the cell wall, in particular, pectins, have a wider range of structural characteristics and a higher molecular weight than would be obtained from ripe plantains (Shiga et al. 2011). The NSPs present are cell wall-derived, and occur naturally in both fresh plantains and processed plantain products (including plantain flour and plantain chips). The cell walls of edible plantain fruits are mainly primary walls in character (excepting fibrous elements associated with skin) and conform to the typical description of type I cell walls where neutral xyloglucans and acidic pectins dominate. The relative levels of acidic

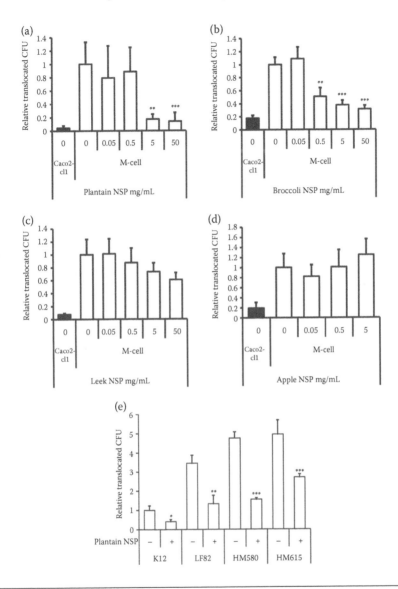

Figure 13.2 Plantain and broccoli nonstarch polysaccharides (NSP) block the translocation of *E. coli* across M-cells *in vitro*. (a) Crohn's disease mucosa-associated *E. coli* HM605 translocation through M-cells is inhibited by the presence of plantain NSP at 5 and 50 mg/mL ($N = 6$). (b) Broccoli NSP inhibits bacterial translocation across M-cells at 0.5, 5, and 50 mg/mL ($N = 3$). (c) Neither leek NSP nor (d) apple NSP inhibited HM605 translocation across M-cells (both $N = 2$, each at least $n = 5$ replicates). Translocation is measured as CFU expressed relative to M-cell translocation in the absence of fibers. (e) Plantain NSP (5 mg/mL) inhibits translocation across M-cells for a wide range of *E. coli* ($N = 3$). Translocation is measured as CFU expressed relative to M-cell translocation of *E. coli* K12. For all, $*P < 0.05$; $**P < 0.01$; $***P < 0.001$; ANOVA. (From Roberts, C. L., A. V. Keita, S. H. Duncan et al. 2010. Translocation of Crohn's disease *Escherichia coli* across M-cells: Contrasting effects of soluble plant fibres and emulsifiers. *Gut* 59:1331–9. With permission.)

Table 13.1 Some Characteristics of Green and Ripe Plantain Sourced from Ecuador[a]

| | | Starch Content | Free Sugar Content | NSP Content | | |
				Total	Soluble	Insoluble
Plantain	Green	40	3	18.8	6.1	12.7
	Ripe	26	18	15.3	4.4	10.9

Note: All values are shown as g/100 g fresh weight peeled fruit. Green is defined as ripeness stage 1, ripe is defined as ripeness stage 7.

[a] Flour produced from locally grown cultivars *Musa* AAB (Horn) var. Dominico.

and neutral polysaccharides present are dependent on cultivar and ripeness, and so it is essential that any bioactivity testing is performed on a reproducible soluble fiber source.

The yield of soluble nonstarch fiber from green plantain is 6–7% dry matter with a ratio of acidic to neutral polysaccharides of approximately 9:1. The preparation used in our studies is substantially free of low-molecular-weight sugars such as glucose and fructose, with the molecular weight distribution of the polysaccharides being between ~800 and ~5000 kDa. In soluble plantain NSP, the matrix polysaccharides are largely of a pectic nature (acidic), with smaller quantities of varied neutral polysaccharides also present (Englyst and Cummings 1986). Acidic polysaccharides comprise a group of pectin polysaccharides with associated arabinans and xylans. The neutral polysaccharides include arabinoxylans, xyloglucans, and mannose-containing polysaccharides, such as galacturonomannans and glucuronomannans. Monosaccharide composition analysis reflects the high quantities of pectin present and the high mannose content is a characteristic of plantain cell walls (Table 13.2).

13.4.3 Soluble Plantain NSP Blocks Adhesion and Translocation of Major Diarrheagenic Pathogens

Although different organisms and different receptors will often be relevant in different hosts, soluble plant fibers contain a wide range of oligosaccharide structures; we felt confident that these specific dietary constituents might have the ability to inhibit a wide range of gut pathogen–host epithelial

Table 13.2 Soluble Nonstarch Polysaccharide (NSP) Composition of Green Plantain (Ripeness Stage 1) Sourced from Ecuador

| Soluble NSP Composition (g/100 g NSP)[a] | | | | | | | |
UA	Glucose	Galactose	Rhamnose	Mannose	Fucose	Xylose	Arabinose
26.8	25.2	8.6	2.4	18.7	2.6	6.7	9.0

[a] Average values obtained from plantains grown over three consecutive seasons. UA, uronic acid.

interactions. We therefore conducted further studies to evaluate soluble plantain NSPs for their ability to inhibit the adherence of a number of different gut pathogens to the intestinal epithelium.

In this work, soluble plantain fiber inhibited the adhesion and invasion of *Salmonella* Typhimurium to intestinal epithelial cells, as well as inhibiting their translocation across M-cells *in vitro*. *S.* Typhimurium can colonize a large number of hosts and cause gastroenteritis and septicemia. Salmonellae first adhere to intestinal epithelial cells before invasion. The mechanism of adhesion is not fully understood but is dependent on the expression of adhesins, including FimH (Guo et al. 2007). Our data with inhibitory soluble fibers (see Figure 13.3) also suggest that lectin–carbohydrate interactions are an important mechanism of adhesion. After the initial contact and the adherence of *Salmonella* to the epithelial cells, the assembly of a type III secretory system (T3SS) is triggered. The T3SS-mediated entry of a number of bacterial effector proteins (e.g., SipC, SipA, SopE/2, SopB, and SptP) causes reorganization of the actin cytoskeleton and the formation of macropinosomes, which engulf the bacteria, allowing entry into the cell (Cossart and Sansonetti 2004). Although *Salmonella* can invade via several routes, including dendritic cells, invasive strains typically enter initially via M-cells, often leading to widespread damage to the FAE (Clark and Jepson 2003). Similarly, plantain NSP also inhibited the adhesion, invasion, and translocation of another common enteric Gram-negative pathogen *Shigella sonnei*, a bacterium that also utilizes a type III secretion system to inject invasion plasmid antigen (Ipa) protein into the invaded cell. Ipa BC protein complex affects the lysis of epithelial cell vacuoles and increases the uptake of *Sh. sonnei* by epithelial cells, including M-cells. As few as 100 bacteria are needed to cause a clinical infection (Niyogi 2005). Our *in vitro* studies demonstrate that soluble plant fibers exhibit inhibitory activity at concentrations ≥5 mg/mL (see Figure 13.3).

While *S.* Typhimurium and *Sh. sonnei* induce their infection via direct invasion of the intestinal epithelium, other diarrheal pathogens exert their pathogenic effect through the release of toxins. Bacteria that cause toxin-mediated diarrhea include *C. difficile*, a major cause of the reported cases of antibiotic-associated diarrhea, and ETEC, the most common cause of traveler's diarrhea. In 2007, there were 8324 death certificates that mentioned *C. difficile*, a 28% increase from 2006 (Office of National Statistics, UK 2008). ETEC strains possess key colonizing factors and harbor heat-labile (LT) and/or the heat-stable (ST) toxins that induce watery diarrhea (Fleckenstein et al. 2010). As per *C. difficile*, a close proximity of ETEC to the host epithelium is also necessary to produce toxic effects (Sears and Kaper 1996) and preventing these interactions should therefore be of therapeutic benefit. We found that soluble plantain NSP exhibits significant inhibitory activity against the interaction of both these diarrheal pathogens to intestinal epithelial cells *in vitro* (see Roberts et al. 2013). We have also reported preliminary data to show that other specific soluble fibers, such as leek and broccoli NSP, are also effective

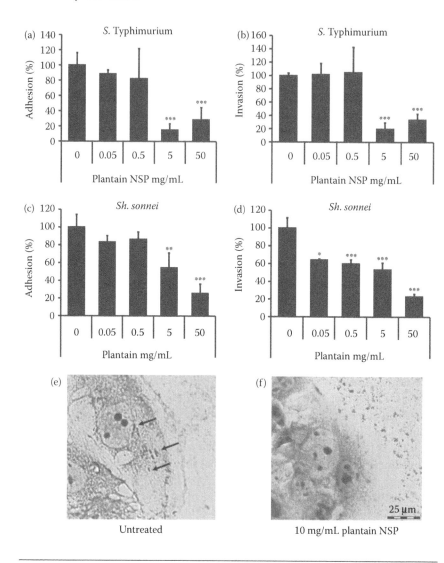

Figure 13.3 Soluble plantain fiber blocks the interaction of *Salmonella* Typhimurium and *Shigella sonnei* with intestinal epithelial cells *in vitro*. (a) Adhesion of and (b) invasion by *S.* Typhimurium LT2 to Caco$_2$ cells are inhibited in the presence of plantain NSP. (c) Adhesion of and (d) invasion by *Sh. sonnei* to confluent Caco$_2$ cell monolayers are inhibited in the presence of plantain NSP. Adhesion and invasion are both expressed relative to control adhesion in the absence of plantain NSP (set at 100%) ($N = 3$, with minimum $n = 3$ replicates for each treatment group; *$P < 0.05$; **$P < 0.01$; ***$P < 0.001$; ANOVA). (e) and (f) Giemsa staining of *Sh. sonnei* infected Caco$_2$ cells (70% confluence), in the (e) absence and (f) presence, of 30 min pretreatment with 10 mg/mL plantain NSP. Solid black arrows indicate intracellular *Sh. sonnei*. (From Roberts, C. L., A. V. Keita, B. N. Parsons et al. 2013. Soluble plantain fibre blocks adhesion and M-cell translocation of intestinal pathogens. *J Nutr Biochem* 24:97–103. With permission.)

in blocking *C. difficile* and ETEC (Simpson et al. 2012 abstract). It is worth noting though that not all adherent gut pathogens can be blocked by soluble plantain NSP. Adherence to Caco2 cells of enteropathogenic *E. coli* (EPEC), a major causative organism of neonatal gastroenteritis, was not inhibited by soluble plantain NSP at any concentration tested (Roberts et al. 2013). Key adhesins, α1-bundlin and intimin, mediating the adhesion of EPEC to intestinal cell lines, including Caco2, appear to be blocked specifically by *N*-acetyl-lactosamine (Hyland et al. 2008), suggesting that oligosaccharides bearing this glycoform are not present within soluble plantain fiber.

The inhibitory effect of soluble plantain fiber observed *in vitro* was also verified in *ex vivo* studies of human FAE and villus epithelium (VE) taken from the resected intestinal tissue of patients undergoing surgery, and mounted in Ussing chambers. Soluble plantain NSP significantly reduced bacterial translocation across isolated FAE and VE tissue of Crohn's mucosa-associated *E. coli* (Roberts et al. 2010) (see Figure 13.4) and *Salmonella enterica* serovar Typhimurium (Roberts et al. 2013). Moreover, we have recently reported soluble plantain NSP to be an effective supplement in poultry feed to reduce salmonellosis in the chicken (Parsons et al. 2012 abstract).

13.5 Conclusions

Our results suggest that there may be potential for soluble dietary fiber to be developed as a prophylaxis against intestinal pathogens causing antibiotic-associated diarrhea and traveler's diarrhea. Soluble plant fibers may also act as a fermentable substrate for bacteria in the large intestine. The modeling of soluble plantain NSP breakdown using mixed fecal microbiota obtained from healthy volunteers has shown that 25–75% of ingested plantain NSP is likely to avoid fermentation in the human colon (Backman 2009, Roberts 2010). Assuming the passage of 1 L of fluid daily into the cecum, we can estimate that readily achievable oral dosing of humans with 5 g soluble plantain NSP twice daily will achieve effective luminal concentrations of ~10 and 7.5 mg/mL in the cecum and rectum, respectively (Roberts et al. 2010). *E. coli*, *C. difficile*, and Salmonellae certainly interact with soluble plantain NSP and use this as an energy source (Roberts et al. 2010, 2013). Bacteroides are also major fermenters of plantain NSP, whereas species tested from key bacteria groups such as Bifidobacteria, Lactobacilli, Streptococci, and Ruminococci cannot easily ferment this soluble dietary fiber source (Backman 2009), suggesting little or no prebiotic effect for soluble plantain NSP.

Evidence supporting our own *in vitro* and *ex vivo* observations of plantain NSP includes a study using banana flakes supplemented to enteral feed to control diarrheal episodes (Emery et al. 1997), and another controlled trial in Bangladesh in which boiled green banana pulp or pectin was shown to be effective in countering persistent childhood diarrhea (Rabbani et al. 2001, 2004). Additional clinical studies also support the beneficial role of soluble

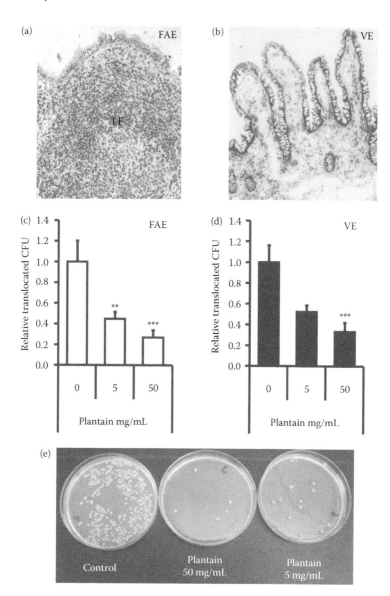

Figure 13.4 Plantain NSP blocks translocation of *E. coli* across the human intestinal epithelium in Ussing chambers. Histology of (a) human villus epithelium [VE] and of (b) an ileal lymphoid follicle [LF] and overlying follicle-associated epithelium [FAE] following Ussing chamber experiments. Magnification ×20. (c) and (d) EGFP-expressing Crohn's disease mucosa-associated *E. coli* HM615 translocation through both FAE ($N = 7$) and VE ($N = 9$) and is inhibited by the presence of plantain NSP. **$P < 0.01$; ***$P < 0.001$; ANOVA. (e) Overnight culture of Ussing chamber serosal medium following 2 h translocation of EGFP-expressing *E. coli* HM615 across isolated human epithelium, in the presence and absence of plantain NSP. (From Roberts, C. L., A. V. Keita, S. H. Duncan et al. 2010. Translocation of Crohn's disease *Escherichia coli* across M-cells: Contrasting effects of soluble plant fibres and emulsifiers. *Gut* 59:1331–9. With permission.)

fiber within the juice of boiled green banana or plantain, both reported to reduce the severity and duration of persistent diarrheas, including shigellosis (Alvarez-Acosta et al. 2009, Rabbani et al. 2009).

Overall, these studies convincingly suggest that soluble plantain fiber may confer a therapeutic benefit in both inflammatory and infective bowel disease patients by preventing bacterial invasion of the mucosa, that is, a "contrabiotic" effect. One could envisage that soluble fiber could easily be formulated with dairy products (e.g., milk, a milk shake, or yoghurt) or a fruit juice (e.g., orange juice or similar) to produce a palatable drink/beverage with the added benefit that it contains soluble fiber and therefore will be highly suitable as a refreshment for sufferers of diarrheal conditions. Such products may also be recommended to a subject in advance of antibiotic therapy in order that the soluble fiber may have a prophylactic effect. Investigation for the use of soluble plantain NSP preparation/supplementation is warranted in clinical trials: (1) as maintenance therapy to prevent relapse in inflammatory bowel disease (Crohn's disease); and (2) trials of the prophylactic use of plantain fiber (vs. placebo) in high-risk patients (e.g., elderly) receiving broad-spectrum antibiotics in antibiotic-associated (*C. difficile*) diarrhea. Such actions of plant NSP on maintaining gut health could be relevant/beneficial not only to man but also play a key role in the prevention of enteric infections in companion animals and in those farm animals that enter the food chain.

Acknowledgments

We thank Professor Jonathan Rhodes, University of Liverpool (Liverpool, UK), for critically reviewing the manuscript, and Dr. Niamh O'Kennedy, Provexis Plc (c/o Rowett Institute for Nutrition & Health, Aberdeen, UK) for the provision and biochemical characterization of the soluble NSP preparations used in our studies.

Funding

H.L.S. is currently supported by the Biotechnology and Biological Sciences Research Council (BBSRC) Industrial CASE award (BB/I016783/1) investigating the role of soluble dietary plant fiber (nonstarch polysaccharides) in the maintenance of intestinal health and the prevention of diarrheal disease. Research on soluble plant fiber was supported by awards from The Wellcome Trust (074949/Z/04/Z), BBSRC (BB/G01969X/1), The Bo and Vera Ax:son Johnsson Foundation, and Provexis plc. B.J.C. also acknowledges support of the European Science Foundation (ESF), in the framework of the Research Networking Programme, The European Network for Gastrointestinal Health Research.

Disclosures

The University of Liverpool with Provexis UK holds a patent for the use of soluble plantain fiber as maintenance therapy for Crohn's disease in addition to a patent pending for its use in antibiotic-associated diarrhea. B.J.C. has received a speaking honorarium from Amgen Inc.

References

Alvarez-Acosta, T., C. Leon, S. Acosta-Gonzalez et al. 2009. Beneficial role of green plantain [*Musa paradisiaca*] in the management of persistent diarrhea: A prospective randomized trial. *J Am Coll Nutr* 28:169–76.

Ananthakrishnan, A. N. 2011. *Clostridium difficile* infection: Epidemiology, risk factors and management. *Nat Rev Gastroenterol Hepatol* 8:17–26.

American Association of Cereal Chemists (AACC). 2001. *Cereal Foods World* 46:112–29.

Anderson, J. W., P. Baird, R. H. Davis et al. 2009. Health benefits of dietary fiber. *Nutr Rev* 67:188–205.

de Araujo, A. N. and L.G Giugliano. 2000. Human milk fractions inhibit the adherence of diffusely adherent *Escherichia coli* (DAEC) and enteroaggregative E-coli (EAEC) to HeLa cells. *FEMS Microbiol Lett* 184:91–4.

Asp, N. G. 1987. Dietary fibre—Definition, chemistry and analytical determination. *Mol Aspects Med* 9:17–29.

Aspholm, M., A. Kalia, S. Ruhl et al. 2006. *Helicobacter pylori* adhesion to carbohydrates. *Methods Enzymol* 417:293–339.

Aune, D., S. M. C. Doris, L. Rosa et al. 2011. Dietary fibre, whole grains, and risk of colorectal cancer: Systematic review and dose-response meta-analysis of prospective. *Brit Med J* 343:d6617.

Backman, R. V. 2009. The effects of plantain non-starch polysaccharide upon the gut bacteria. Doctoral thesis—University of Aberdeen, UK (EThOS/British Library Reference No. 521158).

Bingham, S. A., N. E. Day, R. Luben et al. 2003. Dietary fibre in food and protection against colorectal cancer in the European Prospective Investigation into Cancer and Nutrition (EPIC): An observational study. *Lancet* 361:1496–501.

Blackwood, A. D., J. Salter, P. W. Dettmar, and M. F. Chaplin. 2000. Dietary fibre, physicochemical properties and their relationship to health. *J R Soc Promo Health* 120:242–7.

Borriello, S. P., A. R. Welch, F. E. Barclay, and H. A. Davies. 1988. Mucosal association by *Clostridium difficile* in the hamster gastrointestinal tract. *J Med Microbiol* 25:191–6.

Brownawell, A. M., W. Caers, G. R. Gibson et al. 2012. Prebiotics and the health benefits of fiber: Current regulatory status, future research, and goals. *J Nutr* 142:962–74.

Burkitt, D. P., A. R. Walker, and N. S. Painter. 1972. Effect of dietary fibre on stools and the transit times, and its role in the causation of disease. *Lancet* 30:1408–12.

Buttriss, J. L. and C. S. Stokes. 2008. Dietary fibre and health: An overview. *Nutr Bull* 33:186–200.

Caffall, K. H. and D. Mohnen. 2009. The structure, function, and biosynthesis of plant cell wall pectic polysaccharides. *Carbohyd Res* 344:1879–900.

Campbell, B. J., L. G. Yu, and J. M. Rhodes. 2001. Altered glycosylation in inflammatory bowel disease: A possible role in cancer development. *Glycoconjugate J* 18:851–8.

Cassidy, A., S. A. Bingham, and J. H. Cummings. 1994. Starch intake and colorectal cancer risk: An international comparison. *Br J Cancer* 69:937–42.

Chassiang, B., N. Rolhion, A. de Vallée et al. 2011. Crohn's disease-associated adherent-invasive *Escherichia coli* target murine and human Peyer's patches via long polar fimbriae. *J Clin Invest* 121:966–75.

Clark, M. A. and M. A. Jepson. 2003. Intestinal M cells and their role in bacterial infection. *Int J Med Microbiol* 293:17–39.

Cleary, T. G., J. P. Chambers, and L. K. Pickering. 1983. Protection of suckling mice from the heat-stable enterotoxin of *Escherichia coli* by human milk. *J Infect Dis* 148:1114–9.

Corr, S. C., Y. Li, C. U. Riedel, P. W. O'Toole, C. Hill, and C. G. M. Gahan. 2007. Bacteriocin production as a mechanism for the antiinfective activity of *Lactobacillus salivarius* UCC118. *Proc Natl Acad Sci USA* 104:7617–21.

Cossart, P. and P. J. Sansonetti. 2004. Bacterial invasion: The paradigms of enteroinvasive pathogens. *Science* 304:242–8.

Darfeuille-Michaud, A., C. Neut, N. Barnich et al. 1998. Presence of adherent *Escherichia coli* strains in ileal mucosa of patients with Crohn's disease. *Gastroenterology* 115:1405–13.

Davis, C. D. and J. A. Milner. 2009. Gastrointestinal microflora, food components and colon cancer prevention. *J Nutr Biochem* 20:743–52.

Delahay, R. M. and M. Rugge. 2012. Pathogenesis of *Helicobacter pylori* infection, *Helicobacter* 17(Suppl 1):9–15.

Dumville, J. C. and S. C. Fry. 2000. Uronic acid-containing oligosaccharins: Their biosynthesis, degradation and signalling roles in non-diseased plant tissues. *Plant Physiol Biochem* 38:125–40.

DeVries, J. W. 2003. On defining dietary fibre. *Proc Nutr Soc* 62:37–43.

Emery, E. A., S. Ahmad, J. D. Koethe, A. Skipper, S. Perlmutter, and D. L. Paskin. 1997. Banana flakes control diarrhea in enterally fed patients. *Nutr Clin Pract* 12:72–5.

Englyst, H. N. and J. H. Cummings. 1986. Digestion of the carbohydrates of banana (*Musa paradisiaca sapientum*) in the human small intestine. *Am J Clin Nutr* 44:42–50.

Fleckenstein, J. M., P. R. Hardwidge, G. P. Munson, D. A. Rasko, H. Sommerfelt, and H. Steinsland. 2010. Molecular mechanisms of enterotoxigenic *Escherichia coli* infection. *Microbes Infect* 12:89–98.

Fukuda, S., H. Toh, K. Hase et al. 2011. Bifidobacteria can protect from enteropathogenic infection through production of acetate. *Nature* 469:543–7.

Ganan, M., M. Collins, R. Rastall et al. 2010. Inhibition by pectic oligosaccharides of the invasion of undifferentiated and differentiated Caco-2 cells by *Campylobacter jejuni*. *Int J Food Microbiol* 137:181–5.

Guo, A., M. A. Lasaro, J. C. Sirard, J. P. Kraehenbuhl, and D. M. Schifferli. 2007. Adhesin-dependent binding and uptake of *Salmonella enterica* serovar Typhimurium by dendritic cells. *Microbiology* 153:1059–69.

Ha, M. A., M. C. Jarvis, and J. I. Mann. 2000. A definition for dietary fibre. *Eur J Clin Nutr* 54:861–4.

Hamer, H. M., D. Jonkers, K. Venema, S. Vanhoutvin, F. J. Troost, and R. J. Brummer. 2008. Review article: The role of butyrate on colonic function. *Aliment Pharmacol Ther* 27:104–19.

Havenaar, R. 2011. Intestinal health functions of colonic microbial metabolites: A review. *Benef Microbes* 2:103–14.

Howe, G. R., E. Benito, R. Castelleto et al. 1992. Dietary intake of fiber and decreased risk of cancers of the colon and rectum: Evidence from the combined analysis of 13 case-control studies. *J Natl Cancer Inst* 84:1887–96.

Hull, M. A. 2008. Bile acids and colorectal cancer. In: *Bile Acids: Toxicology and Bioactivity*, eds. Jenkins, G. J. and L. J. Hardie, pp. 84–99. Cambridge: Royal Society of Chemistry Publishing.

Hyland, R. M., J. Sun, T. P. Griener et al. 2008. The bundlin pilin protein of entero-pathogenic *Escherichia coli* is an N-acetyllactosamine-specific lectin. *Cell Microbiol* 10:177–87.

Inan, M. S., R. J. Rasoulpour, L. Yin, A. K. Hubbard, D. W. Rosenberg, and C. Giardina. 2000. The luminal short-chain fatty acid butyrate modulates NF-kappaB activity in a human colonic epithelial cell line. *Gastroenterology* 118:724–34.

Imam, M. Z. and S. Akter. 2011. *Musa paradisiaca* L. and *Musa sapientum* L: A phytochemical and pharmacological review. *J Appl Pharmaceut Sci* 01(05):14–20.

James, S. L., J. G. Muir, S. L. Curtis, and P. R. Gibson. 2003. Dietary fibre: A roughage guide. *Intern Med J* 33:291–6.

Jones, C. H., J. S. Pinkner, R. Roth et al. 1995. FimH adhesin of type 1 pili is assembled into a fibrillar tip structure in the Enterobacteriaceae. *Proc Natl Acad Sci USA* 92:2081–5.

Just, I. and R. Gerhard. 2004. Large clostridial cytotoxins. *Rev Physiol Biochem Pharmacol* 152:23–47.

Just, I., M. Wilm, J. Selzer et al. 1995. The enterotoxin from *Clostridium difficile* (ToxA) monoglucosylates the Rho proteins. *J Biol Chem* 270:13932–6.

Kaczmarczyk, M. M., M. J. Miller, and G. G. Freund. 2012. The health benefits of dietary fiber: Beyond the usual suspects of type 2 diabetes mellitus, cardiovascular disease and colon cancer. *Metabolism* 61:1058–66.

Kelly, C. G. and J. S. Younson. 2000. Anti-adhesive strategies in the prevention of infectious disease at mucosal surfaces. *Expert Opin Investig Drugs* 9:1711–21.

Kim, Y. I. 2000. AGA technical review: Impact of dietary fiber on colon cancer occurrence. *Gastroenterology* 118:1235–57.

Klemm, P., R. M. Vejborg, and V. Hancock. 2010. Prevention of bacterial adhesion. *Appl Microbiol Biotechnol* 88:451–9.

Kumar, V., A. K. Sinha, H. P. Makkar, G. deBoaeck, and K. Becker. 2012. Roles of non-starch polysachharides in human nutrition: A review. *Crit Rev Food Sci Nutr* 52:899–935.

Lattimer, J. M. and M. D. Haub. 2010. Effects of dietary fiber and its components on metabolic health. *Nutrients* 2:1266–89.

Lehmann, F., E. Tiralongo, and J. Tiralongo. 2006. Sialic acid-specific lectins: Occurrence, specificity and function. *Cell Mol Life Sci* 63:1331–54.

Lencer, W. I., T. R. Hirst, and R. K. Holmes. 1999. Membrane traffic and the cellular uptake of cholera toxin. *BBA—Mol Cell Res* 1450:177–90.

Lim, C. C., L. R. Ferguson and G. W. Tannock. 2005. Dietary fibres as "prebiotics": Implications for colorectal cancer. *Mol Nutr Food Res* 49:609–19.

Liu, B., Z. Yu, C. Chen, D. E. Kling, and D. S. Newburg. 2012. Human milk Mucin 1 and Mucin 4 inhibit *Salmonella enterica* Serovar Typhimurium invasion of human intestinal epithelial cells in vitro. *J Nutr* 142:1504–9.

Macfarlane, S., G. T. Macfarlane, and J. H. Cummings. 2006. Review article: Prebiotics in the gastrointestinal tract. *Aliment Pharmacol Ther* 24:701–14.

Martin, H. M., B. J. Campbell, C. A. Hart et al. 2004. Enhanced *Escherichia coli* adherence and invasion in Crohn's disease and colon cancer. *Gastroenterology* 127:80–93.

Newburg, D. S. 2000. Oligosaccharides in human milk and bacterial colonization. *J Pediatr Gastroenterol Nutr* 30:S8–17.

Newburg, D. S., L. K. Pickering, R. H. McCluer, and T. G. Cleary. 1990. Fucosylated oligosaccharides of human milk protect suckling mice from heat-stabile enterotoxin of *Escherichia coli*. *J Infect Dis* 162:1075–80.

Niyogi, S. K. 2005. Shigellosis. *J Microbiol* 43:133–43.

Ofek, I., D. L. Hasty, and N. Sharon. 2002. Anti-adhesion therapy of bacterial diseases: Prospects and problems. *FEMS Immunol Med Microbiol* 38:181–91.

Office of National Statistics, UK. 2008. Deaths involving Clostridium difficile: by communal establishment, 2001 to 2007. http://www.ons.gov.uk/ons/rel/subnational-health2/deaths-involving-clostridium-difficile/communal-establishments–2001-to-2007/index.html (last accessed 31/01/2014).

Olano-Martin, E., M. R. Williams, G. R. Gibson, and R. A. Rastall. 2003. Pectins and pectic-oligosaccharides inhibit *Escherichia coli* O157: H7 Shiga toxin as directed towards the human colonic cell line HT29. *FEMS Microbiol Lett* 218:101–5.

Park, Y., D. J. Hunter, D. Spiegelman et al. 2005. Dietary fiber intake and risk of colorectal cancer: A pooled analysis of prospective cohort studies. *JAMA* 294:2849–57.

Parsons, B. N., P. Wigley, H. L. Simpson et al. 2014. Dietary supplementation with soluble plantain non-starch polysaccharides inhibits intestinal invasion of *Salmonella* Typhimurium in the chicken. *PLoS ONE* 9(2): e87658

Pieters, R. J. 2007. Intervention with bacterial adhesion by multivalent carbohydrates. *Med Res Rev* 27:796–816.

Potter, J. D. 1996. Nutrition and colorectal cancer. *Cancer Causes Control* 7:127–46.

Potter, J. D. and K. Steinmetz. 1996. Vegetables, fruit and phytoestrogens as preventive agents. *IARC Sci Publ* 139:61–90.

Rabbani, G. H., S. Ahmed, I. Hossain et al. 2009. Green banana reduces clinical severity of childhood shigellosis: A double-blind, randomized, controlled clinical trial. *Pediatr Infect Dis J* 28:420–5.

Rabbani, G. H., T. Teka, S. K. Saha et al. 2004. Green banana and pectin improve small intestinal permeability and reduce fluid loss in Bangladeshi children with persistent diarrhea. *Dig Dis Sci* 49:475–84.

Rabbani, G. H., T. Teka, B. Zaman, N. Majid, M. Khatun, and G. J. Fuchs. 2001. Clinical studies in persistent diarrhea: Dietary management with green banana or pectin in Bangladeshi children. *Gastroenterology* 121:554–60.

Raninen, K., J. Lappi, H. Mykkanen, and K. Poutanen. 2011. Dietary fiber type reflects physiological functionality: Comparison of grain fiber, inulin, and polydextrose. *Nutr Rev* 69:9–21.

Roberts, C. L., A. V. Keita, S. H. Duncan et al. 2010. Translocation of Crohn's disease *Escherichia coli* across M-cells: Contrasting effects of soluble plant fibres and emulsifiers. *Gut* 59:1331–9.

Roberts, C. L., A. V. Keita, B. N. Parsons et al. 2013. Soluble plantain fibre blocks adhesion and M-cell translocation of intestinal pathogens. *J Nutr Biochem* 24:97–103.

Roche, N., J. Angstrom, M. Hurtig, T. Larsson, T. Boren, and S. Teneberg. 2004. *Helicobacter pylori* and complex gangliosides. *Infect Immun* 72:1519–29.

Rose, D. J., M. T. DeMeo, A. Keshavarzian, and B. R. Hamaker. 2007. Influence of dietary fiber on inflammatory bowel disease and colon cancer: Importance of fermentation pattern. *Nutr Rev* 65:51–62.

Ruiz-Palacios, G. M., L. E. Cervantes, P. Ramos, B. Chavez-Munguia, and D. S. Newburg. 2003. *Campylobacter jejuni* binds intestinal H(O) antigen (Fuc alpha 1, 2Gal beta 1, 4GlcNAc), and fucosyloligosaccharides of human milk inhibit its binding and infection. *J Biol Chem* 278:14112–20.

Sansonetti, P. J. and A. Phalipon. 1999. M cells as ports of entry for enteroinvasive pathogens: Mechanisms of interaction, consequences for the disease process. *Semin Immunol* 11:193–203.

Schroten, H., F. G. Hanisch, R. Plogmann et al. 1992. Inhibition of adhesion of S-fimbriated *Escherichia coli* to buccal epithelial cells by human milk fat globule membrane components: A novel aspect of the protective function of mucins in the nonimmunoglobulin fraction. *Infect Immun* 60:2893–9.

Scott, K. P., S. H. Duncan, and H. J. Flint. 2008. Dietary fibre and the gut microbiota. *Nutr Bull* 33:201–11.

Sears, C. L. and J. B. Kaper. 1996. Enteric bacterial toxins: Mechanisms of action and linkage to intestinal secretion. *Microbiol Rev* 60:167–215.

Sengupta, S., J. G. Muir, and P. R. Gibson. 2006. Does butyrate protect from colorectal cancer? *J Gastroen Hepatol* 21:209–18.

Sharon, N. 2006. Carbohydrates as future anti-adhesion drugs for infectious diseases. *BBA Gen Subjects* 1760:527–37.

Shiga, T. M., C. A. Soares, J. R. Nascimento, E. Purgatto, F. M. Lajolo, and B. R. Cordenunsi. 2011. Ripening-associated changes in the amounts of starch and non-starch polysaccharides and their contributions to fruit softening in three banana cultivars. *J Sci Food Agric* 91:1511–6.

Simpson, H. L., C. L. Roberts, J. M. Rhodes, and B. J. Campbell. 2012. Soluble plant fibres, particularly leek and plantain, inhibit adherence of diarrhoea-associated pathogens *C difficile* and enterotoxigenic *Escherichia coli* to intestinal epithelial cells. *Gut* 61(Suppl. 2):A85 (abstract).

Tiralongo, J. and A. P. Moran. 2010. Bacterial lectin-like interactions in cell recognition and adhesion. In: *Microbial Glycobiology*, eds. H. Otto, J. B. Patrick and M. von Itzstein, pp. 549–65. San Diego: Academic Press.

Ulluwishewa, D., R. C. Anderson, W. C. McNabb, P. J. Moughan, J. M. Wells, and N. C. Roy. 2011. Regulation of tight junction permeability by intestinal bacteria and dietary components. *J Nutr* 141:769–76.

Vinolo, M. A., H. G. Rodrigues, R. T. Nachbar, and R. Curi. 2011. Regulation of inflammation by short chain fatty acids. *Nutrients* 3:858–76.

Voth, D. E. and J. D. Ballard. 2005. Clostridium difficile toxins: Mechanism of action and role in disease. *Clin Microbiol Rev* 18:247–63.

Wagner, C. and M. Hensel. 2011. Adhesive mechanisms of *Salmonella enterica*. In: *Bacterial Adhesion*, eds. D. Linke and A. Goldman, pp. 17–34. The Netherlands: Springer.

CHAPTER 14

Polysaccharide-Based Structures in Food Plants

Gut and Health Effects

JOHN A. MONRO

Contents

14.1 Introduction   347
14.2 Polysaccharide-Based Structures and Nutritional Properties
in the Foregut   350
    14.2.1 Effects of Structure on Enzyme Access to Substrates   350
14.3 Polysaccharide-Based Structures and Hindgut Function   358
    14.3.1 Fecal Bulking Effects   358
    14.3.2 Influence of Plant Tissue Structure on Fecal Parameters   358
14.4 Retaining Polysaccharide-Based Food Structures for Health:
Minimal Processing   360
14.5 Conclusion   362
14.6 Summary   363
References   363

14.1 Introduction

Carbohydrate is almost universally the major dietary source of metabolic energy. Nearly all of it is obtained from plants, and nearly all of it requires digesting before it is available for human metabolism. However, plants have developed a range of structures, nearly all based on the ability of polysaccharides to form multimolecular complexes, which obstruct digestion when the plant is consumed as food. These structures make an important contribution to the properties of dietary fiber that transcends the effects of isolated nondigestible polysaccharides. The elimination of the structural impediments to digestion that dietary fiber imposes so as to maximize the accessibility of starch to the digestive enzymes in the gut has been an important aim of food processing for thousands of years. But, it has also generated its own challenges for human health.

Overcoming polysaccharide-based food structures, to increase energy availability, has until recently been a matter of survival. But, nowadays, thanks to agricultural advances, and to modern food technologies, natural barriers to digestion have been lowered or removed to the extent that diets often contain a surfeit of highly digestible carbohydrate. In addition, refinement has led to a deficiency of the native structures, and of the nonstarch polysaccharides from which they were constructed, which formerly acted to modulate digestion in ways favorable to health as well as providing roughage that sustained large bowel function. As a result, diet-related scourges of the modern world—obesity, metabolic syndrome, diabetes, constipation, and colorectal cancer to name a few—are now reaching epidemic proportions (Buttris and Stokes 2008, Slattery et al. 2004, Zimmet et al. 2001). As polysaccharide-based plant structures in plant foods can have a critical role in determining the proportion of carbohydrate that is made available by food processing and digestion, it is of fundamental importance to dietary management in health and disease (Poutanen 2012).

Polysaccharide-based food structure exists in a wide range of forms and at a number of levels of organization or morphology (Table 14.1) (McDougall et al. 1996). At the molecular level, the polymeric nature of polysaccharides coupled with their multiple –OH groups gives them a capacity for extensive alignments linked by noncovalent bonds, making them well suited to form the fibers that are the structural basis of most food plants. In solution, their high degree of polymerization gives them a large hydrodynamic volume with the capacity to interact at relatively low concentrations (Dikeman and Fahey 2006). The –OH groups also confer a strong water-binding capacity. Some polysaccharides, such as pectins, also bear charged groups. The combined capacities to form between-chain linkages and to bind water confer on polysaccharides an ability to form an enormous range of structures, from pseudocrystals to fibers to colloids, gels, and viscous solutions, not only after extraction, but within the "free space" of cell wall structures (BeMiller 2007).

All such manifestations of polysaccharide structure—fibers, gels, viscous solutions, and hydrated cell walls—have important roles to play in the properties of dietary fibers that have an impact on health (Brownlee 2011). Furthermore, the health benefits of fiber are affected by the higher-level organizations of cell walls into plant tissues that have specific functional roles in the plant. For instance, the cellular structure of undigested plant tissue fragments, which were originally "designed" to protect starch in the seed, may

Table 14.1 Polysaccharide-Based Nondigestible Structures in Plants That Contribute to the Properties of Non-digested Food Residues as Dietary Fiber

Structural Entity	Function in Plant	Common Properties
a. Polysaccharides		
b. Polysaccharide aggregates		
Starch	Storage	Pseudocrystalline
Pectin	Support/hydration	Hydrated network
Hemicellulose	Support/hydration	Pseudocrystalline/amorphous matrix
Cellulose	Structure/support	Crystalline microfibrillar
c. Subcellular structures		
Starch granules	Storage	Densely packed pseudocrystalline with surface pores
Cell walls	Structure and adhesion	Digestion resistant, porous, and hydrated, depending on encrusting substances such as lignin
d. Cells		
Epidermis	Protection	Cellulosic and waxed
Parenchyma	Support/metabolism	Thin walled
Collenchyma	Support/protection	Thick-walled cellulose
Sclerenchyma/fibers	Support	Thick-walled cellulose, lignified
Xylem vessels	Support	Thick-walled cellulose and lignified cavities
e. Multicellular-tissues		
Epidermis/seed	Protection	Resistant, waxed, and coherent
coats	Protection	Coherent, thick walled, and cellulosic with protective agents such as polyphenolics
Endosperm (cereals)	Storage	Thin walled, hard, and dense until gelatinized
Cotyledon (pulses)	Storage/support	Thicker walls than the endosperm

play an important role in creating hydrated volume and mechanical stimulation. In the form of colonic roughage, they are essential to the functioning and protection against disorders of the large bowel. Wheat bran is the obvious example (Gelinas 2013).

This chapter discusses the various forms of polysaccharide-based plant structures that are consumed in food, the importance of them in determining carbohydrate digestibility and bowel function, their impact on human health, and how food-processing methods that alter them can be used to improve the nutritional properties of foods.

14.2 Polysaccharide-Based Structures and Nutritional Properties in the Foregut

14.2.1 Effects of Structure on Enzyme Access to Substrates

14.2.1.1 Starch The contribution of polysaccharide properties and polysaccharide-based structures to the nutritional attributes of foods, and to the beneficial properties of dietary fibers, can be seen very clearly in the impact that the plant storing starch as granules, and protecting it in seeds, has on digestion. Starch is the source of most food energy and is the plant polysaccharide, and is the only class of polysaccharide that is digestible by human enzymes. Nonetheless, the molecular structure of starch favors the formation of supramolecular structures that inhibit digestion. Starch solely consists of α-D-glucose units $\alpha(1-4)$ linked into long linear amylose chains, or into shorter amylose chains connected to the longer chains at $\alpha(1-6)$-linked branch points in the amylopectin form of starch. Most starch (~70%) is branched (amylopectin) and has a molecular weight of 50–500 million, and a degree of polymerization in millions, depending on the plant species (French 1984, James et al. 2003, Thomas and Atwell 1998). The long, regular strings of glucose units in both amylose and amylopectin allow H-bonded interactions between starch chains, resulting in pseudocrystalline regions that resist digestion by sterically hindering amylase access. Therefore, they may substantially contribute to dietary fiber loading of the colon, because any starch that is not digested in the time available for intestinal transit to the colon is, by definition, dietary fiber.

Above the molecular scale of amylose and amylopectin, native starch is packed by plants into compact granules that impose further restrictions on enzyme access (Ayoub et al. 2006, Gallant et al. 1997). Starch granules characteristically consist of concentric rings of alternating amorphous and pseudocrystalline structures laid down during granule growth (Figure 14.1). The amorphous regions are rich in branches at $\alpha(1-6)$ glycosidic bonds, while in the pseudocrystalline regions, the starch is highly organized as tightly packed short branches, approximately 10–20 glucose subunits in length (Gallant et al. 1997, Ratnayake and Jackson 2007, Waigh et al. 2000). The high degree of organization of the pseudocrystalline region is revealed by the Maltese cross birefringence pattern typical of native starch, and, because of their precise packing, the pseudocrystalline regions are far more resistant to digestion by α-amylase than the amorphous regions (Donald 2004). Furthermore, the highly organized starch granule as a whole may be relatively resistant to digestion, thanks to protein and lipid, together coating the granule surface to form a barrier resistant to water and digestive enzymes (Debet and Gidley 2006).

Although covered with a resistant coating, almost all types of starch granules bear surface pores that lead through channels to near the center (hilum) of the granule (Huber and BeMiller 2000). The pores may be well

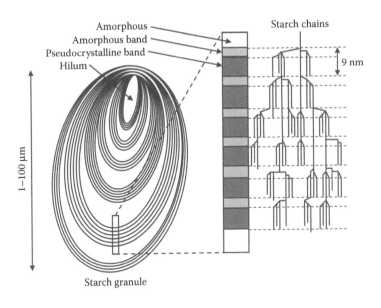

Amorphous
Amorphous band
Pseudocrystalline band
Hilum
Starch chains
9 nm
1–100 μm
Starch granule

Figure 14.1 The tightly organized arrangement of starch in starch granules allows dense storage of energy while making the raw starch granule resistant to digestion.

developed, as in maize, or nearly absent and much smaller, as in potato and tapioca (Juszczak et al. 2003). They may play an important role in digestion by allowing the penetration of water and enzymes into the center of the granules (Copeland et al. 2009). However, digestion remains relatively slow while the starch is in its well-organized natural (ungelatinized) state.

In some forms of raw starch, for instance, potato starch, digestion is so slow that a large proportion of the starch reaches the colon undigested. Therefore, by definition, it must be classified as dietary fiber (type 2 resistant starch). However, upon heat gelatinization, it is rapidly converted into the available carbohydrates (Figure 14.2).

14.2.1.2 Seeds At a higher organizational level than the starch granule, polysaccharide-based structures in the form of cell walls and tissues may determine the amount of potentially digestible starch that enters the colon as dietary fiber. Encapsulations by cell walls, by protective tissues, and by undigested starch gel on the surface of cell clusters maintained by cell wall adhesion, are all ways in which polysaccharide-based structures can act as a hindrance to the digestion of starch in seed particles. Added to the encapsulated starch (RS2), the seed coat itself is a valuable source of highly resilient cell walls constructed from nonstarch polysaccharides. Since they have evolved to resist biological attack, seed coats are usually relatively resistant to fermentation in the colon; so, make a valuable contribution to hindgut bulk, as in the case of wheat bran and pea hulls (Poutanen 2012).

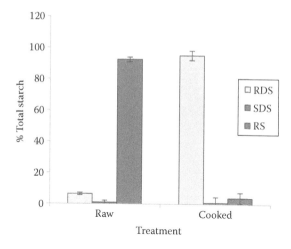

Figure 14.2 Effects of food structure at the molecular level—dependence of digestibility of starch *in vitro* on its molecular form: rapidly digested (RDS), slowly digested (SDS), and digestion-resistant starch (RS) in potatoes digested raw (pseudocrystalline, intact starch granules), or freshly cooked (starch dispersed after gelatinizing).

Cereal seeds of *Graminae* have evolved as dry, hard structures. The structural integrity of the cereal kernel and its protection from the environment is maintained by the starch/protein concretion of the endosperm, combined with the tough surrounding testa or seed coat (the bran in wheat). In cereals, the cell walls of the endosperm are thin and fragile, and the seed coat is the primary polysaccharide-based structure that effectively protects the endosperm from digestion. Even after cooking, if the cereal seed coat remains intact, the starch may be almost completely inaccessible for digestion, but is slowly digested if the seed is cut, and rapidly digested if the seed is crushed (Figure 14.3).

In pulses, the starch-containing reserve tissues of the cotyledons differ in structure from the endosperm of cereals. The internal cell walls retain a supporting function and may remain robust, especially in species in which the cotyledons become seed leaves after germination (Berg et al. 2012). The thick and resistant cell walls of pulses may retard the gelatinization of starch by confining it within the cell lumen (Tovar et al. 1990, 1992). When the starch is densely packed within resilient clusters of intact cells with robust cell walls, swelling is constrained. In addition, an encapsulating layer of gel from unconstrained starch in the outer cell layers of pulse fragments, supported by hydrated pectic polysaccharides of the cell walls, may impede water and enzyme penetration. However, partly because they are pectin rich compared with cereals, as processing is prolonged, the cell walls of pulses will degrade enough for the cells to separate. Then the starch has more freedom to swell and disperse, and digestion is more rapid.

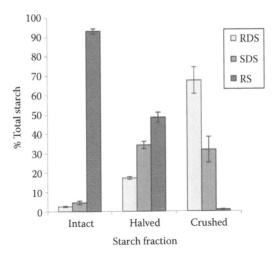

Figure 14.3 Influence of tissue structure on digestion revealed by the effect of cutting and crushing of cooked wheat kernels on *in vitro* digestion of starch. Individual whole hydrated kernels ($n = 5$/treatment) were cooked and digested either intact (intact), after they had been transversely cut into half (cut) or crushed to 1 mm thickness (crushed). RDS, rapidly digested; SDS, slowly digested; RS, resistant starch. Error bars are the standard deviations.

The effects of different cell structures in pulses and cereal products on the starch digestion, and of more relevance to this chapter—the delivery of dietary fiber, such as type 1 resistant starch—can be seen in the different relationships between resistant starch content and particle size in the two grain types (Figure 14.4). The resistant starch in pulses increases much more rapidly as a function of particle size than in cereals. This no doubt reflects the barrier action, in pulses, of the robust cell walls that are virtually absent from cereal endosperm, in which the cell walls are thin and fragile. The progressive increase in inaccessible (resistant) starch with increasing particle size is a very clear trend.

The hardness of cereal endosperm has its advantages in food processing, because it means that the endosperm shatters into digestible particles as the seed is dismembered by the crushing and shearing action of roller mills. After further processing, it produces a highly digestible, highly glycemic product that makes little contribution to dietary fiber requirements, unless the bran or a supplementary fiber source is included. As a result, the digestion of starch in processed cereal products is much more rapid than in pulses consumed as cooked grains (Figure 14.5). The contrasting difference between processed cereals and pulses provides a clear demonstration of the valuable role of polysaccharide-based structures in modulating the glycemic impact of foods.

In domestic cooking, the robust cell walls of pulses are often able to survive moist heat enough to remain annealed, so that cohesive plant cell clusters

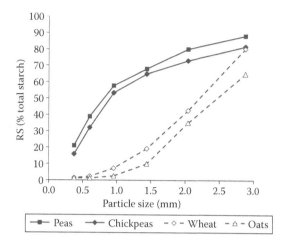

Figure 14.4 Effect of particle size reduction in cereals (wheat and oats) and pulses (peas and chickpeas) on the resistant starch (RS) load as a function of particle size. RS, starch remaining after 120 min *in vitro* pancreatic digestion.

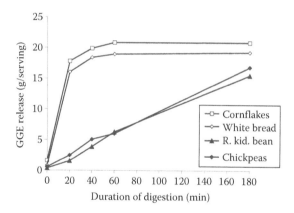

Figure 14.5 Structure-dependent digestion patterns: GGE release associated with different types of food structure: Porous, no intact cell walls (white bread and cornflakes) based on crushed and dispersed endosperm, compared with robust and intact plant cell walls encapsulating starch (chickpeas and red kidney beans) (GGE = glycemic glucose equivalent (g)). (Reprinted from *Food Chem*, 135, Mishra, S. and J. Monro. Wholeness and primary and secondary food structure effects on *in vitro* digestion patterns determine nutritionally distinct carbohydrate fractions in cereal foods, 1968–74, 2012b. With permission from Elsevier.)

with encapsulated starch remain after cooking. This makes pulses some of the most slowly digested of carbohydrate sources, with a typically low glycemic effect compared with other carbohydrate foods (Venn and Mann 2004). Kidney beans and chickpeas, for instance, show a digestion pattern *in vitro* that is typical of pulses, with a slow linear digestion that is usually incomplete

(Mishra and Monro 2012b) (Figure 14.5). *In vivo* pulses may load the colon with fermentable starch (type 1 resistant starch), which is partly responsible for their reputation for causing flatulence.

The penetration of digestion through layers of intact cells underlying the cut surfaces may be a relatively slow process. Recent detailed studies of the release of nutrients from cut nut fragments have shown that cell walls form a very effective barrier against the intestinal environment. After 3 h of simulated gastric plus duodenal digestion of almond fragments, the intracellular contents had been lost from only the first layer of cells, at the fracture surface (Mandalari et al. 2008). After 12 h of digestion, the loss of nutrients had extended to only three to five cell layers deep. There was no evidence of cell wall fracture; so, any enzyme penetration into the food particles could occur only by diffusion through the cell walls.

14.2.1.3 Fruit and Vegetables In nonstarchy leaves, roots, and stems eaten as food, polysaccharide-based supporting structures such as xylem fibers and vessels also have their own influence on digestion. Even the thin-walled parenchyma cells of fruit have a contribution to make through effects of the particles they provide in the intestinal lumen.

In most fruits, available carbohydrates are in the form of soluble sugars—glucose, fructose, and sucrose—that are highly soluble and mobile. Therefore, the only direct influences to reduce the rate of sugar availability from fruits are those that delay the transfer of sugars from the intestinal lumen to the gut wall, as the capacity to absorb at the gut wall is seldom limiting in healthy subjects. Nevertheless, there are several ways in which polysaccharide-based structures can reduce nutrient uptake. First, chewed fruit, in which clusters of cells remain intact as fragments of tissue, release nutrients more slowly than the same fruit that has been consumed as a pulp (Palafox-Carlos et al. 2011, Tydeman et al. 2010a, b). Second, even when the fruit or vegetable has been reduced to a pulp, digested *in vitro*, and the polysaccharides soluble in the digestion medium have been removed, the cell wall fragments of the disperse parenchyma remnants are able to substantially reduce the rate of diffusion of sugars (Figure 14.6). Such retardation can be regarded as a structural effect, as cell wall fragments, with their enmeshed hydrated pectic polysaccharides, increase the length of diffusion pathways. At the gut wall, such reduced diffusion will reduce the rate of blood glucose loading, leading to attenuation of the *in vivo* glycemic response. Third, in addition to reduced diffusion, cell wall fragments reduce mixing, which is the main mechanism for bulk transfer of sugars from the gut lumen to the gut wall (Lentle and Janssen 2011).

14.2.1.4 Interactions between Foods In real diets, diverse foods are often consumed together, or in close enough succession to become mixed in the gut. In such conditions, different polysaccharide structures from different food

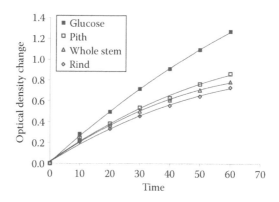

Figure 14.6 Retardation of diffusion by cell wall remnants of broccoli tissue after *in vitro* digestion. Glucose diffusion was retarded by about 40% by the pith (parenchyma cells) and rind (cortex containing parenchyma, fiber, and vascular cells). The tissue remnants (cell walls) were at bed density after settling for 16 h by gravity. All the solutions contained 10% glucose (w/v) at the beginning of dialysis. The mean between the duplicate range was <0.1 OD units.

sources may interact to amplify their individual properties. As an example, when cell wall residues from *in vitro* digestion were added to a solution made slightly viscous via the presence of soluble polysaccharide, the mixing of the combined solution was reduced far more than the sum of the reductions due to the soluble polysaccharide and cell wall alone (Mishra and Monro 2012a) (Figure 14.7).

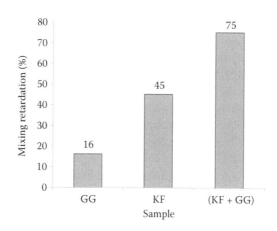

Figure 14.7 Retardation of mixing caused by 0.25% guar gum, by insoluble remnants of kiwifruit digested *in vitro* (KF), and by the kiwifruit remnants in 0.25% guar solution (KF + GG). The kiwifruit was at bed density after being allowed to gravity settle for 16 h, and the guar was added to a concentration of 0.25% to obtain the KF + GG sample. Mean SD ± 4.5%. (Reprinted from *Food Chem* 135, Mishra, S. and J. Monro. Kiwifruit remnants from digestion *in vitro* have functional attributes of potential importance to health, 2188–94, 2012a. With permission from Elsevier.)

The effect of cell wall remnants interacting with viscous polysaccharide can be understood in terms of polysaccharide and particle structure. Long polysaccharide chains occupy large hydrodynamic volumes and create viscosity through their interactions in solution, involving entanglement and/or formation of transient junction zones when polysaccharide chains align (Dikeman and Fahey 2006). In the presence of hydrated cell wall fragments, the hydrated polysaccharides that are part of the cell wall will capture a proportion of the available water so that the soluble polysaccharide becomes more concentrated in the free solution space that remains available, so that interchain contact increases. In addition, the particles provide relatively large polysaccharide-bearing surfaces with which the soluble polysaccharides can interact, as well as interacting with themselves.

Hydrated cell wall fragments not only reduce the rate of processes involved in the transfer of digestion products to the gut wall, but also reduce the activity of digestive enzymes. Digestion of particulate high-starch foods by pancreatic amylase was greatly reduced by the presence of fruit cell wall fragments at realistic concentrations (Figure 14.8). Taking only digestion rate into account (i.e., excluding any effects of diffusion and mixing on nutrient transfer), fruit cell walls reduced the estimated glycemic index of several carbohydrate foods from high (>70) to low (<55) glycemic index category. Reductions in the coefficients of mass transfer measured from the rate at which carbohydrate passed from the unstirred digesta into a stirred dialysis chamber were similar to the reductions in digestion, while the viability of the digestive enzyme was not reduced; so, it is likely that cell wall structures were influencing enzyme activity through their microrheological effects. Therefore, it appears that the impact of polysaccharide structures in the form of cell wall remnants, on the rate of nutrient availability from digestion in the gut, will

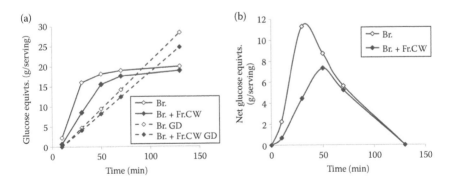

Figure 14.8 *In vitro* digestion curves of white bread (Br) and white bread plus fruit cell walls (Br + Fr. CW) (graph a). The dashed lines represent theoretical blood glucose disposal (Br.GD and Br + Fr.GD). The differences between the lines of glucose disposal and the digestion curves (net glucose equivalents) provide simulated blood glucose response curves (graph b). The relative areas under the curves show the estimated suppression of the blood glucose response by the cell walls.

result from a combination of reduced digestion rate, reduced diffusion rate, and reduced mixing.

14.3 Polysaccharide-Based Structures and Hindgut Function

Polysaccharide-based plant structures in the form of digestion-resistant remnants of cell walls play an essential role in maintaining large bowel health and function and are able to influence colonic fermentation in a number of interrelated ways. The cell wall fibrous (celluloses) and matrix (hemicellulosic and pectic) polysaccharides that comprise digestion-resistant structures provide essential fermentable substrates for bacteria. But from a physical viewpoint, polysaccharide-based structures that survive fermentation also make a major contribution to fermentation and large bowel function. They act as supports on which societies ("consortia") of bacteria proliferate as biofilms, in which metabolic interactions between species of bacteria determine the metabolic products, such as the type of short-chain fatty acid produced from fermentable substrates (Macfarlane and Dillon 2007).

14.3.1 Fecal Bulking Effects

One of the most important functions of food structure in the large bowel is to provide hydrated bulk in the distal colon (Buttris and Stokes 2008). Bulk in the colorectal region induces a defecation response that has a number of beneficial effects beyond giving the host a sense of well-being. It removes stagnant fecal matter in which carbohydrate substrates are depleted, and protein putrefaction is giving rise to nitrogenous products that increase the risk of colorectal cancer (Paturi et al. 2012). It leads to replenishment of distal colonic polysaccharide that resident bacteria ferment, producing butyric acid, which protects against colorectal cancer (Ou et al. 2013). In resilient plant tissues such as lignified xylem vessels and fibers, and in seed coats such as wheat bran, persistent plant structure in the form of robust cells occupies volume and provides water-bearing cavities (Monro and Mishra 2010), which will reduce the chemical activity of toxins by dilution. The colonic water load also helps to promote fecal softening and distribute pressure, thereby reducing the likelihood of disorders such as hemorrhoids and diverticulitis (Anderson et al. 2009, Burkitt 1984) (Table 14.2).

14.3.2 Influence of Plant Tissue Structure on Fecal Parameters

The influence of the cell and cell wall type in the distal colon has been clearly shown in a comparison of the effects of the pith versus rind (cortex) from broccoli stems and on fecal bulking in the rat (Monro and Mishra 2010). The pith consists of thin-walled unlignified parenchyma cells that are extensively fermented in the hindgut. In contrast, the rind has embedded in it vascular and supporting structures, such as vascular bundles rich in lignified xylem vessels and fibers that resist fermentation and provide cavities and volume that confers a high water-holding capacity in the fecal mass.

Table 14.2 Some of the Interacting Effects of Polysaccharide-Based Structures in the Small and Large Intestines and Their Consequences for Physiology and Disease Risk

Structural Aspects	Physiological Effects	Reduced Disease Risk
Small Intestine		
Particle resilience	Delayed gastric emptying	Diabetes
Increased viscosity	Reduced digestion rates	Cardiovascular disease
Decrease in diffusion rate	Reduced absorption rates	Obesity
Reduced mixing	Reduced postprandial glycemia	
Reduced digestive activity	Reduced postprandial lipidemia	
	Prolonged satiety	
	Distributed nutrient absorption	
Large Intestine		
Resilient plant tissue structure	Increased colonic water load	Constipation
Water-holding cavities	Fecal softening and pressure distribution	Hemorrhoids Diverticular disease
Water-binding capacity	Toxin dilution	Colitis
Increased bulk	Defecation activated and bacterial substrates replenished	Colorectal cancer
Encapsulation of starch		Allergies
Fermentable substrates for bacteria	Fermentation displaced distally	Inflammatory bowel disease
Physical supports for bacterial consortia and biofilms	Short-chain fatty acids—butyrate Increased gut immunity Improved gut barrier integrity	

Changes in fecal parameters as a result of consuming broccoli pith and rind were measured by incorporating the two tissue types at 12.5% dry weight into low-fiber rat diets in place of sucrose, and measuring fecal dry matter output, its water-holding capacity, and calculated hydrated fecal output per 100 g diet, which has been shown to be an accurate model of fecal-bulking capacity in humans (Monro 2004). Changes in fecal parameters over the baseline markedly differed between the pith and rind (Table 14.3) and reflected the structure of the two tissues. Dry matter increases reflected resistance to fermentation and were much higher for the rind than the pith. Increases in fecal water-holding capacity, which reflected the cellular structure of the rind compared with the pith (confirmed by microscopy), were also much greater for the rind than the pith. The combination of increased dry matter and increased water-holding capacity gave the rind a much greater efficacy in terms of dilution by colonic water ("water load," Table 14.3) and the creation of hydrated bulk, which is a stimulus for laxation (Table 14.3).

Table 14.3 Increases in Fecal Parameters (%) over Baseline Values as a Result of Including Dietary Fiber Sources of Different Structure (Parenchymatous Pith versus Fibrous Rind) by Substitution of 12.5% Sucrose in a Low-Fiber Baseline Diet

Fecal Parameter	Broccoli Pith		Broccoli Rind		Wheat Bran	
(Per 100 g Diet)*	Mean	± SD	Mean	± SD	Mean	± SD
Dry matter	21	±1.2	111	±3.8	90	±4.0
Water-holding capacity	10	±0.5	53	±3.8	39	±2.2
Water load	33	±3.0	224	±19.7	165	±14.5
Hydrated fecal output	29	±2.3	189	±13.8	142	±10.8

Source: From Monro, J. A. and S. Mishra. 2010. *Food Digestion* 1:47–56.

Table 14.4 Different Glycemic Impact (GGE) and Estimated Glycemic Index (GI$_{est}$) Values for White Bread and Grain Bread Due to Carbohydrate Structure in the Grain Bread Having the Combined Effect of Retarding Digestion, Retaining Water, and Replacing Starch

Bread Type	GGE/100 g (g)	GGE/Serving (g)	GI$_{est}$(%)
White bread	34.3	20.9	73.2
Grain bread (25% kernels >2 mm diameter)	18.1	13.4	52.7

Note: Digestion curves on which the calculations were based are shown in Figure 14.9.

14.4 Retaining Polysaccharide-Based Food Structures for Health: Minimal Processing

Appreciation of the importance of food structure in determining rates of carbohydrate availability has led to the adoption of reduced or minimal processing technologies with the aim of sparing the natural relationship between digestible and nondigestible food components, and/or preserving the structure of the nondigestible components.

Tissue structure can be retained by consuming whole foods, in which the incomplete comminution by chewing allows some food structure to survive, and reduces the rate of availability of nutrients, such as glucose from starch digestion. The much slower availability of nutrients from fruit consumed as pieces than from fruits consumed as a puree is an example (Tydeman et al. 2010a).

In cooked food, the retention of tissue structure is a strategy commonly used in the baking industries to reduce both the rate and the extent of carbohydrate digestion, when fragments of intact kernels are included in grain breads (Table 14.4). The effectiveness of substituting partially intact kernels for flour in bread products is revealed by the raised *in vitro* glycemic impact (g. glucose equivalents [GGEs] per weight of bread) and estimated glycemic index values due to increases in digestion rates when kernel-rich breads were homogenized to remove grain structure. Homogenizing increased starch availability for digestion in the grain bread but not in the white bread, showing the role of kernel intactness (Figure 14.9). However, even after homogenizing, the grain bread had a substantially lower digestion profile than the white bread. The diluting effect of the undigestible seed coat (bran) and the greater water retention by intact granules were also ways in which structure contributed to the lower glycemic potency of the grain bread before homogenizing.

Arguments in favor of increasing the proportion of dietary carbohydrate consumed as whole grains in which native structure is partially retained are that "wholeness," in the sense of intactness, is associated with a reduced blood glucose loading (Venn and Mann 2004). The digestive advantages of minimal processing extend beyond benefits of reducing the rate and extent of starch digestion in the foregut for glycemic control. In the hindgut, minimally processed cereal and pulse products provide more resistant starch and nonstarch polysaccharide to act as fermentable substrates for the colonic microbiota, and greater colonic bulking to stimulate colonic transit, than is supplied by refined finely milled products. Increasing the particle size is significantly associated with decreasing glycemic response (Fardet 2006) and increased colonic fermentation (Bird et al. 2000), which is consistent with the results of *in vitro* analyses of grain starch digestibility.

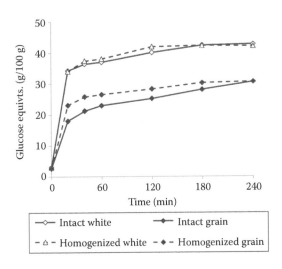

Figure 14.9 The role of structure in the glycemic impact of "grain" bread containing 25% partially intact (>2 mm diameter) kernels compared with white bread, indicated by glucose release during *in vitro* digestion. Homogenizing increased carbohydrate release in the grain bread, and not in the white bread. Even after homogenizing, the glycemic impact of the grain bread remained relatively low due to the presence of dietary fiber and retained water. The mean between-duplicate range was <5%.

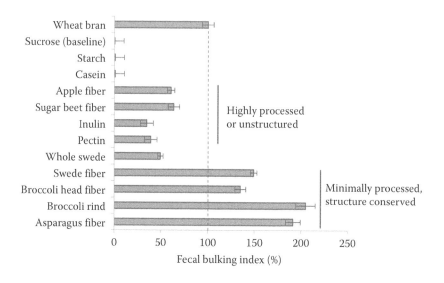

Figure 14.10 Minimally processed vegetable dietary fiber sources prepared by cold-water maceration of vegetable tissues retain a high fecal bulking capacity compared with isolated polysaccharides (pectin and inulin) and highly processed cell wall preparations (sugar beet fiber and commercial apple fiber).

In non-cereals too, minimal processing may provide benefits in the large bowel when retention of hydrated polysaccharides in the cell wall matrix, as well as the cellular structure, is maintained. Vegetable fibers prepared by cold-water maceration, in which only a small proportion of the pectic polysaccharides are extracted, and subsequently milled to 1.0 mm, that is, not to a fine powder, exhibit a strong fecal bulking capacity, greater than that of wheat bran (Figure 14.10). Nonstarch polysaccharide extracts and highly processed commercial dietary fibers such as sugar beet fiber, apple fiber, pectin, and inulin, which have typically had heat treatments before being milled to a fine powder, were much less effective (Figure 14.10).

14.5 Conclusion

It is evident from the foregoing discussion that the retention of polysaccharide-based structure in plant foods can confer a number of nutritional and health benefits. These benefits arise from much more than the provision of dietary fiber *per se*; the physical effects of polysaccharide-based food structures on associated nutrients and the intrinsic properties of the structures themselves are important. Nutrition and health will clearly benefit from the increased attention of food processors to the preservation of natural fibers and of the natural structures in which they occur in plant foods for human consumption.

14.6 Summary

The importance of both digestible polysaccharide (starch) and nondigestible polysaccharides (dietary fiber) in human nutrition and health is now well established. Digestible polysaccharides are important as the most abundant and accessible form of dietary energy consumed by humans. Nondigestible polysaccharides and the structures based on them, on the other hand, are important in determining the availability of potentially digestible carbohydrate in the foregut, and the proportion of it that reaches the colon undigested, as dietary fiber. Research and analysis of dietary fiber has tended to focus on the types of polysaccharides involved, or on dietary fiber as a food component measured as a total nondigestible polysaccharide conglomerate in finely milled samples. Dietary fiber exists in nature in many different structures. The important nutritional role of these structures is often ignored, or intentionally eliminated by the methods prescribed for food analysis. However, dietary fiber structure at the molecular, cellular, tissue, and whole food levels can modulate both the rate and extent of carbohydrate digestion from foods in a number of ways, as well as contributing in its own right to nutrition and gut function. Through their effects on energy availability from the diet, polysaccharide-based plant structures are relevant to energy sufficiency, and increasingly to problems of energy excess such as obesity, metabolic syndrome, and diabetes. In the large bowel, polysaccharide-based plant structures have an essential role in protecting against large bowel disorders, such as constipation and colorectal cancer, by acting as substrates for the colonic microbiota and by providing resilient structures that contribute to bulk, hydration, and stimulation; so, promote regularity and bowel transit. This chapter has discussed the various forms of polysaccharide-based plant structures in food plants and presents experimental results to illustrate the ways in which they may exert their benefits on nutrition and gut health.

References

Anderson, J. W., P. Baird, and R. H. Davis, Jr. et al. 2009. Health benefits of dietary fiber. *Nutr Rev* 67:188–205.

Ayoub, A., T. Ohtani, and S. Sugiyama. 2006. Atomic force microscopy investigation of disorder process on rice starch granule surface. *Starch-Starke* 58:475–9.

BeMiller, J. N. 2007. *Carbohydrate Chemistry for Food Scientists*. 2nd edition. St. Paul (MN): American Association of Cereal Chemists.

Berg, T., J. Singh, A. Hardacre, and M. J. Boland. 2012. The role of cotyledon cell structure during *in vitro* digestion of starch in navy beans. *Carbohydr Polym* 87:1678–88.

Bird, A. R., T. Hayakawa, Y. Marsono et al. 2000. Coarse brown rice increases fecal and large bowel short-chain fatty acids and starch but lowers calcium in the large bowel of pigs. *J Nutr* 130:1780–7.

Brownlee, I. A. 2011. The physiological roles of dietary fibre. *Food Hydrocolloid* 25:238–50.

Burkitt, D. 1984. Fiber as protective against gastrointestinal-diseases. *Am J Gastroenterol* 79:24952.

Buttris, J. L. and C. S. Stokes. 2008. Dietary fibre and health: An overview. *Nutr Bull* 33:186–200.

Copeland, L., J. Blazek, H. Salman, and M. C. Tang. 2009. Form and functionality of starch. *Food Hydrocolloid* 23:1527–34.

Debet, M. R. and M. J. Gidley. 2006. Three classes of starch granule swelling: Influence of surface proteins and lipids. *Carbohydr Polym* 64:452–65.

Dikeman, C. L. and G. C. Fahey. 2006. Viscosity as related to dietary fiber: A review. *Crit Rev Food Sci Nutr* 46:649–63.

Donald, A. M. 2004. Understanding starch structure and functionality. In *Starch in Food: Structure, Function and Applications*, ed. A. E. Eliasson, pp. 154–84. Cambridge: Woodhead Publishing Limited.

Fardet, A., F. Leenhardt, D. Lioger, A. Scalbert, and C. Rémésy. 2006. Parameters controlling the glycemic response to breads. *Nutr Res Rev* 19:18–25.

French, D. 1984. Organisation of starch granules. In *Starch Chemistry and Technology*, ed. R. L. Whistler, J. N. BeMiller, and E. F. Paschall, pp. 183–247. Orlando: Academic Press.

Gallant, D. J., B. Bouchet, and P. M. Baldwin. 1997. Microscopy of starch: Evidence of a new level of granule organization. *Carbohydr Polym* 32:177–91.

Gelinas, P. 2013. Preventing constipation: A review of the laxative potential of food ingredients. *Int J Food Sci Technol* 48:445–67.

Huber, K. C. and J. M. BeMiller. 2000. Channels of maize and sorghum starch granules. *Carbohydr Polym* 41:269–76.

James, M. G., K. Denyer, and A. M. Myers. 2003. Starch synthesis in the cereal endosperm. *Curr Opin Plant Biol* 6:215–22.

Juszczak, L., T. Fortuna, and F. Krok. 2003. Non-contact atomic force microscopy of starch granules surface. Part I. Potato and tapioca starches. *Starch-Starke* 55:1–7.

Lentle, R. G. and P. W. M. Janssen. 2011. *The Physical Processes of Digestion*. New York: Springer.

Macfarlane, S. and J. F. Dillon. 2007. Microbial biofilms in the human gastrointestinal tract. *J Appl Microbiol* 102:1187–96.

Mandalari, G., R. M. Faulks, G. T. Rich et al. 2008. Release of protein, lipid, and vitamin E from almond seeds during digestion. *J Agric Food Chem* 56:3409–16.

McDougall, G., I. Morrison, D. Stewart, and J. Hillman. 1996. Plant cell walls as dietary fibre: Range, structure, processing and function. *J Sci Food Agric* 70:133–50.

Mishra, S. and J. Monro. 2012a. Kiwifruit remnants from digestion *in vitro* have functional attributes of potential importance to health. *Food Chem* 135:2188–94.

Mishra, S. and J. Monro. 2012b. Wholeness and primary and secondary food structure effects on *in vitro* digestion patterns determine nutritionally distinct carbohydrate fractions in cereal foods. *Food Chem* 135:1968–74.

Monro, J. A. 2004. Adequate intake values for dietary fibre based on faecal bulking indexes of 66 foods. *Eur J Clin Nutr* 58:32–9.

Monro, J. A. and S. Mishra. 2010. Digestion-resistant remnants of vegetable vascular and parenchyma tissues differ in their effects in the large bowel of rats. *Food Digestion* 1:47–56.

Ou, J., F. Carbonero, E. G. Zoetendal et al. 2013. Diet, microbiota, and microbial metabolites in colon cancer risk in rural Africans and African Americans. *Am J Clin Nutr* 98:11–120.

Palafox-Carlos, H., J. F. Ayala-Zavala, and G. A. Gonzalez-Aguilar. 2011. The role of dietary fiber in the bioaccessibility and bioavailability of fruit and vegetable anti-oxidants. *J Food Sci* 76:R6–15.

Paturi, G., T. Nyanhanda, C. A. Butts, T. D. Herath, J. A. Monro, and J. Ansell. 2012. Effects of potato fiber and potato-resistant starch on biomarkers of colonic health in rats fed diets containing red meat. *J Food Sci* 77:H216–23.

Poutanen, K. 2012. Past and future of cereal grains as food for health. *Trends Food Sci Technol* 25:58–62.

Ratnayake, W. S. and D. S. Jackson. 2007. A new insight into the gelatinization process of native starches. *Carbohydr Polym* 67:511–29.

Slattery, M. L., K. P. Curtin, S. L. Edwards, and D. M. Schaffer. 2004. Plant foods, fiber, and rectal cancer. *Am J Clin Nutr* 79:274–81.

Thomas, D. J. and W. A. Atwell. 1998. *Starches*. St. Paul (MN): Eagen Press.

Tovar, J., A. Defrancisco, I. M. Bjork, and N. G. Asp. 1990. Relationship between microstructure and *in vitro* digestibility of starch in precooked leguminous seed flours. *Food Struct* 10:19–26.

Tovar, J., Y. Granfeldt, and I. M. Bjorck. 1992. Effect of processing on blood-glucose and insulin responses to starch in legumes. *J Agric Food Chem* 40:1846–51.

Tydeman, E. A., M. L. Parker, R. M. Faulks et al. 2010a. Effect of carrot (*Daucus carota*) microstructure on carotene bioaccessibility in the upper gastrointestinal tract. 2. *In vivo* digestions. *J Agric Food Chem* 58:9855–60.

Tydeman, E. A., M. L. Parker, M. S. J. Wickham et al. 2010b. Effect of carrot (*Daucus carota*) microstructure on carotene bioaccessibilty in the upper gastrointestinal tract. 1. *In vitro* simulations of carrot digestion. *J Agric Food Chem* 58:9847–54.

Venn, B. J. and J. I. Mann. 2004. Cereal grains, legumes and diabetes. *Eur J Clin Nutr* 58:1443–61.

Waigh, T. A., K. L. Kato, A. M. Donald, M. J. Gidley, C. J. Clarke, and C. Riekel. 2000. Side-chain liquid-crystalline model for starch. *Starch-Starke* 52:450–60.

Zimmet, P., K. Alberti, and J. Shaw. 2001. Global and societal implications of the diabetes epidemic. *Nature* 414:782–7.

CHAPTER **15**

Dietary Polysaccharides for the Modulation of Obesity via Beneficial Gut Microbial Manipulation

KANTHI KIRAN KONDEPUDI, MAHENDRA BISHNOI,
KOTESWARAIAH PODILI, PADMA AMBALAM, KOUSHIK
MAZUMDER, NIDA MURTAZA, RITESH K. BABOOTA, and
RAVNEET K. BOPARAI

Contents

15.1 Introduction   367
    15.1.1 Obesity and Role of Gut Microbes   368
    15.1.2 Antiobesity Medications and Side Effects   369
    15.1.3 Alternate and Safe Approaches   369
15.2 Functional Foods in Obesity and Related Complications   370
    15.2.1 Dietary Fibers, Colonic Fermentation, and Formation
        of Short-Chain Fatty Acids   370
15.3 Conclusion   378
References   378

15.1 Introduction

Increase in body mass index (BMI), defined as a person's weight in kilograms divided by the square of the height in meters (kg/m^2), leads to obesity, which is classified as class I for BMI between 30 and 35, associated with a moderate risk of mortality; class II for BMI between 35 and 39.9 associated with a high risk of mortality; and class III for BMI ≥ 40 associated with a very high risk of mortality (González-Castejón and Rodriguez-Casado 2011). Obesity became globally pandemic and is rising alarmingly in developing countries such as India. It is staggering that 62% of the American population is overweight and

26% of them are obese as per WHO reports. From an Indian perspective, 7.3% of the Indian population is overweight and 1.2% is obese (Chatterjee 2002). As per the National Health Family Survey data, in India, Punjab is the "heaviest" state with 30% of males and 38% of females being obese (National Survey 2007). The World Health Organization's World Health Statistics showed that 2.8 million people die across the world annually due to obesity and its associated complications (WHO-World Health Statistics 2012). Obesity is associated with multiple comorbidities such as type 2 diabetes and cardiovascular complications such as hypertension, hyperlipidemia, arteriosclerosis, and cancer. Obesity is an uncontrolled adipose tissue development (hypertrophy or hyperplasia of adipocytes) with high levels of lipid accumulation. For adipose tissue types, their development, secretome, and physiology have been described elsewhere (Delzenne et al. 2011, Gregor and Hotamisligil 2007, Rosen and Mac Dougald 2006, Stephens 2012).

15.1.1 Obesity and Role of Gut Microbes

Gut microbes are believed to contain greater proportions of beneficial microbes and less pathogenic ones under normal health conditions. Beneficial microbes metabolize endo- and xenobiotics, ferment nutrients, and secrete bioactive molecules that affect the host's physiology and metabolism (Delzenne et al. 2011). This "microbial organ" is the largest and most well-studied microbial community of adult humans and resides in the colon; it consists of 10^{13}–10^{14} bacterial cells that make more than 10 times the human cells. The complex human gut microbiome represents more than 100 times the human genome (The Human Microbiome Consortium 2012, Segata et al. 2013). Firmicutes and Bacteroidetes are the dominant phyla and Proteobacteria, Fusobacteria, Verrucomicrobia, and Actinobacteria are the subdominant phyla in the human gut as evidenced by metagenomic analysis (Tilg and Kaser 2011). Metabolic functions of gut microbes influence the metabolic status of humans and these kinds of studies became a major topic for obesity research (Delzenne et al. 2011). If the balance between beneficial and pathogenic microbes is disturbed (dysbiosis), pathogenic microbes will dominate and this may lead to a pathophysiological condition. Obesity is one such condition where bacterial dysbiosis in the gut is considered as one of the contributing factors. Fewer Bacteroidetes and more Firmicutes and lipopolysaccharide (LPS)-secreting Gram-negative pathogens colonize the gut of obese individuals (Ouchi et al. 2011). Certain gut bacteria that secrete LPS such as *Escherichia coli* and an endotoxin-producing *Enterobacter cloaca* B29 were recently reported to contribute to obesity development (Cani et al. 2007, Fei and Zhao 2013). LPS and other endotoxins translocate via toll receptors into the circulation and cause low-grade inflammation and metabolic endotoxemia (Ouchi et al. 2011). On the other hand, there are gut microbes that could alleviate metabolic complications. Very recently, the oral administration of live *Akkermansia muciniphila*, a mucin-degrading bacteria isolated from the mucus layer, was found to reverse the complications associated with high-fat-diet-induced metabolic disorders in mice through enhanced intestinal levels of endocannabinoids that control inflammation, the gut barrier, and gut peptide secretion (Everard et al. 2013). Studies on human gut microbial composition in 123 nonobese and 169 obese Danish individuals showed a difference in the number of gut microbial genes and bacterial richness (Le Chatelier et al. 2013). Marked adiposity, insulin resistance, and dyslipidemia, as well as a more pronounced inflammatory phenotype, were observed in individuals with low bacterial richness (23% of the population) who also gained more weight compared to those with high bacterial richness. These variations in the gut microbiome may allow for the identification of individuals in the general adult population who may be at increased risk of progressing to adiposity-associated comorbidities (Cotillard et al. 2013, Le Chatelier et al. 2013). A balance between good and pathogenic bacteria is, therefore, essential for gut health. Food ingredients such as dietary fibers (DFs) and prebiotics may bring significant changes in the gut microbial composition and their gene richness. This could, in turn, regulate gene expression in host tissues, including the colon, small intestine, liver, adipose tissue, and muscle, and help to improve the overall metabolic health.

15.1.2 Antiobesity Medications and Side Effects

Antiobesity medications reduce or control weight by altering appetite, metabolism, or the consumption of calories (Kennett and Clifton 2010). Fen-phen, a combination of fenfluramine (a serotonin-releasing agent) and phentermine (norepinephrine-, dopamine-, and a serotonin-releasing agent), fenfluramine (a serotonin reuptake inhibitor), sibutramine (noradrenaline and a serotonin reuptake inhibitor), rimonabant (a cannabinoid-1 receptor antagonist), and orlistat (a pancreatic lipase inhibitor) are associated with serious and multiple side effects (Kennett and Clifton 2010). Lorcaserin (a serotonin receptor agonist; trade name Belviq, Arena Pharmaceuticals, Nancy Ridge Drive, San Diego, California) and a combination of phentermine (increases noradrenaline, dopamine, and serotonin) and topiramate (acts on the brain receptor associated with satiety; trade name Qsymia) have been recently approved by the US-FDA (FDA News release 2012).

15.1.3 Alternate and Safe Approaches

The potential side effects of antiobesity medications (Carter et al. 2012) are suggestive of the need for safer ways of prevention or treatment of obesity. Diet and physical activity are the safer options. Bioactive food ingredients are deemed important as they could modify the pathways and gene/protein expressions in a beneficial way (Baboota et al. 2013). Owing to the involvement of certain pathogenic gut microbial groups for the development of obesity and beneficial microbial groups that could alleviate obesity, intentional gut microbial manipulation using diets rich in DFs is of high relevance for the regulation of the obesity pandemic.

15.2 Functional Foods in Obesity and Related Complications

Many definitions are in vogue to define "functional foods" (FF). However, there is no standard or commonly accepted definition to date. FFs are similar to conventional foods but additionally impart beneficial health effects such as reducing the risk of chronic diseases. They contain bioactive compounds (FF ingredients), which are of several classes such as polyphenols, proteins, DFs, probiotics, prebiotics, omega fatty acids, and so on. Many of them are derived from edible as well as medicinal plants, and algal and microbial sources, and some are derived from animal sources. Novel FF ingredients are in great demand. More details on FF ingredients and their role in alleviating obesity and comorbidities are described elsewhere (Baboota et al. 2013, Choudhary and Grover 2012, Serrano et al. 2012). This chapter focuses mainly on various plant-derived DFs/polysaccharides and their role in managing obesity through beneficial gut microbial manipulation.

15.2.1 Dietary Fibers, Colonic Fermentation, and Formation of Short-Chain Fatty Acids

As per the American Association of Cereal Chemists (AACC)-approved definition, "a dietary fiber is the edible parts of plants or analogous carbohydrates that are resistant to digestion and absorption in the human small intestine with complete or partial fermentation in the large intestine. Dietary fiber includes polysaccharides, oligosaccharides, lignin, and associated plants substances. Dietary fibers promote beneficial physiological effects including laxation, and/or blood cholesterol attenuation, and/or blood glucose attenuation." The Commission of the European Communities (2008) defines DFs as "carbohydrate polymers with three or more monomeric units, which are neither digested nor absorbed in the small intestine." DFs act by reducing energy density in foods as it adds substantially more weight to foods than calories. DFs, in general, are categorized into soluble and insoluble fibers. Insoluble fibers bulk the feces and promote the excretion of bile acids with a decrease in intestinal transit time (i.e., laxative effect). Soluble viscous fibers slow down glucose absorption by delaying gastric emptying as it increases the total transit time of the food material while soluble nonviscous fibers are good substrates for microbial fermentation in the large bowel (Cummings and Stephen 2007, Wong et al. 2006). The physical effects of DF include reduction in total energy consumption due to maximal sensory stimulation in the mouth due to longer chewing times, slower gastric emptying, slower rate of nutrient absorption, and reduction in the energy density of the diet. Therefore, increasing DF consumption is related to weight management. In the recent past, there has been an increase in research on the identification of bioactive DFs for modulating various disorder, including weight gain and obesity. Pectins, β-glucan, xylan, arabinoxylan, inulin, resistant starch (RS), and gum arabic (GA) are some of the well-studied DFs. DFs are also rich in whole-grain cereals and their intake significantly lowers the risk from metabolic disorders and gastrointestinal diseases, boosts the immune system, and stimulates the growth of beneficial microbes in the colon (Anderson et al. 2009). Therefore, the general consensus among public health authorities and nutritionists is that DFs provide health benefits when incorporated in regular diets (Férnandez-López et al. 2007). Several studies showed that DF consumption significantly enhances weight loss (Slavin 2013). Colonic microbial fermentation of DFs generates acetate, propionate, or butyrate, short-chain fatty acids (SCFA), whose molar ratio in a healthy colon is anticipated to be 60:20:20 (Bergman 1990). SCFAs are involved in various physiological processes and provide beneficial health effects. SCFAs may reduce the risk of metabolic disorders via binding to G-protein-coupled receptors, GPR41 and GPR43, also known as free fatty acid receptor 3 (FFAR3) and 2 (FFAR2) (Ulven 2012). These are highly expressed in human intestinal mucosa, immune cells, and liver and adipose tissue (Brahe et al. 2013). These receptors could be potential targets for the treatment of metabolic disorders as they form a link among gut, immunity, and metabolism (Maslowski et al. 2009, Ulven 2012). In addition, SCFAs are recognized as potential mediators of intestinal inflammatory response (Meijer et al. 2010). Propionate suppresses proinflammatory markers (Al-Lahham et al. 2010) and enhances appetite (Arora et al. 2011). Butyrate, the prime among SCFAs, acts as a fuel for colonocytes, promotes health, and acts as an epigenetic regulator through histone deacetylase inhibition (Canani et al. 2012). Therefore, a good SCFA profile in the colon is crucial for its health. This could be achieved by incorporating DF or combinations in the regular diet (Slavin 2013). Here, we describe the occurrence, structure, and role in obesity management of RS, arabinoxylan, inulin, β-glucan, pectin, GA, and fucoidans.

15.2.1.1 Resistant Starch A fraction of the dietary as retrograded starch, identified in the large bowel that resists digestion by the human digestive enzymes, was designated as resistant starch (Englyst and Englyst 2005). It will not be hydrolyzed in the small intestine but is fermented in the colon (David and Cyril 2000). Four basic types of RS have been reported (Topping et al. 2008): RS1 is composed of starch granules attached to the cell walls of plant material; RS2 is native granular starch with a B-type x-ray pattern, such as that found in potato and high-amylose maize; RS3 is crystallized starch and maltodextrins made by a retrogradation process; and RS4 is a chemically modified starch (esterified or transglycosylation product). RS is a linear molecule of α-(1 → 4)-D-glucan, derived from the retrograded amylose fraction (Tharanathan 2002). Whole grains, legumes, cooked and chilled pasta, potatoes, rice, and unripe bananas contain RS in different proportions (Fuentes-Zaragoza et al. 2010). RS formation can be controlled by regulating moisture content, pH, temperature, duration of heating, repeated heating–cooling cycles, and so on, which may yield RS as much as 30%. RS provides many technological properties, such as better appearance, texture, and mouth feel than conventional fibers (Charalampopoulos et al. 2002). Owing to its increased expansion, enhanced crispiness, and reduced oil "pick up" in deep-fat-fried foods, in contrast to the traditional DF, it imparts improved eating qualities, gritty texture, and strong flavor (Tharanathan 2002). Owing to the low water-holding capacity, RS serves as a functional ingredient that can enhance texture in the final product (Baixauli et al. 2008). Foods such as bread, cakes, muffins, pasta, and battered foods have been enriched with RS (Sanz et al. 2009).

The health benefits of RS are well established and mainly attributed to colonic microbial fermentation through the formation of SCFA (Weaver et al. 1992), stool bulking giving a mild laxative effect (Phillips et al. 1995), reducing intestinal pH, and the production of potentially harmful secondary bile acids, ammonia, and phenols (Birkett et al. 1996), enhancing the growth of healthy bacteria in the bowel—the "prebiotic effect" (Topping et al. 2003), and preventing the degradation of the mucous layer within the colon. The mucous layer is believed to protect colon cells (Toden et al. 2006).

RS may protect from T2DM possibly by reducing the glycemic index of a food by displacing digestible carbohydrate (Jenkins and Kendall 2000). Diet containing high RS has been shown to reduce body weight gain, fat pad weight, and glycemic response, along with improved insulin sensitivity in diet-induced obese rats (Aziz et al. 2009). Higgins et al. (2011) showed that 13% high-amylose maize starch reduced adiposity but not weight regain in high-fat-diet-induced obesity in rats. In obesity-prone and obesity-resistant phenotypes of male Sprague-Dawley rats, obesity-prone rats showed less weight when fed for 4 weeks with 4%, 12%, and 16% RS compared to the control. SCFA levels were significantly high in cecal contents of animals fed with RS. Glucagon-like peptide-1 and peptide YY levels were significantly high in plasma, whereas gastric inhibitory polypeptide was decreased in animals fed with >8% RS. Insulin sensitivity was not affected by RS in any of the groups (Belobrajdic et al. 2012). In another study, feeding RS to rats showed altered gut microbial composition with a significant enhancement in Bacteroidetes and Actinobacteria, which was linked to changes in SCFA and gene expression (Gsta2 and Ela1) in the colon (Young et al. 2012). RS2 intervention in mice altered the gut weight and proglucagon expression levels, and the mice were colonized by higher levels of Bacteroidetes and Bifidobacterium, Akkermansia, and Allobaculum species in a dose-dependent manner of the DF (Tachon et al. 2013). RS significantly enhances the butyrogenic bacteria such as *Roseburia* and *Facecalibacterium* due to the anti-inflammatory action of butyrate or by the bacteria itself (Brahe et al. 2013). In a study with high fat diet (HFD)-induced obese rats, oral administration of RS, sodium butyrate, or a combination of RS and SB in separate groups decreased the abdominal fat. The decrease was greater when the animals were fed with the combination of RS and SB than SB or RS alone. RS was associated with increased butyrate production in the cecum and increased serum PYY and GLP-1, which otherwise was not noticed in the group fed with oral SB. This signifies that colonic fermentation of DFs to SCFA may be more beneficial than oral administration of SCFAs (Vidrine et al. 2013).

Food products prepared with refined grains contain less or almost no RS. Therefore, it is important to incorporate RS that could elicit favorable metabolic effects in obese and nonobese individuals.

15.2.1.2 Arabinoxylans   Several epidemiological studies have indicated that a diet containing whole-grain cereals can protect against metabolic disorders. The effect is mainly attributed to the fibers and micronutrients in the outer layer of the cereal grain. Arabinoxylans (AXs) are emerging nonstarch DFs distributed in high quantities in whole-grain cereals, including wheat, rye, barley, oat, rice, sorghum, maize, and millet. Their use as food ingredients is gaining importance.

Depending on the source, AXs exhibit different molecular features, which are determinants of their functional properties. In cereal grains, arabinoxylans are the main nonstarchy polysaccharides and they are located in the cell walls of the endosperm, aleurone layer, bran, and husk (Fincher and Stone 1986). AXs are covalently linked to each other or to other cell wall components and are insoluble in aqueous media. Different extraction methods have been reported for the extraction of AXs from various plant tissues (Faurot et al. 1995, Fincher and Stone 1974, Izydorczyk et al. 1991), which involve the removal of protein and starch by enzymatic treatment followed by alkaline extraction.

Structurally, AXs are heteropolymers consisting of a linear β-$(1 \rightarrow 4)$-D-xylopyranose backbone, which is branched by short carbohydrate chains, mainly D-glucuronic acid or 4-O-methyl glucuronic acids, L-arabinose, and/or various oligosaccharides containing L-arabinose, D-xylose, D- or L-galactose, and D-glucose (Andersson and Aman 2001, Izydorczyk and Biliaderis 1995). The pattern of attachment of arabinose and uronic acid residues to the xylan backbone has been a matter of continuous research. One of the unique features of arabinoxylans is the presence of hydroxycinnamic acids, mainly ferulic acid, and to a lesser extent, dehydrodiferulic acid, p-coumaric acid, and sinapic acid are covalently attached via ester linkage to C(O)-5 of the arabinofuranosyl residue (Ebringerova and Heinze 2000, Rao and Muralikrishna 2001).

The frequency and nature of substitution differ greatly among AX from different origins. Clear differences in the arabinose-to-xylose ratio, an indicator of the average degree of substitution (avDAS), can be found between AX in wheat endosperm (avDAS ~0.5–0.7) and that in bran tissues, whereas the aleurone and seed coat contain less branched AX (avDAS 0.1–0.4) and the outer pericarp contains highly branched AX (avDAS 1.1–1.3) (Andersson and Aman 2001, Cleemput et al. 1993, Gruppen et al. 1993, Izydorczyk and Biliaderis 1995, Maes and Delcour 2002). The distribution of the arabinosyl residues along the xylan backbone is probably of greater importance than the degree of substitution, since it determines the conformation and ability of arabinoxylans to interact with the other cell wall components. The chain conformation and intermolecular matrix association have a direct bearing on the functional properties of AX. The degree of substitution with hydroxycinnamic acids also varies with tissue locations, and the aleurone layer in wheat bran contains 10-fold higher hydroxycinnamic acids attached to arabinoxylans than endosperm tissues (Barron et al. 2007). Furthermore, AX from the endosperm of rice, maize, and sorghum contains more arabinose, galactose, and glucuronic acid residues than those from wheat, rye, and barley. In the food industry, AX has several applications. In a randomized, single-blind, controlled, crossover intervention trial on seven female and four male adults, AX supplementation (15 g) for 6 weeks, with a 6-week washout period in between, resulted in lower postprandial responses in serum glucose, insulin, triglycerides, and total plasma ghrelin with no difference in plasma acylated ghrelin (Garcia et al. 2007). Neyrinck et al. (2011) studied the mechanism of action of wheat AX in HFD-induced obese mice. Upon dietary intervention with AX, adiposity, body weight gain, serum and hepatic cholesterol, and insulin resistance were all reduced significantly. Adipocyte size was significantly decreased and high levels of rumenic acid were detected in the white adipose tissue by gut bacterial metabolism of arabinoxylan. HFD feeding significantly altered the total bacterial clustering as indicated by DGGE fingerprints between control and HFD groups. There was a drop in *Roseburia* spp. and *Bacteroides–Prevotella* spp. numbers and an increase in the number of bifidobacteria among the HFD animals as revealed by qPCR analyses. Further, AX supplementation rectified the high fat (HF) diet-induced dysbiosis with a specific increase in *Bifidobacterium animalis* ssp. *lactis*. It also improved the gut barrier function through increased expression of tight-junction proteins and proglucagon and lowered the circulating inflammatory markers. Expression of genes associated with adipocyte differentiation, fatty acid uptake, fatty acid oxidation and inflammation, and key lipogenic enzyme activity was significantly decreased in the subcutaneous adipose tissue (Neyrinck et al. 2011). Changes associated in the human gut microbes upon AX intervention and its implications on obesity need to be studied.

15.2.1.3 Pectin   Pectins are found in plant cell walls as well as in the outer skin and rind of fruits and vegetables. Orange rind contains 30% pectin, apple peels contain 15% pectin, and onion skin contains 12% pectin, respectively. Pectins are building blocks of galacturonic acid interspersed with rhamnose units and are branched with chains of pentose and hexose units (Ridley et al. 2001). Soluble in hot water and forming gels on cooling, pectin can therefore be used as gelling and thickening agents in the food industry. Pectin lowers cholesterol as it binds to the cholesterol and bile acids in the gut and promotes their excretion (Mudgil and Barak 2013). Pectin was found to significantly delay gastric emptying time and increased satiety; however, postprandial release of cholecystokinin and pancreatic polypeptide was not modified (Di Lorenzo et al. 1988, Sanaka et al. 2007). Sánchez et al. (2008) reported that methoxylated apple pectin decreased body weight, total cholesterol, and triacylglycerols in Zucker fatty rats. Therefore, pectin incorporation in the diet may induce satiety and delay gastric emptying and hence be useful as an adjuvant in the treatment of overeating disorders.

15.2.1.4 Inulin Fructans are the nondigestible polymers composed of fructose residues with or without a terminal glucose moiety. Fructans are classified into short-chain-length fructans, called *fructooligosaccharides*, longer-chain-length fructans with β-(2 → 1) linkages, called *inulins*, fructans with β-(2 → 6) linkages, called *levans*, and fructans containing both linkages, called *graminans* (Tungland and Meyer, 2002). Inulins are composed of β-(2 → 1)-linked fructose residues and are produced and stored as reserve carbohydrates by various dicotyledonous plants. Inulin-type fructans (ITF) are naturally distributed in onion, banana, chicory, and artichokes; they promote gut health, ameliorate plasma lipid profiles, and enhance mineral absorption (Han et al. 2013; Kelly 2008). Welch et al. (2008) found that ITF enhance satiety, decrease energy intake, and regulate body weight in human and animal studies. In another study, inulin supplementation in the diet reduced liver and abdominal fat weight, whereas cellulose supplementation decreased feed intake, abdominal fat, and BW compared to control in hens (Mohiti-Asli et al. 2012). ITF treatment (0.2 g/day per mouse) blunted the HF diet-induced accumulation of large adipocytes and decreased PPARγ-activated differentiation factors and overexpression of GPR43 in the subcutaneous adipose tissue. ITF modulated the gut microbiota through increased bifidobacteria at the expense of *Roseburia* spp. and *Clostridium* cluster XIVa (Dewulf et al. 2011).

In a double-blind placebo-controlled study, Dewulf et al. (2012) observed that the intervention with ITF in obese women decreased the fat mass, plasma lactate, and phosphatidylcholine levels. ITF also suppressed the number of pathobionts and significantly increased the numbers of *Bifidobacteria* and *Faecalibacterium prausnitzii* with decreased circulatory LPS levels (Dewulf et al. 2012).

15.2.1.5 Fucoidan Fucoidans are polysaccharides extracted from brown algae and have been shown to exert various health benefits (Vo and Kim 2013). They have been isolated from brown algae, *Cladosiphon okamuranus*, *Fucus vesisulosus*, and the sporophyll of *Undaria pinnatifida*, and have shown *in vitro* and *in vivo* antiadipogenic efficacy (Han and Gushiken 2004, Kim et al. 2009, 2012, Park et al. 2011). Fucoidans are acidic and sulfated polymers of L-fucose in combination with xylose, galactose, and mannose. The type I chains contain the repeating α-L-fucopyranose moieties linked by the 1 → 3 glycosidic bond while in type II, the α-L-fucopyranose moieties are linked by alternating 1 → 3 and $1 \rightarrow 4$ glycosidic bonds. Sulfation occurs at the C2, C3, and C4 positions (Holtkamp et al. 2009).

Han and Gushiken (2004) observed that fucoidan from *Cladosiphon okamuranus* tokida (Okinawamozuku) could inhibit the pancreatic lipase activity *in vitro* and plasma triacylglycerol levels in rats at a dose of 250 mg/kg of the body weight. This indicated that fucoidan may inhibit the intestinal absorption of dietary fat by inhibiting its hydrolysis. Further, it has been shown that feeding 30, 50, or 100 g/kg fucoidan to high-fat-diet-induced obese mice prevented the body and parametrial adipose tissue weight with a significant reduction in hepatic triacylyglycerol contents. In another study, Kim et al. (2009) showed that fucoidan could inhibit adipocyte differentiation through the down-regulation of the expression of aP2, ACC, and PPARγ. Fucoidans promoted lipolysis by enhancing the expression of lipases and caused a reduction in lipid accumulation and glucose uptake into the adipocytes (Park et al. 2011). It significantly decreased the expression of PPARγ, C/EBPα, ap2, and inflammation-related genes. Kim and Lee (2012) showed a significant reduction in the lipid accumulation and generation of reactive oxygen species in adipocytes. Supplementation of 1% or 2% of fucoidan in the high-fat diet had significantly decreased the body weight gain, food efficiency ratio, and relative liver and epididymal fat mass in mice. Triglyceride, total cholesterol, and low-density lipoprotein levels in the plasma were significantly decreased and liver steatosis was significantly improved. Fucoidan supplementation down-regulated the expression of epididymal adipose tissue-associated genes such as PPARγ, FABP, and acetyl-CoA carboxylase (Kim et al. 2013). Jeong et al. (2013) studied the effect of low-molecular-weight fucoidan (LMWF) using obese diabetic mice (leptin receptor-deficient db/db mice) and the mechanisms involved in endoplasmic reticulum (ER) stress-responsive skeletal muscle cells (L6 myotubes). LMWF significantly decreased the body weight parameters by decreasing the lipid, glucose, triglyceride, cholesterol, and low-density lipoprotein levels in the serum. The ER stressor greatly decreased the phosphorylation levels of AMPK and Akt with a marked reduction in glucose uptake and fatty acid oxidation. In L6 myotubes, LMWF markedly reduced the ER stress-induced upregulation of the mammalian target of the rapamycin–p70S61 kinase network and improved the action of insulin via AMPK stimulation. AMPK activation by LMWF suggests that controlling the ER stress-dependent pathway by LMWF could be a potential therapeutic strategy for ameliorating ER stress-mediated metabolic dysfunctions. In addition to antiobesity efficacy, fucoidans have been shown to be beneficial as they have anticoagulant, anticancer, antioxidant, antiallergic, anti-inflammatory, and antiviral activities. Owing to the innumerable biological activities and health benefit effects, extensive studies of fucoidans in clinical studies will discover novel biological properties and their application in pharmaceutical, nutraceutical, cosmeceutical, and functional food industries.

15.2.1.6 β-Glucan β-Glucans are a heterogeneous group of nonstarch polysaccharides consisting of glucose polymers linked by a β-glycosidic bond. β-Glucans exhibit variations in terms of the frequency and length of branching, degree of branching, molecular weight, polymer charge, and/or solution conformation (random coil or triple or single helix), and solubility. These factors play a significant role and impart different biological activities. The structure of β-glucan depends on both the source and the method of isolation. Prokaryotes and some eukaryotes consist of the simplest glucan, which is linear and unbranched β-(1 → 3)-D-glucan, whereas nonlignified cell walls of cereal grains, barley, oats, or wheat consist of linear β-(1 → 3;1 → 4)-D-glucans. Yeast, fungi, and algae consist of glucans with β-(1 → 4;1 → 6) or β-(1 → 3;1 → 6) branches. Some cyclic and (1 → 3;1 → 6) β-glucans have been isolated from various bacteria. Glucans act as signal molecules and play an important role in plant–microbe interactions (El Khoury et al. 2012).

The β-linkages in the β-glucan make them nondigestible by escaping the human digestive enzymes. However, they are highly fermentable in the cecum and colon by the gut microbial consortia. A maximum growth rate and cell proliferation rate of human intestinal bacteria with maximum lactic acid productions have been reported with β-glucans (Kedia et al. 2008). Among the different fibers, the health benefits of β-glucans have been most extensively studied and the health claims with β-glucan-containing foods have been allowed in countries such as Canada, the United States, Sweden, Finland, and the United Kingdom (Ripsin et al. 1992).

β-Glucans were found to be the most effective against infectious diseases and cancer due to their immunostimulation property (Brown and Gordon 2003, Daou and Zhang 2012, Estrada et al. 1997). However, their immunological potency varies with the molecular mass, solution conformation, backbone structure, degree of branching, as well as the cell type that is targeted (Sonck et al. 2010).

In a randomized study, 14 healthy volunteers were fed with isocaloric breakfasts containing 3% β-glucan-enriched bread (βGB) or a control bread (CB). βGB showed a significantly higher reduction of hunger and increase of fullness and satiety than CB, a 19% reduction of energy intake, a 23% lower plasma ghrelin, and a 16% higher total of PYY. Glucose response was also attenuated by βGB versus CB (Vitaglione et al. 2009).

In a study conducted by Peng et al. (2013), whole oat (0.04 g β-glucan/g) supplementation did not affect appetite. However, it significantly reduced body weight, fat, and food efficiency and lowered serum glucose, free fatty acids, triacylglycerols, cholesterol, and low-density lipoprotein-cholesterol/high-density lipoprotein-cholesterol in HFD-induced obese rats. Liver triacylglycerols and cholesterol, as well as fatty acid synthase, glycerol 3-phosphate acyltransferase and hydroxymethylglutaryl-CoA reductase activities, were significantly reduced with 30% oat supplementation. Expressions of oxidation markers PPARα, CPT-1, and phosphorylated-AMPK were stimulated upon supplementation with 15% and 30% (Peng et al. 2013).

15.2.1.7 Gum Arabic GA is a complex polysaccharide indigestible by both humans and animals. GA, derived from exudates of *Acacia senegal* or *Acacia seyal* trees, consists of a mixture of polysaccharides (major component) plus oligosaccharides and glycoproteins (Babiker et al. 2012). Its composition varies with the source, climate, and soil. The U.S. Food and Drug Administration (FDA) has approved GA since the 1970s (Anderson 1986). In a randomized, placebo-controlled, double-blind trial, Babiker et al. (2012) evaluated the effect of GA on BMI and body fat percentage on healthy females. Volunteers were divided into test and placebo groups of 60 each. The test group received 30 g/day of GA, whereas the placebo group received 1 g/day of pectin for 6 weeks. The GA-fed group showed a significant reduction in BMI and body fat percentage as compared to the placebo. GA ingestion caused a significant reduction in BMI and body fat percentage among healthy adult females. These results showed that GA could be exploited for the prevention or treatment of obesity and for the development of novel food products containing GA.

15.3 Conclusion

The above discussions suggest that DFs lower the body fat and body weight and modulate the gut microflora through prebiotic action. Other beneficial effects include improved immune functions (more anti-inflammatory markers and less proinflammatory markers), gut barrier function, regulation of gut hormones (increases satiety), and alteration of gene expression in liver and adipose tissues. SCFA, especially butyrate, generated due to colonic fermentation modulates the host's health by stimulating immune regulators, modulating several diseases, and also epigenetically regulating gene expression. Hence, careful dietary manipulation of gut-associated microflora should be a top priority for the prevention or management of obesity and comorbidities. Further research should be channeled to identify novel DFs, determine the optimal levels of supplementation of a single fiber or a combination of different fibers in diets, and identify their role in modulating gut microbes and their interaction with host genes targeting specific lifestyle disorders. The knowledge thus obtained would be useful in the formulation and development of new functional food products with health-enhancing characteristics.

References

Al-Lahham, S. H., H. Roelofsen, M. Priebe et al. 2010. Regulation of adipokine production in human adipose tissue by propionic acid. *Eur J Clin Invest* 40:401–7.

Anderson, D. M. 1986. Evidence for the safety of gum arabic (*Acacia senegal* (L.) Willd.) as a food additive—A brief review. *Food Addit Contam* 3:225–30.

Andersson. R. and P. Aman. 2001. Cereal arabinoxylans: Occurrence, structure and properties. In: *Advanced Dietary Fiber Technology*, eds. B. V. McCleary, and L. Prosky. pp. 301–14. Oxford: Blackwell Science Ltd.

Anderson, J. W., P. Baird, R. H. Davis Jr. et al. 2009. Health benefits of dietary fiber. *Nutr Rev* 67:188–205.

Arora, T., R. Sharma, and G. Frost. 2011. Propionate. Anti-obesity and satiety enhancing factor? *Appetite* 56:511–5.

Aziz, A. A., L. S. Kenny, B. Goulet, and S. Abdel-Aal. 2009. Dietary starch type affects body weight and glycemic control in freely fed but not energy-restricted obese rats. *J Nutr* 139:1881–9.

Babiker, R., T. H. Merghani, K. Elmusharaf, R. M. Badi, F. Lang, and A. M. Saeed. 2012. Effects of gum arabic ingestion on body mass index and body fat percentage in healthy adult females: Two-arm randomized, placebo controlled double-blind trial. *Nutr J* 11:111. doi: 10.1186/1475-2891-11-111.

Baboota, R. K., M. Bishnoi, P. Ambalam et al. 2013. Functional food ingredients for the management of obesity and associated co-morbidities—A review. *J Func Foods* 5:997–1012.

Baixauli, R., A. Salvador, S. Martinez-Cervera, and S. M. Fiszman. 2008. Distinctive sensory features introduced by resistant starch in baked products. *Food Sci Technol* 41:1927–33.

Barron, C., A. Surget, and X. Rouau. 2007. Relative amounts of tissues in mature wheat (*Triticum aestivum* L.) grain and their carbohydrate and phenolic acid composition. *J Cereal Sci* 45:88–96.

Belobrajdic, D. P., R. A. King, C. T. Christophersen, and A. R. Bird. 2012. Dietary resistant starch dose-dependently reduces adiposity in obesity-prone and obesity-resistant male rats. *Nutr Metab (Lond)* 9:93.

Bergman, E. N. 1990. Energy contributions of volatile fatty acids from the gastrointestinal tract in various species. *Physiol Rev* 70:567–90.

Birkett, A., J. Muir, J. Phillips, G. Jones, and K. O'Dea. 1996. Resistant starch lowers fecal concentrations of ammonia and phenols in humans. *Am J Clin Nutr* 63:766–72.

Brahe, L. K., A. Astrup, and L. H. Larsen. 2013. Is butyrate the link between diet, intestinal microbiota and obesity-related metabolic diseases? *Obes Rev* 14:950–59.

Brown, G. D. and S. Gordon. 2003. Fungal β-glucans and mammalian immunity. *Immunity* 19:311–5.

Canani, R. B., M. Di Costanzo, and L. Leone. 2012. The epigenetic effects of butyrate: Potential therapeutic implications for clinical practice. *Clin Epigenetics* 4:4.

Cani, P. D., J. Amar, M. A. Iglesias et al. 2007. Metabolic endotoxemia initiates obesity and insulin resistance. *Diabetes* 56:1761–72.

Carter, R., A. Mouralidarane, S. Ray, J. Soeda, and J. Oben. 2012. Recent advancements in drug treatment of obesity. *Clin Med* 12:456–60.

Charalampopoulos, D., R. Wang, S. S. Pandiella, and C. Webb. 2002. Application of cereals and cereal components in functional foods: A review. *Int J Food Microbiol* 79:131–41.

Chatterjee, P. 2002. India sees parallel rise in malnutrition and obesity. *Lancet* 360:1948.

Choudhary, M. and K. Grover. 2012. Development of functional food products in relation to obesity. *Funct Foods Health Dis* 2:188–97.

Cleemput, G., S. P. Roels, M. Vanoort et al. 1993. Heterogeneity in the structure of water soluble arabinoxylans in European wheat flours of variable bread-making quality. *Cereal Chem* 70:324–9.

Commission of the European Communities. 2008. Draft commission directive: Amending directive 90/496/EEC. http://www.food.gov.uk/multimedia/pdfs/consultation/cwd (accessed July 15, 2013).

Cotillard, A., S. P. Kennedy, L. C. Kong et al. 2013. Dietary intervention impact on gut microbial gene richness. *Nature* 500:585–8.

Cummings, J. H. and A. M. Stephen. 2007. Carbohydrate terminology and classification. *Eur J Clin Nutr* 61:S5–S18.

Daou, C. and H. Zhang. 2012. Oat beta glucan: Its role in health promotion and prevention of diseases. *Comp Rev Food Sci Food Safety* 11:355–65.

David, J. A. J. and W. C. K. Cyril. 2000. Resistant starches. *Curr Opin Gastroenterol* 16:178–83.

Delzenne, N. M., A. M. Neyrinck, F. Bäckhed, and P. D. Cani. 2011. Targeting gut microbiota in obesity: Effects of prebiotics and probiotics. *Nat Rev Endocrinol* 7:639–46.

Dewulf, E. M., P. D. Cani, A. M. Neyrinck et al. 2011. Inulin-type fructans with prebiotic properties counteract GPR43 overexpression and PPARγ-related adipogenesis in the white adipose tissue of high-fat diet-fed mice. *J Nutr Biochem* 22:712–22.

Dewulf, E. M., P. D. Cani, S. P. Claus et al. 2012. Insight into the prebiotic concept: Lessons from an exploratory, double blind intervention study with inulin-type fructans in obese women. *Gut* 62:1112–21.

Di Lorenzo, C., C. M. Williams, F. Hajnal, and J. E. Valenzuela. 1988. Pectin delays gastric emptying and increases satiety in obese subjects. *Gastroenterology* 95:1211–5.

Ebringerova, A. and T. Heinze. 2000. Xylan and xylan derivatives-biopolymers with valuable properties, 1—Naturally occurring xylans structures, isolation procedures and properties. *Macromol Rapid Commun* 21:542–56.

El Khoury, D., C. Cuda, B. L. Luhovyy, and G. H. Anderson. 2012. Beta glucan: Health benefits in obesity and metabolic syndrome. *J Nutr Metab* 2012:851362. doi: 10.1155/2012/851362.

Englyst, K. N. and H. N. Englyst. 2005. Carbohydrate bioavailability. *Brit J Nutr* 94:1–11.

Estrada, A., C. H. Yun, A. Van Kessel, B. Li, S. Hauta, and B. Laarveld. 1997. Immunomodulatory activities of oat beta-glucan *in vitro* and *in vivo*. *Microbiol Immunol* 41:991–8.

Everard, A., C. Belzer, L. Geurts et al. 2013. Cross-talk between Akkermansia muciniphila and intestinal epithelium controls diet-induced obesity. *PNAS* 110: 9066–71.

Faurot, A. L., L. Saulnier, S. Berot et al. 1995. Large scale isolation of water soluble and insoluble pentosans from wheat flour. *Lab Wiss Tech* 28:436–44.

FDA News Release. 2012. http://www.fda.gov/NewsEvents/Newsroom/Press Announcements/ucm309993.htm http://www.fda.gov/NewsEvents/Newsroom/PressAnnouncements/ucm312468.htm (accessed September 6, 2013).

Fei, N. and L. Zhao. 2013. An opportunistic pathogen isolated from the gut of an obese human causes obesity in germfree mice. *Int Soc Microbial Ecol* 7:880–4.

Férnandez-López, J., M. Viuda-Martos, E. Sendra, E. Sayas-Barberá, C. Navarro, and J. A. Perez-Alvarez. 2007. Orange fibre as potential functional ingredient for dry-cured sausages. *Eur Food Res Technol* 226:1–6.

Fincher, G. B. and B. A. Stone. 1974. A water soluble arabinogalactan-peptide from wheat endosperm. *Aus J Biol Sci* 27:117–32.

Fincher G. B. and B. A. Stone 1986. Cell walls and their components in cereal grain technology. In: *Advances in Cereal Science and Technology*, ed. Y. Pomeranz. pp. 207–295. St Paul: American Association of Cereal Chemists Inc.

Fuentes-Zaragoza, E., M. J. Riquelme-Navarrete, E. Sánchez-Zapata, and J. A. Pérez-Álvarez. 2010. Resistant starch as functional ingredient: A review. *Food Res Int* 43:931–42.

Garcia, A. L., B. Otto, S. C. Reich et al. 2007. Arabinoxylan consumption decreases postprandial serum glucose, serum insulin and plasma total ghrelin response in subjects with impaired glucose tolerance. *Eur J Clin Nutr* 61:334–41.

González-Castejón, M. and A. Rodriguez-Casado. 2011. Dietary phytochemicals and their potential effects on obesity: A review. *Pharmacol Res* 64:438–55.

Gregor, M. F. and G. S. Hotamisligil. 2007. Thematic review series: Adipocyte biology. Adipocyte stress: The endoplasmic reticulum and metabolic disease. *J Lip Res* 48:1905–14.

Gruppen, H., F. J. M. Kormelink, and A. G. J. Voragen. 1993. Water unextractable cell wall materials from wheat flour, 3-A structural model for arabinoxylans. *J Cereal Sci* 18:111–28.

Han, K. H., H. Tsuchihira, Y. Nakamura et al. 2013. Inulin type fructans with different degrees of polymerization improve lipid metabolism but not glucose metabolism in rats fed a high fat diet under energy restriction. *Dig Dis Sci* 58:2177–86.

Han, L. K., K. Gushiken, and H. Okuda. 2004. Anti-obesity effects of fucoidan prepared from *Cladosiphon okamuranus tokida* (Okinawamozuku). *Jap J Const Med* 66:55–60.

Higgins, J. A., M. R. Jackman, I. L. Brown et al. 2011. Resistant starch and exercise independently attenuate weight regain on a high fat diet in a rat model of obesity. *Nutr Metab* (Lond) 8:49.

Holtkamp, A. D., S. Kelly, R. Ulber, and S. Lang. 2009. Fucoidans and fucoidanases-focus on techniques for molecular structure elucidation and modification of marine polysaccharides. *Appl Microbiol Biotechnol* 82:1–11.

Izydorczyk, M. S. and C. G. Biliaderis. 1995. Cereal arabinoxylans: Advances in structure and physicochemical properties. *Carbohydr Polym* 28:33–48.

Izydorczyk, M. S., C. G. Biliaderis, and W. Bushuk. 1991. Comparison of structures and comparison of water soluble pentosans from different wheat varieties. *Cereal Chem* 68:139–44.

Jenkins, D. J. and C. W. Kendall. 2000. Resistant starches. *Curr Opin Gastroenterol* 16:178–83.

Jeong, Y. T., Y. D. Kim, Y. M. Jung et al. 2013. Low molecular weight fucoidan improves endoplasmic reticulum stress-reduced insulin sensitivity through AMP-activated protein kinase activation in L6 myotubes and restores lipid homeostasis in a mouse model of type 2 diabetes. *Mol Pharmacol* 84:147–57.

Kedia, G., J. A. V´azquez, and S. S. Pandiella. 2008. Evaluation of the fermentability of oat fractions obtained by debranning using lactic acid bacteria. *J Appl Microbiol* 105:1227–37.

Kelly, G. 2008. Inulin type prebiotics: A Review. *Alt Med Rev* 13:315–29.

Kennett, G. A. and P. G. Clifton. 2010. New approaches to the pharmacological treatment of obesity: Can they break through the efficacy barrier? *Pharmacol Biochem Behavior* 97:63–83.

Kim, K. J. and B. Y. Lee. 2012. Fucoidan from the sporophyll of *Undaria pinnatifida* suppresses adipocyte differentiation by inhibition of inflammation-related cytokines in 3T3-L1 cells. *Nutr Res* 32:439–47.

Kim, M. J., U. J. Chang, and J. S. Lee. 2009. Inhibitory effects of fucoidan in 3T3-L1 adipocyte differentiation. *Marine Biotechnol* (NY) 11:557–62.

Kim, M. J., J. Jeon, and J. S. Lee. 2013. Fucoidan prevents high-fat diet-induced obesity in animals by suppression of fat accumulation. *Phytother Res* 28:137–43.

Le Chatelier, E., T. Nielsen, J. Qin et al. 2013. Richness of human gut microbiome correlates with metabolic markers. *Nature* 500:541–6.

Maes, C. and J. A. Delcour. 2002. Structural characterization of water extractable and unextractable arabinoxylans in wheat bran. *J Cereal Sci* 35:315–26.

Maslowski, K. M., A. T. Vieira, A. Ng et al. 2009. Regulation of inflammatory responses by gut microbiota and chemoattractant receptor GPR43. *Nature* 461:1282–6.

Meijer, K., P. de Vos, and M. G. Priebe. 2010. Butyrate and other short chain fatty acids as modulators of immunity: What relevance for health? *Curr Opin Clin Nutr Metab Care* 13:715–21.

Mohiti-Asli, M., M. Shivazad, M. Zaghari, S. Aminzadeh, M. Rezaian, and G. G. Mateos. 2012. Dietary fibers and crude protein content alleviate hepatic fat deposition and obesity in broiler breeder hens. *Poultry Sci* 91:3107–14.

Mudgil, D. and S. Barak. 2013. Composition, properties and health benefits of indigestible carbohydrate polymers as dietary fiber: A review. *Int J Biol Macromol* 61:1–6.

Neyrinck, A. M., S. Possemiers, C. Druart et al. 2011. Prebiotic effects of wheat arabinoxylan related to the increase in *Bifidobacteria*, *Roseburia* and *Bacteroides/Prevotella* in diet induced obese mice. *PLoS One* 6:e20944.

NFHS-3. 2007. *National Health Survey 3*. International Institute of Population Sciences, Mumbai.

Ouchi, N., J. L. Parker, J. J. Lugus, and K. Walsh. 2011. Adipokines in inflammation and metabolic disease. *Nat Rev Immunol* 11:85–97.

Park, M. K., U. Jung, and C. Roh. 2011. Fucoidan from marine brown algae inhibits lipid accumulation. *Marine Drugs* 9:1359–67.

Peng, C. H., H. C. Chang, M. Y. Yang, C. N. Huang, S. J. Wang, and C. J. Wang. 2013. Oat attenuate non-alcoholic fatty liver and obesity via inhibiting lipogenesis in high fat-fed rat. *J Funct Foods* 5:53–61.

Phillips, J., J. G. Muir, A. Birkett et al. 1995. Effect of resistant starch on fecal bulk and fermentation-dependent events in humans. *Am J Clin Nutr* 62:121–30.

Rao, M. V. S. S. T. S. and G. Muralikrishna. 2001. Non-starch polysaccharides and bound phenolic acids from native and malted finger millet (Ragi, *Eleusine coracana*, Indaf–15). *Food Chem* 72:187–92.

Ridley, B. L., M. A. O'Neill, and D. Mohnen. 2001. Pectins: Structure, biosynthesis, and oligogalacturonide-related signaling. *Phytochem* 57:929–67.

Ripsin, C. M., J. M. Keenan, D. R Jacobs et al. 1992. Oat products and lipid lowering: A meta-analysis. *J Am Med Assoc* 267:3317–25.

Rosen, E. D. and O. A. Mac Dougald. 2006. Adipocyte differentiation from the inside out. *Nat Rev Mol Cell Biol.* 7:885–96.

Sanaka, M., T. Yamamoto, H. Anjiki, K. Nagasawa, and Y. Kuyama. 2007. Effects of agar and pectin on gastric emptying and post-prandial glycaemic profiles in healthy human volunteers. *Clin Exp Pharmacol Physiol* 34:1151–5.

Sánchez, D., B. Muguerza, L. Moulay, R. Hernández, M. Miguel, and A. Aleixandre. 2008. Highly methoxylated pectin improves insulin resistance and other cardio-metabolic risk factors in Zucker fatty rats. *J Agri Food Chem* 56:3574–81.

Sanz, T., A. Salvador, R. Baixauli, and S. M. Fiszman. 2009. Evaluation of four types of resistant starch in muffins. II. Effects in texture, colour and consumer response. *Eur Food Res Technol* 229:197–204.

Segata, N., D. Boernigen, T. L. Tickle, X. C. Morgan, W. S. Garrett, and C. Huttenhower. 2013. Computational metaòmics for microbial community studies. *Mol Sys Biol* 9:666.

Serrano, José C. E., A. Cassanyé, and M. Portero-Otin. 2012. Trends in functional food against obesity. In: *Scientific, Health and Social Aspects of the Food Industry*, ed. Dr. Benjamin Valdez, ISBN: 978-953-307-916-5, InTech, Available from: http://www.intechopen.com/books/scientific-health-and-social-aspects-ofthe-food-industry/trends-in-functional-food-against-obesity (accessed August 31, 2013).

Slavin, J. 2013. Fiber and prebiotics: Mechanisms and health benefits. *Nutrients* 5:1417–35.

Sonck, E., E. Stuyven, B. Goddeeris, and E. Cox. 2010. The effect of β-glucans on porcine leukocytes. *Vet Immun Immunopathol* 135:199–207.

Stephens, J. M. 2012. The fat controller: Adipocyte development. *PLOS Biol* 10:e1001436.

Tachon, S., J. Zhou, M. Keenan, R. Martin, and M. L. Marco. 2013. The intestinal microbiota in aged mice is modulated by dietary resistant starch and correlated with improvements in host responses. *FEMS Microbiol Ecol* 83:299–309.

Tharanathan, R. N. 2002. Food-derived carbohydrates: Structural complexity and functional diversity. *Crit Rev Biotechnol* 22:65–84.

The Human Microbiome Project Consortium. 2012. Structure, function and diversity of the healthy human microbiome. *Nature* 486:207–14.

Tilg H. and A. Kaser. 2011. Gut microbiome, obesity, and metabolic dysfunction. *J Clin Invest* 121:2126–32.

Toden, S., A. R. Bird, D. L. Topping, and M. A. Conlon. 2006. Resistant starch prevents colonic DNA damage induced by high dietary cooked red meat or casein in rats. *Cancer Biol Ther* 5:267–72.

Topping, D., B. H. Bajka, A. R. Bird et al. 2008. Resistant starches as a vehicle for delivering health benefits to the human large bowel. *Microb Ecol Health Dis* 20:103–8.

Topping, D. L., M. Fukushima, and A. R. Bird. 2003. Resistant starch as a prebiotic and synbiotic: State of the art. *Proc Nutr Soc* 62:171–6.

Tungland, B. C. and D. Meyer. 2002. Nondigestible oligo- and polysaccharides (dietary fiber): Their physiology and role in human health and food. *Comp Rev Food Sci Food Safety* 1:90–109.

Ulven, T. 2012. Short-chain free fatty acid receptors FFA2/GPR43 and FFA3/GPR41 as new potential therapeutic targets. *Front Endocrinol (Lausanne)* 3:111.

Vidrine, K., J. Ye, R. J. Martin et al. 2013. Resistant starch from high amylose maize (HAM-RS2) and dietary butyrate reduce abdominal fat by a different apparent mechanism. *Obesity* (Silver Spring) 22(2):344–8.

Vitaglione, P., R. B. Lumaga, A. Stanzione, L. Scalfi, and V. Fogliano. 2009. Beta glucan bread reduces energy intake and modifies plasma ghrelin and peptide YY concentrations in the short term. *Appetite* 53:338–44.

Vo, T. S. and S. K. Kim. 2013. Fucoidans as a natural bioactive ingredient for functional foods. *J Funct Foods* 5:16–27.

Weaver, G. A., J. A. Krause, T. L. Miller, and M. J. Wolin. 1992. Cornstarch fermentation by the colonic microbial community yields more butyrate than does cabbage fibre fermentation; cornstarch fermentation rates correlate negatively with methanogenesis. *Am J Clin Nutr* 55:70–7.

Welch, R. W., M. T. Kelly, A. M. Gallagher, J. M. Wallace, and M. B. E. Livingstone. 2008. The effects of inulin-type fructans on satiety and energy intake: Human studies. *Agro Food Industry Hi-Tech* 19:S4–S6.

Wong, J. M. W., R. De Souza, C. W. C. Kendall, A. Emam, and D. J. A. Jenkins. 2006. Colonic health: Fermentation and short chain fatty acids. *J Clin Gastroenterol* 40:235–43.

World Health Statistics. 2012. http://www.who.int/gho/publications/world_health_statostocs/WHS2012_IndicatorCompendium.pdf (accessed September 3, 2013).

Young, W., N. C. Roy, J. Lee et al. 2012. Changes in bowel microbiota induced by feeding weanlings resistant starch stimulate transcriptomic and physiological responses. *Appl Environ Microbiol* 78:6656–64.

CHAPTER 16

Fructooligosaccharides, Diet, and Cancer Prevention

Myths or Realities?

NOUREDDINE BENKEBLIA

Contents

16.1 Introduction   385
16.2 FOS and Fructans and Health Benefits   386
16.3 Prebiotic Effects   387
16.4 FOS, Fructans, and Cancer   389
        16.4.1 Cancer and Diet   389
16.5 Conclusions   392
Acknowledgments   393
References   393

16.1 Introduction

During the last century, a number of relevant scientific research data and population-based epidemiological studies demonstrated the role of diet in preventing and even controlling many noncommunicable diseases (NCDs) (Popkin 2006a). Moreover, specific dietary components that increase or decrease the probability of these diseases in individuals have also been identified.

On the other hand, rapid changes in diet and lifestyles, consequent to industrialization, urbanization, economic development, and market globalization, have taken place over the past decades, and these changes significantly impacted the health and nutritional status (Kaput et al. 1994). Since the Second World War, standards of living have improved, and food availability has expanded and diversified and have impacted negatively in terms of inappropriate dietary patterns, and decreased physical activities associated with a sedentary lifestyle (Popkin 2006b). Because of these changes in dietary and lifestyle patterns, chronic NCDs, including obesity, diabetes mellitus, cardiovascular diseases (CVDs), hypertension and stroke, and many types of cancers, are increasing and these have become significant causes of death in both developing and newly developed countries (Forman and Bulwer 2006, Popkin et al. 2006, Reddy and Katan 2004, WHO 2003).

Considering the concepts of "let food be your medicine" (*Hippocrates*) and prevention is a more effective strategy than treatment of NCDs diseases, specific nutrients have shown real projective actions against these diseases. These nutrients are found in many foods called "functional foods." Functional foods refer to any food that contains significant amounts of bioactive components, often called "phytochemicals" because they are mainly of plants origin," and they may provide desirable health benefits beyond basic nutrition and play important roles in the prevention of chronic diseases. However, the key question is whether any of these purified bioactive components has the same health benefit, as does the whole food or mixture of foods in which the phytochemical is present. However, the additive and synergistic effects of phytochemicals are responsible for their potent health benefits, and these preventive actions can be attributed to their complex mixture in whole foods (Craig 1997, Craig and Beck 1999, Dillard and German 2000, Lila and Raskin 2005, Liu 2003).

16.2 FOS and Fructans and Health Benefits

Fructooligosaccharides (FOS), as fructan molecules, have a history of more than 150 years. Some review articles have reported on some historical aspects including a little on the general background on fructan research (Meier and Reid 1982, Pollock and Cairns 1991, Pontis and Del Campillo 1985). First and prior to the contemporary science of fructans, ancient peoples used fructan-containing plants as food, feed, or medicine.

Generally, it is recommended to eat an average of 400 g of fruits and vegetables per day, and scientific advances linking diet and health have fostered unprecedented attention on the role of nutrition in health promotion and disease prevention. This is unfortunate as considerable evidence indicates that adequate fruits and vegetables consumption has a role in preventing many chronic diseases, including heart diseases, stroke, and several cancers (Appel et al. 1997, Block et al. 1992, Cherbut 2002, Flamm et al. 2001, Hertog et al. 1996, Johnsen et al. 2003, Joshipura et al. 1999, Ness and Powles 1997, Olsen and Gudmand-Heyer 2000, WCRF-AICR 2013). Because of the great interest of consumers in diet food and also because FOS are not yet being marketed widely throughout the world as food ingredients or additives, cultivated crops, such as banana, wheat, barley, asparagus, and Jerusalem artichoke remain the main source of FOS (Mitsuoka 1987, Spiegel 1994, Tashiro et al. 1992). In *Allium* species, onion and garlic are considered as a major source of FOS since FOS constitute 25–35% of total nonstructural carbohydrate (Darbyshire and Steer 1990), while leek and shallot are a minor source (Campbell et al. 1997a, Van Loo et al. 1995). Thus, FOS are presently produced industrially and used as food ingredients, while in Japan they are considered as food and are found in more than 500 food products, including soft drinks, cookies, cereals, and candies, resulting in significant daily consumption (Spiegel 1994, Tomomatsu 1994).

In fact, the use of FOS in the human diet has increased since the initial commercial production of a specific oligofructan (Neosugar®) in Japan in 1983. The benefits of adding FOS to the human diet were first reported by the NSG (Neosugar Study Group) at a series of conferences held in Japan to highlight research with Neosugar in 1982, 1983, and 1984. The reports given have linked biochemical–nutritional–health changes in humans resulting from eating Neosugar, and these results were confirmed later by Buddington et al. (1996). Although this history started with Neosugar, it has become evident that many of the conclusions could be extended to other FOS (Farnworth 1993). FOS and fructans have numerous physiological actions (Scheppach 2001), and Tomomatsu (1994) enumerated health benefits attributed to oligosaccharides:

- Encourage proliferation of bifidobacteria and reduce detrimental bacteria
- Reduce toxic metabolites and detrimental enzymes
- Prevent pathogenic and autogenous diarrhea
- Prevent constipation
- Protect liver function
- Reduce serum cholesterol
- Reduce blood pressure
- Have an anticancer effect
- Produce nutrients

Thus, these physiological effects are the basis for associating FOS intake with reduced diseases and prevention. However, only some predominant effects will be developed in the section below (see Section 16.3).

16.3 Prebiotic Effects

The large bowel is by far the most colonized region of the gastrointestinal tract, with ca 10^{12} bacteria per gram of gut content. Through the fermentation process, colonic bacteria, most of which are anaerobes, produce a wide variety of compounds that may affect gut as well as systemic physiology. Thus, fermentation of carbohydrates reaching the large bowel produces short-chain carboxylic acids—mainly acetate, propionate, and butyrate—and lactate, which allow the host to salvage part of the energy of nondigestible oligosaccharides, and which may also play a role in regulating both cell division and cellular metabolism. In addition to their selective effects on bifidobacteria and lactobacilli, FOS influence many aspects of bowel function through fermentation, and are mildly laxative (Cummings 1997). Indeed, FOS constitute a carbon source for microbial flora of bowel and the ability of bifidobacteria to utilize FOS was well demonstrated (Biedrzycka and Bielecka 2004, Bouhnik et al. 2004, Gibson and Roberfroid 1995, Marx et al. 2000, Mitsuoka 1996, Muramatsu et al. 1994). These works also reported that the majority of *Bifidobacterium* strains fermented all FOS and even low polymerized inulin. Biedrzycka and Bielecka (2004) claimed that the results of *in vitro* studies indicate the specificity of *Bifidobacterium* except *B. bifidum* to utilize short-chain FOS and oligofructose (OF), but not HP-inulin. However, according to van Laere et al. (1997), the main factors affecting the susceptibility of FOS to fermentation are chemical structure, the degree of polymerization, and possible linear or branched structure, as well as solubility in water. Generally, FOS with short chain length, unbranched nature, and high solubility in water are well and preferentially fermented. Nevertheless, discrepancies in the capability of different *Bifidobacterium* species to metabolize FOS may be due to the differences in the expression of fructan-hydrolyzing enzymes, since the latter have not been extensively investigated (see also Chapter 4) (Figure 16.1).

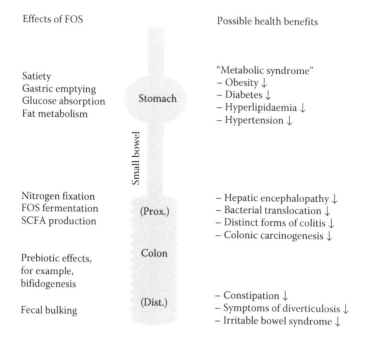

Figure 16.1 Potential physiological effects of FOS (left column) and possibly related health benefits (right column). (SCFA, short-chain fatty acids) (From Scheppach, W., H. Luehrs, and T. Menzel. 2001. *Br J Nutr* 85(Suppl. 1):S23–30. With permission.)

16.4 FOS, Fructans, and Cancer

Initial research demonstrated that FOS have anticarcinogenic and tumor growth inhibitory effects (Taper 1998, Taper and Roberfroid 1999). However, the most surprising activity of FOS is the capacity to significantly reduce the number of metastases (Taper and Roberfroid 2000a,b). Moreover, FOS also have potential in cancer chemotherapy and have been shown to mitigate the therapeutic effects of all six investigated cytotoxic drugs representative of the different groups of cytotoxic drugs, classically used in human cancer treatment (Taper and Roberfroid 2002). Indeed, studies have demonstrated that risk factors for some cancers include both hereditary and environmental factors and dietary patterns, which represent controllable risk factors for the development of these cancers. For example, much attention was focused on a decrease in colon cancer risk through an increased intake in dietary fiber; recently, this has included interest in the consumption of FOS (Brady et al. 2000). However, because factors involved in the initiation and promotion of colon cancer might be separated in time from actual tumor development, it is difficult to choose "outcomes" or "end points" that are definitive indicators of efficacy of FOS, since studies that have explored the cause–effect relationship directly have used animal models.

Beside these encouraging results regarding FOS and inulin in experimental animals, making the same recommendations to humans could most probably help to prevent some major cancers. Nevertheless, to justify claims of enhanced function or reduction in the risk of cancers, and other diseases as well, most of the available information must be confirmed in humans by means of relevant nutrition studies focusing on well-validated endpoints. Moreover, such studies will be of more value if they are based on sound mechanistic hypotheses (Roberfroid 2000).

16.4.1 Cancer and Diet

Colorectal cancer (CRC) and colon cancer are the third most common form of cancer, and the second cause of death in many developing countries, such as the United States. In recent years, scientific data suggest that the ingestion of probiotics (Jacobsen et al. 1999), prebiotics (fructans, FOS, and xylooligosaccharides [XOS]), or synbiotics (combinations of both) represents a novel new approach in the prevention of these types of diseases. Probiotics and prebiotics affect the intestinal microflora by promoting the growth of beneficial bacteria such as lactobacillus and bifidobacteria (Gibson and Wang 1994, Gibson and Roberfroid 1995, Kleessen et al. 2001), and inhibiting the levels of pathogenic microorganisms (Carmen et al. 2005, Makras and De Vuyst 2006). This approach has the potential to inhibit or retard the development and progression of neoplasia via mechanisms such as decreasing intestinal inflammation, enhancing immune function and antitumorigenic activity, and reduction in bacterial enzymes that hydrolyze precarcinogenic compounds such as β-glucuronidase. Therefore, probiotics and prebiotics have the potential to impact significantly on the development, progression, and treatment of CRC and may have a valuable role in cancer prevention (Geier et al. 2006).

16.4.1.1 Animal Studies   Several animal studies on the relationship between fructans and cancer are available. A daily intake of 50–100 g/kg of long-chain inulin and OF statistically significantly reduced preneoplastic lesions (Reddy et al. 1997, Rowland et al. 1998), while inulin significantly reduced the propagation phase of the carcinogen (Rowland et al. 1998), while 150 g OF or inulin/kg significantly reduced intramuscularly implanted tumor cell carcinoma (Taper et al. 1997). On the other hand, immune system stimulation and a significant reduction in the numbers of spontaneously developing tumors associated with the oral intake of OF were also observed (Perdigon et al. 1993, Pierre et al. 1997).

Recent publications reported on the scientific evidence from a large number of studies conducted over the last decade that examined the effects of garlic on CRC, where levels of evidence have been ranked from level I to level V, according to study designs (Ngo et al. 2007). One randomized controlled trial (RCT, level II) reported a statistically significant 29% reduction in both the size and number of colon adenomas in CRC patients taking aged garlic extract. Five of eight cases with control/cohort studies (level III) suggested a protective effect of high intake of raw/cooked garlic and two of eight of these studies suggested a protective effect for distal colon. A published meta-analysis (level III) of seven of these studies confirmed this inverse association, with a 30% reduction in relative risk. Eleven animal studies (level V) demonstrated a significant anticarcinogenic effect of garlic and/or its active constituents. On balance, there is consistent scientific evidence derived from RCT of animal studies reporting protective effects of garlic on CRC despite great heterogeneity of measures of intakes among human epidemiological studies.

The inhibitory effect of XOS and other FOS on precancerous colon lesions was also estimated and results showed that both XOS and FOS markedly reduced the number of aberrant crypt foci (ACF) in the colon, suggesting that XOS and FOS dietary supplementation may be beneficial to gastrointestinal health, and XOS were more effective than FOS (Hsu et al. 2004).

Similar and synergistic effect was observed when long-chain inulin or OF and bifidobacteria are administered simultaneously (Gallaher et al. 1996, Gallaher and Khil 1999), although the effect of other oligosaccharides in reducing colon cancer risk in carcinogen-treated rats is uncertain (Gallaher and Khil 1999).

Overall, synbiotics supplementation in carcinogen-treated rats primarily modulated immune function, coinciding with a reduced number of colon tumors, and inulin-based enriched with OF (100 g/kg per day) combined with synbiotics may contribute to the suppression of colon carcinogenesis by modulating the gut-associated lymphoid tissue (Roller et al. 2004). On the other hand, the growth of induced mammary tumor cell lines was significantly inhibited by supplementing the diet with OF (Taper and Roberfroid 1999).

More interestingly, the incorporation of inulin or OF in the basal diet of animals showed encouraging results by: (i) reducing the incidence of induced mammary tumors; (ii) inhibiting the growth of transplantable malignant tumors; (iii) decreasing the incidence of lung metastases of a malignant tumor implanted intramuscularly; (iv) significantly potentiating the effects of subtherapeutic doses of six cytotoxic drugs commonly utilized in human cancer treatment; and moreover (v) potentiating the effects of radiotherapy on the solid form of transplantable liver tumors (TLT) to a statistically much high level (Taper and Roberfroid 2000a, Taper and Roberfroid 2005).

From the review of the available experimental data, it is concluded that fat most probably has no modulating effect but that unbalanced diets rich in lipids could act as a positive modulator of chemically induced carcinogenesis by virtue of their capacity to cause a break in metabolic and proliferative homeostasis. Thus, vegetable carbohydrates and fibers as well as restriction in caloric intake could act as negative modulators of the same process because they could restore this homeostasis. It is thus supposed that to maintain dietary balance by increasing nondigestible carbohydrates and/or reducing calorie intake is the most effective way to negatively modulate chemically induced carcinogenesis in animals (Roberfroid 1991). Beside these encouraging results regarding FOS and inulin in experimental animals, however, to make the same recommendations to humans could most probably help prevent some major cancers.

16.4.1.2 Human Studies The effects of nutrition on tumor incidence and growth are a subject of priority interest (Williams and Dickinson 1990, Roberfroid 1991), and among the most frequently investigated dietary compounds, the nondigestible carbohydrates play a major role in nutritional prevention (Roberfroid 1991). FOS were used in various experimental models to study their cancer risk-reducing capacity. Initial research demonstrated that FOS have anticarcinogenic and tumor growth inhibitory effects (Taper et al. 1998, Taper and Roberfroid 1999). However, the most surprising activity of FOS is the capacity to significantly reduce the number of metastases (Taper and Roberfroid 2000a). Moreover, FOS also have potentiation of cancer chemotherapy and have been shown to potentiate the therapeutic effects of all six investigated cytotoxic drugs representatives of the different groups of cytotoxic drugs classically used in human cancer treatment.

FOS and fructans benefit the gastrointestinal tract via fermentation and the proliferation of desirable bacterial species, and promote the growth of bifidobacteria *in vivo* (Hidaka 1986, 1991). XOS are also used by several species of bifidobacteria (Okazaki et al. 1990), and the differences in the colonic microflora have been considered an important contributing factor to the incidence of colon cancer. Recent studies suggest that bifidobacteria are associated with the suppression of potentially pathogenic and putrefactive bacteria in adults (Hidaka 1986, 1991, Homma 1988, Reddy et al. 1997), and the incidence of colon cancer and the population of *Clostridium perfringens* decrease as the population of bifidobacteria increases (Kubota 1990). Jenkins et al. (1999) reported that inulin and OF markedly increase the colonic bifidobacteria population, thus modifying the intestinal microflora. In fact, bifidobacteria have the ability to suppress some pathogenic bacteria, such as *Escherichia coli*, because of their capacity to metabolize oligo- and polysaccharides, while other intestinal bacteria cannot (Yazawa et al. 1978).

To date, the exact chemopreventive effects of FOS and fructans still remain unclear and additional animal and human studies are required to define the exact role of these dietary fibers and the short-chain fatty acid (SCFA) products of their fermentation, for example, acetate, propionate, and butyrate, in reducing the risk of colon cancer. Therefore, FOS, OF, and XOS are considered beneficial to gastrointestinal health by promoting bifidobacteria growth, and consequently supplying SCFAs that in their turn lower the colonic pH (Campbell et al. 1997b).

The suggested hypothesis is that indigestible dietary fibers are fermented by colonic bacteria, resulting mainly in the formation of SCFA, which are recognized for their potential to act on secondary chemoprevention by slowing growth and activating apoptosis in colon cancer cells. More clearly, butyrate activates the GSTs (glutathione-S-transferases), and functional consequences of this activation include a reduction of DNA damage caused by carcinogens such as hydrogen peroxide or 4-hydroxynonenal (HNE) in butyrate-treated colon cells (Williams and Dickinson 1990, Scharlau et al. 2009).

However, all these interesting findings suggest that FOS, fructans, and other oligosaccharides significantly modify the population and metabolic characteristics of the gastrointestinal bacteria, which might in turn modulate enteric functions and provide resistance to CRCs (Buddington et al. 2002).

16.5 Conclusions

In conclusion, and after reviewing their health benefits, it is presently admitted that FOS, fructans, and other OFs fit well within the current concept of the class of dietary material and could be labeled as "functional foods" since their vast health benefits are continuously appreciated. It is also likely that owing to their specific properties, FOS affect several functions and contribute to reducing the risk of many diseases. Thus, they may contribute in a significant way to well-being by their specific effects on several physiological functions. However, and bearing in mind their superior functional properties, such as prebiotic effects and modulation of colonic microflora, improvement of the gastrointestinal physiology, or the prevention of some cancers, some further basic research on their real utilization in the human feeding are needed. Having more and more improved technical tools, such as genetic and molecular biology, the methodology can be reversed, showing the consequences under the administration of FOS. Therefore, the last "consensus" is revealing that the available data, based on research with inulin-type fructans and originating from animal and human models, are demonstrating that these prebiotics may reduce the risk of carcinogenesis processes.

Finally, it might be concluded that prebiotics, probiotics, and synbiotics can reduce some cancer risks. Numerous animal studies have shown that they prevent the development of chemically induced colon tumors; however, the question is: can they prevent these diseases in humans? This question needs to be answered and ascertained in long-term prospective studies with cancer development as an endpoint (Pool-Zobel and Sauer 2007).

Acknowledgments

The author thanks Dr. Karl Aiken for his critical reading of the manuscript and for his comments.

References

Appel, L. J., T. J. Moore, E. Obarzanek et al. 1997. A clinical trial of the effects of dietary patterns on blood pressure. *New Engl J Med* 336:1117–24.

Biedrzycka, E. and M. Bielecka. 2004. Prebiotic effectiveness of fructans of different degrees of polymerization. *Trends Food Sci Technol* 15:170–5.

Block, J., B. Patterson, and A. Subar. 1992. Fruits, vegetables and cancer prevention: A review of the epidemiological evidence. *Nutr Cancer* 18:1–29.

Bouhnik, Y., L. Raskine, G. Simoneau et al. 2004. The capacity of nondigestible carbohydrates to stimulate fecal bifodobacteria in healthy humans: A double-bind, randomized, placebo-controlled, parallel-group, dose-response relation study. *Am J Clin Nutr* 80:1658–64.

Brady, L. J., D. D. Gallaher, and F. F. Busta. 2000. The role of probiotic cultures in the prevention of colon cancer. *J Nutr* 130:410S–4.

Buddington, K. K., J. B. Donahoo, and R. K. Buddington. 2002. Dietary oligofructose and inulin protect mice from enteric and systemic pathogens and tumor inducers. *J Nutr* 132:472–7.

Buddington, R. K., C. H. Williams, S. C. Chen, and S. A. Witherly. 1996. Dietary supplement of neosugar alters fecal flora and decreases activities of some reductive enzymes in human subjects. *Am J Clin Nutr* 63:709–16.

Campbell, J. M., L. L. Bauer, G. C. Fahey, A. J. C. L. Hogarth, B. W. Wolf, and D. E. Hunter. 1997a. Selected fructooligosaccharides (1-kestose, nystose, and 1^F-β-fructofuranosylnystose) composition of foods and feeds. *J Agric Food Chem* 45: 3076–82.

Campbell, J. M., G. C. Jr. Fahey, and B. W. Wolf. 1997b. Selected indigestible oligosaccharides affect large bowel mass, cecal and fecal short-chain fatty acids, pH and microflora in rats. *J Nutr* 127:130–6.

Carmen, C. M., G. Miguel, H. Manuel, S. Yolanda, and S. Seppo. 2005. Adhesion of selected *Bifidobacterium* strains to human intestinal mucus and the role of adhesion in enteropathogen exclusion. *J Food Prot* 68:2672–8.

Cherbut, C. 2002. Inulin and oligofructose in the dietary fiber concept. *Br J Nutr* 87(Suppl. 2):S159–62.

Craig, W. J. 1997. Phytochemicals: Guardians of our health. *J Am Diet Assoc* 97:S199–S204.

Craig, W. and L. Beck. 1999. Phytochemicals: Health protective effects. *Can J Diet Pract Res* 60:78–84.

Cummings, J. H., M. B. Roberfroid, H. Andersson et al. 1997. A new look at dietary carbohydrate: Chemistry, physiology and health. *Eur J Clin Nutr* 57:417–23.

Darbyshire, B. and B. T. Steer. 1990. Carbohydrate biochemistry. In *Onions and Allied Crops, Vol. 3. Biochemistry, Food Science, and Minor Crops*, ed. H. D. Rabinowitch and J. L. Brewster, pp. 1–16. Boca Raton, FL: CRC Press.

Dillard, C. J. and J. B. German. 2000. Phytochemicals: Nutraceuticals and human health. *J Sci Food Agric* 80:1744–56.

Farnworth, E. R. 1993. Fructans in human and animal diet. In *Science and Technology of Fructans*, ed. M. Suzuki, and N. J. Chatterton, pp. 257–272. Boca Raton, FL: CRC Press.

Flamm, G., W. Glinsman, D. Kritchevsky, L. Prosky, and M. Roberfroid. 2001. Inulin and oligofructose as dietary fiber: A review of the evidence. *Crit Rev Food Sci Nutr* 45:353–62.

Forman, D. and B. E. Bulwer. 2006. Cardiovascular disease: Optimal approaches to risk factor modification of diet and lifestyle. *Curr Treat Options Cardiovasc Med* 8:47–57.

Gallaher, D. D. and J. Khil. 1999. The effect of synbiotics on colon carcinogenesis in rats. *J Nutr* 129:1483S–7.

Gallaher, D. D., W. H. Stallings, L. L. Blessing, F. F. Busta, and L. J. Brady. 1996. Probiotics, cecal microflora, and aberrant crypts in the rat colon. *J Nutr* 126:1362–71.

Geier, M. S., R. N. Butler, and G. S. Howarth. 2006. Probiotics, prebiotics and synbiotics: A role in chemoprevention for colorectal cancer? *Cancer Biol Ther* 5:1265–9.

Gibson, C. R. and M. Roberfroid. 1995. Dietary modulation of the human colonic microbiota. Introducing the concept of prebiotics. *J Nutr* 125:1401–12.

Gibson, G. R. and X. Wang. 1994. Regulatory effects of bifidobacteria on the growth of other colonic bacteria. *J Appl Bacteriol* 77:412–20.

Hertog, M. G., G. B. Bueno de Mesquita, A. Fehily, P. M. Sweetnam, P. C. Elwood, and D. Kroumhout. 1996. Fruit and vegetable consumption and cancer mortality in the Caerphilly study. *Epidemiol Biomarker Prev* 5:673–7.

Hidaka, H., T. Eida, T. Takizawa, T. Tokunage, and Y. Tashiro. 1986. Effects of fructooligosaccharides on intestinal flora and human health. *Bifidobact Microflora* 5:37–50.

Hidaka, H., Y. Tashiro, and T. Eida. 1991. Proliferation of bifidobacteria by oligosaccharides and their useful effect on human health. *Bifidobact Microflora* 10:65–79.

Homma, N. 1988. Bifidobacteria as a resistance factor in human being. *Bifidobact Microflora* 7:35–43.

Hsu, C.-K., J.-W. Liao, Y.-C. Chung, C.-P. Hsieh, and Y.-C. Chan. 2004. Xylooligosaccharides and fructooligosaccharides affect the intestinal microbiota and precancerous colonic lesion development in rats. *J Nutr* 134:1523–8.

Jacobsen, C. N., V. Rosenfeldt Nielsen, A. E. Hayford et al. 1999. Screening of probiotic activities of forty-seven strains of *Lactobacillus* spp. by *in vitro* techniques and evaluation of the colonization ability of five selected strains in humans. *Appl Environ Microbiol* 65:4949–56.

Jenkins, D. J., C. W. Kendall, and V. Vuksan. 1999. Inulin, oligofructose and intestinal function. *J Nutr* 129:1431S–3.

Joshipura, K. J., A. Ascherio, J. Mansun et al. 1999. Fruit and vegetable intake in relation to risk of ischaemic stroke. *J Am Med Assoc* 282:1233–9.

Johnsen, S. P., K. Overvad, C. Stripp, A. Tjonneland, S. E. Husted, and H. T. Sorensen. 2003. Intake of fruit and vegetable and the risk of ischaemic stroke in a cohort of Danish men and woman. *Am J Clin Nutr* 78:57–64.

Kaput. J., D. Swartz, E. Paisley, H. Mangian, W. L. Daniel, and W. J. Visek. 1994. Diet-disease interactions at the molecular level: An experimental paradigm. *J Nutr* 124(8 Suppl):S1296–305.

Kleessen, B., L. Hartmann, and M. Blaut. 2001. Oligofructose and long-chain inulin: Influence on the gut microbial ecology of rats associated with a human faecal flora. *Br J Nutr* 86:291–300.

Kubota, Y. 1990. Fecal intestinal flora in patients with colon adenoma and colon cancer. *Nippon Shokakibyo Gakkai Zasshi* 87:771–9.

Lila, M. A. and I. Raskin. 2005. Health-related interactions of phytochemicals. *J Food Sci* 70:R20–7.

Liu, R. H. 2003. Health benefits of fruit and vegetables are from additive and synergistic combinations of phytochemicals. *Am J Clin Nutr* 78:S517–20.

Makras, L. and L. De Vuyst. 2006. The *in vitro* inhibition of Gram-negative pathogenic bacteria by bifidobacteria is caused by the production of organic acids. *Int Dairy J* 16:1049–57.

Marx, S. P., S. Winkler, and W. Hartmeier. 2000. Metabolization of β-(2,6)-linked fructooligosaccharides by different bifidobacteria. *FEMS Microbiol Lett* 182:163–9.

Meier, H. and J. S. Reid. 1982. Reserve polysaccharides other than starch in higher plants. In *Encyclopedia of Plant Physiology*, ed. F. A. Loewus and W. Tanner, pp. 418–471. Berlin: Springer Verlag.

Mitsuoka, T. 1996. Intestinal flora and human health. *Asia Pacific J Clin Nutr* 5:2–9.

Mitsuoka, T., H. Hidaka, and T. Eida. 1987. Effects of fructo-oligosaccharides on intestinal microflora. *Nahrung* 31:427–36.

Muramatsu, K., S. Onodera, K. Kikuchi, and N. Shiomi. 1994. Substrate specificity and subsite affinities of β-fructofuranosidase from *Bifidobacterium adolescentis* G1. *Biosci Biotechnol Biochem* 58:1642–5.

Ness, A. R. and J. W. Powles. 1997. Fruits and vegetables, and cardiovascular disease: A review. *Int J Epidemiol* 26:1–13.

Ngo, S. N. T., D. B. Williams, L. Cobiac, and R. J. Head. 2007. Does garlic reduce risk of colorectal cancer? A systematic review. *J Nutr* 137:2264–9.

Okazaki, M., S. Fujikawa, and N. Matsumoto. 1990. Effect of xylooligosaccharide on the growth of bifidobacteria. *Bifidobact Microflora* 9:77–86.

Olsen, M. and E. Gudmand-Heyer. 2000. Efficacy, safety, and tolerability of fructooligosaccharides in the treatment of irritable bowel syndrome. *Am J Clin Nutr* 72:1570–5.

Perdigon, G., M. Medici, M. E. Bibas Bonet de Jorrat, M. Valverde de Budeguer, and A. Pesce de Ruiz Holgado. 1993. Immunomodulating effects of lactic-acid bacteria on mucosal and tumoral immunity. *Int J Immunother* 9:29–52.

Pierre, F., P. Perrin, M. Champ, F. Bornet, K. Meflah, and J. Menanteau. 1997. Short-chain fructo-oligosaccharides reduce the occurrence of colon tumors and develop gut-associated lymphoid tissue in min mice. *Cancer Res* 57:225–8.

Pontis, H. G. and E. Del Campillo. 1985. Fructan. In *Biochemistry of Storage Carbohydrates in Green Plants*, ed. P. M. Dey and R. A. Dixon, 205–227. London: Academic Press.

Pollock, C. J. and A. J. Cairns. 1991. Fructan metabolism in grasses and cereals. *Annu Rev Plant Physiol Plant Mol Biol* 42:77–101.

Pool-Zobel, B. L. and J. Sauer. 2007. Overview of experimental data on reduction of colorectal cancer risk by inulin-type fructans. *J Nutr* 137:2580S–4.

Popkin, B. M. 2006a. Global nutrition dynamics: The world is shifting rapidly toward a diet linked with noncommunicable diseases. *Am J Clin Nutr* 84:289–98.

Popkin, B. M. 2006b. The nutrition transition: An overview of world patterns of change. *Nutr Rev* 62(Suppl. 2):S140–3.

Popkin, B. M., S. Kim, E. R. Rusev, S. Du, and C. Zizza. 2006. Measuring the full economic costs of diet, physical activity and obesity-related chronic diseases. *Obes Rev* 7:271–93.

Reddy, D. S., R. Hamid, and C. V. Rao. 1997. Effect of dietary oligo- fructose and inulin on colonic preneoplastic aberrant crypt foci inhibition. *Carcinogenesis* 18:1371–4.

Reddy, K. S. and M. B. Katan. 2004. Diet, nutrition and the prevention of hypertension and cardiovascular diseases. *Public Health Nutr* 7:167–86.

Roberfroid, M. 1991. Dietary modulation of experimental neoplastic development: Role of fat fiber content and caloric intake. *Mut Res* 259:351–62.

Roberfroid, M. B. 2000. Prebiotics and probiotics: Are they functional foods? *Am J Clin Nutr* 71(Suppl.):1682S–7.

Roller, M., A. P. Femia, G. Caderni, G. Rechkemmer, and B. Watz. 2004. Intestinal immunity of rats with colon cancer is modulated by oligofructose-enriched inulin combined with *Lactobacillus rhamnosus* and *Bifidobacterium lactis*. *Brit J Nutr* 92:931–8.

Rowland, I. R., C. J. Rumney, J. T. Coutts, and L. Lievense. 1998. Effect of *Bifidobacterium longum* and inulin on gut bacterial metabolism and carcinogen induced aberrant crypt foci in rats. *Carcinogenesis* 2:281–5.

Scharlau, D., A. Borowicki, N. Habermann et al. 2009. Mechanisms of primary cancer prevention by butyrate and other products formed during gut flora-mediated fermentation of dietary fibre. *Mut Res/Rev Mut Res* 682:39–53.

Scheppach, W., H. Luehrs, and T. Menzel. 2001. Beneficial health effects of low-digestible carbohydrate consumption. *Br J Nutr* 85(Suppl. 1):S23–30.

Spiegel, J. E., R. Rose, P. Karabell, V. H. Franks, and D. F. Schmitt. 1994. Safety and benefits of fructooligosaccharides as food ingredients. *Food Technol* 1:85–9.

Taper, H. S. and M. Roberfroid. 1999. Influence of inulin and oligofructose on breast cancer tumor growth. *J Nutr* 129(Suppl. 7):1488S–91.

Taper, H. S. and M. Roberfroid. 2002. Inulin/oligofructose and anticancer therapy. *Br J Nutr* 87(Suppl. 2):S283–6.

Taper, H. S. and M. B. Roberfroid. 2000a. Non-toxic potentiation of cancer chemotherapy by dietary oligofructose or inulin. *Nutr Cancer* 38:1–5.

Taper, H. S. and M. Roberfroid. 2000b. Inhibitory effect of dietary inulin and oligofructose on the development of cancer metastases. *Anticancer Res* 20:4291–4.

Taper, H. S. and M. B. Roberfroid. 2005. Possible adjuvant cancer therapy by two pre-biotics—inulin or oligofructose. *In Vivo* 19:201–4.

Taper, H., N. Delzenne, and M. B. Roberfroid. 1997. Growth inhibition of transplant-able mouse tumors by non-digestible carbohydrates. *Int J Cancer* 71:1109–12.

Taper, H., S. Lemort, and M. Roberfroid. 1998. Inhibition effects of dietary inulin and oligofructose on the growth of transplantable mouse tumor. *Anticancer Res* 18:4123–6.

Tashiro, Y., T. Eida, and H. Hidaka. 1992. Distribution and quantification of fructooli-gosaccharides in food materials. *Sci Rep Meiji Seiki Kaisha* 31:35–40.

Tomomatsu, H. 1994. Health effects of oligosaccharides. *Food Technol* 10:61–5.

Van Laere, K. M. J., M. Bosveld, H. A. Schols, C. Beldman, A. G. J. Voragen. 1997. Fermentative degradation of plant cell wall derived oligosaccharides by intes-tinal bacteria. In *Proceedings of the International Symposium on Non Digestible Oligosaccharides: Healthy Food for the Colon?* 4–5 December, Wageningen, 37–46.

Van Loo, J., P. Coussement, L. De Leentheer, H. Hoebregs, and G. Smits. 1995. On the presence of inulin and oligofructose as natural ingredients in the western diet. *Crit Rev Food Sci Nutr* 35:525–52.

Yazawa, K., K. Imai, and Z. Tamura. 1978. Oligosaccharides and polysaccharides spe-cifically utilizable by bifidobacteria. *Chem Pharm Bull* 26:3306–11.

WCRF-AICR (World Cancer Research Fund—American Institute of Cancer Research). 2013. Food, nutrition and the prevention of cancer: A global perspective. http://www.dietandcancerreport.org (accessed: 8 May, 2013).

WHO (World Health Organization). 2003. Diet, nutrition, and the prevention of chronic diseases. Report of a Joint WHO/FAO Expert Consultation, WHO Technical Report Series 916.

Williams, C. M. and J. W. Dickinson. 1990. Nutrition and cancer. Some biochemical mechanism. *Nutr Res Rev* 3:45–100.

CHAPTER 17

Polymers of the Plant Cell Wall or "Fiber"

*Their Analysis in Animal Feeding and Their Role in
Rabbit Nutrition and Health*

THIERRY GIDENNE

Contents

17.1 Introduction   400
17.2 Plant Cell Wall Polymers in Feeds for Monogastric Animals:
Definition, Analysis, and Physicochemical Properties   401
    17.2.1 Definition in Animal Feeding: Dietary Fiber Concept
Is Evolving   401
    17.2.2 Biochemical Characteristics of Dietary Fiber   402
    17.2.3 Methods for Fractionating and Estimating Dietary Fiber
Fractions in Animal Feeds   405
17.3 Nutritional Role of Dietary Fiber for Growing Rabbit   409
    17.3.1 Fiber Level in the Feed and Intake Regulation   409
    17.3.2 Fiber Digestion in Rabbit: A Main Source of Energy
through Microbial Activity   411
    17.3.3 Role of Dietary Fiber in the Rabbit Cecal Ecosystem   413
    17.3.4 Role of Dietary Fiber in the Digestive Health of Young
Rabbit   414
    17.3.5 Dietary Fiber Recommendations to Reduce the Risk of
Digestive Disorders in Weaned Rabbit   422
17.4 General Conclusions   423
References   423

17.1 Introduction

Dietary fiber concepts historically differ in animal feeding as compared to human nutrition and health. For the latter, this is a rather modern concept, mainly developed in the 1960s (Hipsley 1953) to deal with several pathologies (colorectal cancer, etc.), regularly revisited (Trowell 1978, De Vries 1999, Elleuch et al. 2011), and often restricted to the polysaccharides of the plant cell wall of the fruit and legumes. In contrast, animal nutritionists deal with other "less refined" fiber sources, often from whole plants (forages, by-products of seeds processing, etc.), and recover a larger range of chemical components, including other polymers, such as polyphenolic (lignins, tannins) or polylipidic compounds (cutins) and so on. Thus, two centuries ago, Heinrich Einhof developed the so-called Weende method (which in fact was setup at Möglin in 1806, Germany, and not at the Weende agronomy station) to isolate a "crude fiber" residue (Van Soest and Mc Queen 1973) to assess the nutritional value of ruminant feeds (forages and grasses). Over the years, many systems of analysis have been proposed for the replacement of crude fiber, but none have been successful in dislodging Weende procedure as the official method, and it is still used in animal feeding, for example, for quality checking of fiber sources.

Now, these two concepts are converging, and dietary fiber is generally defined as the polysaccharides and associated substances resistant to mammal enzyme digestion and absorption that can be partially or totally fermented in the gut. Champ et al. (2003) provide a concise synopsis of various views regarding the classification of dietary fibers. The overall tendency is toward an extension of the definition by including resistant starches as well as nondigestible oligosaccharides, and it was recently revisited by De Vries (2010) to reach an official enzymatic-gravimetric method that recovers total dietary fiber (TDF) in feeds. However, today, this topic is still subjected to very active research because of the complexity of the physical structure and chemical composition of the plant cell walls, and in the wide and different physiological effects of the different constituents.

The importance of dietary fiber in animal feeding is due to its influence on the passage rate and mucosa functionality, and its role as a substrate for gut microbiota that relates to performances and digestive health (Montagne et al. 2003). Our review will consider briefly the definition and structure of the different classes of fiber and cell wall constituents, followed by a description of some analytical methods employed for animal feeds. In addition, as an example, the nutritional role and impact of fiber intake on digestive health will be described for the growing rabbit, since, as a monogastric herbivore, this animal is a very pertinent research model and is of interest to meat production in Western Mediterranean, Eastern Europe, and Asian countries (China, Vietnam, etc.).

17.2 Plant Cell Wall Polymers in Feeds for Monogastric Animals: Definition, Analysis, and Physicochemical Properties

17.2.1 Definition in Animal Feeding: Dietary Fiber Concept Is Evolving

Briefly recall that the terms "cell wall" and "dietary fiber" refer to a common plant structure, and are often imprecisely used in various contexts. The term "plant cell walls" should be employed when describing the structure of the plant cell, which is extremely complex, and not uniform: the type, size, and shape of the wall are closely linked to the function of the cell within the plant (skeletal tissue, seeds, etc.). The plant cell walls consist of a series of polymers often associated and/or substituted with glycoproteins (extensin), phenolic compounds, and acetic acid, together with, in some cells, the phenolic polymer lignin. Cutin and silica are also found in the walls and/or in the middle lamella. A growing plant cell is gradually enveloped by a primary wall that contains few cellulosic microfibrils and some noncellulosic components, such as pectic substances. During plant ageing, some cells develop a thick secondary cell wall consisting of cellulose embedded in a polysaccharide + lignin matrix (Mc Dougall et al. 1996). Globally, the wall is formed of cellulose microfibrils (the backbone) embedded in a matrix of lignins, hemicelluloses, pectins, and proteins (Figure 17.1).

The concept of dietary fiber is larger than the cell wall botanical definition, since, in animal nutrition, it includes not only the polysaccharides (cellulose, hemicelluloses, pectic substances, etc.) but also oligosaccharides, gums, resistant starch, and inulin. According to their botanical origin, they may be associated with lignins and other noncarbohydrate components (e.g., polyphenols, waxes, saponins, cutin, phytates, and resistant protein). Dietary fiber is often defined by nutritionists as the feed components resistant to mammal enzyme digestion and absorption, and that can be partially or totally fermented in the gut. This "catch-all" definition

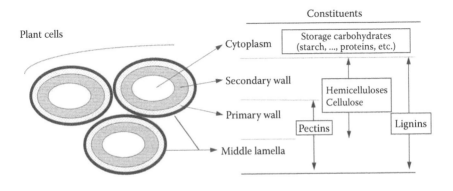

Figure 17.1 Schematic representation of plant cell walls and their main constituents.

thus includes resistant starch, oligosaccharides, fructans, protein linked to the cell wall, and so on (De Vries and Rader 2005). Another approximation is the dietary fiber for polygastric animals defined by Mertens (2003) as the indigestible or slowly digesting organic matter of feeds that occupies space in the gastrointestinal tract, mainly insoluble fiber. It excludes rapidly fermenting and soluble carbohydrates (oligosaccharides, fructans, etc.), and thus seems unsuitable for monogastric animals. Accordingly, depending on the feeds classically used for one animal species or feeding system, the dietary fiber concept differs largely. An even broader definition may include synthetic nondigestible oligosaccharides (DP > 3, fructo-oligosaccharides, polydextrose, etc.). Each definition is convenient for its own paradigm sourcing from the botanical origin of fibers that differed totally according to the final target for their physiological effects: human (legumes, cereals, fruits, etc.), ruminant (forages, straws, etc.), or monogastric animal (brans or by-products of cereals or seeds). For the latter, we will detail the biochemical characteristics of the main sources of dietary fiber in the following section.

17.2.2 Biochemical Characteristics of Dietary Fiber

The biochemical features of dietary fiber are highly variable, depending on many factors such as molecular weight, nature of monomers, and type of linkages. Accordingly, the biochemical features of fiber are one of the main factors responsible for variations in their physiological effects, and thus it is of importance to describe them. With the exception of lignin, the cell wall constituents are predominantly polysaccharides composed of neutral and/or acidic sugars.

There are two main groups of dietary fiber components according to their location, chemical structure, and properties (Figures 17.1 and 17.2):

- Cell wall components
  - Water-soluble nonstarch polysaccharides (part of β-glucans, arabinoxylans, pectic substances, etc.)
  - Water-insoluble polymers: lignins, cellulose, hemicelluloses, and pectic substances
- Cytoplasm components
  - Oligosaccharides, fructans, inulin, resistant starch, and mannans

Water-soluble polysaccharides and oligosaccharides include several classes of molecules with a degree of polymerization ranging from about 15 to more than 2000 (β-glucans). Most of them are insoluble in ethanol (80% v/v). Examples include soluble hemicelluloses such as arabinoxylans (in wheat, oat, and barley ≈ 20–40 g kg^{-1} DM) and β-glucans (in barley or oat ≈ 10–30 g kg^{-1} DM), oligosaccharides such as α-galactosides (in lupin, pea, or soya seeds, 50–80 g kg^{-1} DM), and soluble pectic substances (pulps of fruits or beets, from 100 to 400 g kg^{-1} DM). Because of their highly variable structure,

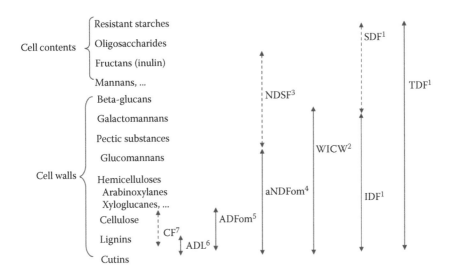

Figure 17.2 Dietary fiber fractions and their quantification by some gravimetric methods pertinent in animal feed analysis. 1: Soluble dietary fiber and total dietary fiber (Mc Cleary et al. 2010, AOAC procedures 985.29 and 991.43, including resistant starch); 2: Water insoluble cell wall (Carré and Brillouet 1989); 3: Neutral detergent soluble fiber (Hall et al. 1997); 4: Neutral detergent fiber assayed with a heat-stable amylase and expressed free of ash; 5: Acid detergent fiber expressed free of ash; 6: Acid detergent lignin. (Adapted from Mc Cleary, B. V., J. W. De Vries, J. L. Rader et al. 2010. *J Assoc Off Anal Chem Int* 93:221–33; Carré, B. and J. M. Brillouet. 1989. *J Assoc Off Anal Chem* 72:463–7; Hall, M. B et al. 1997. *J Sci Food Agric* 74:441–9.)

no satisfactory method is at present available to determine precisely these compounds in animal feeds.

Pectic substances are a group of polysaccharides present in the middle lamellae and closely associated with the primary cell wall, especially in the primary cells (young tissues) of dicotyledonous plants, such as in legume seeds (40–140 g kg^{-1} DM in soybean, pea, faba bean, white lupin), and also in fruits and pulps. Pectic substances correspond to several classes of polymers, including pectins (rhamnogalacturonan backbone and side chains of arabinose and galactose or xylose) and neutral polysaccharides (arabinans, galactans, arabinogalactans) frequently associated with pectins. Their extraction requires the use of a chelating agent such as ammonium oxalate or ethylene diamine tetraacetic acid (EDTA) (present in the solution for determining neutral detergent fiber (NDF), so they are not completely recovered in NDF analysis as described below). Pectins of the middle lamellae serve as an adhesive in plant tissue, cementing plant cells together.

In the cell wall, the cellulose is the major structural polysaccharide and the most widespread polymer on earth. It is a homopolymer (in contrast to hemicelluloses and pectins), formed from linear chains of $\beta[1 \rightarrow 4]$-linked D-glucopyranosyl units (whereas starch is formed of $\alpha[1 \rightarrow 4]$-linked D-glucopyranosyl chains). The degree of polymerization is usually around 8000–10,000. Individual glucan chains aggregate (hydrogen bonding) to form microfibrils, and could serve as the backbone of the plant. Thus, cellulose is only soluble in a strong acid solutions (i.e., 72% sulfuric acid) where it is hydrolyzed. Quantitatively, cellulose represents 400–500 g kg^{-1} DM in the hulls of legumes and oilseeds, 100–300 g kg^{-1} DM in forages and beet pulps, and 30–150 g kg^{-1} DM in oilseeds or legume seeds. Most cereal grains contain small quantities of cellulose (10–50 g kg^{-1} DM) except in oats (100 g kg^{-1} DM).

The hemicelluloses are a group of several polysaccharides, with a lower degree of polymerization than cellulose. They have a β[1 → 4]-linked backbone of xylose, mannose, or glucose residues that can form extensive hydrogen bonds with cellulose. Xyloglucans are the major hemicelluloses of the primary cell wall in dicotyledonous plants (in vegetables, in seeds), whereas mixed linked glucans (β[1 → 3,4]) and arabinoxylans are the predominant hemicelluloses in cereal seeds (the latter two include partly water-soluble and water-insoluble polymers, described above). Hemicelluloses include other branched heteropolymers (units linked β[1 → 3], β[1 → 6], α[1 → 4], α[1 → 3]) such as highly branched arabinogalactans (in soybean), galactomannans (seeds of legumes), or glucomannans. Polymers formed of linear chains of pentose (linked β[1 → 4]) such as xylans (in secondary walls), or hexose such as mannans (in palm kernel meal) are also considered as hemicelluloses. Pentosans such as xylans and arabinoxylans are soluble in weak basic solutions (5–10%), or in hot dilute acids (5% sulfuric acid). Hexosans such as mannans, glucomannans, or galactans can only be dissolved in strong basic solutions (17–24%). Quantitatively, hemicelluloses constitute 100–250 g kg^{-1} of the DM in forages and agro-industrial byproducts (brans, oilseeds, and legume seeds, hulls, and pulps) and about 20–120 g kg^{-1} DM of grains and roots.

Lignins are polyphenolic compounds of the cell wall. They can be described as highly branched and complex three-dimensional network (high molecular weight), built up from three phenylpropane units (conyferilic, coumarilic, and sinapyilic acids). A lignin network tends to fix the other polymers in place, exclude water and make the cell wall more rigid and resistant to various agents, such as bacterial enzymes. Most concentrate feeds and young forages contain less than 50 g lignin kg^{-1}. The degree of lignifications of the plant cell wall may reach 120 g kg^{-1} with ageing in forages, or up to 590 g kg^{-1} in grape seed meal.

Other constituents are also present in cell walls, but frequently in smaller quantities. Minerals, such as silica, are essentially in graminaceous leaves. Phenolic acids are chemically linked to hemicelluloses and lignin in graminaceous plants. Some proteins are linked to cell walls through intermolecular bonds from amino acids such as tyrosine, and thus resist standard extractions. In addition, plant epidermal cells may be covered by a complex lipid (cutin for aerial parts, suberin for underground structures), which could encrust and embed the cell walls, making them impermeable to water. Other phenolic compounds can also be mentioned, that is, condensed tannins, which may exist in higher plants. They form cross-linkages with protein and other molecules. They could be included in the sum of indigestible polysaccharides + lignin. However, condensed tannins, lignins, and indigestible proteins are closely related because indigestible complexes of these substances are common in plants (Van Soest 1994).

17.2.3 Methods for Fractionating and Estimating Dietary Fiber Fractions in Animal Feeds

Because of the wide diversity of plant cell types, and of cell walls accordingly, that constitutes the different plant tissues, it implies that the quantitative analysis of the different fiber fractions could be only approached by a combination of methods. The fractionation methods are thus varied and were developed according to the material tested. There is no global method used, and the choice of the method to investigate the fiber depends on the composition of each particular dietary fiber fraction. Detailed reviews have been published on this subject (De Vries and Rader 2005, Hall 2003, Mertens 2003). The methods mentioned here (Figure 17.2) describe the techniques of fractionation that are sufficiently precise and pertinent in a "routine" laboratory in charge of controlling the quality of the feed sources and give chemical parameters for implementing the databases for feed formulation.

17.2.3.1 Crude Fiber and Dietary Fiber Fractionation with Van Soest Procedures
The crude fiber method (AOAC 962.10) must be mentioned because it is highly reproducible, quick, simple, cheap, and frequently used all over the world. This technique extracts a fibrous residue after an acidic hydrolysis followed by a basic hydrolysis. The main drawback of crude fiber lies in the high variability in the chemical composition of its residue, as depending on the feed, it can dissolve up to 60% cellulose, 80% pentosans, and 95% lignin. For these reasons, this criterion is not able to explain the physiological effects exerted by most of the fiber sources on the animal digestive physiology. Since the crude fiber criterion is cheap and precise, it is commonly used to verify the lignocellulose concentration of a raw material to be compared with values in tables of feed composition.

The main alternative to crude fiber is the sequential procedure of Van Soest developed in 1967 and successively updated (Mertens 2003). The NDF method was designed to isolate insoluble dietary fiber (IDF) components in the plant cell walls by using a hot neutral detergent solution: cellulose, hemicelluloses, and lignins (Mertens et al. 2002), as pectin substances are partially solubilized. This method is criticized due to its variability among laboratories, especially when it is compared with the results obtained with other feed constituents. It is partially due to the different procedures that can be used to perform it (with heat-stable amylase and/or sodium sulfite or not, ash-free or not), but usually described with the same reference (Uden et al. 2005). The acid detergent fiber

(ADF) (AOAC 973.18) method isolates cellulose and lignin, the worst digested fibrous fractions, by a hot acid detergent solution. For complex feeds (such as for monogastrics), it is designed to be done after NDF analysis, as if it is performed directly it also retain pectins. As crude fiber, it was used to predict dietary energy value for some species, such as pigs or rabbits (Wiseman et al. 1992). Final step is the isolation of the acid detergent lignin (ADL) residue by using a strong acid solution at room temperature (Robertson and Van Soest 1981) which correspond to the lignin fraction. The main advantages of this sequential methodology are that is possible to obtain an approximate estimation of lignin (ADL), cellulose (ADF-ADL), and hemicelluloses (NDF-ADF) content, and that it is relatively quick, simple, and economical, and has an acceptable reproducibility when used a standardized methodology (EGRAN, 2001) and improves the fractionation of the cell wall.

These methods have been complemented by the estimation of the fiber dissolved by the neutral detergent solution (NDSF: neutral detergent soluble fiber; Hall et al. 1997) that mainly includes fructans, galactans, β-glucans, and pectic substances. The NDSF is obtained gravimetrically as the difference between ethanol/water insoluble residue and starch and NDF after correction for protein and ash. Therefore, the NDSF measurement may be affected by the accumulation of errors in the measurement of the different components, as well as the error linked to the value used for protein correction (Hall 2003). Now, the determination of NDSF is not adapted for routine analysis in animal feeding.

17.2.3.2 Concepts of Water-Insoluble Cell Wall, Total Dietary Fiber, and Soluble Dietary Fiber Parallel to the difficulties to estimate the water-soluble polysaccharides, the concept of dietary fiber has emerged, first in human nutrition, and has now been extended to other mammals (De Vries 2010, Trowell 1978), and assayed in the feeding of monogastric animals, such as rabbits, because of the high dietary fiber content (>50%). For instance, in poultry feeding, the concept of water-insoluble cell wall (WICW) (Figure 17.2) was developed to simply and precisely predict the metabolizable energy content of a feed (Carré 1990). WICW is a criterion obtained through a simple enzymatic-gravimetric procedure. It corresponds to lignins and polysaccharides that are water-insoluble (Carré and Brillouet 1989) and not digested by poultry.

Currently, TDF is primarily analyzed by enzymatic-gravimetric methods based on AOAC procedures 985.29 and 991.43 that solubilize the different fiber fractions with enzymes and solvents and measure the weight of residues after these treatments (reviewed by Bach Knudsen 2001, De Vries 2010, Elleuch et al. 2011). Recently, these procedures (Figure 17.2) have been updated to include nondigestible oligosaccharides and resistant starch (Mc Cleary et al. 2010). IDF could be quantified by the above-mentioned AOAC method for TDF, by avoiding the recovery of water-soluble structural polysaccharides. IDF should correspond to polysaccharides that are slowly hydrolyzed and fermented in the gut, that is, mostly lignins (indigestible), hemicelluloses, and cellulose. Conversely, IDF should not include "soluble" polysaccharides, which are rapidly fermented (e.g., pectins and β-glucans), and highly digested (at similar levels compared to starch or proteins).

When calculating the difference between the residual TDF and any measurement of "insoluble fiber" (NDF, WICW, etc.), you can estimate this "soluble" fiber fraction content (SDF). According to Van Soest et al. (1991), "soluble fiber" may be obtained by subtracting the content of NDF after correction for ash and protein from the TDF value, thus including nonstarch polysaccharides (NSP), that is, fructans, galactans, β-glucans, and pectins. One of the problems for calculating a difference between two methods (e.g., TDF and NDF) is that for some raw materials we obtained negative values (such as for sunflower meals, Table 17.1). Soluble fiber content may also be calculated by difference as organic matter–(protein + fat + soluble sugars + starch + NDF).

It is also possible to determine "directly" the soluble fiber content of a feed according to the AOAC Prosky enzymatic-gravimetric procedure (AOAC procedure 993.19, Megazyme 2005, Prosky et al. 1992); the carbohydrates are solubilized in phosphate buffer or MES (4-morpholine-ethanoesulfonic acid)/TRIS buffer; α-glucans are hydrolyzed by amyloglucosidase; insoluble fiber is separated by filtration; solubilized dietary fiber is precipitated with an ethanol solution from the solvent extract and measured gravimetrically after correction for protein and ash contents. Inaccuracies in the SDF determination may arise from the partial degradation of carbohydrates, the incomplete extraction and/or precipitation with the addition of ethanol, the interference by other substances, and differences in the nature of the analyzed feed (Hall et al. 1997, Theander et al. 1994).

Besides, let us recall that for a biochemist the solubility of polysaccharide is related to its structure; they can be set regularly (insoluble) or irregularly (soluble) on the backbone or as side chains. For example, the presence of a substitution group such as COOH increases solubility. But since the soluble and insoluble nature of dietary fibers involves differences in their technological functionality and physiological effects, the term "soluble" is frequently indifferently used for biochemical or physiological properties, and this provides some confusion for nonadvertised readers.

17.2.3.3 Other Approaches for Cell Wall Polysaccharide Analysis Another approach is to estimate dietary fiber from the sum "NSP + lignin." There are several methods available to estimate total, soluble, and insoluble NSP (Bach Knudsen 2001, De Vries and Rader 2005), where the nonfibrous components are extracted by solubilization, by enzymatic hydrolysis, or by combining both procedures. Once isolated, the fiber residue can be quantified gravimetrically (weighing the residue) or chemically (hydrolyzing the residue and determining its single constituents: sugars and lignin). According to these procedures, there are three types of methodologies: chemical-gravimetric,

Table 17.1 Cell Wall Constituents (% DM) According to Several Methods of Analysis in Some Raw Materials Used in Rabbit Feeds

Ingredients	Wheat Straw	Wheat Bran	Dehydrated Lucerne	Sugar Beet Pulp	Sunflower Meal	Soybean Hulls	Grape Pomace
aNDFom[a]	80	45	45	46	42	62	64
ADFom[b]	54	11	34	22	31	44	54
ADL[c]	16	3	8	2	10	2	34
NDSF[d]	—	3	18	30	—	22	—
Crude fiber[e]	40	10	27	19	26	36	26
WICW[f]	84	45	47	58	39	72	69
TDF[g]	85	46	48	68	41	—	72
IDF[g]	82	45	42	55	37	—	68
INSP[h]	55	36	33	64	26	55	36
Rhamnose	<1	<1	<1	11	<1	11	<1
Arabinose	2	8	2	18	3	4	<1
Xylose	18	16	6	2	5	7	8
Mannose	<1	<1	<1	1	1	6	2
Galactose	<1	<1	<1	4	1	2	2
Glucose	33	9	19	19	11	29	19
Uronic acids	2	2	7	18	5	6	5
SNSP[i]	1	3	3	10	1	2	1
Crude protein	3	15	16	9	34	11	13

[a] Neutral detergent fiber assayed with a heat-stable amylase and expressed free of ash.
[b] Acid detergent fiber expressed free of ash.
[c] Acid detergent lignin (Van Soest et al. 1991).
[d] NDSF, neutral detergent soluble fiber (Hall et al. 1997, Hall 2003).
[e] According to the Weende method (AOAC procedure 993.19: official method 962.10).
[f] Water-insoluble cell wall, including lignin (Carré and Brillouet 1989).
[g] Mc Cleary et al. (2010).
[h] Insoluble nonstarch polysaccharides, not including lignin, determined by direct monomeric analysis of cell wall polysaccharides (Englyst 1989, Barry et al. 1990).
[i] Water-soluble nonstarch polysaccharides (Brillouet et al. 1988, Englyst 1989).

enzymatic-gravimetric, and enzymatic-chemical. By this way, TDF can be quantified (NSP and lignin) and separated into insoluble and soluble fiber (in aqueous solution), and its monosaccharide composition is obtained. The combination of the monosaccharide composition of fiber with additional chemical information may allow describing better fiber structure that influences its physicochemical properties, and accordingly, the effect exerted in the animal on the digestive physiology and digestibility. However, these methodologies are complex, expensive, with a relatively low reproducibility (especially for monomers determination), and are difficult to implement as routine analysis.

17.2.3.4 Conclusions about Methods for Fiber Analysis The determination of the fiber content of a compound feed or a raw material is highly variable, depending on the analytical method of estimation. The choice of which definition should be used by the nutritionist thus depends on the type of information required (to relate to digestive processes, to predict the nutritive value).

They can be determined using sophisticated extraction techniques, and examples of their concentration in some feedstuffs are given in Table 17.1.

Finally, the enzymatic-gravimetric determination using the Van Soest procedures is still (NDF, ADF, ADL) the most simple, low-cost, rapid, and reproducible method, for analyzing the fiber fractions that are slowly digested in the gut. Now, to examine the effects of the highly digested fractions of the dietary fiber (water-insoluble pectins, β-glucanes, water-soluble pectins, oligosaccharides, etc.), new criteria are assayed. One approach is to estimate this "soluble" fraction by difference, from TDF and another criterion for insoluble fiber (NDF, etc.). Although these "soluble" fiber fractions remain hard to analyze in the feed, their effects on the digestive physiology of the animal are presently subjected to much research, and the results are summarized for the rabbit in the following section.

17.3 Nutritional Role of Dietary Fiber for Growing Rabbit

Plant polymers are the major fraction in rabbit diets and account classically for at least 40–50% (Table 17.2). The importance of fiber is due to its influence on intake, rate of passage, and its role as a substrate for microbiota. But, for the growing rabbit, one of the main challenges is to provide fiber recommendations for the prevention of digestive troubles without too large an impairment in performance (growth, feed efficiency).

The concepts of dietary fiber, fiber quantification, and characterization of the different fractions have thus been largely discussed, and have promoted changes in fiber recommendations for the growing rabbit.

17.3.1 Fiber Level in the Feed and Intake Regulation

One of the main dietary components implicated in feed intake regulation, after weaning, is the digestible energy (DE) concentration. The domestic rabbit (fed a pelleted balanced diet) is able to regulate its DE intake (and thus its growth) when the dietary DE concentration is between 9 and 11.5 MJ kg^{-1} (Figure 17.3). But a higher correlation is obtained with the lignocellulose level of the diet, when the dietary fiber level is between 10% and 25% ADF. However, the incorporation of fat into the diet, while maintaining the dietary fiber level, increases the dietary DE level, but leads to a slight reduction in the intake.

Finally, the voluntary feed intake is more related to the dietary ADF level because of the low digestion of this fraction, and probably because the ADF level also corresponds to a "ballast" value that limits the intake. For

Table 17.2 Fiber Levels and Other Main Constituents in Commercial Pelleted Feeds Used for the Growing Rabbit in Conventional Breeding

Chemical Criteria (g kg^{-1} as Fed)	Mean Range
Total dietary fiber[a] (TDF)	450–600
Neutral detergent fiber (aNDFom)	280–460
Acid detergent fiber (ADFom)	150–230
Acid detergent lignin (ADL)	35–65
Crude fiber	120–180
Soluble fiber[b]	35–120
Other Constituents	
Starch	80–130
Sugars	30–60
Crude protein	140–190
Ether extract	20–40

Source: Data from Mc Cleary, B. V., J. W. De Vries, J. L. Rader et al. 2010. *J Assoc Off Anal Chem Int* 93:221–33.
[a] Mc Cleary et al. (2010).
[b] Calculated as OM-CP-EE-aNDFom-starch-sugars.

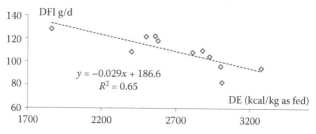

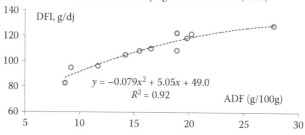

Figure 17.3 Voluntary feed intake of the rabbit, after weaning, according to the ADF or the digestible energy content of a pelleted feed. DFI: daily feed intake measured between weaning (4 weeks) and 11 weeks of age.

instance, the replacement of starch with digestible fiber fractions (hemi-celluloses or pectins), without changing the ADF level, did not greatly affect the intake (Gidenne et al. 2004, Perez et al. 2000). Further research is required to assay the effects of other fiber fractions, such as the most "soluble" ones.

In return, when the dietary fiber level is very high (>25% ADF), the animal cannot increase its intake sufficiently to meet its energetic needs, thus leading to a lower growth rate, but without digestive problems.

17.3.2 Fiber Digestion in Rabbit: A Main Source of Energy through Microbial Activity

It is acknowledged that polysaccharides of the cell wall are hydrolyzed and then fermented only by bacterial enzymes. Accordingly, in monogastric mammals, fiber became an energy source only from the activity of the micro-biota, which takes place mainly in the large intestine: the cecum and proximal colon for the rabbit. However, the extent of the fiber digestion is rather different according to the fraction, ranging from 10% for cellulose to 90% for soluble fiber (TDF-NDF). Obviously, the digestion of fiber is lower than that of protein or starch, and increasing the dietary fiber level led to a reduction in the digestive efficiency.

For the adult rabbit that is fed a high-fiber diet, the energy provided by the cecal volatile fatty acid (VFA) absorption could represent up to 50% of the maintenance energy (Gidenne 1994, Marty and Vernay 1984). But increasing the fiber intake (and lowering that of starch) either increases or has no effect on the fibrolytic activity and cecal VFA concentration (ranging from 80 to 100 mM), while a lower butyrate molar proportion is generally registered. Since the fiber digestibility is frequently not affected by the dietary fiber con-centration, it may be assumed that the quantity of fiber entering the cecum is not a limiting factor for the fermentation processes, as the digesta retention time in the cecum is relatively short, allowing, predominantly, degradation of the more easily digestible fiber fractions such as pectins or hemicelluloses. The quality of fiber, particularly their fermentability, is able to modulate the microbial activity. For instance, increasing the levels of pectins through the incorporation of beet pulps in a diet increases the VFA concentration in the cecum. In a collaborative study, García et al. (2002) reported that the cecal VFA level decreased with the degree of lignification of NDF, and that the dietary uronic acids concentration (provided mainly by pulps) is positively correlated to the cecal VFA and pH. In association with changes in microbial activity, it is suspected that the dietary fiber supply would be able to modulate the microbial population balance, as suggested by Combes et al. (2013).

Though, the extent of fiber degradation is ultimately determined by the time necessary for the microbiota to hydrolyze and ferment polysaccha-rides. Because the retention time in the ceco-colic segment of the rabbit is relatively short (8–12 h, Gidenne 1997), only the most rapidly fermentable cell wall polysaccharides are highly digested (pectins, soluble fiber fractions, etc.), whereas lignocellulose is degraded only to a small extent. For instance, when wheat bran and beet pulp replace starch (with constant level of ADF), the whole tract digestibility of the diet was not reduced (Gidenne and Bellier 2000, Gidenne and Perez 2000). The utilization for the growth of this fiber fraction is particularly high and comparable to that of starch, since the replacement in a complete diet of 10 points of starch by hemicelluloses (NDF-ADF) and pectins does not affect the feed efficiency in the growing rabbit (Gidenne and Perez 2000).

However, it must be stated that for some diets, the level of digestible cellulose is higher than that of digestible hemicelluloses. Lignins and cutin are considered almost totally nondegradable, although positive values for lignin digestibility have been obtained, which might indicate a solubilization rather than digestion. In rabbit feeding, the two main raw materials that increase the digestible hemicelluloses level in the diet are sugar beet pulp (low lignified and with a high hemicelluloses/cellulose ratio, 1.1 compared to alfalfa, 0.4) and wheat bran (with the highest hemicelluloses/cellulose ratio, 3.2). Uronic acids, an important constituent of pectins (and depending on the source of fiber also of hemicelluloses) and more soluble than other cell wall components, are the substrates that are more easily fermented. It would suggest that other components of soluble fiber (pentosans, mannans, galactans, etc.) might have a similar or even higher degradability than uronic acids.

While the fibers are mainly degraded in the large intestine, there are some evidences that some components of structural carbohydrates are degraded prior to entering the cecum of rabbits. This has also been observed in other nonruminant species such as pigs and poultry. The extent of prececal fiber digestion in rabbits varies from 5% to 43% for NDF (Gidenne and Ruckebusch 1989, Merino and Carabaño 1992) and from 0% to 37% for NSP (Carabaño et al. 2001, Gidenne 1992). It must be pointed out that the values obtained using NDF with respect to those obtained with NSP might be overestimated due to solubilization and filtration of cell wall components, which would be considered digested. When NSP were analyzed, it was found that arabinose and uronic acids, typical monomers of pectic substances, were largely digested before the ileum (from 0.2 to 0.5). On the contrary, glucose and xylose, the major monomers in most fiber sources, showed a much lower ileal digestibility (0–0.2). These results imply that around 0.4 (from 0.2 to 0.8) of total digestible fiber (including water-soluble NSP) is degraded before the cecum, which is similar to that observed in pigs (Bach Knudsen 2001). It could be explained from the cecotrophy practice of the rabbit: soft feces very rich in live microbiota are ingested daily and thus would provide fibrolytic enzymes that have been observed in the stomach and the small intestine (Marounek et al. 1995).

17.3.3 Role of Dietary Fiber in the Rabbit Cecal Ecosystem

Most of the effects exerted by fiber on the rabbit digestive physiology depend on their hydrolysis and fermentation by the digestive microbiota. However, it is difficult to study the influence of any dietary component on the microbiota, as the traditional cultivation techniques allow to work with around one-fourth of the intestinal microbiota. For this reason, other indirect techniques have been used as the volatile fatty acid concentration, the microbial nitrogen synthesized, or the fibrolytic activity. The cecal microbial population secretes enzymes capable of hydrolyzing the main components of the dietary fiber. Greater enzymatic activity for degrading pectins and hemicelluloses than for degrading cellulose has been detected in several studies (Jehl and Gidenne 1996, Marounek et al. 1995). These results are parallel to the fecal digestibility of the corresponding dietary fiber constituents in rabbits (Table 17.3), and are also consistent with the smaller counts of cellulolytic bacteria in the rabbit cecum as compared to xylanolytic or pectinolytic bacteria (Boulahrouf et al. 1991).

The cecal VFA profile is specific to the rabbit, with a predominance of acetate (77 mmol 100 mL^{-1} as average, and ranging from 65 to 87) followed by butyrate (17 mmol 100 mL^{-1} as average, and ranging from 6 to 28) and then by propionate (6 mmol 100 mL^{-1} as average, and ranging from 3 to 11). These molar proportions are affected by the fiber level. For instance, the proportion of acetate increases and that of butyrate generally decreases significantly when the fiber level increases, whereas propionic acid proportion was only positively correlated to dietary uronic acid concentration (García et al. 2002).

However, these indirect methods in many circumstances do not seem to reflect adequately the changes produced in the microbiota population. The development of new molecular tools to characterize intestinal microbiota is improving our knowledge about nutrition and digestive microbiota functions in relation to fiber intake. For instance, the cecal microbiota is able to adapt very quickly (within 1 week) to a change in the dietary fiber level (Michelland et al. 2011). Further studies are presently conducted using high-throughput sequencing of the 16S rDNA and would provide new data about the relationship between microbiota and dietary fiber (Combes et al. 2013).

Table 17.3 Digestive Efficacy (%) for Some Dietary Fiber Fractions by the Growing Rabbit

Dietary Fiber Criteria	Mean Range
Neutral detergent fiber (aNDFom)	10–50
Uronic acids	30–85
Soluble fiber (TDF-aNDFom)	70–90
Hemicelluloses (aNDFom-ADF)	15–60
Cellulose (ADFom-ADL)	5–25
Lignin (ADL)	−15–15

17.3.4 Role of Dietary Fiber in the Digestive Health of Young Rabbit

Among the various health troubles related to feeding, the intestinal pathology along with respiratory diseases are the predominant causes of morbidity and mortality in commercial rabbit husbandry. The first of the two mainly occurs in young rabbits, after weaning (4–10 weeks of age), while the second one preferentially affects the adults. In France, enteritis in the growing rabbit induced a mortality rate of 11–12%, even with antibiotherapy strategies. Moreover, digestive disorders are responsible for important morbidity characterized by growth depression and bad feed conversion, and constitute a priority problem to be solved. Till the 1980s, only the crude fiber criterion was used to define the fiber requirements for the growing rabbit, and the value ranges from 6% to 18% according to the authors. Consequently, the precise assessment of the fiber requirements with more "adequate" criteria is essential to reach a low risk of digestive troubles without a too large impairment of the growth and feed efficiency.

17.3.4.1 What Is Digestive Health and How to Measure It? The term "digestive health" thus covers all the parameters that enable the animal to maintain its intestinal balance, in response to various factors such as nutrient intake or exogenous microorganisms. If the digestive balance is not maintained, troubles could appear, such as diarrhea in the young mammal (piglet, rabbit around the weaning period), either because of gut colonization by an identified pathogen (e.g., *E. coli*) or from a multifactorial origin.

However, within a group of young rabbits, animals differently developed the clinical symptoms (diarrhea, impaction) and not all the sick animals died. Several mechanisms of defense could explain the variability in the disease sensibility, such as the gut barrier function and the competitive exclusion between saprophyte and pathogen bacteria. Nutrition and feeding strategies also play an important role in digestive health, in supplying the adequate nutrient quantity and quality to improve (i) mucosa integrity and immune response (avoiding pathogen attachment and colonization) and (ii) the growth/stability of the commensal microbiota (barrier effect).

To develop accurate nutritional strategies, it is necessary to identify the specific nutrients or bioactive components in feeds (or milk) that enhance these mechanisms of defense. These nutritional strategies must be focused around the weaning period, since it is a critical phase for the sensibility to digestive diseases, probably linked to the processes of digestive maturation, including the development of microbiota and the immune system.

The traditional indicator to evaluate the impact of a disease in groups of young domestic mammals is the mortality rate. More recently, a morbidity indicator was developed to assess more precisely the incidence of the clinical symptoms for the growing rabbit (Gidenne 1997), and it could be combined with mortality to obtain the health risk index ("HRi" = morbidity + mortality rate). This approach allows a more precise assessment of the health status.

But these traits show large variations according to many factors. For instance, the mortality rate of rabbits fed the same diet could range from 0% up to 70% according to various factors, such as the litter effect, preventive medication, and age at weaning. Thus, it means that a large number of animals are required to detect a significant difference between two treatments in mortality. For instance, to detect a 5% deviation among two mortality rates, more than 300 animals are required in each group.

When the clinical symptoms (diarrhea, cecal impaction, stomachal borborigmus, etc.) are clear, the morbidity rate is relatively easy to measure but it depends on the frequency of the measurements within a time period. For instance, if the morbidity is checked daily, the measure is more precise and gives a higher value compared to a weekly control (Bennegadi et al. 2001). However, when only a reduction of the growth rate is detectable, a threshold must be defined to class the animal as morbid or not, such that the average minus 2 × standard deviation (signifying the 2.5% of the animals with lower growth rate), or up to 3 SD. But it needs to use a large set of rabbits within a group to define precisely the mean and its range of variation. Moreover, it must be outlined that adequate statistical methods are necessary to treat discrete data (such as mortality or morbidity). For instance, when analyzing models with more than one factor or including more than two levels (within a factor) or to test the interaction between two factors, specific categorical analysis based on a weighted least square analysis must be used instead of a simple Chi square test.

17.3.4.2 Relevance of Fiber Intake Compared to Starch in the Prevention of Digestive Disease Many experiments have been performed to elicit the respective effects of fiber and starch on the incidence of diarrhea in the growing rabbit, but most of them compared variations of the fiber:starch ratio, since, in complete feed formulation, one nutrient is substituted for another one.

Consequently, when a study reported a positive effect of an increased dietary fiber intake on the digestive health, it was in fact difficult to exclude that there was also an effect of a reduced starch intake.

We thus have to deal with two opposite hypotheses: are digestive troubles linked to a carbohydrate overload in the cecum? Or linked to a fiber deficiency? (Or both?). Recently, this question was elicited by studying the ileal flow of starch and fiber in the growing rabbit (5–9 weeks old). With high-starch diets (≥30% starch mainly from wheat), the ileal starch digestibility was very high (>97%), the flow of starch remained under 2 g day^{-1} (intake ≈30 g day^{-1}) at the ileum, while that of fiber was at least 10 times higher (≈20 g NDF day^{-1}) (Gidenne et al. 2000). Thus, an overload of starch appears very unlikely since starch digestion was very efficient already at 5 weeks old. Moreover, a large-scale study using a network of six experimental breeding units (GEC French group) demonstrated through a 2 × 2 factorial design (two level of starch "12 vs. 19%" combined with two ADF levels "15 vs. 19%") that only the fiber level plays a role in digestive trouble occurrence, and not the starch level (Gidenne et al. 2004). Furthermore, by comparing iso-fiber diets but with several starch sources varying in their intestinal digestion (maize, wheat, barley), Gidenne et al. (2005) observed no effect of starch ileal flow on diarrhea incidence in the weaned rabbit. Fiber intake thus plays a major role in determining digestive trouble in the classically weaned rabbit (28–35 days old).

Accordingly, several large-scale studies aimed to validate clearly the relationship between dietary fiber/starch levels and diarrhea incidence for the "classically" weaned rabbit, using an experimental design with a high number of animals per treatment. The relationship between low-fiber diets (<14% ADF) and a higher incidence of diarrhea was clearly established in two studies where the quality of fiber, for example, the proportions of fiber fractions as analyzed through the Van Soest procedure, has been controlled (Bennegadi et al. 2001, Blas et al. 1994). In France, the GEC group performed several large-scale studies (using at least 300 animals per treatment and five experimental sites) to determine the precise fiber recommendations for the prevention of digestive troubles in the growing rabbit. The relevance of Van Soest criteria was studied, since the crude fiber method was too imprecise for this purpose.

17.3.4.3 Primary Importance of Cellulose and Lignins Intake: Impact of Quantity and Quality of the Lignocellulose The favorable effect of ADF supply on the frequency of the digestive disorders and mortality in fattening rabbits was first shown by Maître et al. (1990) using a large-scale design (380 rabbit/diet, in five sites). With a similar design, Gidenne et al. (2004) showed that the health risk index (HRi = mortality + morbidity) increased from 18% to 28% when the dietary ADF content decreased from 19% to 15%.

However, in a second step to improve fiber recommendations, the following question was examined: is a single criterion, such as the supply of lignocellulose, sufficient to define the fiber contributions and the "level of security" of a feed for the growing rabbit? Apart from the quantity of lignocellulose, other studies assessed if the quality of the ADF, that is, the respective effects of lignins and cellulose (according to the Van Soest procedure), had an impact on digestive health.

The nutritional role of lignins was first addressed (Gidenne and Perez 1994, Perez et al. 1994). The intake of lignins (criterion is ADL) involves a sharp reduction of the feed digestibility (Figure 17.4, slope = −1.6), associated with a reduction of the digesta retention time in the whole tract (−20%), and with a rise of the feed conversion ratio. For the latter, the botanical origin of lignins seems to modulate the effects observed. In parallel, a linear relationship ($R^2 = 0.99$; Figure 17.4, $n = 5$ feeds) between an ADL and mortality by diarrhea was outlined for the first time (without major effect of the botanical origin of

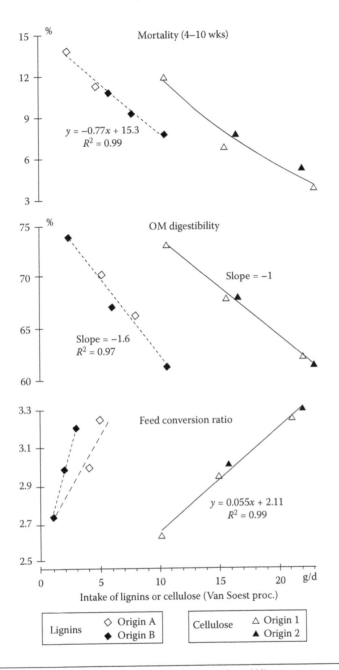

Figure 17.4 Nutritional role of lignins and cellulose in the growing rabbit.

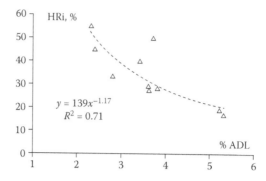

Figure 17.5 In the rabbit, the postweaning digestive troubles incidence is reduced by the dietary lignin level. ADL, acid detergent lignin (Van Soest sequential procedure, EGRAN 2001). HRi, health risk from digestive trouble = mortality + morbidity rate by diarrhea, measured from 28 to 70 days of age, on at least 40 rabbits/diet (data for 10 diets ranging from 14% to 20% ADF level). (Data from Gidenne, T. 2003. *Livest Prod Sci* 81:105–17.)

lignins). The favorable relationship between the dietary ADL level and the HRi was then confirmed with other experiments, as shown in Figure 17.5.

The effects of cellulose intake are less important than for ADL regarding the decrease of the digestibility (Figure 17.4, slope $= -1$) or that of retention time (Gidenne and Perez 1996, Perez et al. 1996). The cellulose (ADF-ADL) also favors digestive health. However, lignins play a specific role since an increase of the ratio lignins/cellulose (L/C) is associated with a lower HRi (Gidenne et al. 2001). Globally, the lignin requirement (ADL) for the growing rabbit can be assumed to be 5–7 g day^{-1}, and that of cellulose from ~11 to 12 g day^{-1}. However, to date, no correct and quick analytical method for lignins is available. Consequently, estimating the amount of lignins in a raw material remains difficult, particularly in tannin-rich ingredients (grape marc, etc.), and caution must be taken to fit requirements.

17.3.4.4 Effects of Fiber Fractions More Digestible than Lignocellulose   A third step in evaluating the fiber requirements for the growing rabbit was to test the following hypothesis: apart from quantity and quality of ADF, is it necessary to specify the effects of more digestible fibers, such as hemicelluloses and pectins or "soluble fiber" (Table 17.3)?

A first approach is to estimate the fiber fraction that is relatively digestible and in a relatively high proportion in feeds (to reduce the analytical error), then to measure the relationship with the digestive health. Digestible fiber "DgF" fraction could be estimated by the sum of the two fractions of hemicelluloses (NDF-ADF, according to the sequential procedure of Van Soest) and water-insoluble pectins. The procedure of the analysis of water-insoluble pectins remains complex; it is nevertheless possible to estimate their value in ingredients from the literature or tables (Bach Knudsen 1997, Maertens et al. 2002). Compared to lignocellulose, the DgF fraction is highly well digested by the rabbit (35–50%, Gidenne 1997).

Although the digestive health of the classically weaned rabbit depends on the level and quality of lignocellulose, it also varies greatly for the same ADF level (Figure 17.6) because the level of more digestible fiber fractions "DgF," that is, [hemicelluloses (NDF-ADF) + water-insoluble pectins], could also vary independently of lignin and cellulose levels. For instance, the ratio DgF/ADF ranged from 0.9 to 1.7 in Figure 17.6. The DgF fraction would play a key role in digestive efficiency and for digestive health, since it is rapidly fermented (compared to ADF), in a delay compatible with the retention time of the ceco-colic segment (9–13 h, Gidenne 1997).

Without changes in ADF dietary level, digestive troubles are rather reduced when DgF replaces starch (Gidenne et al. 2004, Perez et al. 2000). This could originate from the favorable effect of DgF (compare to starch) on cecal fermentative activity (García et al. 2002), and possibly from their moderate effect on the rate of passage (Gidenne et al. 2004).

For the same set of diets as in Figure 17.6, but with an ADF level over 15%, we observed a very close relationship ($R^2 = 0.88$) between the ratio DgF/ADF and the HRi (Figure 17.7). A too high incorporation of DgF with respect to lignins and cellulose should be avoided to minimize the health risk index during fattening. It is thus recommended that the ratio DgF/ADF remain under 1.3 for diets having an ADF level over 15% (see Table 17.4). Therefore, a balanced supply of low- and high-digested fiber fractions is required to reduce the risk of digestive trouble for the rabbit after weaning.

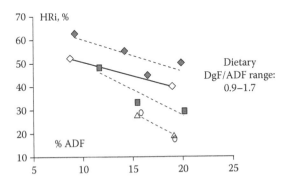

Figure 17.6 The risk of digestive trouble (HRi) in the growing rabbit is jointly dependent on low-digested "ADF" and digestible fiber "DgF." ADF, lignocellulose (Van Soest sequential procedure, EGRAN 2001). DgF, digestible fiber = water-insoluble pectins + hemicelluloses (NDF-ADF); HRi, health risk index from digestive trouble = mortality + morbidity rate by diarrhea, measured from 28 to 70 days of age, on at least 40 rabbits/diet (one point = one diet, $n = 13$; for references, see Gidenne 2003).

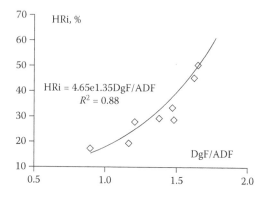

When a sufficient supply of lignocellulose (at least 18%) is provided, it is advisable to replace some starch by digestible fiber fractions. The HRi is improved while the feed efficiency is little modified (Gidenne et al. 2004, Perez et al. 2000, Tazzoli et al. 2009, Trocino et al. 2011). Furthermore, a substitution of protein by DgF also led to a significant improvement in the digestive health status of the growing rabbit, without significant impairment in growth performances (Gidenne et al. 2013, Xiccato et al. 2011).

The favorable effect of supplying lignocellulose was also shown in the young during the weaning period (3–5 weeks old) by Fortun-Lamothe et al. (2005) with a large-scale study (six sites + three reproductive cycles). They reported a lower mortality rate for litters that were fed a diet rich in fiber or when fiber + lipids replaced starch.

Table 17.4 Fiber Requirements to Prevent the Digestive Troubles after Weaning, for the Rabbit Bred in Rational Breeding Systems

Unit[a]	Post weaning (28–42 d old)	End of fattening (42–70 d old)
Lignocellulose "ADFom"	≥190	≥170
Lignins "ADL"	≥55	≥50
DgF[b]/ADF	≤1.3	≤1.3
Cellulose "ADF-ADL"	≥130	≥110
Ratio lignins/cellulose	>0.40	>0.40
Hemicelluloses "NDF-ADF"	>120	>100
SF (TDF-aNDFom)	>7–10%	>7–10%

[a] g kg⁻¹ as fed basis, corrected to a dry matter content of 900 g kg⁻¹.

[b] Digestible fiber fraction = [hemicelluloses (NDF-ADF) + water-insoluble pectins].

17.3.4.5 Impact of Quickly Fermentable Fiber on Digestive Physiology and Health of Growing Rabbit   Another way to analyze the role of cell wall polysaccharides that are rapidly fermented (and highly digested) is to determine the NDSF residue (Hall et al. 1997), which corresponds to the cell wall polysaccharides soluble in neutral detergent solution (=sum of water-soluble and water-insoluble pectins + β-glucans + fructans + oligosaccharides [DP > 15]). Although the level of NDSF is moderate in rabbit feeds, a reduction of its level (12% vs. 8%) could be unfavorable on the digestive health of the early-weaned rabbit (Gomez-Conde et al. 2009). Conversely, a higher level of NDSF improved the mucosal morphology and functionality and its immune response (Gomez-Conde et al. 2007). However, the NDSF criteria remain difficult to analyze, and precision is relatively low for complete feeds with low content of pectins or soluble fiber.

Accordingly, another approach is actually used to assess the content of the quickly fermentable fiber, or soluble fiber "SF" by the difference between the TDF and the aNDFom corrected for protein content. SF would thus be easier to handle in a routine laboratory for feed analysis. It would recover the part of TDF that comprises the nonstarch, non-NDF polysaccharides, including pectic substances, β-glucans, resistant starch, oligosaccharides, fructans, and gums.

But regardless of the advantages and disadvantages of the different methods and calculation procedures, the choice of the method to quantify SF will depend on the correlation with *in vivo* data collected in animals, and particularly the impact on the digestive health.

The soluble fiber level is generally increased in a complete feed by supplying raw materials rich in pectins, such as beet pulps, and thus most of the studies in fact relate "beet pulp level" to performances of physiological data. Accordingly, the SF dietary level is positively related to the fecal digestibility of insoluble fiber fractions (NDF and ADF). As a consequence, the soluble fiber level is likely to affect ileal and, especially, cecal microbiota (Gomez-Conde et al. 2007, 2009) by modifying the amount and type of substrate reaching the cecum. These changes in microbiota may also be related to the modified immune response observed in young rabbits that were fed soluble/insoluble fermentable fiber. The soluble fiber level favors the microbial activity (Trocino et al. 2010) with higher fermentation levels and lower pH, as shown in the meta-analysis of Trocino et al. (2013).

The relationship between mortality by digestive troubles and the SF dietary level is reported in Figure 17.8. To look more precisely at this effect, we selected six studies comparing diets having a similar level NDF, and we observed a very large variation of mortality for the same concentration of SF. Furthermore, for studies having a moderate mortality level (<15%), only two studies out of four relate SF to mortality, and a low number of animals were often used.

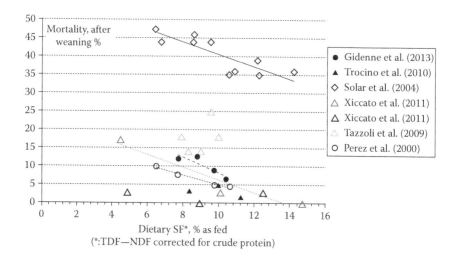

Figure 17.8 Relationship between the dietary soluble fiber level and the postweaning mortality of growing rabbits, for feeds having a similar NDF level within a study. Data from six studies and 31 diets, without antibiotics; within a study, the dietary SF level is varying, but the NDF levels are similar. Mortality: from digestive disorders measured from weaning (28–35 days) to slaughter (63–77 days of age), on at least 30 rabbits/diet. According to studies, SF values were analyzed (TDF-NDF) or calculated by reformulation from feed ingredients.

Accordingly, the criterion that quantifies the quickly fermentable fibers or soluble fibers seemed not to improve the mortality prediction. Thus, it remains very risky to recommend an SF concentration in rabbit feeds in order to reduce the risk of digestive troubles. Nevertheless, it seems that over an SF level of 7%, the mortality rate tended to be lower, and in fact this level is generally reached in feeds that follow the current recommendations for ADF and DgF (Table 17.4). Moreover, the criteria for quickly fermentable fibers correspond to a lower amount of fiber residue than for DgF criteria, and due to a higher analytical error, this could add further imprecision to recommendations.

More research is needed to elucidate the health response of rabbits to soluble fibers intake, with large-scale studies comparing the health of large groups of rabbits (over 100). In perspectives, the effects of the fiber fractions that are rapidly fermented should be precised. The main problem is to obtain a sufficiently robust analytical method (Xiccato et al. 2012) that could be used routinely in a feed control laboratory.

17.3.5 Dietary Fiber Recommendations to Reduce the Risk of Digestive Disorders in Weaned Rabbit

We propose a summary of fiber requirement (Table 17.4) for postweaned and growing rabbits. To reduce the risk of digestive troubles after weaning, for the rabbit bred in rational breeding systems, one criterion is not sufficient for fiber recommendations.

Three key points must be taken into account:

The first criterion to be controlled is the level of ADF that should be over 19% in a complete pelleted feed (Table 17.4).

Second, the quality of lignocelluloses also plays a role in the digestive health, and the minimum level of lignins should be 5% in a feed.

Third, the balance between the low-digested "ADF" and high-digested fiber fraction should be respected; the ratio DgF/ADF should be under 1.3 to avoid too high an intake of highly fermentable polysaccharides (pectins, β-glucans, etc.).

In perspectives, the effects of fiber fractions that are rapidly fermented should be determined, particularly the impact of the "soluble" fiber. Recent studies report a global favorable effect of the soluble fiber, and the range for SF supply in a feed would be 7–10%. However, the concept of SF recovers more or less the same approach than DgF, although the polysaccharides implicated are not exactly the same. The main problem is to obtain a sufficiently robust analytical method (Xiccato et al. 2012) that could be used routinely in a feed control laboratory.

17.4 General Conclusions

The rabbit is a pertinent model to explore the relationships between fiber intake and digestive pathology. The favorable impact of quantity and quality of fiber fractions on the digestive health has been demonstrated. However, the analysis of the cell wall polysaccharides that are quickly fermented remains a challenge for the future. A criterion, such as TDF-aNDFom, needs to be validated in terms of reproducibility and repeatability for feed analyses. It should also be more precisely related to the digestive health of the young rabbit.

References

Bach Knudsen, K. E. 2001. The nutritional significance of "dietary fibre" analysis. *Anim Feed Sci Technol* 90:3–20.

Barry, J. L., C. Hoebler, A. David, F. Kozlowski, and S. Gueneau. 1990. Cell wall polysaccharides determination: Comparison of detergent method and direct monomeric analysis. *Sci Alim* 10:275–82.

Bennegadi, N., T. Gidenne, and L. Licois. 2001. Impact of fibre deficiency and health status on non-specific enteropathy of the growing rabbit. *Anim Res* 50:401–13.

Blas, E., C. Cervera, and J. Fernandez Carmona. 1994. Effect of two diets with varied starch and fibre levels on the performances of 4–7 weeks old rabbits. *World Rabbit Sci* 2:117–21.

Boulahrouf, A., G. Fonty, and P. Gouet. 1991. Establishment, counts and identification of the fibrolytic bacteria in the digestive tract of rabbit. Influence of feed cellulose content. *Curr Microbiol* 22:1–25.

Brillouet, J. M., X. Rouau, C. Hoebler, J. L. Barry, B. Carré, and E. Lorta. 1988. A new method for determination of insoluble cell-walls and soluble non-starchy polysaccharides from plant materials. *J Agric Food Chem* 36:969–79.

Carabaño, R., J. Garcia, and J. C. De Blas. 2001. Effect of fibre source on ileal apparent digestibility of non-starch polysaccharides in rabbits. *Anim Sci* 72:343–50.

Carré, B. and J. M. Brillouet. 1989. Determination of water-insoluble cell-walls in feeds: Interlaboratory study. *J Assoc Off Anal Chem* 72:463–7.

Carré, B. 1990. Predicting the energy value of poultry feeds. In: *Feedstuff Evaluation*, ed. J. Wiseman and D. J. A Cole, 283–300. London: Butterworths.

Champ, M., A. M. Langkilde, F. Brouns, B. Kettlitz, and Y. L. Collet. 2003. Advances in dietary fibre characterisation. 1. Definition of dietary fibre, physiological relevance, health benefits and analytical aspects. *Nutr Res Rev* 16:71–82.

Combes, S., L. Fortun-Lamothe, L. Cauquil, and T. Gidenne. 2013. Engineering the rabbit digestive ecosystem to improve digestive health and efficacy. *Anim Res* 7:1429–39.

De Vries, J. W., L. Prosky, B. Li, and S. Cho. 1999. A historical perspective on defining dietary fiber. *Cereal Foods World* 44:367–9.

De Vries, J. W. and J. I. Rader. 2005. Historical perspective as a guide for identifying and developing applicable methods for dietary fiber. *J AOAC Int* 88:1349–66.

De Vries J. W. 2010. Validating official methodology commensurate with dietary fibre research and definitions. In: *Dietary Fibre, New Frontiers for Food and Health*, ed. J. W. Van der Kamp, J. Jones, B. Mc Cleary, and D. Topping, 29–48. Wageningen: Academic Press.

EGRAN. 2001. Technical note: Attempts to harmonise chemical analyses of feeds and faeces, for rabbit feed evaluation. *World Rabbit Sci* 9:57–64.

Englyst, H. 1989. Classification and measurement of plant polysaccharides. *Anim Feed Sci Technol* 23:27–42.

Elleuch, M., D. Bedigian, O. Roiseux, S. Besbes, C. Blecker, and H. Attia. 2011. Dietary fibre and fibre-rich by-products of food processing: Characterisation, technological functionality and commercial applications: A review. *Food Chem* 124:411–21.

Fortun-Lamothe, L., L. Lacanal, P. Boisot, N. Jehl, A. Arveux, J. Hurtaud, and G. Perrin. 2005. Effects of level and origin of dietary energy on reproduction performance of the does and health status of the young. In: *Proc. 11ème J. Rech. Cunicoles*, ed. G. Bolet, 129–132. Paris: ITAVI Publications.

Garcia, J., T. Gidenne, L. Falcao e Cunha, and J. C. De Blas. 2002. Identification of the main factors that influence caecal fermentation traits in growing rabbits. *Animal* 51:165–73.

Gidenne, T. 1992. Effect of fibre level, particle size and adaptation period on digestibility and rate of passage as measured at the ileum and in the faeces in the adult rabbit. *Brit J Nutr* 67:133–46.

Gidenne, T. 1994. Estimation of volatile fatty acids and of their energetic supply in the rabbit caecum: Effect of the dietary fibre level. In *Proc. VIème Journées de la Recherche Cunicole*, ed. J. M. Perez, 293–299. Paris: ITAVI Publications.

Gidenne, T. 1997. Caeco-colic digestion in the growing rabbit: Impact of nutritional factors and related disturbances. *Livest Prod Sci* 51:73–88.

Gidenne, T. 2003. Fibres in rabbit feeding for digestive troubles prevention: Respective role of low-digested and digestible fibre. *Livest Prod Sci* 81:105–17.

Gidenne, T. and J. M. Perez. 1994. Apports de lignines et alimentation du lapin en croissance. I. Conséquences sur la digestion et le transit. *Ann Zootech* 43:313–22.

Gidenne, T. and J. M. Perez. 1996. Dietary cellulose for the growing rabbit. I. Consequences on digestion and rate of passage. *Ann Zootech* 45:289–98.

Gidenne, T. and R. Bellier. 2000. Use of digestible fibre in replacement to available carbohydrates—Effect on digestion, rate of passage and caecal fermentation pattern during the growth of the rabbit. *Livest Prod Sci* 63:141–52.

Gidenne, T. and Y. Ruckebusch. 1989. Flow and rate of passage studies at the ileal level in the rabbit. *Reprod Nutr Develop* 29:403–12.

Gidenne, T. and J. M. Perez. 2000. Replacement of digestible fibre by starch in the diet of the growing rabbit. I. Effects on digestion, rate of passage and retention of nutrients. *Ann Zootech* 49:357–68.

Gidenne, T., V. Pinheiro, and L. Falcao e Cunha. 2000. A comprehensive approach of the rabbit digestion: Consequences of a reduction in dietary fibre supply. *Livest Prod Sci* 64: 225–37.

Gidenne, T., P. Arveux, and O. Madec. 2001. The effect of the quality of dietary lignocellulose on digestion, zootechnical performance and health of the growing rabbit. *Anim Sci* 73:97–104.

Gidenne, T., L. Mirabito, N. Jehl et al. 2004. Impact of replacing starch by digestible fibre, at two levels of lignocellulose, on digestion, growth and digestive health of the rabbit. *Anim Sci* 78:389–98.

Gidenne, T., N. Jehl, J. M. Perez et al. 2005. Effect of cereal sources and processing in diets for the growing rabbit. II. Effects on performances and mortality by enteropathy. *Anim Res* 54:65–72.

Gidenne, T., V. Kerdiles, N. Jehl et al. 2013. Protein replacement by digestible fibre in the diet of growing rabbits: 2—Impact on performances, digestive health and nitrogen output. *Anim Feed Sci Technol* 183:142–50.

Gomez-Conde, M. S., J. Garcia, S. Chamorro et al. 2007. Neutral detergent-soluble fiber improves gut barrier function in twenty-five-day-old weaned rabbits. *J Anim Sci* 85:3313–21.

Gomez-Conde, M. S., A. Perez de Rozas, I. Badiola et al. 2009. Effect of neutral detergent soluble fibre on digestion, intestinal microbiota and performance in twenty five day old weaned rabbits. *Livest Sci* 125:192–8.

Jehl, N. and T. Gidenne. 1996. Replacement of starch by digestible fibre in the feed for the growing rabbit. 2. Consequences for microbial activity in the caecum and on incidence of digestive disorders. *Anim Feed Sci Technol* 61:193–204.

Hall, M. B., B. A. Lewis, P. J. Van Soest, and L. E. Chase. 1997. A simple method for estimation of neutral detergent-soluble fibre. *J Sci Food Agric* 74:441–9.

Hall, M. B. 2003. Challenges with nonfiber carbohydrate methods. *J Anim Sci* 81:3226–32.

Hipsley, E. H. 1953. Dietary "fibre" and pregnancy taoxaemia. *Br Med J* 22:420–2.

Maertens, L., J. M. Perez, M. Villamide, C. Cervera, T. Gidenne, and G. Xiccato. 2002. Nutritive value of raw materials for rabbits: EGRAN tables 2002. *World Rabbit Sci* 10:157–66.

Maître, I., F. Lebas, P. Arveux, A. Bourdillon, J. Dupperay, and Y. Saint Cast. 1990. Growth and mortality of the growing rabbit according to the level of lignocellulose (ADF-Van Soest). In: *5èmes Journées de Recherches Cunicoles*, ed. F. Lebas. Paris: ITAVI Publications.

Marounek, M., S. J. Vovk, and V. Skrivanova. 1995. Distribution of activity of hydrolytic enzymes in the digestive tract of rabbits. *Brit J Nutr* 73:463–9.

Marty, J. and M. Vernay. 1984. Absorption and metabolism of the volatile fatty acids in the hindgut of the rabbit. *Brit J Nutr* 51:265–77.

Mc Cleary, B. V., J. W. De Vries, J. L. Rader et al. 2010. Determination of total dietary fiber (Codex Definition) by enzymatic-gravimetric method and liquid chromatography: Collaborative study. *J Assoc Off Anal Chem Int* 93:221–33.

Mc Dougall, G. J., I. M. Morrison, D. Stewart, and J. R. Hillman. 1996. Plant cell walls as dietary fibre: Range, structure, processing and function. *J Sci Food Agric* 70:133–50.

Megazyme. 2005. Total dietary fibre assay procedure. For use with AOAC Method 991.43, AACC Method 32-07, 32-21, AOAC Method 985.29, AACC Method 32-05. Megazyme International Ireland Limited, pp. 1–19.

Merino, J. M. and R. Carabaño. 1992. Effect of type of fibre on ileal and fecal digestibility. In: *Proceedings of the 5th World Rabbit Congress*, ed. P. R. Cheeke, Corvallis, USA. *J Appl Rabbit Res* 15:931–7.

Mertens, D. R. 2003. Challenges in measuring insoluble dietary fibre. *J Anim Sci* 81:3233–49.

Mertens, D. R., M. Allen, J. Carmany et al. 2002. Gravimetric determination of amylase-treated neutral detergent fiber in feeds with refluxing in beakers or crucibles: Collaborative study. *J AOAC Int* 85:1217–40.

Michelland, R. J., S. Combes, V. Monteils, L. Cauquil, T. Gidenne, and L. Fortun-Lamothe. 2011. Rapid adaptation of the bacterial community in the growing rabbit caecum after a change in dietary fibre supply. *Animal* 5:1761–8.

Montagne, L., J. R. Pluske, and D. J. Hampson. 2003. A review of interactions between dietary fibre and the intestinal mucosa, and their consequences on digestive health in young non-ruminant animals. *Anim Feed Sci Technol* 108:95–117.

Perez, J. M., T. Gidenne, F. Lebas, I. Caudron, P. Arveux, A. Bourdillon, J. Duperray, and B. Messager. 1994. Dietary lignins in growing rabbits. 2- Consequences on growth performances and mortality. *Annales de Zootechnie* 43:323–32.

Perez, J. M., T. Gidenne, I. Bouvarel et al. 1996. Dietary cellulose for the growing rabbit. II Consequences on performances and mortality. *Ann Zootech* 45:299–309.

Perez, J. M., T Gidenne, I. Bouvarel et al. 2000. Replacement of digestible fibre by starch in the diet of the growing rabbit. II. Effects on performances and mortality by diarrhoea. *Ann Zootech* 49:369–77.

Prosky, L., G. N. Asp, T. F. Scheweizer, J. W. De Vries, and I. Furda. 1992. Determination of insoluble and soluble dietary fiber in foods and food products: Collaborative study. *J Assoc Anal Chem Int* 75:360–7.

Robertson, J. B. and P. J. Van Soest. 1981. The detergent system analysis and its application to human foods. In *The Analysis of Dietary Fiber in Food*, ed. J. Theander, 123–157. New York: Dekker Inc.

Tazzoli, M., L. Carraro, A. Trocino, D. Majolini, and G. Xiccato. 2009. Replacing starch with digestible fibre in growing rabbit feeding. *Italian J Anim Sci* 8 (Suppl. 3):148–250.

Theander, O. 1995. Total dietary fiber determined as neutral sugar residues, uronic acid residues and Klason lignin (the Uppsala method): Collaborative study. *J Assoc Off Anal Chem Int* 78:1030–44.

Theander, O., P. Åman, E. Westerlund, and H. Graham. 1994. Enzymatic/chemical analysis of dietary fiber. *J Assoc Off Anal Chem* 77: 703–709.

Trocino, A., M. Fragkiadakis, G. Radaelli, and G. Xiccato. 2010. Effect of dietary soluble fibre level and protein source on growth, digestion, caecal activity and health of fattening rabbits. *World Rabbit Sci* 18:199–210.

Trocino, A., M. Fragkiadakis, D. Majolini, R. Carabaño, and G. Xiccato. 2011. Effect of the increase of dietary starch and soluble fibre on digestive efficiency and growth performance of meat rabbits. *Anim Feed Sci Technol* 165:265–77.

Trocino, A., J. Garcia, R. Carabaño, and G. Xiccato. 2013. A meta-analysis of the role of soluble fibre in diets for growing rabbits. *World Rabbit Sci* 21:1–15.

Trowell, H. 1978. The development of the concept of dietary fiber in human nutrition. *Am J Clin Nutr* 31:S3–S11.

Uden, P., P. H. Robinson, and J. Wiseman. 2005. Use of detergent system terminology and criteria for submission of manuscripts on new, or revised, analytical methods as well as descriptive information on feed analysis and/or variability. *Anim Feed Sci Technol* 118:181–6.

Van Soest, P. J. 1994. *Nutritional Ecology of the Ruminant*, 2nd ed. New York: Cornell University Press.

Van Soest, P. J. and R. W. Mc Queen. 1973. The chemistry and estimation of fibre. *Proc Nutr Soc* 32:123.

Van Soest, P. J., J. B. Robertson, and B. A. Lewis. 1991. Methods for dietary fiber, neutral detergent fiber, and non starch polysaccharides in relation to animal nutrition. *J Dairy Sci* 74:3583–97.

Wiseman, J., M. J. Villamide, C. de Blas, M. J. Carabaño, and R. M. Carabaño. 1992. Prediction of the digestible energy and digestibility of gross energy of feeds for rabbits. 1. Individual classes of feeds. *Anim Feed Sci Technol* 39:27–38.

Xiccato, G., A. Trocino, D. Majolini, M. Fragkiadakis, and M. Tazzoli. 2011. Effect of decreasing dietary protein level and replacing starch with soluble fibre on digestive physiology and performance of growing rabbits. *Animal* 5:1179–87.

Xiccato, G., A. Trocino, M. Tazzoli et al. 2012. European ring-test on the chemical analyses of total dietary fibre and soluble fibre of compound diets and raw materials for rabbits. In: *10th World Rabbit Congress*, ed. Egyptian Rabbit Science Association, 701–705. Castanet-Tolosan: World Rabbit Science Association (WRSA) Publications.

CHAPTER 18

Role of Dietary Polysaccharides in Monogastric Farm Animal Nutrition

VERONIKA HALAS and LÁSZLÓ BABINSZKY

Contents

18.1 Introduction   430
    18.1.1 Classical and Modern Animal Nutrition   432
    18.1.2 Significance of Carbohydrates in Human and Farm
        Animal Nutrition in General   434
    18.1.3 Aim and Layout of the Chapter   436
18.2 Application of the Total Nutrition Concept in Polysaccharide
    Feeding   436
18.3 Role of Polysaccharides in Monogastric Animal Nutrition   438
    18.3.1 Classification of Polysaccharides in Animal Nutrition   438
    18.3.2 Role of Different Types of Polysaccharides in Monogastric
        Farm Animal Nutrition   441
18.4 Feeding Polysaccharides to Monogastric Animals and Its
    Nutritional Consequences   445
    18.4.1 Digestibility and Metabolism of Different Polysaccharides   445
    18.4.2 Mode of Action of Dietary Fiber in the Digestive Tract   448
    18.4.3 Interaction between Polysaccharides and Other Nutrients   451
    18.4.4 Role of Dietary Fiber in the Function of Intestinal
        Microbiota   454
    18.4.5 Influence of Dietary Polysaccharides on Nutrient and
        Energy Metabolism   455
18.5 Use of Dietary Enzyme Supplementation to Improve the
    Nutritive Value of NSP-Rich Feeds   460
    18.5.1 Objective of Feeding Enzyme Products   460

18.5.2 Most Important Enzyme Products Used in Animal
        Nutrition   462
18.5.3 Use of NSP-Degrading Enzyme Products in Pig and
        Poultry Nutrition   463
18.5.4 Flatulence-Producing Compounds of Soybean Meal   465
18.6 Summary   468
Acknowledgment   469
References   469

18.1 Introduction

According to statistical data, in member countries of the World Health Organization (WHO), 50% of the overall mortality is attributable to cardiovascular diseases and nearly 15% to neoplastic diseases (WHO 2004), the development of which holds nutrition as one of the most important risk factors. By changing our undesirable dietary patterns and consuming foods that are more conforming to the human nutritional expectations, we can hope to achieve an outcome that has an increasing proportion of the population reaching the highest age determined by their genes. Therefore, our modern society has a huge responsibility in the facilitation of people having access to foods of adequate quality, which could result in a further improvement of their quality of life.

In order to enable the agricultural sector supplying the food industry with safe raw materials of adequate quality, we must have a thorough knowledge of the effects exerted by dietary nutrients on health. Therefore, medical science and agricultural science should cooperate more closely than ever before. In addition to agricultural science and medical science, nutritional biologists, geneticists, and other specialists dealing with nutrition will also have an outstanding role in solving this problem in the future.

One of the biggest challenges facing animal agriculture in the twenty-first century is to produce safe and traceable foodstuffs of animal origin in sufficient quantity and quality with the lowest possible impact on the environment. The rapid expansion of the world's human population makes it necessary to produce a steadily increasing quantity of food, which primarily results in an increased demand for raw materials of plant origin, mainly cereals, and also for foods of animal origin with high biological value. This is clearly demonstrated by the fact that the total meat production in the developing world tripled between 1980 and 2002, from 45 to 134 million tons (Thornton 2010). The expanding livestock population requires an increasing volume of feed, which means a substantial utilization of cereals in monogastric animal nutrition. However, it is a well-known fact that industrialization, construction of new motorways, new town construction programs, urbanization, and natural soil erosion result in a continuous shrinking of land area suitable for agricultural production. Owing to limited arable land, sufficient quantities of food raw materials of plant and animal origin can practically only be produced by increasing the efficiency of production. The problem to be solved is aggravated further by climate change as well as the environmental load resulting from the activity of various industrial branches and the agricultural sector, which poses an extremely severe challenge to agriculture and the related food industry.

The production of high-quality, safe, and traceable food in sufficient quantity is an extremely important strategic issue for all countries of the world. This means that, in addition to the quantitative criteria, animal agriculture has to meet the qualitative expectations as well. The quality of foods of animal origin is known to be greatly dependent on the animals' nutrition and feeding, in addition to several other factors. Therefore, animal nutrition often has a key role in increasing the efficiency and ensuring the high quality of production of foods of animal origin. According to statistical data, a total of 625 million tons of industrial concentrate mixes were manufactured for farm animals in 2006 (Gill 2007), and this production volume increased to more than 700 million tons in 2011. It is easy to realize that the quality of this enormous quantity of compound feed decisively influences the animal product quality. The situation is complicated further by the fact that besides the industrially manufactured concentrate mix of the above quantity, in many countries, farm animals are also given feedstuffs of uncertain origin and uncontrolled composition and quality.

Therefore, animal agriculture faces the following important challenges in the twenty-first century:

1. A much more active and conscious participation than ever before is required in the production of a sufficient quantity of high-quality and safe food of animal origin.
2. To achieve the above objective, further improvement of the biological, technological, and economic efficiency of animal nutrition is extremely important.
3. Reconsideration of the interrelationships between animal nutrition, animal protection, and environmental protection is of outstanding importance. This means that, from now on, high-quality, traceable, and safe foods of animal origin should be produced only by the use of technologies that do not cause further pollution of the environment. To this end, such environment-friendly feeding systems have to be developed that would help reduce the emission of harmful substances from animal production establishments into the environment.

It appears from the above that the tasks of modern animal nutrition are not limited to feeding livestock just to meet their nutrient requirements, but it means that this science has a key role in manufacturing good-quality and safe food of animal origin that meet the human nutritional expectations.

We could call this concept "from designed feed to designed food." To attain this objective, it is extremely important to introduce the most recent scientific results into the practice as fast as possible; in other words, to shorten the so-called innovation time, that is, the time it takes from idea to product realization, as much as possible.

18.1.1 Classical and Modern Animal Nutrition

On the basis of the points already discussed, the question arises whether our knowledge of classical nutrition enables us to respond to the challenges of the twenty-first century. The answer to this question is probably no. This is precisely why it is important to integrate the fields closely linked with animal nutrition into the innovation activity. Figure 18.1 illustrates those disciplines of life science and technology by which the classical knowledge of animal nutrition would have to be expanded so that adequate answers to today's challenges can be given.

Examples of such relatively new fields include the following (Babinszky and Halas 2009):

1. Molecular nutrition (the cell-level interpretation of nutrient utilization)
2. Mathematical modeling of growth (the use of mathematics to predict the production of an animal population)
3. Study of the relationship between climate change and animal nutrition
4. Introduction of animal nutrition based on genetic profiling (the relationship between nutrient supply and molecular genetics)
5. Use of the results of nutritional immunology in the practice
6. Use of the results of nutritional microbiology (study of the microbiological processes taking place in the digestive tract and the practical application of the results)
7. Nutritional biotechnology (application of the results of biotechnology in animal nutrition)
8. Development of new and more efficient environment-friendly feeding technologies
9. Use of the "farm-to-fork" ("farm-to-table") food production chain in research and in animal production (elaboration of the "traceability chain")
10. Use of the concept of precision nutrition in animal production

Owing to a lack of space, in the current chapter, we highlight only a few aspects of the scientific background of precision nutrition, which is one of the fastest-developing fields of animal nutrition.

As can be seen in Figure 18.1, precision nutrition applies the research results of both classical nutrition and the new fields of animal nutrition, utilizing large databases with the help of computer technology. Precision nutrition actually means meeting the animals' nutrient and energy requirements

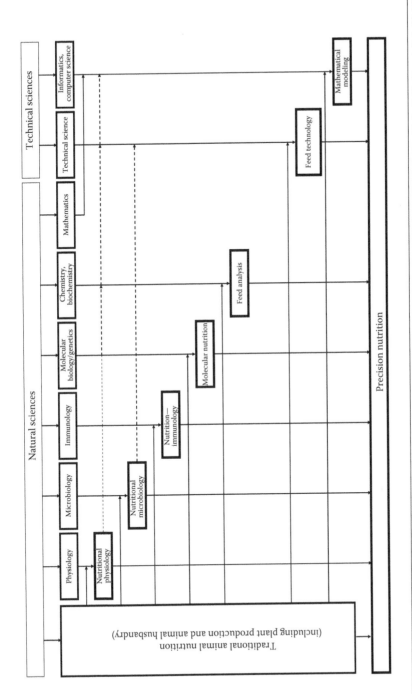

Figure 18.1 Relationship among traditional animal nutrition and other related sciences. (From Babinszky, L. and V. Halas. 2009. *Italian J Anim Sci* 8. (Suppl. 3):7–20. With permission.)

as closely as possible to achieve safe, high-quality, and efficient production that has the least possible impact on the environment (Nääs 2001, Sifri 1997). In the United States, precision nutrition is also called "information intensive nutrition." It should be noted, however, that the use of individual feeding based on computers, different electronic sensors and transponders is an important, but not the only, element of precision nutrition. Namely, it is not sufficient to distribute the concentrate mix in a technically correct way; rather, it is essential to formulate a compound feed that most closely meets the animal's age, live weight, body condition, and health status, a feed that supplies the animal with the energy and nutrients that it needs. This is important, as only in this way can we expect profitable and environment-friendly production and high-quality, safe food raw materials of animal origin.

In addition to the above, studies related to the properties of feeds should also be mentioned. This category includes studies on novel dietary energy and protein sources, interpretation of interactions between dietary nutrients and the search for alternatives of antibiotic growth promoters and possibilities to reduce mycotoxin contamination. In the category of studies on the chemical composition of feeds, one of the most important questions recently has been how we can use the energy sources of the diet (e.g., carbohydrates) in the production of monogastric animals more efficiently than before.

18.1.2 Significance of Carbohydrates in Human and Farm Animal Nutrition in General

The name carbohydrate is derived from the French "hydrate de carbone" and was applied to neutral chemical compounds containing the elements carbon, hydrogen, and oxygen, of which hydrogen and oxygen occur in the same proportion as in water ($C_n(H_2O)_n$). Although Section 18.3.2 discusses the role of carbohydrates in animal nutrition and metabolism in detail, it can be stated here that carbohydrates have an extremely important physiological role in the nutrition of humans and animals. The diet of monogastric animals contains a relatively high number of carbohydrates of very diverse chemical structure in rather high quantity. The most important polymers are *starch, cellulose, hemicellulose, pectins,* and *lignin,* and the major disaccharides are *maltose, sucrose,* and *lactose.*

Carbohydrates are primarily energy-supplying nutrients and fibrous materials that maintain the normal peristalsis (intestinal movement) and provide the bulk and the dry matter content of the feces. It should be mentioned that there are no essential carbohydrates in human nutrition; this means that the human organism can exist, even over a long period of time, without carbohydrate uptake. A good example is the dietary habits of Eskimos who practically do not consume any carbohydrate and still survive, although not for very long, as the uptake of high amounts of fat and protein severely overloads their metabolism. Although this example proves that it is possible to live without carbohydrate uptake, according to the current status of nutrition science, it is not desirable. Namely, a normal, well-balanced nutrition requires the uptake of carbohydrates too. According to the generally accepted position of the current human nutrition science, it is desirable to meet at least half (about 50–65%) of the gross energy (GE) intake from carbohydrates. In addition to the amount of carbohydrates taken up, the ratio of sugar-like to nonsugar-like, that is, complex, carbohydrates in our foods is also very important, as these two categories of carbohydrates differ in their absorption, conversion, and utilization.

Carbohydrate as an energy source plays a key role in a multitude of diverse metabolic processes. Of the latter, meeting the energy requirements of protein deposition is especially important for the production and high quality of food raw materials of animal origin, such as meat. Protein deposition is known to be a process of high energy demand; therefore, an increasing protein intake will result in higher protein deposition if the energy required for this is available in the diet. If the energy intake is not increased proportionally to the protein/amino acid intake, protein deposition cannot be increased further and the deposition curve will reach a certain plateau. In accordance with the so-called linear plateau principle (Bikker 1994), further protein deposition will occur only if, together with the increase of protein intake, the intake of energy is also increased (Figure 18.2). Obviously, protein deposition can only be increased up to the animal's genetically determined maximum protein deposition capacity (PD_{max}).

As farm animals are herbivorous or omnivorous species, feed components of plant origin have a decisive importance in their nutrition. A substantial part, often half but sometimes an even higher proportion, of diets of plant origin is constituted of carbohydrates and, therefore, carbohydrates have a key role in the energy supply of food-producing animals. Owing to the

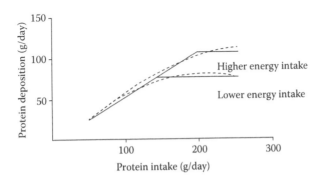

Figure 18.2 Linear-plateau and curvilinear relationship between protein intake and protein deposition in case of two different energy intakes. (From Bikker, P. 1994. Protein and lipid accretion in body components of growing pigs: Effects of body weight and nutrient intake. PhD thesis. Wageningen University, Wageningen, The Netherlands. With permission.)

development of new analytical and experimental methods, over the last few decades, extensive research has been done to explore the role of dietary polysaccharides in monogastric animal nutrition (Souffrant 2001).

18.1.3 Aim and Layout of the Chapter

The aim of the present chapter is to discuss the significance of dietary carbohydrates, particularly polysaccharides, in monogastric farm animal (pig and poultry) nutrition to produce high-quality food raw materials of animal origin.

In this chapter, the following subjects will be discussed in detail:

- Application of the total nutrition concept in polysaccharide nutrition
- Role of polysaccharides in monogastric animal nutrition
- Feeding polysaccharides to monogastric animals and its nutritional consequences
- Use of dietary enzyme supplementation to improve the efficiency of nutrient conversion and the quality of animal products

18.2 Application of the Total Nutrition Concept in Polysaccharide Feeding

To produce foods of animal origin in sufficient quantity and quality, the factors influencing the conversion of dietary nutrients must be known. The concept of total nutrition is an approach to animal nutrition where feed hygiene, food security, food safety, and the maintenance of animal health are all considered as feed objectives (Adams 2001). The total nutrition concept is actually a component of precision nutrition and its essence is that, in addition to nutrients taken in the classical sense of the word, numerous other factors related to the feed and the environment determine the performance of animals in terms of growth potential and health.

To understand total nutrition, we need to understand the links between diet, health, disease, and the environment. In practical circumstances, animals consume a great diversity of different molecules in the feed over and above those from conventional nutrients. According to Adams (2001), the molecules found in diets can be categorized into two major groups, *nutrients* and *nutricines*. Nutrients are generally recognized as feed components such as proteins, carbohydrates, fats, fiber, minerals, vitamins, and so on. Nutricines are dietary components that exert a beneficial effect on health and metabolism, yet are not direct nutrients. The nutricines include antioxidants, emulsifiers, colors, enzymes, flavors, nondigestible oligosaccharides, organic acids, and so on.

The efficiency of nutrient conversion to products of animal origin (meat, eggs, milk, etc.) depends on many factors, for example, on the housing of animals, feed quality, feed intake capacity of animals, rate of digestion and rate of absorption of nutrients, efficacy of nutricines, immune and health status of the livestock, and last but not least on stress (Babinszky 2013). The stress factors can be divided into two major groups (Adams 2001):

1. *Metabolic stress*: oxidation, noninfectious diseases, immune stimulation, immune suppression, formation of harmful intermediate metabolites in the body, and so on
2. *Environmental stress*: pathogens, vaccinations, toxins, heat stress (Babinszky et al. 2011), cold stress, activity (fighting) stress, feed raw materials (Babinszky 1998), and so on

Factors supporting and decreasing the nutritive effect collectively determine the actual nutritive value of a diet by influencing the appetite and feed intake of animals as well as the digestibility, absorption, and metabolism of nutrients (Figure 18.3).

Upon studying the nutritive value of polysaccharides, it can be established that polysaccharides have multiple linkage points with the concept of total nutrition. These linkage points will be discussed in the current chapter. By way of introduction, it is worth stating that carbohydrates (starch, sugars, and fibers) as macronutrients play an important role in animal nutrition as energy sources. A group of carbohydrates provides energy primarily for the host animal, but certain types of carbohydrates also supply energy for the pathogenic and nonpathogenic microbial population colonizing the large intestine of monogastric animals. Many of the fiber components cause environmental stress to the host organism by reducing the digestibility of other nutrients or decreasing the animals' feeling of comfort due to their flatulence-producing effect. To reduce the effect of these stress factors, specific enzymes belonging to the category of nutricines are used. Nondigestible carbohydrates, primarily

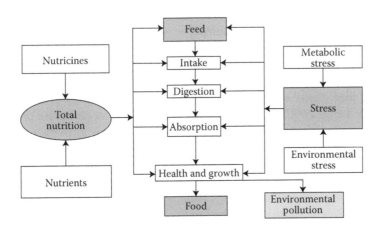

Figure 18.3 Concept of total nutrition. (From Adams, C. A. 2001. *Total Nutrition. Feeding Animals for Health and Growth.* Nottingham: University Press. With permission.)

nondigestible oligosaccharides, also belong to this group of nutricines as they exert a favorable influence on the general health status of the host organism and have often been demonstrated to have a growth-promoting effect.

The digestible nutrient content and primarily the digestible amino acid/digestible energy ratio of the diet have a decisive importance in determining the amount of protein and fat being deposited in the body. According to the linear plateau principle presented earlier, the surplus protein given after the plateau of protein deposition has been reached will not be deposited in the body; rather, it will be used for lipogenesis, which will naturally increase the fat content of the muscles as well. Any deviation from the optimal amino acid/digestible energy ratio will increase fat deposition even if the ratio decreases, as in that case, energy is provided in excess of the energy demand of protein deposition.

In conclusion, the utilization of nutrients taken up is influenced by numerous factors, and thus an accurate determination of the nutritive value of a given compound feed requires a complex approach taking into consideration the concept of total nutrition. Shifts in the ratio of dietary nutrients and changes of different extent in the digestibility of nutrients result in alterations of the qualitative characteristics of meat, shifts in its protein/fat ratio, and increases in the amount of inter- and intramuscular fat as well as a marbled appearance.

18.3 Role of Polysaccharides in Monogastric Animal Nutrition

18.3.1 Classification of Polysaccharides in Animal Nutrition

More than 50% of the feeds of farm animals are composed of carbohydrates. These are typically high-molecular-weight polysaccharides, giant molecules consisting of repeating units (monomers) linked by glycosidic bonds. Carbohydrate units can be compounds consisting of 3, 4, 5, 6, and possibly 7 carbon atoms (triose, tetrose, pentose, hexose, heptose). Trioses and tetroses can usually be found in feed materials in small amounts or not at all, as they are either intermediate compounds or metabolites. Although more than 100 different types of monosaccharides can be found in nature, the polysaccharides of feed plants are predominantly constituted by a total of nine monomers (de Lange 2000). The main carbohydrate blocks of plants are primarily hexoses, although certain cereals may contain as much as 6–9% pentosans (Henry 1987). The best-known pentoses are xylose, arabinose, and ribose. Xylose and arabinose can be found only in plants, while ribose (the sugar component of RNA) is present in all living cells. From a nutritional point of view, the most important hexoses include glucose, fructose, galactose, and mannose. Polysaccharides may be homo- or heteropolysaccharides depending on whether they consist of a single type or multiple types of monomers. Starch and cellulose are examples of homopolysaccharides consisting of glucose building blocks. The physiological properties of carbohydrates only slightly depend on the physical and chemical properties of monomers constituting them. Regarding the digestive-physiological effect, the bonds between monomers and the physical properties of the polymer, such as viscosity or solubility, are much more important (Asp 1996).

Carbohydrates are feed components of diverse composition, and their accurate determination has become possible only with the advent of modern analytical methods utilizing large instruments. Classical feed analysis (the so-called Weende analysis) enabled only the identification of groups having different properties. The grouping of carbohydrates is presented in Figure 18.4. An accurate definition of the terms used during the discussion of this subject is considered essential here; however, this chapter provides only a short discussion of the different methods, as these will be presented in detail in other chapters of the book.

The widely used Weende analysis (proximate analysis) of feed could distinguish between two large groups of carbohydrates: the crude fiber and the so-called nitrogen-free extract (N-free extract), which is the difference of nutrient content determined by various chemical methods on a dry matter basis. The N-free extract includes starch, sugars, oligosaccharides, β-glucans, pectin, a substantial fraction of hemicellulose, and a small amount of cellulose, which are eluted from the sample after acid and then alkaline hydrolysis during crude fiber determination (Henneberg and Stohmann 1859). Crude fiber is the aggregate of carbohydrates of different types and physicochemical properties, and the shortcoming of its use is that it does not contain some of the plant cell wall constituents. During cooking, 90–100% of the hemicellulose and nearly 40% of the cellulose are dissolved, and thus crude fiber has a limited value in evaluating the fiber content of feeds. The determination of fiber fraction according to Van Soest was developed in order to overcome this problem (Van Soest et al. 1991). Initially, this method facilitated the evaluation of ruminant feeds, but today it already provides useful information on pig feeds as well, as it enables not only the quantitative but also the qualitative differentiation of plant cell wall constituents. The fiber fraction determination consists of three main steps: (1) dissolution in a neutral detergent solution; (2) dissolution in an acid detergent solution; and (3) dissolution in 72% sulfuric acid. During boiling in a neutral detergent solution, the soluble cell content is extracted from the sample, and the remaining fraction is called neutral detergent fiber (NDF), which contains hemicellulose, cellulose, lignin, cutin, suberin, and also silicic acid. During boiling in an acid detergent solution buffered to acidic pH, the hemicellulose is dissolved and the remaining fraction is the acid detergent fiber (ADF). The third step, that is, boiling in 72% sulfuric acid, removes the cellulose, and thus only the incrustating substances (lignin, cutin, suberin, silicic acid) are left; however, the latter are chemically not polysaccharides (Jørgensen and Bach Knudsen 2001). A limitation of the determination of fiber fractions is that the amount of nitrogen bound by the NDF fraction interferes with the accuracy of measurement, and

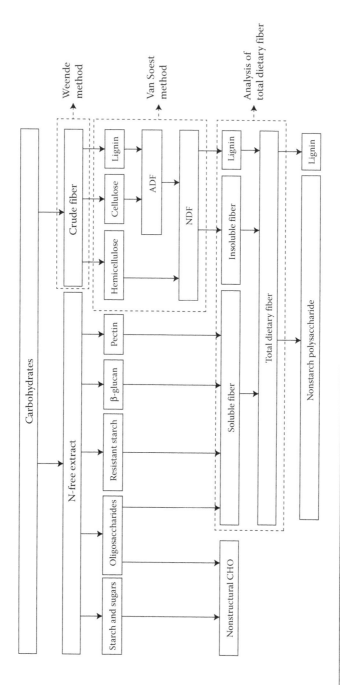

Figure 18.4 Grouping of the polysaccharides of feed and the composition of dietary fiber as measured by different methods. (From Schutte, J. B. 1991. Nutritional value and physiological effects of ᴅ-xylose and ʟ-arabinose in poultry and pigs. PhD thesis, Wageningen University, Wageningen, The Netherlands. With permission.)

also that NDF may contain starch and residual pectin as well. Because of the above-listed shortcomings, the Van Soest method is increasingly being criticized. The total dietary fiber (TDF; including soluble dietary fiber, SDF, and insoluble dietary fiber, IDF) analysis used in human nutrition gives a more reliable method to determine the (nutritive) value of fiber in monogastric animals, as TDF takes into account also those components (pectin, β-glucan, and other soluble sugars), which are washed out from the NDF fraction during analysis (Asp 1996; Bach Knudsen 1997).

Numerous methods have been elaborated for the determination of TDF as well as soluble and insoluble dietary fiber. These methods are based on two different types of measurement procedures: enzymatic-gravimetric and enzymatic-chemical procedures (colorimetric or gas-fluid and high-performance liquid chromatographic determination; AOAC 1995). IDF and SDF collectively account for the quantity of nonstarch polysaccharides (NSP), while the TDF is the sum of IDF, SDF, and lignin (AOAC 1995). The division of carbohydrates into starch and NSP may seem rather arbitrary in view of the fact that the latter is extremely inaccurate from a chemical point of view. Despite this fact, the two large groups defined in this manner make it easier to estimate the nutritive value of carbohydrates in practice, primarily because there is a substantial difference between the two types of carbohydrates in terms of digestibility.

Table 18.1 contains the carbohydrate content and composition of some concentrate components. From the table, it is evident that the by-products have higher fiber content than the conventional feed components. This can be explained by the fact that during processing, the valuable parts (endosperm with or without germ) or certain nutrients (oil, starch) are extracted from the grain and the plant parts left behind become enriched with fiber. The various concentrate components differ from one another not only in their fiber content but also in their fiber composition.

18.3.2 Role of Different Types of Polysaccharides in Monogastric Farm Animal Nutrition

From a nutritional and physiological point of view, carbohydrates have diverse roles: they serve as energy stores, have structural tasks, and perform other special functions.

Plants use primarily starch and, to a lesser extent, sugar polymers (e.g., inulin) as reserve nutrients, which are stored mainly in the seed or in the roots. Concentrate-fed animals meet a substantial proportion of their daily energy demand from starch, which—in animals fed a mixture consisting of corn and soybean—can be absorbed almost completely before the feed reaches the end of the small intestine. Despite this fact, the carbohydrate pool of the animal body is relatively small, as the glycogen contained in the muscles and liver and the blood glucose collectively make up roughly 1% of the organism's nutrients. This limited carbohydrate pool assumes

Table 18.1 Carbohydrates and Lignin in Feedstuffs (g/kg Dry Matter)

	Corn	Wheat	Rye	Barley	Oat	Tapioca	Soybean Meal	Pea	Lupine	Wheat Bran	Soyhull[d]	Sugar Beet Pulp
Total sugars	20	19	32	21	17	21	137	88	104	17	n.a.	32
Starch	690	651	613	587	468	768	27	454	14	222	3	0
β-Glucans	1	8	16	42	28	0	0	0	0	24	n.a.	0
S-NCP[a]	9	25	42	56	40	23	63	52	134	29	138	407
I-NCP[b]	66	74	94	88	110	295	92	76	139	273	650	177
Cellulose	22	20	16	43	82	196	62	53	131	72	47	195
Total NSP[c]	97	119	152	186	232	505	617	180	405	374	835	779
Klarson lignin	11	19	21	35	66	148	16	12	12	75	n.a.	35
Dietary fiber	108	138	174	221	298	653	233	192	416	449	833	814
Analyzed CHO and lignin	823	823	850	834	787	882	400	735	534	704	n.a.	845

Source: Reprinted from *Anim Feed Sci Technol*, 67, Bach Knudsen, K.E., Carbohydrate and lignin contents of plant materials used in animal feeding, 319–38, Copyright (1997), with permission from Elsevier.

[a] Soluble noncellulosic polysaccharides.
[b] Insoluble noncellulosic polysaccharides.
[c] Nonstarch polysaccharides.
[d] According to Dust et al. (2004).

importance if an animal gets into a stressful situation. At such times, the glycogen reserves are mobilized by hormonal effects, providing a rapidly utilizable energy source for "fleeing" (fight or flight phase). The glycogen content of the meat and the rate of mobilization have a significant effect on the eating and technological quality of meat. The stressors affecting the animal immediately before slaughter (rough handling, social stress, etc.) enhance the degradation of glycogen and favor the accumulation of large quantities of lactic acid accompanied by a rapid decrease of the pH value. As a result, certain meat quality parameters, such as juiciness (juice-withholding capacity), color intensity, and frying loss, will deteriorate markedly and result in pale, soft, exudative (PSE) meat. Long-term stress preceding slaughter may also impair meat quality, as, due to the decrease of glycogen reserves, less lactic acid can accumulate in the muscles after slaughter than under normal conditions. The relatively high pH developing in this way fails to provide optimum conditions for the activity of proteases necessary for the conversion of muscle to meat, and this will result in dark, firm, and dry (DFD) meat. In the case of pigs and poultry, primarily the occurrence of PSE meat causes problems. DFD meat is a common anomaly in ruminants, while it rarely occurs in pigs and practically never in poultry.

Structural carbohydrates occur only in plants, insects, and some protozoan organisms (i.e., yeasts). The chitin shell of insects is an N-containing polysaccharide, which is highly resistant to physical impacts from the environment. In the stomach of omnivorous animals (pigs and poultry), but not in that of humans, chitin is degraded by a special enzyme, chitinase. However, chitin as a carbohydrate source has negligible importance in the nutrition of farm animals, as components of plant and—with the exception of countries of the European Union—animal origin are used for the formulation of concentrate mixtures all over the world.

Structural carbohydrates can be found in relatively large quantities in the supporting tissues of plant stalk parts and in the husks of kernels. Besides cellulose, they are usually heteropolysaccharides (hemicellulose, pectin) and carbohydrates of lower molecular weight (e.g., β-glucans). The strength of the supporting tissues is influenced by the lignin content of plants, which reduces the availability of cellulose and decreases the nutritive value of the plant because of the formation of lignocellulose bonds in the lignified plant parts. Although higher living organisms do not have an enzyme system of their own for the digestion of fiber, through the activity of the microbiota living in their digestive tract, a certain part of the structural carbohydrates contained in vegetable foods becomes available to them. The availability of fiber greatly depends on the species and age of the animal consuming it. Owing to the large mass of microbes living in their forestomachs, ruminants have an extremely efficient fiber digestion. In monogastric animals, however, fiber digestion can take place only in the large intestine, and its efficiency decreases in the following order: horse, pig, rabbit, and finally the poultry species.

In order to maintain the intestinal passage and ensure the proper functioning of the digestive system, the feed must contain a certain amount of fiber, the quantity of which differs by animal species and age group. Nondigestible carbohydrates also have an important role in the maintenance of gut health. The results of numerous experiments prove that the microbiota living in the intestinal tract markedly contributes to maintaining the natural resistance and health of the host organism (e.g., Montagne et al. 2003). The large intestinal microflora can be nourished only by substances that have not been absorbed in the small intestine. As the microorganisms living in the large intestine use the enzymatically not degraded carbohydrates as energy sources, the carbohydrates reaching the large intestine may contribute to maintaining a state of eubiosis. Despite this fact, fiber was judged as unfavorable to pig and poultry nutrition over a long period of time, due to the fact that its nutritive value is low and it reduces the digestibility of other nutrients. In Section 18.4.3, the effect of fibers of different type on the digestibility of nutrients will be presented in detail.

Of the structural carbohydrates, the polysaccharides contained by the cell wall of yeasts are mainly mannan polymers linked by $\alpha(1\text{-}6)$ and $\alpha(1\text{-}2)$, and less frequently by $\alpha(1\text{-}3)$ bonds, as well as mannan proteins and β-glucans (for more details, see the review of Kogan and Kocher 2007). As neither the microorganisms living in the intestine nor the host organism itself has a set of enzymes capable of degrading these carbohydrates, they do not represent the nutritive value in the feed. Despite this fact, the feed additives containing mannan and β-glucan extracted from yeasts are also used in practical nutrition as, acting as nutricines, they help maintain eubiosis in the digestive tract and improve the immune responsiveness of animals; in addition, according to some experimental results, they also possess toxin-binding effects (Kogan and Kocher 2007).

Carbohydrates fulfilling a special biological function are typically not polysaccharides but rather complexes constituted by a carbohydrate monomer with N-containing compound (glycoproteins, glycosaminoglycans, aminoglycosides) or some other compound (glycosides). They can be found on the surface of receptors and antigens, participate, among other processes, in the immune response reactions of the organism, and are the building blocks of numerous antimicrobial substances. When they are present in the feed materials, they are mostly regarded as antinutritive factors. Legume seeds contain glycoproteins (lectins) in amounts so high that they can already be harmful to the animal organism. Lectins damage the gut wall, elicit immunological reactions, increase the synthesis of mucosal proteins, and cause impaired absorption of nutrients. If lectins are absorbed from the digestive tract into the blood, they cause disruption of the red blood cells (hemagglutination). This is where their name derives from, as lectins are also called hemagglutinins. Lectins are heat-sensitive compounds, and thus the lectin content of feedstuffs can be markedly reduced by heat treatment.

Glycosides are compounds in which a single, usually toxic, glucan unit is bound to a sugar molecule. They include glucosinolates, tannin, vicin and covicin, saponins, and solanin. Certain feed plants (rape, sorghum, legume seeds, potato) contain large amounts of glycosides. Although glycosides have different mechanisms of action, eventually they cause growth depression (Enneking and Wink 2000; Tripathi and Mishra 2007). In many cases, their concentration in feeds can be reduced by heat treatment or other feed processing procedures; however, the most effective method is to use an intensive selection of feed plants containing high amounts of glycosides.

In summary, compound feeds contain carbohydrates of different composition and physicochemical properties. The relative ratios of starch and sugar to fiber and the antinutritive substance content of the components have a marked influence on the nutritive value of feed.

18.4 Feeding Polysaccharides to Monogastric Animals and Its Nutritional Consequences

18.4.1 Digestibility and Metabolism of Different Polysaccharides

The enzymatic degradability of polysaccharides depends on the type of chemical bonds between the monomers. The α-amylase enzyme present in saliva and pancreatic juice can break only the glycoside bonds of $\alpha(1\text{-}4)$ position, which are typical of starch and sugars. An exception to this is the so-called resistant starch, which is constituted of monomers linked by $\alpha(1\text{-}4)$ bonds but is still inaccessible to amylase because of its physical form. The digestive-physiological effects of resistant starch will be presented in detail in other chapters of this book. Amylase breaks down the polysaccharides into disaccharides (maltose, sucrose), and then the maltase and sucrase enzymes produced by Brunner and Lieberkühn's glands of the small intestine degrade the disaccharides into monosaccharides (glucose, fructose). The digestibility of the dietary starch of poultry and pig feeds (after weaning) is almost complete: 96–98% of the starch is degraded and absorbed before the digesta reach the end of the ileum (Bach Knudsen and Jørgensen 2001), provided that the diet consists of the conventional components such as cereals (corn, barley, wheat), tapioca, and soybean meal. If the diet contains resistant starch or soluble fiber, the ileal digestibility of starch decreases, but it can be improved by heat treatment or enzyme supplementation.

The absorption of so-called intact disaccharides is indicative of mucous membrane damage. If disaccharides enter the blood, the overwhelming majority of them are excreted by the kidney with the urine in unchanged form and, thus, they do not enter the intermediary metabolism. In the first few weeks of their life, suckling animals do not possess sufficient amylase activity, as in this period the mother's milk is their sole nourishment. Lactose—the carbohydrate present in milk—is a special disaccharide consisting of a glucose and a galactose molecule. Lactose is degraded in the small intestine by the enzyme lactase, which is produced in sufficient quantities in piglets up to 2–3 weeks of age. Monosaccharides are absorbed by active transport along the entire length of the small intestine but mostly in the jejunum and ileum. The different carbohydrates have dissimilar rates of absorption; for example, in most animal species, galactose is absorbed more rapidly than glucose, and these are followed by fructose and then pentoses. The rate of absorption of monosaccharides is rather constant and relatively independent of the quantity taken up. Quantitative changes mainly affect the time needed for absorption, rather than the degree of absorption. However, it should be mentioned that in the case of sorbose, mannose, and xylose, the concentration present in the intestine also affects the rate of absorption, probably because their simple diffusion is enhanced parallel to the increase in their concentration.

After absorption, in the intestinal mucosa, the majority of monosaccharides are converted into glucose, which is then transported to the liver via the portal circulation. Therefore, the typical carbohydrate of blood and other tissue fluids is glucose. Occasionally, small amounts of galactose and fructose may also appear in the tissue fluids before they are converted into glucose by the intestinal mucosa or the liver. In the liver, a certain proportion of glucose is transformed into glycogen, and the remainder is transported by the general circulation to the target cells, which then utilize it as an energy source in ATP-yielding transactions. In addition to the liver, the muscle tissue also contains glycogen, and thus the glucose present in the muscle serves not only as an immediately usable source of energy but, through its polymerization, also as reserve nutrient. Glycogen is present in the cytosomes of cells in the form of granules. The stored glycogen plays a role in regulating the blood glucose level and it also constitutes a glucose reserve for muscle function. Glycogen concentration is higher in the liver than in the muscles; despite this fact, much more glycogen is stored in the skeletal muscle, which has a substantially larger total mass than the liver. The functioning of the various tissues depends on blood glucose concentration to varying degrees. The red blood cells and the brain have a high dependence on blood glucose concentration, whereas other tissues, such as the skeletal muscles, can obtain a substantial amount of energy from ketone bodies and fatty acids and, consequently, are less dependent on glucose concentration of the blood.

There is a substantial variation among the different domestic animal species in blood glucose concentration even under postabsorptive conditions. The glucose concentration of the blood shows a certain degree of variability even within a given animal species. The extent of change depends primarily on the time having elapsed since feed intake, the carbohydrate content of the feed, and the condition of the glucose stores. The stability of blood glucose concentration is maintained by a well-regulated mechanism in which the liver and a few hormones, such as insulin, glucagon, adrenaline, and glucocorticoids, play a principal role.

Although the individual NPS have markedly different chemical structure [cellulose, β-glucans of mixed 1-3 and 1-4 bonds, pentosans (arabinoxylans), galactomannans, pectin], their common feature is that the animal organism does not have specific enzymes for their degradation. Therefore, their partial hydrolysis in the digestive tract can only be accomplished through microbial enzyme activity. Although microorganisms can be found in almost all segments of the digestive tract, the conditions prevailing in the large intestine are the most favorable for their colonization because here digestive enzymes are no longer secreted and the large volume of the colon results in a slower passage of digesta, providing sufficient time and constant nutrient supply for the fermentation. Table 18.2 presents the carbohydrate, NSP, and starch and sugar content of some feed ingredients, and the digestibility of NSP measured in pigs. It can be seen that the digestibility of structural carbohydrates fails to reach 50% in most of the feed components; however, in the case of soybean meal and sugar beet pulp, the digestibility of NSP is around 90%. Namely, the composition of dietary fiber determines the extent to which the intestinal microbiota can ferment it. Cellulose, hemicellulose, and resistant starch are only partially digestible, while lignin is not digestible at all, by the intestinal microflora of monogastric animals (Metzler and Mosenthin 2008). β-Glucans, pectin, inulin, and—with the exception of mannan oligosaccharides (MOS)—different oligosaccharides provide an easily fermentable carbohydrate for the gut microflora. In general, it can be stated that the higher the proportion of soluble fiber in the dietary fiber, the higher the digestibility of fiber measured in the feces.

Because of the short large intestine, in poultry species, the bacterial activity is restricted to the cecum, and its role in the host's energy supply is practically negligible as compared to other monogastric species. The pH prevailing in the large intestine is basically determined by the bacterial populations colonizing

Table 18.2 Content of Carbohydrate (CHO), Nonstarch Polysaccharides (NSP), Starch and Sugars (S&S), and the Digestibility of NSP (NSP dig) in Feedstuffs (Reviewed by de Lange 2000 from CVB 1998)

	CHO (%)	NSP (%)	S&S (%)	NSP Dig (%)
Maize	73	10	63	45
Wheat	71	10	61	42
Corn gluten feed	61	39	22	46
Wheat bran	62	47	15	42
Beans (*Phaseolus vulgaris*)	57	16	41	67
Soybean meal	32	22	10	93
Rapeseed meal	44	30	14	49
Sugar beet pulp	71	59	12	87

Source: From Lange, C. F. M. 2000. *Feed Evaluation—Principles and Practice*, 77–92. Wageningen: Wageningen Pers. With permission of Wageningen Academic Publisher.

it, which are characterized by a dynamic balance. The characteristic bacterial species constituting the gut microflora of pigs include *Bacteroides, Prevotella, Eubacterium, Lactobacillus, Fusobacterium, Peptostreptococcus, Selenomonas, Megasphaera, Veillonella, Streptococcus,* and enterobacteria (Russell 1979; Moore et al. 1987), in addition to some yeast species. In poultry, the gut flora represents a much smaller microbial mass, which is constituted mainly by *Clostridium, Bacteroides,* and *Lactobacillus* species (Zhu et al. 2002; Lan et al. 2002). The end-products of microbial fermentation are volatile fatty acids (mainly acetic acid, propionic acid, and butyric acid), which cross the large intestinal wall by passive diffusion. After entering the blood circulation and reaching the liver, acetic acid and butyric acid are used for energy generation and fatty acid synthesis, while propionic acid is utilized for glucose formation through the process of gluconeogenesis. Fermentation also results in the formation of lactic acid, CO_2, NH_3, CH_4, and H_2O (Jørgensen et al. 1996), but the latter plays a role primarily in establishing the environmental conditions of the intestinal milieu.

From the carbohydrate derivatives used for body fat synthesis (glucose and short-chain fatty acids), the body produces primarily saturated fatty acids. As a result of *de novo* fatty acid synthesis, fatty acids of a chain length of 16 and 18 carbon atoms (palmitic acid and stearic acid, respectively) are formed. The body is able to convert stearic acid into oleic acid, which is a monounsaturated fatty acid. Oleic acid can be found in the fat of monogastric animals even if it was not present in their diet. However, essential fatty acids (e.g., linoleic acid and α-linolenic acid), that is, fatty acids of high biological value and having a special role in health protection, cannot be synthesized from dietary polysaccharides. Therefore, if the diet contains exclusively carbohydrate as an energy source, the fatty acid profile of meat will decisively consist of palmitic acid, stearic acid, and oleic acid and thus will not meet the human nutritional expectations.

18.4.2 Mode of Action of Dietary Fiber in the Digestive Tract

Different experimental (surgical) techniques have become available to detect the digestive process in different segments of the gastrointestinal tract in farm animals (Köhler 1992; Laplace et al. 1985; van Leeuwen et al. 1988). These techniques can help to understand the mechanisms governing nutrient digestibility; moreover, they give an insight into the interactions between nutrients during the absorption process. It has been known for a long time that dietary fiber content has an effect on intestinal peristalsis. However, the solubility of fiber influences the digestive processes occurring in the small intestine through different mechanisms of action (Figure 18.5).

Insoluble fibers, which are primarily the NSP constituents of the cell wall, shield the substances inside the cell from the effect of the digestive enzymes. This is known as the "cage effect," and it lowers the digestibility of protein and amino acids particularly. By adding special hydrolyzing enzymes to the diet, the cage effect can be reduced through the partial degradation of

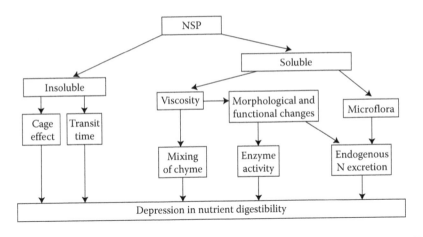

Figure 18.5 Mechanism of action of nonstarch polysaccharides (NSP).

NSP molecules, and thus the nutrients of the plant cell become more available to the digestive enzymes. The mechanism of action and the efficiency of the NSP-degrading enzymes are described in more detail in Section 18.5.3. Besides the cage effect, insoluble fibers affect the digestibility of nutrients, first of all energy, in other ways as well. IDF as part of cellulose and hemicellulose accelerates the intestinal passage (Wilfart et al. 2007). However, the reduction of transit time is typical of the large intestine only (Kesting et al. 1991), and the insoluble fiber content of the diet does not affect the transit time of digesta through the ileum (van Leeuwen et al. 2006). This is proved by the results of numerous studies, which demonstrated that the ileal digestibility* of dietary protein and amino acids did not change if components rich in insoluble fiber, such as wheat bran (up to an inclusion rate of 33%, Graham et al. 1986, or 20%, Wilfart et al. 2007) or wheat straw (up to an inclusion rate of 13.5%, Renteria Flores 2003), were added to the diet. As the efficiency of bacterial fermentation is influenced by the transit time of digesta in the large intestine, and since volatile fatty acids absorbed from the large intestine also contribute to the energy supply of pigs, increasing the IDF content of the diet will lower the digestibility of dietary energy measured along the entire

---

* The digestibility of nutrients should be studied in that segment of the digestive tract which is the main site of their absorption. Dietary proteins are broken down in the small intestine and absorbed as amino acids until the end of ileum, whereas the limited amounts of amino acids and other N-containing substances absorbed from the hind gut cannot participate in protein synthesis and are excreted via urine. Therefore, in monogastric farm animal nutrition, the so-called ileal digestibility of amino acids is routinely determined and the diets are formulated according to the ileal digestible amino acid (ID AA) requirement of monogastric animals and the ileal digestible amino acid content of feedstuffs (see more details in Babinszky 2008). The digestibility of fats and energy should be determined by feces collection, as the nutrients providing energy can be absorbed along the entire length of the digestive tract.

length of the digestive tract (Wilfart et al. 2007). A further consequence of rapid transit through the large intestine is that the feeding of diets containing insoluble fiber will result in a lower rate of water reabsorption, and thus the feces will be more dilute than in animals consuming a low amount of fiber (Graham et al. 1986).

The mechanism of action of soluble fibers is completely different from that of insoluble fibers. In the presence of soluble fibers (β-glucans, pentosans, pectins), the viscosity of the intestinal content increases (Mosenthin et al. 2001; Noblet and Le Goff 2001). Owing to the decreased intensity of intestinal contractions, this increased viscosity slows down the transit of digesta through the small intestine (Cherbut et al. 1990); however, this does not favor the digestive processes after all. This can be explained, on the one hand, by the fact that, during passage through the small intestine, a certain part of the water contained in the chyme forms a hydration sphere around the intestinal content due to the reduced intestinal motorics, and this makes it difficult for the digestive enzymes to enter the intestinal lumen (Simon 1999). Furthermore, with the reduction of intestinal peristalsis, the mixing of enzymes with the intestinal content will also decrease, thus the efficiency of digestion will be lower if a diet containing a high amount of SDF is fed (Johnston et al. 2003). Feeding a diet of high NSP content prolongs the gastric emptying time (van Leeuwen et al. 2006); in addition, the passage of digesta through the digestive tract will gradually become slower as the viscosity increases; therefore, feed mixtures of high NSP content will usually result in a reduced feed intake (Van der Klis and Van Voorst 1993).

Besides influencing the transit time of digesta and decreasing the mixing of feed with digestive enzymes, the higher viscosity of the intestinal content also influences the proliferation of cells in the digestive tract. In rats, Ikegami et al. (1990) observed dramatic morphological and structural changes as a result of the higher-viscosity intestinal content due to NSP substances: the mass of the small intestine, cecum, and pancreas increased, the secretion of pancreatic enzymes was enhanced, while the activity of the enzymes produced was also augmented. Similar results were obtained by Simon (2001) in an experiment conducted with chickens, in which the morphological parameters of the jejunum were studied. As a result of feeding high-viscosity (oat-based) diets, the intestinal villi became shortened and their thickness also increased, which resulted in the reduction of absorptive surface as compared to the control group fed a corn- and wheat-based diet. These morphological changes were attributable to the abrasive effect of the fiber-rich mixture; however, the organism tried to compensate for this by the enhanced protein synthesis of the intestinal epithelium. This is indicated by the observation that in chicks that were fed a high-viscosity diet, the proliferation of jejunal epithelial cells was about 10% higher than in birds fed the control diet (Simon 2001).

Data from the literature clearly indicate that the high fiber content of the diet increases the excretion of endogenous proteins (Nyachoti et al. 1997;

Schulze et al. 1994). The degree of this increase is greatly influenced by the solubility of the fiber. In the experiment conducted by de Lange et al. (1989), a 4% pectin supplementation increased endogenous protein excretion by 21%, while in the study of Libao-Mercado et al. (2006), a 6% pectin supplementation resulted in 50% higher endogenous protein excretion. The endogenous protein measured during these studies had substantial threonine content, which indicates endogenous excretion resulting from the abrasion of intestinal epithelial cells. The increase of endogenous protein excretion is not necessarily harmful. Dietary fiber increases the intestinal secretion of mucin, which is fundamentally important for the integrity of intestinal function (Montagne et al. 2003). According to some research results, soluble fiber not only results in the increased abrasion of intestinal epithelial cells and mucin, but it also limits the reabsorption of endogenous substances (Grala et al. 1998; Mosenthin et al. 1994; Nyachoti et al. 1997). Although the intestinal microflora is localized primarily in the large intestine, the elevated soluble fiber content of the diet increases the bacterial mass present in the terminal segment of the small intestine (Lien et al. 1997). This further increases the quantity of protein and amino acids of nondietary origin in the ileal chyme (digesta) and decreases the apparent ileal digestibility of dietary protein and amino acids (see more detail in Babinszky 2008).

By lowering the efficiency of digestion, high-fiber diets decrease the absorption of nutrients, which leads to reduced animal performance and less efficient feed conversion. When using feed components rich in soluble fiber, the excretion of endogenous nitrogen, particularly threonine, may reach an extent that already limits the synthesis of body proteins (Myrie at al. 2008), thus lowering the efficiency of meat production in a complex manner.

18.4.3 Interaction between Polysaccharides and Other Nutrients

The use of purified NSP sources in experiments might assist to separate the NSP-specific effects from the ingredient-specific effects (Owusu-Asiedu et al. 2006). However, in practical feeding, purified fiber is rarely used. There are numerous publications in which pigs were fed with a natural source of fiber containing both soluble and insoluble fractions; therefore, the results usually refer to the effect of "mixed" fiber.

Tables 18.3 and 18.4 present the results of some experiments studying the effect of dietary fiber content on the digestibility of protein, amino acids, and fat in pigs. From the data presented in the table, it is clear that the increase of fiber content was usually associated with a lower ileal digestibility of protein and amino acids and a reduced fecal digestibility of fat. This depressive effect of fiber on digestibility is more expressed when feed components rich in soluble fiber are used. The results of several studies indicate that the digestibility of amino acids markedly decreases already when low amounts of a feed component rich in soluble fiber are present in the concentrate; however, above a certain inclusion rate, the depressive effect of fiber on digestibility does not

Table 18.3 Some Literary Data on the Effect of Different Types of Fibers on the Digestibility of Crude Protein and Amino Acids

Authors	Fiber Source	Fiber Type	Protein	Amino Acids	BW
			Effect of Fiber on Digestibility of		
Mosenthin et al. (1994)	Citrus pectin	Pectin 75 g/kg	ID ↓	FD and ID ↓ for all AAs[a]	70 kg
Bach Knudsen and Hansen (1991)	Wheat by-products	NSP 30–54 g/kg, lignin 4–8 g/kg	FD ↓ and ID Ø or ↓		40–50 kg
	Oat by-products	NSP 34–96 g/kg, lignin 9–13 g/kg	FD and ID ↓		40–50 kg
Schultze et al. (1994)	Purified NDF from wheat bran	NDF 0, 60, 120, 180 g/kg	ID ↓		25 kg
Lenis et al. (1996)	Purified NDF from wheat bran	NDF 18 versus 805 g/kg	FD and ID ↓	ID ↓ for all AAs[a]	27 kg
Dilger et al. (2004)	Soyhulls	NDF 27–76 g/kg	FD and ID Ø	ID[b] ↓ for Arg, His, Iso, Lys, Phe, Asp, Ser, Tyr; ID[b] Ø for the rest of AAs	35 kg
Yin et al. (2000)	Wheat by-products	Insoluble NSP 75–184 g/kg	FD and ID ↓	ID ↓ for all AAs[a] except for Arg	26 kg
Wilfart et al. (2007)	Wheat bran	IDF 132–229 g/kg DM; SDF 32–41 g/kg DM	FD ↓ and ID Ø		30 kg
Dégen et al. (2011)	Soyhulls up to 10%	NDF 135–179 g/kg	ID ↓	ID ↓ for Lys, Met, Cys, Thr, Trp, Agr, Ile, Val	35 kg

Source: Reprinted from Dégen, L., V. Halas, and L. Babinszky. 2007. Effect of dietary fiber on protein and fat digestibility and its consequences on diet formulation for growing and fattening pigs: A review. *Acta Agr Scand A–An* 57:1–9, Copyright (2007), with permission from Taylor & Francis Ltd, www.tandfonline.com.

Note: BW, body weight; FD, fecal digestibility; ID, ileal digestibility (both refer to apparent digestibility); ↓, reducing effect; Ø, no effect.

[a] Arg, His, Iso, Leu, Lys, Met, Phe, Thr, Try, Val, Ala, Asp, Cys, Glu, Gly, Pro, Ser, Tyr.

[b] Both apparent and true ileal digestibility.

Table 18.4 Literary Data on the Effect of Different Types of Fibers on the Digestibility of Crude Fat

Authors	Fiber Source	Fiber Type	Effect of Fiber	Body Weight
Freire et al. (1998)	Wheat bran	NDF 100 versus 160 g/kg	Fecal digestibility ↓	5 kg
Le Goff and Noblet (2001)	77 Different diets	NDF 112–394 g/kg	Fecal digestibility ↓	61 and 234 kg
Noblet and Perez (1993)	114 Different diets	NDF 44–261 g/kg	Fecal digestibility ↓	45 kg
Mroz et al. (1996)	Soybean hulls, cellulose	NDF 87–355 g/kg, ADF 35–286 g/kg	Ileal dig. Ø; fecal dig. ↓	40 kg
Bakker et al. (1995)	Soyhulls, cellulose	NDF 91–380 g/kg; CF 29–258 g/kg	Fecal digestibility ↓	60 and 90 kg
Wilfart et al. (2007)	Wheat bran	IDF 132–229 g/kg DM SDF 32–41 g/kg DM	Fecal digestibility ↓	30 kg
Högberg and Lindberg (2004)	Insoluble:soluble fiber ratio 7.3 to 2.4	NSP 95–250 g/kg DM	Ileal dig. Ø; fecal dig. ↑	3–9 weeks old
Dégen et al. (2009)	Wheat bran up to 60%	Crude fiber 30–112 g/kg	Fecal digestibility Ø or ↑ depending on fat supplementation	40 kg

Source: Reprinted from Dégen, L., V. Halas, and L. Babinszky. 2007. Effect of dietary fiber on protein and fat digestibility and its consequences on diet formulation for growing and fattening pigs: A review. *Acta Agr Scand A-An* 57:1–9, Copyright (2007), with permission from Taylor & Francis Ltd, www.tandfonline.com.

Note: ↓, reducing effect; Ø, no effect.

increase further (Dégen et al. 2011; Dilger et al. 2004). The studies of Dégen et al. (2011) demonstrated a linear-plateau relationship between dietary fiber content and the ileal digestibility of amino acids.

The mode of action of dietary fiber on fat digestibility depends on the solubility of the fiber. Soluble NSP depresses the digestibility of fat by means of changing the viscosity of the digesta. Pasquier et al. (1996) found that the extent of *in vitro* lipolysis with gastric and pancreatic lipase was significantly decreased by an emulsion prepared in the presence of high-viscosity guar gum when compared with those obtained without fiber or with a low- or medium-viscosity guar gum. Insoluble NSP reduces the transit time of the digesta in the total tract due to the faster flow in the hindgut and may result in a shorter time for digestive enzyme action, with particular concern for lipase (Dégen et al. 2007). However, the passage time in the small intestine is either not affected or even prolonged (Kesting et al. 1991), which raises the question whether insoluble fiber interferes with ileal fat digestibility (Högberg and Lindberg 2004; Mroz et al. 1996). It was reported that certain fibrous constituents absorb sterolic derivatives such as bile acids in the digesta, thus preventing absorption and enhancing fecal excretion of these derivatives as reviewed by Kreuzer et al. (2002). This mechanism explains the decreased fat digestibility, because of less emulsification in the small intestine due to the binding of bile acid.

Owing to the fact that dietary fiber dilutes the energy content of feed, fat supplementation is often used when fiber-rich feedstuffs are included in diet formulation. However, there might be an interaction between dietary fat and fiber, leading to a lower digestibility of nutrients (Bakker et al. 1995; Dégen et al. 2009; Key and Mathers 1993) and an underestimation of the energy value of the feed (Bakker 1996).

It can be concluded from the literature that the effect of dietary fiber on protein and fat digestibility has been studied extensively. Increasing dietary fiber decreases the digestibility of protein, amino acid, and fat. On the other hand, increasing dietary fat content reduces fermentation in the hindgut and results in a lower fiber digestibility. Thus the feeding value, that is, the digestible protein and amino acid, digestible fiber, and digestible fat content of a compound feed, cannot be computed additively from the feed ingredients due to the fact that dietary fiber reduces the digestibility coefficient of nutrients. Moreover, owing to the fat × fiber interaction, the extent of depression in fiber and fat digestibility cannot be determined precisely.

18.4.4 Role of Dietary Fiber in the Function of Intestinal Microbiota

Several chapters in this book discuss the effect of dietary fiber on gut health and eubiosis; therefore, in the present chapter, the role of fiber in the function of intestinal microbiota in pigs and poultry is overviewed briefly. Historically, dietary fiber was defined as the skeletal remains of plant cells in the diet, which is resistant to hydrolysis by the digestive enzymes of humans (Trowell et al. 1976); thus, it escapes small intestinal digestion and is available for the gut microbes. Fermentation of carbohydrates leads to the production of short-chain fatty acids that improve the proliferation of epithelial cells. Moreover, volatile fatty acids, particularly butyric acid, have a key role in signaling proinflammatory cytokines and therefore in the defense mechanisms of the gut tissue. Fermentable carbohydrate from potato starch (resistant starch) increased the count of lactobacilli while decreasing the number of coliforms in the ileum, enhanced acetic and butyric acid production in the colon, and reduced ammonia concentration both in the ileum and in the colon of piglets 7 days after weaning (Bikker et al. 2006). Although soluble dietary fibers are degraded by the gut flora to a higher extent than insoluble fibers, several studies have found that SDF destroys the eubiosis. High-viscosity digesta increases the rate of bile acid excretion by the feces, withholding it from reabsorption, while bile acids inhibit the growth of various intestinal microbes, including lactobacilli and bifidobacteria (Kurdi et al. 2006). According to a review by Montagne et al. (2003), development of swine dysentery, higher *E. coli* count in pigs, and higher *Salmonella* count in poultry were found after feeding diets with high SDF. Whitney et al. (2006) reported reduced severity of intestinal infections caused by *Lawsonia intracellularis* when feeding diets containing distiller's dried grains with solubles (DDGS), which is high in hemicellulose. It seems that piglet and poultry diets rich in insoluble fiber protect more efficiently against pathogenic bacteria than diets high in soluble fiber (Montagne et al. 2003).

Some specific components, such as inulin and oligosaccharides such as fructo- and galacto-oligosaccharides, have particular prebiotic effects (Hathaway 2000; Pettigrew 2000). By definition, prebiotics are nondigestible components of food or feed that stimulate the growth and/or activity of beneficial bacteria in the digestive system, thus promoting gut and general health of the host (Gibson and Roberfroid 1995). MOS have recently been assigned to nutricines (Halas and Nochta 2012), considering that they are not direct nutrients either for the intestinal microbiota or for the host, but potentially have positive effects on the health and performance of farm animals. Mannans assist in maintaining intestinal integrity (Iji et al. 2001), the digestive and absorptive functions of the gut (Nochta et al. 2010), and they may also boost the specific immunity of weaning pigs (Nochta et al. 2009). Moreover, recent results suggest that MOS enhance the disease resistance of swine by promoting antigen presentation, thus enhancing the shift from an innate to an adaptive immune response (Che et al. 2011, 2012).

18.4.5 Influence of Dietary Polysaccharides on Nutrient and Energy Metabolism

18.4.5.1 Energy Flow within the Body In order to facilitate an understanding about the effect of polysaccharides on the utilization of nutrients and energy, and eventually on product (meat) quality, a brief overview on formation of

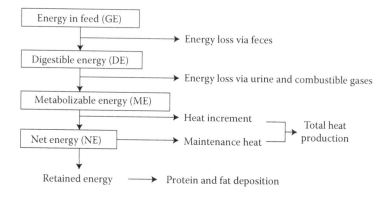

Figure 18.6 Energy flow within the body.

dietary energy in the organism is presented below (Figure 18.6). The energy flow demonstrates that a certain proportion of dietary energy is lost for the animal during the digestive and metabolic processes; therefore, the GE of the feed or ration does not provide relevant information about the nutritive value of the compound feed.

The GE is practically the combustion heat of the feed, which is equivalent to the total combustion heat of different energy-containing nutrients present in the feed or feed component. The average GE of dietary proteins, fats, and carbohydrates are 23.7, 38.9, and 17.5 kJ/g, respectively, but the values may slightly differ depending on the building blocks of the macronutrients.

A certain proportion of total or GE taken up with the feed is excreted with the feces, and the energy retained in the body is called digestible energy (DE). Taking into consideration the digestive characteristics, on average 20–25% of the energy taken up by pigs and poultry species fed concentrate mixes is excreted with the feces. However, the digestibility of dietary energy is greatly influenced by the species and age of the animal, the composition, antinutritive substance content, and processing of the feed, and the use of certain feed additives. In general, it can be stated that the digestibility of energy improves with age. In poultry species, a change in the efficiency of digestion can be observed only up to 2–4 weeks of age, and the extent of that change is greatly influenced by the quality of morphological maturation of the intestinal epithelium during the first 7–10 days after hatching (Batal and Parsons 2002). In pigs, the increase in energy digestibility from piglet to adult age (sow, breeding boar) is clearly the result of the improving fiber digestion. The DE content of fiber-rich feed components (e.g., wheat bran, DDGS) is about 10–15% higher when determined in sows than in growing pigs (Sauvant et al. 2004).

As dietary fiber markedly reduces the absorption of other nutrients and thus also the digestibility of energy, mixtures containing high-fiber components usually have lower DE content. Insoluble fibers depress the digestibility of energy primarily because of the cage effect and the faster intestinal passage.

This depressive effect is greater than that caused by soluble fibers. Although soluble fibers depress the ileal digestibility of energy more than insoluble fibers, as a consequence of fermentation occurring in the large intestine, the nutrients that have remained undigested until then will result in a substantial energy surplus (Figure 18.7) and will eventually provide more DE for the pig than components rich in insoluble fiber (Högberg and Lindberg 2004). In the practice, fat supplementation is used to compensate for the lower energy content. However, the question arises whether the fat × fiber interaction influences the digestibility of energy. In a recent study, Dégen et al. (2009) have found that although the fat × fiber interaction greatly influences the digestibility of nutrients, primarily of fat and fiber, the digestibility of energy contained by concentrate mixes is determined decisively by the fiber content if the latter is supplied by wheat bran. In conclusion, of several studies there might be interaction between dietary fiber and fat; however, it certainly depends on the solubility of fiber and saturation of supplemented fat.

A certain proportion of DE taken up with the diet is lost by excretion *via* the urine and with the intestinal gases (primarily methane). The energy retained in the body is called metabolizable energy (ME). When calculating the ME, theoretically, the energy lost by skin surface abrasion (skin and hairs) would also have to be taken into consideration; however, this does not have practical importance. The energy excreted in the urine is mostly in the form of unused and catabolized proteins; therefore, the efficiency of protein

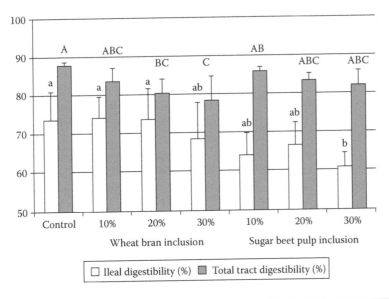

Figure 18.7 Effect of dietary wheat bran or sugar beet pulp inclusion on the ileal and fecal digestibility of energy (%) in growing pigs. [a,b]Means of ileal digestibility data with different superscript differ significantly ($P < 0.05$). [A,B,C]Means of total tract digestibility data with different superscript differ significantly ($P < 0.05$). (From V. Halas, unpublished data.)

utilization greatly influences the dietary ME content. If the protein content and amino acid composition of the diet correspond to the requirements of animals of a given age and body weight, the dietary ME content is about 94–96% of the dietary DE. Gas production is negligible in poultry species, as the short large intestinal segment limits bacterial activity. Thus, the dietary carbohydrate content cannot influence the DE to ME conversion in poultry but it can have an effect on it in pigs, as the fermentation of nondigestible carbohydrates yields methane in addition to acetic acid. The energy lost with methane is on average 0.4% of the dietary energy in growing pigs (20–60 kg), while in sows this value is 1.5%, and it may even reach 3% when high-fiber diets are fed (Noblet and van Milgen 2004).

The ME is still not utilizable for the body in its entirety, as the heat increment generated during the metabolism of nutrients represents a further energy loss. The energy remaining after deducting the heat increment from the ME is termed net energy (NE). This term indicates that the NE is the proportion of dietary energy that can be used by the body without any further loss, for maintenance and for production (weight gain, conceptus development, milk, egg, and wool production). The heat increment is the sum of ATP use during nutrient metabolism, the energy consumption during absorption and excretion, and the heat generated during fermentation. When the fermentable carbohydrate content of the diet is increased, in addition to methane production mentioned above, the greater heat loss also decreases the utilization efficiency of the energy taken up by the organism.

18.4.5.2 Influence of Dietary Polysaccharides on Energy Utilization and Protein and Fat Deposition In the distribution of NE, a priority can be observed, namely, the requirements of maintenance are met first. The energy requirements of maintenance are equivalent with the energy utilization of a nonproducing, nonworking, and nonfasting animal in a thermoneutral environment. It includes the energy (ATP) use of all the processes necessary for the maintenance of life (maintenance of homeostasis, muscle tone, circulation, respiration, brain and nerve tissue, absorption, and transport of nutrients). The maintenance energy requirement (MEm) is usually expressed as a function of the so-called metabolic body weight (body weight $kg^{0.75}$), since the animal's heat production changes proportionally to the body surface rather than the body mass. The value of MEm depends on the animal's age and species, the level of production, the composition of feed, the keeping conditions, environmental factors (temperature, type of management), and also on the animal's activity. In poultry and pigs, the energy utilization associated with motion may increase the energy requirement by as much as 5–25%. Experiments with pigs have demonstrated that the composition of feed and the type of carbohydrate fed influence the animals' activity. Animals consuming a compound feed with high levels of NSP were calmer than those that were fed a diet rich in starch (Schrama et al. 1996). On the other hand, it is also true that, in animals that were fed a high-NSP diet, the so-called resting heat production (i.e., the heat production not related to activity) was higher than in pigs fed the high-starch diet, and thus there was no notable difference between the two groups in total heat production.

The results of experiments conducted with pigs (Anugwa et al. 1989) and broilers (Simon 2001) indicate that higher fiber content and viscosity of the feed are accompanied by an increase in the relative weight of the digestive tract. As the maintenance energy requirement is markedly influenced by digestive tract weight (Nyachoti et al. 2000), the long-term feeding of diets with high soluble fiber content is likely to result in increased maintenance energy requirement and, thus, the energy taken up with the feed will be less efficiently utilized for supporting the productive processes.

Only the energy provided in excess of the maintenance requirement can be used for production (milk, eggs) and for weight gain in growing animals. During gain, the energy requirement of protein synthesis/deposition has priority, and only the energy that remains after meeting this requirement will be incorporated into body fat. Carbohydrates and fats are used for energy generation and fat production, while absorbed amino acids are utilized primarily for protein synthesis in the body. In the energy-yielding transactions, the energy efficiency of ATP generation, that is, the ratio of ATP produced (kJ)/substrate (kJ), varies: on average, it is 58% for amino acids, 66% for fat, 68–70% for glucose, and only 50% for fermentable fiber (Black 1995). It appears that the body gives priority to carbohydrates for meeting the energy requirement of protein synthesis. Namely, the findings of some studies with pigs show that the extra energy supply derived from starch and, to a smaller extent, fermentable NSP supports protein deposition more efficiently than the energy that was derived from fat (Halas and Babinszky 2010; van Milgen et al. 2001).

The energy efficiency of fat production is the highest when the body uses fatty acids for the deposition of body fat; in the case of saturated fatty acids, the efficiency of transformation reaches 90% (Black 1995; van Milgen et al. 2001). The results of experiments with broiler chickens and pigs also confirm that the unsaturated, and especially the polyunsaturated, fatty acids are incorporated into the animal body much less efficiently than the saturated fatty acids (Crespo and Esteve-Garcia 2002; Halas and Babinszky 2010; Kloareg el al. 2007; van Heugten et al. 2007). The energy efficiency of carbohydrates during fat production also depends on whether the substrate provided by them is glucose resulting from enzymatic degradation or volatile fatty acids produced by fermentation. The energy efficiency of starch and glucose was 80–84%, while that of fermentable NSP varied between 58% and 62% in the different experiments (Halas and Babinszky 2010; Noblet et al. 1994; van Milgen et al. 2001).

In addition to the fat-producing effect of nutrients, it is an interesting question whether the dietary energy source influences the partitioning of body fat. Results of certain studies have shown that backfat thickness decreases when pigs are fed a fiber-rich diet (Scipioni et al. 1991), while it increases when a high-fat diet is fed (de la Llata et al. 2001; Mersmann et al. 1984). To answer this question, the relative partitioning of fat deposition should be studied in the course of feeding when isocaloric addition of different energy sources added to a basal ration. In the study of Halas et al. (2010), the percentage partitioning of body fat did not change when 200 kJ DE/kg$^{0.75}$ extra energy was supplied daily from fermentable NSP, starch, and vegetable oil (Table 18.5). The results indicate that the partitioning of fat in the body depends primarily on energy supply, and that the fat content of meat is not influenced by the energy source.

Thus, the energy source present in the diet determines the efficiency of energy-producing processes and body fat synthesis. Although the GE of polysaccharides is independent of their chemical structure, it is determined in the course of digestion whether they can be utilized as glucose or as volatile fatty acids. These two pathways are markedly different in terms of energy efficiency, as fermentable carbohydrates provide much less NE for productive processes than does starch. In animal production, the objective is to have the least possible loss during nutrient conversion and, therefore, over a long period of time, there was a reluctance to use fiber-rich components in the nutrition of monogastric animals. However, the growing human population and the available quantity of industrial by-products suitable for feeding purposes create a situation in which it becomes necessary to use fiber-rich feed components in intensive animal production.

18.5 Use of Dietary Enzyme Supplementation to Improve the Nutritive Value of NSP-Rich Feeds

18.5.1 Objective of Feeding Enzyme Products

The use of enzyme products of microbial origin in pig and poultry nutrition is a possible tool facilitating economical, environment-friendly, and high-quality animal production. So far, more than 50 different types of enzyme products have been authorized for use in the European Union. These products contain either a single or multiple enzymes.

A wide variety of specific enzymes responsible for the hydrolysis of dietary nutrients are produced in the digestive tract of animals. Thus, the question may arise, what effect, if any, do exogenous enzymes have on the production of animals?

Simon (1999) summarized the objectives of using microbial enzymes as follows:

- *Diminishing the effect of antinutritive substances present in the feed.* Essentially this is the primary objective of supplementing grain-based diets with NSP-hydrolyzing enzymes. The primary substrates of NSP enzymes are the substances constituting the soluble NSP fraction; therefore, β-glucanase-containing enzyme

Table 18.5 Effect of Feeding Level and Energy Source on the Relative Partitioning of Body Fat (%)

| | Low Feeding Level | | | | High Feeding Level | | | | | P-Value | |
	Control	Add fNSP	Add dStarch	Add dFat	Control	Add fNSP	Add dStarch	Add dFat	RMSE	FL	ES
Lean	25.9	23.5	26.4	27.0	22.5	22.4	22.6	21.7	3.2	<0.01	0.677
Viscera	9.4	7.3	10.4	11.6	10.1	11.8	11.0	10.3	2.4	0.075	0.483
Hide and subcutaneous fat	46.1	51.1	47.3	47.3	61.2	58.3	58.3	61.0	6.4	<0.01	0.917
Leftover	18.4	11.7	14.2	14.0	6.0	8.2	8.6	8.5	3.6	<0.01	0.745

Source: From Halas, V. et al. 2010. *Br J Nutr* 103:123–33. With permission.
Note: Add fNSP, Add dStarch, Add dFat are 200 kJ DE/kg$^{0.75}$/d extra energy above the control from fermentable NSP, digestible starch and digestible fat, respectively.

products are used primarily in barley-based concentrate mixes, while xylanase-containing products are applied in wheat-, triticale-, and rye-based compound feeds. Through the partial hydrolysis of β-glucans and pentosans, these enzymes lower the viscosity of the digesta and prevent the antinutritive effect of NSP fractions.

- *Hydrolyzing and rendering utilizable those substrates for which the animal organism does not have a suitable digestive enzyme.* In this case, the objective is to improve the bioavailability. An example of this purpose of utilization is the use of phytase, an enzyme that releases phosphorus from phytic acid and makes it absorbable and utilizable for the body.
- *Reduction of phosphorus and nitrogen emission.* This aspect is important especially in areas with high livestock density, where phosphorus and nitrogen emission results in extensive pollution of the environment. Supplementing feeds with phytase enzyme is one of the possible means of reducing the phosphorus excretion of pigs and poultry. However, it should be noted that the most efficient way of regulating nitrogen excretion is the optimization of amino acid supply. The use of different enzymes as feed supplements can decrease the nitrogen emission from animals only in a relatively low degree.
- Recently, an increasing number of studies have reported that exogenous enzymes may be regarded as an alternative to the use of antibiotic growth promoters. However, the results of some these studies still await confirmation.

18.5.2 Most Important Enzyme Products Used in Animal Nutrition

Today, the feed industry manufactures a wide variety of enzyme products for the animal production sector. However, only a few enzymes and their mixtures are used in nutrition. These include the following:

β-Glucanase: β-Glucanase occurs extensively in nature, and it degrades β-glucans, the main constituents of plant cell walls. Barley contains especially high amounts of β-glucan. The β-glucanase enzyme is also needed for degrading the wall of cells present in the aleurone layer and endosperm of barley. It is used in both pig and poultry nutrition.

Xylanase: Xylanase degrades polysaccharides belonging to the group of pentosans, such as hemicellulose, which is actually a xylan formed D-xylose with beta bonds. This enzyme can be used successfully in poultry and pig diets containing high levels of fiber and saturated fatty acids.

Pectinase: Pectinase degrades pectin, which is a constituent of plant cell wall and is produced as a polymer of methyl-D-galacturonate. It is used primarily in poultry nutrition.

Cellulase: Cellulase is practically indigestible for mammals, with the exception of ruminants. In the feed industry, it can primarily be applied in monogastric animals when high-fiber feed components are used.

Proteinases (proteases): Proteases belong to the most important industrial enzymes, constituting approximately 40% of the total quantity of enzyme products marketed. Proteases produced by fungi have long been used as feed additives and their beneficial effects against digestive disorders and dyspepsia have been known for a long time. In the future, proteases will primarily be used in piglet nutrition as a feed additive.

Amylase: Amylase degrades starch granules that serve as reserve material in feed components of plant origin. As its production in the body of animals is often insufficient, amylase is manufactured also on an industrial scale. It is most effective when used in the diets of poultry and early-weaned piglets.

Lipase: Lipase is responsible for the degradation of oils and fats. It is produced by the pancreas but numerous microorganisms can also synthesize it. As a result, its industrial-scale production has also become possible.

Phytase: It can be produced industrially, as numerous bacteria and fungi produce phytase. It has practical importance in decomposing phosphorus, which is stored in plants in the form of phytate phosphorus. Lacking their own enzyme, monogastric animals need phytase to transform phosphorus occurring as phytate chelate into an available and utilizable form. Phytase is used in both pig and poultry nutrition.

18.5.3 Use of NSP-Degrading Enzyme Products in Pig and Poultry Nutrition

Numerous papers have reported the favorable effects obtained by the enzyme supplementation of grain (primarily barley, wheat, triticale, and rye)-based pig diets. The majority of these studies were conducted with young animals (suckling and/or weaned piglets), but the literature contains data on the use of enzymes in growing and finishing pigs and in sows as well. Summarizing the relevant scientific results, it can be stated that the highest number of studies have been conducted with β-glucanase, xylanase, and protease. Less papers have been published on studies with amylase, cellulase, and lipase.

From the data available in the literature, it can be observed that while in earlier studies usually a single enzyme was added to the diet of pigs, recent works increasingly study the collective effect exerted by the combinations of two, three, or more enzymes.

The results of these experiments demonstrate that the use of enzyme products often results in improved nutrient digestibility, and this improvement is also reflected in the production parameters as well (Thacker 1993). The results of studies performed by Thacker (1993) with β-glucanase are summarized in Tables 18.6 and 18.7.

Table 18.6 Effect of β-Glucanase Supplementation on the Digestibility of Dry Matter, Crude Protein, and Energy in Growing Pigs

Digestibility (%)	Control Group	β-Glucanase Group
Dry matter	80.5	82.7
Crude protein	75.1	77.7
Energy	77.9	80.8

Source: From Thacker, P. A. 1993. In *Recent Developments in Pig Nutrition 2*, 295–306. Nottingham: Nottingham University Press. With permission.

The data presented in Tables 18.6 and 18.7 demonstrate that, when added to diets containing high levels of barley, β-glucanase improves the digestibility of dry matter, protein, and energy and increases the performance of growing pigs.

The effect of xylanase on the ileal digestibility of nutrients was studied in pigs that were fed a wheat-, triticale-, and soybean-based concentrate mix in the 10–30, 30–60, and 60–100 kg live weight categories (Table 18.8, L. Babinszky and J. Tossenberger, unpublished data). The data presented in Table 18.8 show that the addition of xylanase to the diet improved the ileal digestibility of nutrients in both weaned piglets and growing pigs. However, this favorable effect could no longer be observed in the 60–100 kg live weight category. These data also indicate that the enzyme supplementation can be expected to exert its beneficial effects primarily in animals of the younger age category.

NSP-degrading enzymes are also used in broiler nutrition, as a supplement to concentrates containing high levels of wheat or barley. As has already been mentioned, NSP-degrading enzymes exert their favorable effect by decreasing the viscosity of digesta, which is expected to result in improved nutrient digestibility. According to observations, the viscosity of digesta in animals fed the enzyme-supplemented diet may decrease from 12.6 to 5.9 cPs.

Some research results indicate that, in addition to improving the digestibility of nutrients, the NSP-degrading enzymes also change the microbiological composition of the digestive tract (Bedford 1996). The change of the microbe population may influence animals' general health status as well. The improved digestibility of nutrients and the more favorable health status may

Table 18.7 Effect of β-Glucanase on the Performance of Growing Pigs

Item	Control Group	β-Glucanase Group
Average body weight gain (g/day)	740	769
Average feed intake (kg/day)	2.32	2.35
Feed conversion ratio (kg/kg)	3.13	3.10

Source: From Thacker, P. A. 1993. In *Recent Developments in Pig Nutrition 2*, 295–306. Nottingham: Nottingham University Press. With permission.

Table 18.8 Effect of Xylanase Supplementation on the Ileal Digestibility of Nutrients (%)

Item	Control Group	Xylanase Group
	Treatments	
Live weight: 10–30 kg		
Dry matter	67.7[a]	74.7[b]
Energy	70.0[a]	76.7[b]
Crude protein	67.1[a]	75.9[b]
Crude fat	58.9[a]	63.3[a]
N-free extract	75.8[a]	81.2[b]
Live weight: 30–60 kg		
Dry matter	68.0[a]	73.7[b]
Energy	70.8[a]	75.7[b]
Crude protein	68.4[a]	75.0[b]
Crude fat	37.9[a]	39.3[a]
N-free extract	75.6[a]	80.6[b]
Live weight: 60–100 kg		
Dry matter	72.2[a]	75.8[a]
Energy	74.7[a]	77.5[a]
Crude protein	76.6[a]	79.0[a]
Crude fat	39.2[a]	41.7[a]
N-free extract	78.0[a]	80.8[a]

Source: L. Babinszky and J. Tossenberger, unpublished data.

[a,b] Means in each row with different superscript differ significantly ($P < 0.05$).

collectively improve the performance of animals too. The effect of β-glucanase on the digestibility of nutrients is shown in Table 18.9. As shown by the data presented in the table, β-glucanase added to the diet significantly ($P < 0.05$) improved the digestibility of crude protein, crude fat, and starch.

Numerous experiments have confirmed the beneficial effect of enzyme mixtures if an enzyme combination corresponding to the substrate, that is, the type of cereal included in the concentrate, was used. The data presented in Table 18.10 also support this observation. The feeding value of wheat varieties having a low ME level due to their high arabinoxylan content can be improved by the addition of appropriate enzyme mixtures to the diets of monogastric animal species such as pigs and poultry.

18.5.4 Flatulence-Producing Compounds of Soybean Meal

It is well known that legume seed meals contain various antinutritional compounds (trypsin inhibitor, glycinin antigen, lectin, oligosaccharides, saponins, etc.). Many of the antinutritional components present in soybean meal can be destroyed or inactivated by heat processing methods (Kim and Baker 2003). Other antinutritional components such as saponins and flatulence-producing compounds are not inactivated by heat processing. Flatulence-producing

Table 18.9 Fecal Digestibility of Nutrients in Broiler Chicks Fed a High-Viscosity Barley Diet with or without β-Glucanase[a]

Dietary Treatment	Crude Protein Digestibility (%)	Crude Fat Digestibility (%)	Starch Digestibility (%)
High-viscosity barley	77.1[b]	72.3[c]	95.8
High-viscosity barley + β-glucanase	83.7[c]	86.2[b]	97.9
SEM (together)	0.99	1.41	0.92

Source: Reprinted from M. Almirall et al. 1995. *Journal of Nutrition* 125:947–55, Copyright (1995). With permission from American Society for Nutrition.

[a] *Trichoderma longibrachiatum* (Finnfeeds International, Marlborough, Wiltshire, England).

[b,c] Different letters within a column differ significantly ($P < 0.05$).

compounds in soybean meal include oligosaccharides and NSP. These carbohydrate polymers are poorly digested by the endogenous enzymes of the host animals. They can increase both osmolarity in the gut and the gut passage rate, which can cause reduced nutrient digestibility. Moreover, these undigested carbohydrates can be utilized by microorganisms in the colon, and this can cause increased intestinal gas formation, nausea, and discomfort to pigs. Common flatulence-producing compounds in soybean meal and other

Table 18.10 Effects of a Glucanase Product (Avizyme TX) on the Performance of Broiler Chickens Fed with Wheat of Different ME Content

Treatments	Weight Gain (g/day)	Feed Intake (g/day)	Feed Conversion Efficiency (kg Feed/ kg Body Weight)	Apparent ME[a] (MJ/ kg DM)
Control with corn	63[a]	122	1.94[a]	16.65[a]
Low-ME wheat	44[b]	110	2.52[b]	12.02[c]
Low-ME wheat + enzyme	57[ab]	112	1.98[a]	14.94[b]
Normal wheat	55[ab]	111	2.03[a]	13.83[b]
Normal wheat + enzyme	62[a]	119	1.94[a]	14.86[b]
SEM (together)	4.7	8.1	0.021	0.20

Source: Reprinted from *J Nutr*, 125, Choct, M. et al. Annison: Non-starch polysaccharide-degrading enzymes increase the performance of broiler chickens fed wheat of low apparent metabolizable energy, 485–92, Copyright (1995), with permission from Elsevier.

[a] Avizyme TX Finnfeeds International, Marlborough, England (xylanase: 2000 U/kg, β-glucanase: 300 U/g, pectinase: 15 U/g).

[b,c] Different letters within a column differ significantly ($P < 0.05$).

legume seed meals are the oligosaccharides, that is, α-1,6-galactosides, and also β-1,4-mannans and ß-galactomannans (Kim and Baker 2003). Enzyme supplements to reduce these flatulence-producing compounds in legume seed meals have been developed and used by nutritionists.

Primarily, the α-1,6-galactosidase and β-1,4-mannanase enzymes are suitable for eliminating the harmful effects of these components. According to Pettey et al. (2000), Schneider et al. (2003), and Kim and Baker (2003), β-1,4-mannanase supplements positively affect the efficiency of feed utilization in nursery and growing pigs but not finishing pigs (Figure 18.8).

According to Reid (1984), complete hydrolysis of ß-galactomannans requires three enzymes: α-1,6-galactosidase, β-1,4-mannanase, and β-1,4-mannosidase. Benefits of supplementing this multiple enzyme mixture were observed during the late nursery phase, the grower period, and the finisher period too (Kim et al. 2001). According to this study, in the late nursery phase, the enzyme mixture improved the digestibility of GE by 7%, the lysine, threonine, and tryptophan digestibility by 3%, and the feed efficiency by 11% during the rearing period.

Summarizing the research results obtained on enzyme feeding, it can be stated that the nutritive value of feeds can be increased by enzyme supplementation; however, the efficiency of the latter depends on the species and age of the animal and the feed components used. Before using enzyme products, it is expedient to determine the NSP content of feed components, and the actual activity of the enzyme product to be used should also be known. The relevant experimental data indicate that the enzyme supplementation of pig and poultry diets containing high levels of cereals reduces the viscosity of digesta and prevents the antinutritive and gas-forming effect of the NSP fractions. As a result, the digestibility of nutrients and the efficiency of animal production will improve.

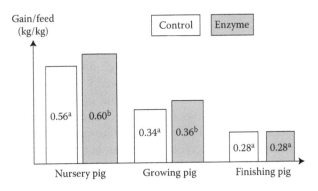

Figure 18.8 Gain/feed of pigs fed diets either with or without β-1,4-mannanase supplement. [a,b] Means of gain/feed data with different superscript differ significantly ($P < 0.05$). (Adapted from Kim, S. W. and D. H. Baker. 2003. *Pig News Info* 24:91–6. With permission.)

18.6 Summary

The most important statements of this chapter can be summarized as follows. The polysaccharides present in the diet may represent nutrient (energy) sources, nutricines (supporting eubiosis, boosting immune response) and antinutritive factors (depressing digestibility, acting as flatulence factors) for the animals. Therefore, the carbohydrate supply of livestock should be evaluated on the basis of the total nutrition concept, relying on the knowledge of precision nutrition. From the digestive-physiological point of view, carbohydrates can be divided into two well-distinguishable groups: (1) starch and sugars, for the degradation of which there is a suitable enzyme system in the digestive tract, and (2) non-starch polysaccharides, commonly known as fiber, which are utilized in the animal organism through the intestinal microbiota. Starch plays a very important role in the energy supply of animals (and humans), while fiber is regarded as having a health-preserving effect both in human dietetics and in animal nutrition. Acting as ballast material, fiber facilitates the development of satiety; moreover, as a consequence of its low energy content and poor utilization, the energy intake can be decreased substantially. It has been known for a long time that the different energy sources of the feed (starch, fiber, saturated or unsaturated fatty acids) result in fat deposition of different degree in the body. Experimental data show that at the same level of energy supply, even if it comes from different energy sources, there is no difference in the amount of fat incorporated into meat. Dietary polysaccharides adversely affect the fatty acid composition of meat, as palmitic acid, stearic acid, and, to a lesser extent, oleic acid are formed from them. Therefore, an unbalanced carbohydrate feeding will result in a meat composition that does not meet the human nutritional expectations.

Intensive animal production requires the intake of substantial amounts of nutrients and energy, which can be accomplished when feeding a high-starch diet but can hardly, or not at all, be achieved with fiber-rich nutrition. Increasing the fiber content is known to reduce the energy density of the ration and depress the digestibility of other nutrients. Thus, as compared to compound feeds of normal fiber content, high-fiber diets will result in the absorption of less protein, amino acid, and energy from the digestive tract. Certain special fiber components, mainly found in legume seeds, are flatulence producing when fed in large quantities, causing marked discomfort to animals. The negative effect of fiber on digestion can be diminished by the use of special carbohydrate-degrading enzymes, but the efficiency of enzyme supplementation is influenced by the animal's species and age and the composition of feed. For the effective use of enzymes, it should be kept in mind that it is always the specific feed component (substrate) that determines what type of enzyme should be applied and in what concentration in order to ensure the successful production of high-quality food materials of animal origin. It is essential to mention that, like the use of any feed additive, the feeding of enzyme products should also be based on economic efficiency calculations in order to ensure profitable production.

Acknowledgment

The support of TÁMOP-4.2.1/B-10/1-2010-0002 program is gratefully acknowledged.

References

Adams, C. A. 2001. *Total Nutrition. Feeding Animals for Health and Growth.* Nottingham: University Press.

Almirall, M., M. Franchesch, A. M. Perez-Vendrell, J, Brufau, and E. Esteve-Garcia. 1995. The differences in intestinal viscosity produced by barley and β-glucanase alter digesta enzyme activities and ileal nutrient digestibilities more in broiler chicks than in cocks. *J Nutr* 125:947–55.

AOAC. 1995. *Official Methods of Analysis of AOAC International.* 16th Edition. Washington, DC: Association of Official Agricultural Chemists.

Anugwa, N. O. L., V. H. Varel, J. Dickson, W. G. Pond, and L. P. Krook. 1989. Effects of dietary fiber and protein concentration on growth, feed efficiency, visceral organ weights and large intestine microbial populations of swine. *J Nutr* 119:879–86.

Asp, N. G. 1996. Dietary carbohydrates: Classification by chemistry and physiology. *Food Chem* 57:9–14.

Babinszky, L. 2008. The concept of ileal digestible amino acid and ileal protein in swine and poultry nutrition. In *Veterinary Nutrition and Dietetics*, ed. S.Gy. Fekete, 119–146. Veszprém: OOk Press.

Babinszky, L. and V. Halas. 2009. Innovative swine nutrition: Some present and potential applications of latest scientific findings for safe pork production. *Italian J Anim Sci* 8. (Suppl. 3):7–20.

Babinszky, L. 2013. Application of the total nutrition concept in swine feeding to produce high quality pork. In *Proceedings of the 20th KRMIVA International Symposium on Animal Nutrition.* Opatia, Croatia, 46–48.

Babinszky, L., V. Halas, and M. W. A. Verstegen. 2011. Impacts of climate change on animal production and quality of animal food products. In *Climate Change. Socioeconomic Effects*, ed. J. A. Blanco and H. Kheradmand, 165–190. Rijeka: InTech Publisher.

Babinszky, L. 1998. Dietary fat and milk production (Chapter 8). In *The Lactating Sow*, ed. M. W. A. Verstegen, P. J. Moughan, and J. W. Schrama, 143–157. Wageningen: Wageningen Pers.

Bach Knudsen, K. E. 1997. Carbohydrate and lignin contents of plant materials used in animal feeding. *Anim Feed Sci Technol* 67:319–38.

Bach Knudsen, K. E. and I. Hansen. 1991. Gastrointestinal implications in pigs of wheat and oat fractions. *Br J Nutr* 65:217–32.

Bach Knudsen, K. E. and H. Jørgensen. 2001. Intestinal degradation of dietary carbohydrates from birth to maturity. In *Digestive Physiology of Pigs*, ed. J. E. Lindberg and B. Ogle, 109–120. Wallingford: CABI Publishing.

Bakker, G. C. M. 1996. Interaction between carbohydrates and fat in pigs—Impact on energy evaluation of feeds. PhD thesis, Wageningen University, The Netherlands.

Bakker, G. C. M., R. Jongbloed, M. W. A. Verstegen et al. 1995. Nutrient apparent digestibility and the performance of growing fattening pigs as affected by incremental additions of fat to starch or non-starch polysaccharides. *Anim Sci* 60:325–35.

Batal, A. B. and C. M. Parsons. 2002. Effects of age on nutrient digestibility in chicks fed different diets. *Poult Sci* 81:400–7.

Bedford, M. R. 1996. The effect of enzymes on digestion. *J Appl Poult Res* 5:370–8.

Bikker, P., A. Dirkzwager, J. Fledderus et al. 2006. The effect of dietary protein and fermentable carbohydrates levels on growth performance and intestinal characteristics in newly weaned piglets. *J Anim Sci* 84:3337–45.

Bikker, P. 1994. Protein and lipid accretion in body components of growing pigs: Effects of body weight and nutrient intake. PhD thesis. Wageningen University, Wageningen, The Netherlands.

Black, J. L. 1995. The evolution of animal growth models. In *Modelling Growth in the Pig*, EAAP Publication No. 78, ed. P. J. Moughan, M. W. A. Verstegen, and M. I. Visser-Reyneveld, 3–9. Wageningen: Wageningen Pers.

Che, T. M., R. W. Johnson, K. W. Kelley et al. 2012. Effects of mannan oligosaccharide on cytokine secretions by porcine alveolar macrophages and serum cytokine concentrations in nursery pigs. *J Anim Sci* 90:657–68.

Che, T. M., R. W. Johnson, K. W. Kelley et al. 2011. Mannan oligosaccharide improves immune responses and growth efficiency of nursery pigs experimentally infected with porcine reproductive and respiratory syndrome virus. *J Anim Sci* 89:2592–602.

Cherbut, C., E. Albina, M. Champ et al. 1990. Action of guar gums on the viscosity of digestive contents and on the gastrointestinal motor function in pigs. *Digestion* 46:205–13.

Choct, M., R. J. Hughes, R. P. Trimble et al. 1995. Non-starch polysaccharide-degrading enzymes increase the performance of broiler chickens fed wheat of low apparent metabolizable energy. *J Nutr* 125:485–92.

Crespo, N. and E. Esteve-Garcia. 2002. Nutrient and fatty acid deposition in broilers fed different dietary fatty acid profiles. *Poult Sci* 81:1533–42.

CVB. 1998. *Central Veevoeder Bureau*, The Netherlands: Lelystad.

de la Llata, M., S. S. Dritz, M. D. Tokach et al. 2001. Effects of dietary fat on growth performance and carcass characteristics of growing and finishing pigs reared in a commercial environment. *J Anim Sci* 79:2643–50.

de Lange, C. F. M., W. C. Sauer, R. Mosenthin et al. 1989. The effect of feeding different protein-free diets on the recovery and amino acid composition of endogenous protein collected from the distal ileum and feces in pigs. *J Anim Sci* 67:746–54.

de Lange, C. F. M. 2000. Characterisation of the non-starch polysaccharides. In *Feed Evaluation—Principles and Practice*, ed. P. J. Moughan, M. W. A. Verstegen, and M. I. Visser-Reyneveld, 77–92. Wageningen: Wageningen Pers.

Dégen, L., V. Halas, and L. Babinszky. 2007. Effect of dietary fiber on protein and fat digestibility and its consequences on diet formulation for growing and fattening pigs: A review. *Acta Agr Scand A-An* 57:1–9.

Dégen, L., V. Halas, J. Tossenberger et al. 2011. Dietary impact of NDF from different sources on the apparent ileal digestibility of amino acids. *Acta Agraria Kaposvariensis* 15:1–11.

Dégen, L., V. Halas, J. Tossenberger et al. 2009. The impact of dietary fiber and fat levels on total tract digestibility of energy and nutrients in growing pigs and its consequence for diet formulation. *Acta Agr Scand A-An* 59:150–60.

Dilger, R. N., J. S. Sands, D. Ragland et al. 2004. Digestibility of nitrogen and amino acids in soybean meal with added soyhulls. *J Anim Sci* 82:715–24.

Dust, J. M., A. M. Gajda, E. A. Flickinger et al. 2004. Extrusion conditions affect chemical composition and *in vitro* digestion of select food ingredients. *J Agric Food Chem* 52:2989–96.

Enneking, D. and M. Wink. 2000. Towards the enlimination of anti-nutritive factors in grain legumes. In *Linking Research and Marketing Opportunities for Pulses in the 21st Century*, ed. R. Knights, 671–683. Dordrecht/Boston/London: Kluwer Academic Press.

Freire, J. P. B., J. Peiniau, L. F. Cunha et al. 1998. Comparative effects of dietary fat and fibre in Alentejano and Large White piglets: Digestibility, digestive enzymes and metabolic data. *Livest Prod Sci* 53:37–47.

Gibson, G. R. and M. B. Roberfroid. 1995. Dietary modulation of the human colonic microbiota: Introducing the concept of prebiotics. *J Nutr* 125:1401–12.

Gill, C. 2007. World feed panorama: Bigger cities, more feed. *Feed Int* 28:5–9.

Graham, H., K. Hasselman, and P. Åman. 1986. The influence of wheat bran and sugar-beet pulp on the digestion of dietary components in cereal-based pig diet. *J Nutr* 116:242–51.

Grala, W., M. W. A. Verstegen, A. J. M. Jansman et al. 1998. Nitrogen utilization in pigs fed diets with soybean and rapeseed products leading to different ileal endogenous nitrogen losses. *J Anim Sci* 76:569–77.

Halas, V. and L. Babinszky. 2010. Efficiency of fat deposition from different energy sources in pigs using multivariate regression analysis. *Acta Agr Scand A-An* 60:38–46.

Halas, V., L. Babinszky, J. Dijkstra et al. 2010. Efficiency of fat deposition from non-starch polysaccharides, starch and unsaturated fat in pigs. *Br J Nutr* 103:123–33.

Halas V. and I. Nochta. 2012. Mannan oligosaccharides in nursery pig nutrition and their potential mode of action. *Animals* 2:261–74.

Hathaway, M. 2000. Alternatives to in-feed antibiotics. *Proceedings of Minnesota Nutrition Conference*, Bloomington, Minnesota.

Henneberg, W. and F. Stohmann. 1859. Über das Erhaltungsfutter volljahrigen Rindviehs. *J Landwitrsch* 34:485–551.

Henry, R. J. 1987. Pentosan and (1-3),(1-4)-beta-glucan in endosperm and whole grain of wheat, barley, oats and rye. *J Cereal Sci* 6:253–8.

Högberg, A. and J. E. Lindberg. 2004. Influence of cereal non-starch polysaccharides on digestion site and gut environment in growing pigs. *Livest Prod Sci* 87:121–30.

Ikegami, S., F. Tsuchihashi, H. N. Tsuchihashi et al. 1990. Effect of viscous indigestible polysaccharides on pancreatic-biliary secretion and digestive organs in rats. *J Nutr* 120:353–60.

Iji, P. A., A. A. Saki, D. R. Tivey. 2001. Intestinal structure and function of broiler chickens on diets supplemented with a mannan oligosaccharide. *J Sci Food Agr* 81:1186–92.

Johnston, L. J., S. Noll, A. Renteria et al. 2003. Feeding by-products high in concentration of fiber to nonruminants. In *Proceedings of the 3rd National Alternative Feeds Symposium Western Regional Coordinating Committee*, Kansas City, 1–26.

Jørgensen, H., X. Q. Zaho, and B. Eggum. 1996. The influence of dietary fibre and environmental temperature on the development of the gastrointestinal tract, digestibility, degree of fermentation in the hind-gut and energy metabolism in pigs. *Br J Nutr* 75:363–78.

Kesting, U., E. Schnabel, and G. Bolduan. 1991. Colon capacity of the sow [Zur Dickdarmkapazitat der Sau, in German]. In: *Digestive physiology of the Hindgut. Adv AnimPhys Anim Nutr* 22:84–8.

Key, F. and J. C. Mathers. 1993. Complex carbohydrate digestion and large bowel fermentation in rats given wholemeal bread and cooked haricot beans (*Phaseolus vulgaris*) fed in mixed diets. *Br J Nutr* 69:497–509.

Kim, S. W., I. Mavromichalis, and R. A. Easter. 2001. Supplementation of alpha-1,6-galactosidase and beta-1,4-mannanase to improve soybean meal utilization by nursing pig. *J Anim Sci* 79 (Suppl. 2):Abstract 106.

Kim, S. W. and D. H. Baker. 2003. Use of enzyme supplements in pig diets based on soyabean meal. *Pig News Info* 24:91–6.

Kloareg, M., J. Noblet, and J. van Milgen. 2007. Deposition of dietary fatty acids, de novo synthesis and anatomical partitioning of fatty acids in finishing pigs. *Br J Nutr* 97:35–44.

Kogan, G. and A. Kocher. 2007. Role of yeast cell wall polysaccharides in pig nutrition and health protection. *Livest Sci* 109:161–5.

Köhler, T. 1992. Evaluation of techniques to collect ileal digesta in pigs. PhD thesis. Wageningen University, The Netherlands.

Kreuzer, M., H. Hanneken, M. Wittmann et al. 2002. Effects of different fibre sources and fat addition on cholesterol and cholesterol-related lipids in blood serum, bile and body tissues of growing pigs. *J Anim Physiol Anim Nutr* 86:57–73.

Kurdi, P., K. Kawanishi, K. Mizutani et al. 2006. Mechanism of growth inhibition by free bile acids in Lactobacilli and Bifidobacteria. *J Bacteriol* 188:1979–86.

Lan, P. T., H. Hayashi, M. Sakamoto et al. 2002. Phylogenetic analysis of cecal microbiota in chicken by the use of 16S rDNA clone libraries. *Microbiol Immunol* 46:371–82.

Laplace, P. J., B. Darcy-Vrillon, Y. Duval-Iflah, and P. Raibaud. 1985. Proteins in the digesta of the pig: Amino ac composition of endogenous, bacterial and fecal fractions. *Reprod Nutr Dévé* 25:1083–99.

Le Goff, G. and J. Noblet. 2001. Comparative total tract digestibility of dietary energy and nutrients in growing pigs and adult sows. *J Anim Sci* 79:2418–27.

Lenis, N. P., P. Bikker, J. van der Meulen et al. 1996. Effect of dietary neutral detergent fiber on ileal digestibility and portal flux of nitrogen and amino acids and on nitrogen utilization in growing pigs. *J Anim Sci* 74:2687–99.

Libao-Mercado, A. J., S. Leeson, S. Langer et al. 2006. Efficiency of utilizing ileal digestible lysine and threonine for whole body protein deposition in growing pigs is reduced when dietary casein is replaced by wheat shorts. *J Anim Sci* 84:1362–74.

Lien, K. A., W. C. Sauer, and M. Fenton. 1997. Mucin output in ileal digesta of hogs fed a protein-free diet. *Z Ernaehrungswiss* 36:182–90.

Mersmann, H. J., W. G. Pond, and J. T. Yen. 1984. Use of carbohydrate and fat as energy source by obese and lean swine. *J Anim Sci* 54:894–902.

Metzler, B. U. and R. Mosenthin. 2008. A review of interactions between dietary fiber and the gastrointestinal microbiota and their consequences on intestinal phosphorus metabolism in growing pigs. *Asian-Aust J Anim Sci* 21:603–15.

Montagne, L., J. R. Pluske, and D. J. Hampson. 2003. A review of interactions between fibre and the intestinal mucosa, and their consequences on digestive health in young non-ruminant animals. *Anim Feed Sci Tech* 108:95–117.

Mosenthin, R., E. Hambrecht, and W. C. Sauer. 2001. Utilization of different fibres in piglet feeds. In *Recent Development in Pig Nutrition 3*, ed. P. C. Grasworthy and J. Wiseman, 300–320. Nottingham: Notthingham University Press.

Mosenthin, R., W. C. Sauer, and F. Ahrens. 1994. Dietary pectin's effect on ileal and fecal amino acid digestibility and exocrine pancreatic secretions in growing pigs. *J Nutr* 124:1222–9.

Moore, W. E. C., L. V. H. Moore, E. P. Cato et al. 1987. Effect of high-fiber and high-oil diets on the fecal flora of swine. *Appl Environ Microbiol* 53:1638–44.

Mroz, Z., G. C. M. Bakker, A. W. Jongbloed et al. 1996. Apparent digestibility of nutrients in diets with different energy density, as estimated by direct and marker methods for pigs with or without ileo-cecal cannulas. *J Anim Sci* 74:403–12.

Myrie, S. B., R. F. Bertolo, W. C. Sauer et al. 2008. Effect of common antinutritive factors and fibrous feedstuffs in pig diets on amino acid digestibilities with special emphasis on threonine. *J Anim Sci* 86:609–19.

Nääs, I. 2001. Precision animal production. *Agr Eng Int GIGR J Sci Res Dev* 3:1–10.

Noblet, J., H. Fortune, X. S. Shi et al. 1994. Prediction of net energy value of feeds for growing pigs. *J Anim Sci* 72:344–54.

Noblet J. and G. Le Goff. 2001. Effect of dietary fibre on the energy value of feeds for pigs. *Anim Feed Sci Technol* 90:35–52.

Noblet, J. and J. M. Perez. 1993. Prediction of digestibility of nutrients and energy values of pig diets from chemical analysis. *J Anim Sci* 71:3389–98.

Noblet, J. and J. van Milgen. 2004. Energy value of pig feeds: Effect of pig body weight and energy evaluation system. *J Anim Sci* 82:E229–38.

Nochta, I., V. Halas, J. Tossenberger et al. 2010. Effect of different levels of mannan oligosaccharide supplementation on the apparent ileal digestibility of nutrients, N-balance and growth performance of weaned piglets. *J Anim Physiol Anim Nutr* 94:747–56.

Nochta, I., T. Tuboly, V. Halas et al. 2009. The effect of different levels of dietary mannanoligosaccharide on specific cellular and humoral immune response in weaned piglets. *J Anim Physiol Anim Nutr* 93:496–504.

Nyachoti, C. M., C. F. M. de Lange, B. W. McBride et al. 1997. Significance of endogenous gut protein losses in the nutrition of growing pigs: A review. *Can J Anim Sci* 77:149–63.

Nyachoti, C. M., C. F. M. de Lange, McBride et al. 2000. Dietary influence on organ size and *in vitro* oxygen consumption by visceral organs of growing pigs. *Livest Prod Sci* 65:229–37.

Owusu-Asiedu, A., J. F. Patience, B. Laarveld et al. 2006. Effects of guar gum and cellulose on digesta passage rate, ileal microbial populations, energy and protein digestibility, and performance of grower pigs. *J Anim Sci* 84:843–52.

Pasquier, B., M. Armand, C. Castelain et al. 1996. Emulsification and lipolysis of triacylglycerols are altered by viscous dietary fibers in acidic gastric medium *in vitro*. *Biochem J* 314:269–75.

Pettey, L. A., S. D. Carter, B. W. Senne et al. 2000. Effects of Hemicell addition to corn-soy bean meal diets on growth performance, carcass traits, and apparent nutrient digestibility of finishing pigs. *J Anim Sci* 77 (Suppl. 1):Abstract 73.

Pettigrew, J. E. 2000. Bio-Mos effects on pig performance: A review. In *Biotechnology in the Feed Industry*. Proceedings Alltech, 16th Annual Symposium, 31–44.

Reid, J. S. G. 1984. Galactomannans. In *Biochemistry of Storage Carbohydrates in Green Plants*, eds. P.M. Dey and R.A. Dixon, 265–288. London: Academic Press.

Renteria Flores, J. A. 2003. Effects of soluble and insoluble dietary fiber on diet digestibility and sow performance. PhD Dissertation, University of Minnesota, St. Paul, MN.

Russell, E. G. 1979. Types and distribution of anaerobic bacteria in the large intestine of pigs. *Appl Environ Microbiol* 37:187–93.

Sauvant, D., J. M. Perez, and G. Tran. 2004. Tables of composition and nutritional value of feed materials: Pigs, poultry, cattle, sheep, goats, rabbits, horses, fish. Wageningen: Academic Publishers.

Schneider, J. D., S. D. Carter, T. Morrilo et al. 2003. Effects of ractopamine and β-mannanase addition to corn- soybean meal diets on growth performance and carcass traits of finishing pigs. *J Anim Sci* 81 (Suppl. 2):Abstract 44.

Schrama, J. W., M. W. A. Verstegen, P. H. J. Verboeket et al. 1996. Energy metabolism in relation to physical activity in growing pigs as affected by type of dietary carbohydrate. *J Anim Sci* 74:2220–5.

Schulze, H., P. van Leeuwen, M. W. A. Verstegen et al. 1994. Effect of level of dietary neutral detergent fiber on ileal apparent digestibility and ileal nitrogen losses in pigs. *J Anim Sci* 72:2362–8.

Schutte, J. B. 1991. Nutritional value and physiological effects of D-xylose and L-arabinose in poultry and pigs. PhD thesis, Wageningen University, Wageningen, The Netherlands.

Scipioni, R., L. Sardi, D. Barchi et al. 1991. Elevate quantita di insilati nell'alimentazione del suino pesante: effeti sulle performance di accresimento e di macellazione. *Riv Suinicolt* 32:71–8.

Sifri, M. 1997. Precision nutrition for poultry. *J Appl Poult Res* 6(4):461.

Simon, O. 1999. Microbial enzymes as feed additives in poultry nutrition. In *Use of Growth Promoters in Animal Nutrition. Proceedings of the 8th International Symposium on Animal Nutrition*, ed. L. Babinszky, 61–81. Kaposvár: University Press.

Simon, O. 2001. The influence of feed composition on protein metabolism in the gut. In *Gut Environment of Pigs*, ed. A. Piva, K. E. Bach Knudsen, and J. E. Linberg, 32–62 Nottingham: Nottingham University Press.

Souffrant, W. B. 2001. Effect of dietary fibre on ileal digestibility and endogenous nitrogen losses in the pig. *Anim Feed Sci Technol* 90:93–102.

Thacker, P. A. 1993. Novel approaches to growth promotion in the pig. In *Recent Developments in Pig Nutrition 2*, ed. D. J. A. Cole, W. Haresign, and P. C. Garnsworthy, 295–306. Nottingham: Nottingham University Press.

Thornton, P. K. 2010. Livestock production: Recent trends, future prospects. *Philos T Roy Soc B* 365:2853–67.

Tripathi, M. K. and A. S. Mishra. 2007. Glucosinolates in animal nutrition: A review. *Anim Feed Sci Technol* 132:1–27.

Trowell, H., D. A. T Southgate, T. M. S. Wolever et al. 1976. Dietary fibre redefined. *Lancet* 307:967.

Van der Klis, J. D. and A. Van Voorst. 1993. The effect of a soluble polysaccharide (carboxy methyl cellulose) on the physico-chemical conditions in the gastrointestinal tract of broilers. *Br Poult Sci* 34:971–83.

Van Leeuwen, P., J. Huisman, M. W. A. Verstegen, M. J. Baak, D. J. van Kleef, E. J. van Verden, and L. A. den Hartog. 1988. A new technique for collection of ileal chyme in pigs. *Proceeding of IVth International Seminar on Digestive Physiologie in the Pig.* 20–30, Jablona, Poland.

Van Heugten, E., J. J. C. G. Van den Borne, M. W. A. Verstegen et al. 2007. Measurement of fatty acid oxidation in swine using 13C labelled fatty acids. In *Proceedings of the 2nd International Workshop on Energy and Protein Metabolism and Nutrition.* EAAP publication No 124, ed. I. Ortigues-Marty, N. Miraux, and W. Brand-Williams, 235–236. Wageningen: Wageningen Academic Publishers.

van Leeuwen, P., A. H. van Gelder, J. A. de Leeuw et al. 2006. An animal model to study digesta passage in different compartments of the gastro-intestinal tract (GIT) as affected by dietary composition. *Curr Nutr Food Sci* 2:97–105.

van Milgen, J., J. Noblet, and S. Dubois. 2001. Energetic efficiency of starch, protein, and lipid utilization in growing pigs. *J Nutr* 131:1309–18.

Van Soest, P. J., J. B. Robertson, and B. A. Lewis. 1991. Methods for dietary fibre, neutral detergent fibre and non-starch polysaccharides in relation to animal nutrition. *J Dairy Sci* 74:3583–97.

Whitney, M. H., G. C. Shurson, and R. C. Guedes. 2006. Effect of including distillers dried grains with solubles in the diet, with or without antimicrobial regimen, on the ability of growing pigs to resist a *Lawsonia intracellularis* challenge. *J Anim Sci* 84:1870–9.

WHO. 2004. World Health Organization. *The World Health Report 2004—Changing History.* http://www.who.int/whr/2004/annex/topic/en/annex_2_en.pdf (accessed: June 23, 2013).

Wilfart A., L. Montagne, H. Simmins et al. 2007. Digesta transit in different segments of the gastrointestinal tract of pigs as affected by insoluble fibre supplied by wheat bran. *Br J Nutr* 98:54–62.

Yin, Y. L., J. D. G. McEvoy, H. Shulze et al. 2000. Apparent digestibility (ileal and overall) of nutrients and endogenous nitrogen losses in growing pigs fed wheat (var. Soissons) or its by products without or with xylanase supplementation. *Livest Prod Sci* 62:119–32.

Zhu, X. Y., T. Zhong, Y. Pandya et al. 2002. 16S rRNA-based analysis of microbiota from the cecum of broiler chickens. *Appl Environ Microbiol* 68:124–37.

Index

A

AACC, *see* American Association of
    Cereal Chemists (AACC)
AB, *see* All-bran (AB)
Aberrant crypt foci (ACF), 390
Acetylated starches, 114–115
ACF, *see* Aberrant crypt foci (ACF)
Acid detergent fiber (ADF), 405, 439
Acid detergent lignin (ADL), 405
Adequate intake (AI), 318
ADF, *see* Acid detergent fiber (ADF)
Adipocytes, 264
ADL, *see* Acid detergent lignin (ADL)
AG, *see* Arabinogalactan (AG)
Agaricus blazei, 176–177; *see also*
    Mushroom polysaccharides
Agave, 46–47, 49; *see also* Fructan
    A. angustifolia Haw, 52–53
    A. cantala, 53
    A. fourcroydes, 53
    agavins, 48, 50
    age and fructan content, 53
    A. potatorum Zucc, 53
    A. tequilana, 49, 50, 52
    carbohydrates in, 50
    economically important, 52
    enzymes and fructan content in, 53
    territories used for, 51
Agave fructan
    on calcium and magnesium
        absorption, 67–68
    classification, 52

fermentable inulin-type fructan
    effect, 66
functions of, 53
future potential 68
GLP-1, 67
hunger hormone, 65
inulins with SDP, 66
lipid and glucose metabolism
    modulation, 64–65
on mice health, 63–64
satiety hormone homeostasis, 65
in stem, 51
structures, 54
values of, 50
Agavins, 48, 50
AG proteins, *see* Arabinogalactan-
    proteins (AG proteins)
AI, *see* Adequate intake (AI)
AICR, *see* American Institute for
    Cancer Research (AICR)
Akkermansia muciniphila, 368–369
Aktivated barley, 251
All-bran (AB), 305
Allium species, 76–77; *see also*
    Fructooligosaccharides in
    Allium species
    edible, 78, 91
    FOS content in, 90–91
    high-FOS *Allium* breeding,
        89–90
α-D-Galacturonic acid (GalA),
    33, 333
α-Glucanotransferases, 121–122

American Association of Cereal
    Chemists (AACC), 370
American Institute for Cancer Research
    (AICR), 306
AML, see Amylose leaching (AML)
AMP-activated protein kinase (AMPK),
    278
AMPK, see AMP-activated protein kinase
    (AMPK)
Amylase, 463
    α-amylase, 118–119, 445
    β-amylase, 119–120
Amylopectin, 209
Amylose, 209
Amylose leaching (AML), 112
Animal agriculture; see also Dietary
        polysaccharides
    challenges in, 430–431
    modern animal nutrition, 432–434
    precision nutrition, 432
    significance of carbohydrates,
        434–436
Annealing, 112
Antimicrobial activity 163
Antiobesity medications, 369
Antioxidant
    capacity of apple, 37–38, 39
    dietary fiber, 33
    phenolic acids, 220
Antiviral activity 162–163
AOAC, see Association of Official
        Analytical Chemist (AOAC)
Apple, 36
    antiatherogenic effect of, 39
    antioxidant capacity of, 37–38, 39
    cholesterol-lowering, 37
    immunomodulation, 38
    nutrients in peel, 37
    polyphenols in, 36, 39
Arabinogalactan (AG), 214
Arabinogalactan-proteins (AG proteins),
        221; see also Nonstarch
        polysaccharide (NSP)
    beneficial roles, 222
    health implications, 221
    structure of, 222
Arabinoxylans (AXs), 208, 216, 373; see
        also Nonstarch polysaccharide
        (NSP)
    backbone of, 216
    effect of structure on physicochemical
        characteristics of, 219–220

nutraceutical importance of, 220–221
    in rice endosperm cell walls, 217
    rye water-insoluble, 218
    structure of, 216
    wheat water-unextractable, 217
Area under the curve (AUC), 269
Association of Official Analytical
        Chemist (AOAC), 37
AUC, see Area under the curve (AUC)
Auricularia auricula, 178–179; see also
        Mushroom polysaccharides
Autotransporter adhesins, 331
avDAS, see Average degree of substitution
        (avDAS)
Average degree of substitution (avDAS),
        373–374
AXs, see Arabinoxylans (AXs)

B

Back transfer reaction, 4
Bacterial adhesins, 331–332
Bacterial toxins, 332
Bacteroidetes, 278
BAR, see Bio-array resource (BAR)
Barley β-glucan, 235
BBC, see Bran buds with corn (BBC)
BBP, see Bran buds with psyllium (BBP)
BCG, see Calmette-Guerin bacillus (BCG)
Belviq, 369
β-Fructofuranosidase, 135, 142
βGB, see β-Glucan-enriched bread (βGB)
β-Glucan, 150, 234, 253, 376–377; see also
        Mushroom polysaccharides;
        Nonstarch polysaccharide
        (NSP)
    Aktivated barley, 251
    in barley, 235
    on blood lipids, 243–244, 248–253
    cholesterol reduction, 163
    in cholesterol reduction, 248–253
    effect of MW, 249
    food products with barley, 237–240
    on glycemic and insulin response,
        240–248
    health benefits of barley, 240
    immune response against, 215–216
    lentinan, 174
    Mws of, 215
    in oats, 249
    properties of, 236
    Prowashonupana, 234

structural analysis of, 215
structure of, 214, 234
β-Glucanase, 462
  effect on pigs, 464
  on fecal digestibility, 466
β-Glucan-enriched bread (βGB), 376
Bioaccessible compounds, 35–36
Bioactive dietary constituents, 32; *see also*
      Dietary fiber; Phenol
  substances of mushrooms, 150
Bio-array resource (BAR), 7
Bioavailability, 36
Biological response modifiers (BRMs),
      160, 172, 215; *see also*
      Mushroom polysaccharides
BMI, *see* Body mass index (BMI)
Body mass index (BMI), 278, 367
Body weight (BW), 302
Bran buds with corn (BBC), 305
Bran buds with psyllium (BBP), 305
Brazilian Cerrado, 132; *see also* Fungal
      enzymes in FOS production
BRMs, *see* Biological response modifiers
      (BRMs)
Butyrate, 328, 330
  production, 285
Butyrogenic bacteria, 372
BW, *see* Body weight (BW)

C

Cage effect, 448
Calmette-Guerin bacillus (BCG), 163
Cancer prevention, 91–92
Cannabinoid receptor 1 (CB₁), 280
Carbohydrate (CHO), 245, 434, 468; *see*
      also Dietary polysaccharides;
      Polysaccharide-based
      structures
  in animal nutrition, 438
  content in feedstuffs, 446
  crude fiber, 439
  in feedstuffs, 442
  functional, 59–60
  monomer with N-containing
      compound, 444
  N-free extract, 439
  nondigestible, 444
  for protein deposition, 435
  roles, 441
  significance of, 434–436
  structural, 443

Cardiovascular disease (CVD), 76,
      250, 386
  prevention, 162
CB, *see* Control bread (CB)
CB₁, *see* Cannabinoid receptor 1 (CB₁)
CCK, *see* Cholecystokinin (CCK)
CD14, 279
Cellulase, 462
Cellulose, 33, 235, 403–404
  microfibrils, 34
Cell walls
  in cereals, 352
  constituents, 408
  in pulses, 352
Cereal endosperm in food processing,
      353
Cerrado, 132; *see also* Brazilian Cerrado
  enzymes source for 6-FOS synthesis,
      137
  vegetation, 134
Cetyl trimethyl ammonium bromide
      (CTAB), 211
CGTase, *see* Cyclomaltodextrin
      glucanotransferase
      (CGTase)
Chicory (*Cichorium intybus* L.), 5, 7
Chicory fructan, 260, 290–291; *see also*
      Glucose metabolism disorders;
      Gut microbes
  biosynthesis, 7, 23
  on blood glucose, 266–272
  caloric value of, 289
  dietary fiber and diabetes, 265–266
  and fat storage, 286–287
  1-FFT activity, 8
  for glucose metabolism
      disorders, 265
  glycemic index reduction by, 290
  on gut barrier function, 286
  and gut-derived peptides, 287–288
  and gut microbiota modulation, 282
  inulin, 5, 261
  on leptin, 287
  on microbiota modulation, 283–284
  as prebiotic ingredients, 282–286
  and SCFA production, 285
  on serum glucose, 272–276
  sugar substitution by, 290
Chitin, 443
Chive (*Allium schoenoprasum*), 77
CHO, *see* Carbohydrate (CHO)
Cholecystokinin (CCK), 246

Cholesterol reduction
by apple, 37
by β-glucan, 163, 248–253
by mushroom polysaccharides, 192
Chronic disease prevention, 90
Chronic idiopathic constipation (CIC),
309
CIC, see Chronic idiopathic constipation
(CIC)
Cold-water swelling (CWS), 111
Colonic bacteria, 387
Colorectal cancer (CRC), 389
Constipation, 309
Constipation-predominant irritable
bowel syndrome (IBS-C),
309
treatment of, 321
Contrabiotic effect, 328, 331, 341
Control bread (CB), 376
Conventionalization, 278
Cool paste viscosity (CPV), 115
Cordyceps mushrooms, 178; see also
Mushroom polysaccharides
Coriolous versicolor, 177; see also
Mushroom polysaccharides
Correlated spectroscopy (COSY), 154
COSY, see Correlated spectroscopy
(COSY)
CPV, see Cool paste viscosity (CPV)
CRC, see Colorectal cancer (CRC)
C-reactive protein (CRP), 249, 313
Crosslinking in starch, 113–114
CRP, see C-reactive protein (CRP)
Crude fiber, 439; see also Carbohydrate
fractionation, 405
CTAB, see Cetyl trimethyl ammonium
bromide (CTAB)
CVD, see Cardiovascular disease (CVD)
CWS, see Cold-water swelling (CWS)
Cyclodextrin glycosyltransferase,
120–121
Cyclomaltodextrin glucanotransferase
(CGTase), 119

D

DAEC, see Diffusely adherent E. coli
(DAEC)
Dahlia variabilis (DVS), 52
Dark, firm, and dry meat (DFD meat),
443
DC, see Dendritic cells (DC)

DDGS, see Distiller's dried grains with
solubles (DDGS)
DE, see Digestible energy (DE)
Degenerative diseases, 213
Degree of polymerization (DP), 4, 47,
212, 260
Degree of substitution (DS), 115
Dendritic cells (DC), 187
Deoxyribonucleic acid (DNA), 214
DFD meat, see Dark, firm, and dry meat
(DFD meat)
DgF, see Digestible fiber (DgF)
Diabetes mellitus; see also Glucose
metabolism disorders; Obesity
dietary fiber and, 265–266
effect of β-glucan, 240
type 2, 263–264
Diabetes Prevention Program (DPP), 264
Dietary enzyme supplementation,
460; see also Dietary
polysaccharides; Nonstarch
polysaccharide (NSP)
amylase, 463
in animal nutrition, 462–463
β-glucanase, 462, 464, 466
cellulase, 462–463
feeding enzyme products, 460, 462
flatulence-producing compounds,
465–467
lipase, 463
NSP-degrading enzyme products,
463–465
pectinase, 462
phytase, 463
proteases, 463
xylanase, 462, 465
Dietary fiber for rabbit, 409, 423; see also
Dietary fiber
cellulose and lignins intake, 416–418
commercial feed constituents, 410
DgF estimation, 418
digestion in rabbit, 411–412
digestive health, 414
digestive troubles and DgF, 419–420
disease prevention, 415–416
fecal digestibility, 413
fermentable fiber and physiology,
421–422
intake regulation, 410, 409–411
rabbit cecal ecosystem, 413
recommendations for risk reduction,
422–423

Dietary fiber fractionation, 405
    cell wall polysaccharide analysis,
        407–408
    crude fiber method, 405
    fiber analysis methods, 409
    NDF method, 405
    soluble fiber content estimation, 407
    Van Soest procedures, 405–406
    WICW, 406
Dietary fiber in gastroenterology, 302,
        318, 321
    cohort studies, 307
    colonic functions, 303–305
    constipation, 309–310
    DF properties, 317
    diseases prevention, 305–308,
        316–318, 319–320
    diverticular disease, 305, 312–313
    enteral formula, 314
    hemorrhoids complications, 310–311
    irritable bowel syndrome, 311–312
    prebiotic oligosaccharides, 314–316
    prebiotics and acute pancreatitis,
        313–314
    recommendations, 302–303
Dietary fibers (DFs), 32, 233, 302, 369,
        400, 454; see also Dietary
        fiber for rabbit; Dietary fiber
        fractionation; Nonstarch
        polysaccharide (NSP); Plant cell
        wall polymers; Soluble dietary
        plant NSP
    antioxidant, 33
    biochemical characteristics of,
        402–405
    components, 402, 440
    compounds, 234
    on crude fat digestibility, 453
    determination, 439
    for diabetes, 265–266
    digestion, 443–444
    fractions and quantification, 403
    health benefits, 32, 39, 329–331, 371
    insoluble vs. soluble fiber, 329
    matrix components, 329
    NSP component, 330
    and obesity, 370, 378
    pectic substances, 403
    physical effects of, 370
    and polysaccharide structure, 348
    on protein and amino acid
        digestibility, 452

source of, 328
Weende method, 400
Dietary polysaccharides, 430, 468–469;
        see also Animal agriculture;
        Carbohydrate; Dietary enzyme
        supplementation; Dietary
        fibers (DFs); Nonstarch
        polysaccharide (NSP); Obesity;
        Oligosaccharides (OS); Total
        nutrition
    carbohydrate in feedstuffs, 442, 446
    carbohydrate monomer, 444
    classification of, 438–441
    digestibility, 445–448
    disaccharide absorption, 445
    energy flow within body, 455–458
    on energy utilization and protein and
        fat deposition, 458–460, 461
    fiber digestion, 443–444
    glycogen, 443, 446
    glycosides, 445
    grouping, 440
    ileal digestibility, 449
    interaction with other nutrients,
        451–454
    on intestinal microbiota, 454–455
    lignin in feedstuffs, 442
    mode of action, 448–451
    in monogastric animal nutrition, 438
    monosaccharides absorption, 446
    nutritional consequences, 445
    starch, 441, 446
    TDF determination methods, 441
    Weende analysis, 439
Diet in disease prevention, 385; see also
        Fructooligosaccharide (FOS)
Differential scanning calorimetry (DSC),
        108
Diffusely adherent *E. coli* (DAEC), 333
Digestible energy (DE), 409, 456
Digestible fiber (DgF), 418
    digestive troubles and, 419–420
    fermentable fiber, 421–422
Digestion of starch, 122
Dimethyl sulfoxide (DMSO), 116, 157
1,1-Diphenyl-dipicrylhydrazyl (DPPH),
        190
Diseases prevention by mushroom, 60
    antimicrobial activity, 163
    antiviral activity, 162–163
    CVD prevention, 162
    tumor therapy, 161–162

Dissolved oxygen (DO), 183
Distiller's dried grains with solubles
    (DDGS), 455
DM, *see* Dry matter (DM)
DMSO, *see* Dimethyl sulfoxide (DMSO)
DNA, *see* Deoxyribonucleic acid (DNA)
DO, *see* Dissolved oxygen (DO)
DP, *see* Degree of polymerization (DP)
DPP, *see* Diabetes Prevention Program
    (DPP)
DPPH, *see* 1,1-Diphenyl-dipicrylhydrazyl
    (DPPH)
Dry matter (DM), 81
DS, *see* Degree of substitution (DS)
DSC, *see* Differential scanning
    calorimetry (DSC)
DVS, *see* *Dahlia variabilis* (DVS)

E

EAEC, *see* Enteroaggregative *E. coli*
    (EAEC)
eCB, *see* Endocannabinoid system (eCB)
Ectomycorrhizal mushrooms,
    181; *see also* Mushroom
    polysaccharides
Edible mushroom, 178
EDTA, *see* Ethylene diamine tetraacetic
    acid (EDTA)
EFSA, *see* European Food Safety
    Authority (EFSA)
Elasticity increment (IE), 159
Electrospray ionization-mass
    spectrometry (ESI-MS), 213
Endocannabinoid system (eCB), 280
Endo-inulinases, 132; *see also* Inulin
    activity, 136
Endoplasmic reticulum (ER), 376
Enteroaggregative *E. coli* (EAEC), 333
Enteropathogenic *E. coli* (EPEC), 339
Enterotoxigenic *E. coli* (ETEC), 331
Enterotoxins, 332
Enterotypes, 278
Enzyme
    β-2, 6-linked FOS production, 137
    source of 6-FOS synthesis, 137
EPEC, *see* Enteropathogenic *E. coli*
    (EPEC)
EPIC, *see* European Prospective
    Investigation into Cancer and
    Nutrition (EPIC)
ER, *see* Endoplasmic reticulum (ER)

ESI-MS, *see* Electrospray ionization-mass
    spectrometry (ESI-MS)
ETEC, *see* Enterotoxigenic *E. coli* (ETEC)
Ethylene diamine tetraacetic acid
    (EDTA), 403
European Food Safety Authority (EFSA),
    164, 253
European Prospective Investigation into
    Cancer and Nutrition (EPIC),
    305
Exo-inulinases, 132; *see also* Inulin

F

FAB-MS, *see* Fast atom bombardment-
    mass spectrometry (FAB-MS)
FAE, *see* Follicle-associated epithelium
    (FAE)
Fast atom bombardment-mass
    spectrometry (FAB-MS), 213
Fasting-induced adipose factor (Fiaf), 278
    suppression, 278
FDA, *see* U. S. Food and Drug
    Administration (FDA)
1-FEH, *see* Fructan exohydrolase (1-FEH)
Fenfluramine, 369
Fen-phen, 369
FF, *see* Functional foods (FF)
FFA, *see* Free fatty acids (FFA)
FFAR3, *see* Free fatty acid receptor 3
    (FFAR3)
1F-Fructofuranosyl nystose, 81
1-FFT, *see* Fructan: fructan
    1-fructosyltransferase (1-FFT)
Fiaf, *see* Fasting-induced adipose factor
    (Fiaf)
Fibers, 75–76
    fraction determination method,
        439, 441
Fimbriae, 331
Finger millet, 218
Firmicutes phyla, 278
FNB, *see* Food and Nutrition Board
    (FNB)
Follicle-associated epithelium (FAE), 333
Food and Nutrition Board (FNB), 32
FOS, *see* Fructooligosaccharide (FOS)
Free fatty acid receptor 3 (FFAR3), 371
Free fatty acids (FFA), 262
Free sugars, 208
Fructan: fructan 1-fructosyltransferase
    (1-FFT), 2, 48

activity in roots, 5–6
regulation, 7
Fructan, 2, 47, 105–106, 260;
    see also Fructan
    biosynthesis modification;
    Fructooligosaccharide
    (FOS); Heterologous fructan
    production; Plant fructan;
    Tailor-made fructan
agavins, 48, 50
bacterial biosynthesis, 2
against bacteriostatic compounds, 2
bcacterial growth in, 58
catalytic breakdown of, 5
classification, 52, 260
for commercial production of, 5
definition, 47
degradation by temperature, 6
degree of polymerization, 48
as energy storage molecule, 2
enzymes, 53
fructan structures, 54
fructosyltransferases regulation, 7
to improve organoleptic properties,
    132
level in wheat, 6
neo-series, 2
plant fructan, 2
relevance of, 48–49
shortest, 4
stability in storage organs, 20–21
storage, 106
from transfructosylating activity on
    sucrose, 133
types of, 48
Fructan analytical tools, 55
    fructan derivatization to methylated
        alditol acetates, 56
    GC-MS, 55
    HPAECPAD, 55 56
    MALDI-TOF-MS, 56–57
    MIR spectroscopy, 58, 59
    NMR, 57–58
    TLC, 55
Fructan biosynthesis modification; *see
    also* Heterologous fructan
    production
    to alter fructan type, 9
    for higher mDP and Yield, 9
    in other plants, 10–11
Fructan exohydrolase (1-FEH), 2
    degradation of inulin, 4

in fructan-accumulating plants, 20
inhibited by sucrose, 6
regulation, 7
Fructan prebiotic activity, 60–61
on bacterial growth, 62
in vitro study, 61
measuring, 63
mice studies 63
Fructooligosaccharide (FOS), 49,
    105–106, 131, 316, 386; *see also*
    Fructan; Fungal enzymes in
    FOS production
animal studies, 390–391
β-fructofuranosidases, 135
cancer and diet, 389
in edible *Allium* species, 81
history of, 77–78
HPAEC/PAD profiles of, 136, 138
in human diet, 387
human studies, 391–392
occurrence, 140
physiological effects of, 388
prebiotic effects, 387–388
Fructooligosaccharides in *Allium* species,
    75; *see also Allium* species
biosynthesis pathway, 85, 86
chemistry, 79
distribution of, 85, 86
in edible *Allium* species, 81
enzymatic synthesis of, 87, 88–89
1F-Fructofuranosyl nystose, 81
1-Kestose, 81
mechanism of hydrolysis, 86
Nystose, 81
soluble carbohydrate separation, 84
structure, 79, 80, 82, 83
Fructosyltransferases (FTs), 48, 132
induction, 4
FTases genes, 144
FTs, *see* Fructosyltransferases (FTs)
Fucoidans, 375–376
Functional foods (FF), 386
in obesity, 370
Fungal enzymes in FOS production,
    134, 138, 139; *see also*
    Fructooligosaccharide (FOS)
β-2, 6-linked, 137
β-fructofuranosidase, 142
endo-inulinase activity, 136
enzyme production, 142, 144
FTases genes, 144
hydrolytic activity, 140

Fungal enzymes *(Continued)*
   industrial processes, 143
   inulin hydrolysis, 143
   6-kestose production, 139
   limitation, 140
   microbial β-fructofuranosidases, 135
   sucrose into FOS, 139–140
   sugar utilization, 135
   transferase to hydrolase activity,
      136–137
   transfructosylating activity, 141–142
   two-step process, 142

G

GA, *see* Gum arabic (GA)
GalA, *see* α-D-Galacturonic acid
   (GalA)
Galacto-oligosaccharides (GOS), 315
Ganoderan, 154, 174; *see also* Mushroom
   polysaccharides
   as adjuvant cancer therapy, 188
   chemical structures of, 175
Ganoderma; *see also* Mushroom
   polysaccharides
   lucidum, 174
   tsugae, 176
Garlic (*Allium sativum*), 77; *see also*
   Allium species
Gas chromatography (GC), 153
Gas chromatography–mass spectrometry
   (GC–MS), 55, 153, 213
Gas liquid chromatography–mass
   spectrometry (GLC–MS), 218
Gastric inhibitory peptide (GIP), 246
GC, *see* Gas chromatography (GC)
GC–MS, *see* Gas chromatography–mass
   spectrometry (GC–MS)
GE, *see* Gross energy (GE)
Gelatinization, 108, 159
Gelatinization temperature range
   (GTR), 113
Gelatinization transition temperature
   (GTT), 112
6G-FFT, *see* 6G-fructan:fructan
   fructosyltransferase (6G-FFT)
6G-fructan:fructan fructosyltransferase
   (6G-FFT), 48
GGEs, *see* g. Glucose equivalents (GGEs)
g. Glucose equivalents (GGEs), 360
Ghrelin, 65
GI, *see* Glycemic index (GI)

GIP, *see* Gastric inhibitory peptide
   (GIP); Glucose-dependent
   insulinotropic polypeptide
   (GIP)
GLC–MS, *see* Gas liquid
   chromatography–mass
   spectrometry (GLC–MS)
GLP-1, *see* Glucagon-like peptide 1
   (GLP-1)
GLP-2, *see* Glucagon-like peptide-2
   (GLP-2)
Glucagon, 262
Glucagon-like peptide-1 (GLP-1), 65, 66,
   263, 281
   impact of chicory fructan on, 287–288
Glucagon-like peptide-2 (GLP-2), 280
   impact of chicory fructan on, 287
Glucan-protein complex, 155
Glucoamylase, 120
Glucomannans, 33
Glucose, 261
   dietary disposal, 262
   endogenous, 262
   polysaccharides, 235
Glucose-dependent insulinotropic
   polypeptide (GIP), 263
Glucose metabolism disorders, 261;
   see also Diabetes mellitus;
   Chicory fructan; Gut microbes
   Fiaf suppression, 278
   glucose disposal, 261–262
   IFG, 264
   IGT, 240, 264
   insulin resistance, 264–265
   metabolic syndrome, 265
   microbiota profile in populations
      suffering from, 276–277
   postprandial blood glucose level
      regulation, 262–263
   type 2 diabetes, 263–264
Glutathione-*S*-transferases (GSTs), 392
Glycemic index (GI), 270
Glyco-calyx, 208
Glycogen, 446
Glycogenesis, 262
Glycosides, 445
God's mushroom, *see Agaricus—blazei*
GOS, *see* Galacto-oligosaccharides (GOS)
GPR, *see* G-protein-coupled receptors
   (GPR)
G-protein-coupled receptors (GPR),
   281, 371

Graminans, 48, 375
Green onion, *see* Scallion (*Allium fistulosum*)
Grifola frondosa, 177; *see also* Mushroom polysaccharides
Grifolan, 177; *see also* Mushroom polysaccharides
Gross energy (GE), 435
GSTs, *see* Glutathione-S-transferases (GSTs)
GTR, *see* Gelatinization temperature range (GTR)
GTT, *see* Gelatinization transition temperature (GTT)
Gum arabic (GA), 370, 377
Gut-derived peptides, 280–281
Gut microbes, 368–369; *see also* Chicory fructan; Glucose metabolism disorders
    bacteroidetes, 278
    diet and composition of, 281–282
    eCB and CB$_1$, 280
    enterotypes, 278
    Firmicutes phyla, 278
    fructan on, 283–284
    and glucose metabolism disorders, 276–277
    gut-derived peptides, 280–281
    metabolic endotoxemia inflammation, 278–280
    in nutrient harvest regulation, 277–278
    of pigs, 448
    in regulation of fat storage, 278
Gut peptide, *see* Glucagon-like peptide-1 (GLP-1)

H

Hairy region of pectins, *see* Rhamnogalacturonan I regions (RGI)
HDL, *see* High-density lipoprotein (HDL)
Health benefits of FOS, 90, 95
    attributed to oligosaccharides, 91
    cancer prevention, 91–92
    on glycemia and insulinemia, 94–95
    lipids metabolism, 92–93
    mineral absorption, 94
    prebiotic effects, 93–94
    to prevent chronic diseases, 90

Health risk index (HRi), 414
Heat-labile toxin (LT), 337
Heat-moisture-treatment, 112, 113
Heat-stable toxin (ST), 337
Hemagglutinins, 444
Hemicelluloses, 33
Heteroglycans, 179; *see also* Mushroom polysaccharides
Heterologous fructan production, 11; *see also* Fructan biosynthesis modification; Tailor-made fructan
    using bacterial genes, 11, 17
    fructan pathway in nonfructan plants, 18–19
    in genetically engineered crops, 12–16
    using plant genes, 17
    6-SFT in nonfructan plants, 18
    1-SST into nonfructan plants, 17–18
Heteronuclear multiple bond coherence (HMBC), 154
Heteronuclear multiple quantum coherence (HMQC), 154
Heteropolysaccharides, 150, 155
HF, *see* High-fat (HF)
HFCS, *see* High-fructose corn syrup (HFCS)
HFD, *see* High fat diet (HFD)
HG, *see* Homogalacturonan (HG)
High-amylose starch prebiotic, 122
High-density lipoprotein (HDL), 162, 248, 265
High-fat (HF), 287, 374
High fat diet (HFD), 372
High-fructose corn syrup (HFCS), 266
Highmolecular-weight (High-MW), 122, 249
High-MW, *see* Highmolecular-weight (High-MW)
High-performance anion exchange chromatography-pulsed amperometric detection (HPAEC-PAD), 4, 55, 56
High-performance liquid chromatography (HPLC), 153
Himalaya-292, 234; *see also* β-Glucan
HIV, *see* Human immunodeficiency virus (HIV)
HMBC, *see* Heteronuclear multiple bond coherence (HMBC)
HMOs, *see* Human milk oligosaccharides (HMOs)

HMQC, *see* Heteronuclear multiple
  quantum coherence (HMQC)
HNE, *see* 4-Hydroxynonenal (HNE)
HOMA IR, *see* Homeostasis model
  assessment-estimated insulin
  resistance (HOMA IR)
HOMA$_{IR}$, *see* Homeostatic model
  assessment for insulin
  resistance (HOMA$_{IR}$)
Homeostasis model assessment-
  estimated insulin resistance
  (HOMA IR), 246
Homeostatic model assessment for
  insulin resistance (HOMA$_{IR}$),
  265
Homogalacturonan (HG), 33
Homoglycan, *see* Homopolysaccharide
Homopolysaccharide, 150, 156
Hot aqueous extraction, 155
HPAEC-PAD, *see* High-performance
  anion exchange
  chromatography-pulsed
  amperometric detection
  (HPAEC-PAD)
HPLC, *see* High-performance liquid
  chromatography (HPLC)
H. pylori adhesin BabA, 332
HRi, *see* Health risk index (HRi)
HT29, *see* Human intestinal epithelial
  cell cultures (HT29)
Human immunodeficiency virus
  (HIV), 163
Human intestinal epithelial cell cultures
  (HT29), 318
Human milk oligosaccharides (HMOs),
  302, 314–316
Hunger hormone, *see* Ghrelin
Hydrolysis
  of FOS, 86
  of inulin, 143
  of starch-based products, 118
4-Hydroxynonenal (HNE), 392

I

IBS, *see* Irritable bowel syndrome (IBS)
IBS-C, *see* Constipation-predominant
  irritable bowel syndrome
  (IBS-C)
ICU, *see* Intensive care unit (ICU)
ID AA, *see* Ileal digestible amino acid
  (ID AA)

IDF, *see* Insoluble dietary fiber (IDF)
IE, *see* Elasticity increment (IE)
IFG, *see* Impaired fasting glucose (IFG)
IFN-γ, *see* Interferon-γ (IFN-γ)
IGT, *see* Impaired glucose intolerance
  (IGT)
II, *see* Insulinemic index (II)
IL-6, *see* Interleukin-6 (IL-6)
Ileal
  break, 281
  digestibility, 449
Ileal digestible amino acid (ID AA),
  449
Impaired fasting glucose (IFG), 264;
  see also Glucose metabolism
  disorders
Impaired glucose intolerance (IGT),
  240, 264; *see also* Glucose
  metabolism disorders
Incretins, 263
Information intensive nutrition, 434
Infrared (IR), 212
Innovation time, 432
Insoluble dietary fiber (IDF), 405, 441
Insoluble fiber, 302, 329, 448; *see also*
  Dietary fiber
Insulin, 262; *see also* Diabetes mellitus;
  Glucose metabolism disorders
  resistance, 264–265
Insulinemic index (II), 270
Insulin receptor (IR), 265
Insulin receptor substrate-1 (IRS-1), 279
Intensive care unit (ICU), 313
Interferon-γ (IFN-γ), 187
Interleukin-6 (IL-6), 279
Inulin, 2, 260, 375; *see also* Fructan;
  Levan
  accumulation, 5–6
  from *Agave tequilana*, 49
  chicory, 261
  degradation, 4
  fructosyl unit in, 132
  hydrolysis, 143
  in nature, 260
  neoseries, 48
  polymer length in chicory, 5
  under stress condition, 6–7
  uses, 4–5
Inulinases, 132
Inulin-type fructan (ITF), 375
Invasion plasmid antigen (Ipa), 337
Ipa, *see* Invasion plasmid antigen (Ipa)

IR, *see* Infrared (IR); Insulin receptor (IR)
Irritable bowel syndrome (IBS), 311, 321
   diagnostic criteria, 311
   fiber effects on, 312
IRS-1, *see* Insulin receptor substrate-1 (IRS-1)
ITF, *see* Inulin-type fructan (ITF)

J

Juiciness, 443

K

1-kestose, 4, 81, 83
   tetra and oligosaccharides from, 87
6-Kestose production, 139
Krestin; *see also* Polysaccharide-K (PSK)
KS-2, 174; *see also* Mushroom polysaccharides

L

Lactose, 445
Laxative effect, 370
L/C, *see* Lignins/cellulose (L/C)
LDL, *see* Low density lipoproteins (LDL)
LDP, *see* Long degree of polymerization (LDP)
Leaky gut, 279
Lectins, 444
Leek (*Allium porum*), 77
Legume seed meals, 465
Lentinan, 154, 174; *see also* β-Glucan; Mushroom polysaccharides
   antimicrobial activity, 190
   against cancer, 161
   as hypocholesterolemic agent, 192
   immunostimulating properties, 186–187
Lentinula edodes, *see Lentinus edodes*
Lentinus edodes, 173; *see also* Mushroom polysaccharides
Leptin, 287
Levan, 2, 48, 260, 375; *see also* Fructan; Inulin
   fructosyl unit in, 132
   by levansucrase, 2
   neoserie, 48
   in *Streptococci*, 2
Light transmittance (LT), 116

Lignins, 404
Lignins/cellulose (L/C), 418
Linear inulin with β (2–1)-fructofuranosyl linkages, 48
Lingzhi mushroom; *see also Ganoderma—lucidum*
Lipase, 463
Lipogenesis, 262
Lipopolysaccharide (LPS), 265, 368
   in acute and chronic infections, 279
   metabolic endotoxemia, 279
Lipoprotein lipase (LPL), 278
LMWF, *see* Low-molecular-weight fucoidan (LMWF)
Long degree of polymerization (LDP), 48
Lorcaserin, 369
Low density lipoproteins (LDL), 38, 92, 162, 215, 248
Low-molecular-weight fucoidan (LMWF), 376
LPL, *see* Lipoprotein lipase (LPL)
LPS, *see* Lipopolysaccharide (LPS)
LT, *see* Heat-labile toxin (LT); Light transmittance (LT)

M

Macropinosomes, 337
MAE, *see* Microwave-assisted extraction (MAE)
Maintenance energy requirement (MEm), 458
Maitake mushroom, *see Grifola frondosa*
MALDI-TOF-MS, *see* Matrix-assisted laser desorption–ionization-time-of-flight-mass spectrometry (MALDI-TOF-MS)
Mannan oligosaccharides (MOS), 447
Mathematical growth modeling, 432; *see also* Animal agriculture
Matrix-assisted laser desorption–ionization-time-of-flight-mass spectrometry (MALDI-TOF-MS), 55, 218
Maximum protein deposition capacity (PD_{max}), 435
M cells, *see* Microfold cells (M cells)
mDP, *see* Mean degree of polymerization (mDP)
ME, *see* Metabolizable energy (ME)

Mean degree of polymerization (mDP), 4
Medicinal mushrooms, 156, 195; *see also*
    Mushroom polysaccharides
MEm, *see* Maintenance energy
    requirement (MEm)
MES, *see* 4-Morpholine-ethanoesulfonic
    acid (MES)
Metabolic endotoxemia, 279
Metabolic syndrome, 265; *see also*
    Glucose metabolism disorders
Metabolizable energy (ME), 457
Microbial β-fructofuranosidases, 135
Microbial polysaccharides, 172; *see also*
    Mushroom polysaccharides
Microfold cells (M cells), 333
Microwave-assisted extraction (MAE), 152
Microwaves hyphenated with
    ultrasounds, 152
Midinfrared spectroscopy (MIR
    spectroscopy), 58
MIR spectroscopy, *see* Midinfrared
    spectroscopy (MIR
    spectroscopy)
MMNO, *see* N-Methyl morpholine–N-
    oxide (MMNO)
Molecular nutrition, 432; *see also* Animal
    agriculture
Molecular weight (MW), 209, 236
4-Morpholine-ethanoesulfonic acid
    (MES), 407
MOS, *see* Mannan oligosaccharides (MOS)
Mushroom polysaccharides, 171, 195–196
    AAP, 178–179
    αβ-glucan, 155, 156, 189
    antimicrobial properties, 190–191
    antioxidant properties, 154, 188–190
    antitumor properties, 186–188
    applications of, 193–195
    cholesterol-lowering effect, 192
    extraction and purification, 182
    ganoderan, 154, 174
    gelation of, 159
    glucan–protein complex, 155
    grifolan, 177
    health regulations, 163
    heteroglycans, 179
    heteropolysaccharides, 155
    homopolysaccharides, 156
    hot aqueous extraction, 155
    hypocholesterolemic effect, 192
    hypoglycemic effects, 191
    hypolipidemic effects, 191, 192

    immunostimulation, 186, 189
    isolation of, 181
    issues in, 173
    KS-2, 174
    lentinan, 154, 174
    medicinal properties of, 185
    medium for, 184
    microwave-assisted extraction, 152
    molecular weight of, 157
    pleuran, 176
    prebiotic properties, 193
    pressurized liquid extraction, 151, 152
    production of bioactive, 179–185
    PSK, 177
    PSPC, 177
    renaturing, 160
    schizophyllan, 156, 174
    shear rate, 159
    solid–gel transformations, 159
    storage modulus as function of
        time, 140
    structure of, 153–156, 175
    supercritical fluid extraction, 151–152
    synergistic effects, 193
    types of bioactive, 173–179
    ultrasonic-assisted extraction, 152, 153
    viscosity of, 158
    water solubility, 155, 157–158
Mushrooms, 150, 164; *see also* Diseases
    prevention by mushroom;
    Mushroom polysaccharide
    Agaricus blazei, 176–177
    biologically active substances of, 150
    Cordyceps, 178
    Coriolous versicolor, 177
    cultivation of, 181
    Ganoderma lucidum, 174
    Ganoderma tsugae, 176
    Grifola frondosa, 177
    Lentinus edodes, 173
    medicinal, 156, 195
    Pleurotus ostreatus, 176
    Tremmella mushrooms, 178
    worldwide production, 180
MW, *see* Molecular weight (MW)

N

N-acetylneuraminic acid (NeuAc), 332
Natural killer cell (NK cell), 187, 216
nc-AFM, *see* Noncontact atomic force
    microscopy (nc-AFM)

NCDs, *see* Noncommunicable diseases
(NCDs)
NDF, *see* Neutral detergent fiber (NDF)
NDO, *see* Nondigestible carbohydrates
(NDO)
NE, *see* Net energy (NE)
Neokestose, 83
Neolevan fructan, trisaccharide
precursor in, 132
Neosugar, 387; *see also*
Fructooligosaccharide (FOS)
Neosugar Study Group (NSG), 91
Net energy (NE), 458
NeuAc, *see* N-acetylneuraminic acid
(NeuAc)
NeuGc, *see* N-Glycolylneuraminic acid
(NeuGc)
Neutral detergent fiber (NDF), 403, 439
method, 405
N-free extract, *see* Nitrogen-free extract
(N-free extract)
N-Glycolylneuraminic acid (NeuGc), 331
Nitrogen-free extract (N-free extract),
439; *see also* Carbohydrate
NK cell, *see* Natural killer cell (NK cell)
N-Methyl morpholine–N-oxide
(MMNO), 211
NMR, *see* Nuclear magnetic resonance
(NMR)
NNRs, *see* Nordic Nutrition
Recommendations (NNRs)
NOESY, *see* Nuclear Overhauser effect
spectroscopy (NOESY)
Noncommunicable diseases (NCDs), 385
Noncontact atomic force microscopy
(nc-AFM), 110
Nondigestible carbohydrates (NDO), 92
Nonectomycorrhizal mushrooms,
181; *see also* Mushroom
polysaccharides
Nonstarch polysaccharide (NSP), 210,
224, 328, 347, 407, 441; *see also*
Arabinogalactan-proteins (AG
proteins); Arabinoxylans (AXs);
β-Glucan; Dietary enzyme
supplementation; Dietary
fiber; Dietary polysaccharides;
Pectins; Polysaccharide-based
structures; Soluble dietary
plant NSP; Starch
action mechanism, 449
in cereals and pulses, 210

classification of, 211
degree of polymerization, 212
digestibility, 446, 454
in feedstuffs, 446
health benefits of, 213–214
isolation, 211
purification, 211–212
structural analysis, 212–213
Nordic Nutrition Recommendations
(NNRs), 302
NSG, *see* Neosugar Study Group (NSG)
NSP, *see* Nonstarch polysaccharide (NSP)
Nuclear magnetic resonance (NMR), 55,
154, 212
Nuclear Overhauser effect spectroscopy
(NOESY), 154
Nutricines, 436
Nutrients, 436
Nutritional biotechnology, 432; *see also*
Animal agriculture
Nystose, 81, 83

O

Oat β-glucan, 249
Obesity, 367, 378; *see also* Dietary
polysaccharides; Diabetes
mellitus
antiobesity medications, 369
arabinoxylans, 373–374
β-glucans, 376–377
comorbidities, 368
dietary fiber, 370–371
fucoidans, 375–376
functional foods in, 370
GA, 377
inulins, 375
pectins, 374–375
resistant starch, 371–373
and role of gut microbes, 368–369
safe approaches, 369
SCFA, 371
Odds ratios (ORs), 303
OF, *see* Oligofructose (OF)
OGTT, *see* Oral glucose tolerance test
(OGTT)
Oleic acid, 448
Oligofructose (OF), 388
Oligosaccharides (OS), 302; *see also*
Dietary polysaccharides;
Fructooligosaccharide (FOS)
benefits, 387

Oligosaccharides (*Continued*)
  in blocking bacterial gut infections,
    332–333
  in human milk, 302, 314–316
  undigestible, 208–209
Onions (*Allium cepa*), 77
Oral glucose tolerance test (OGTT),
    246, 264
Orlistat, 369
ORs, *see* Odds ratios (ORs)
OS, *see* Oligosaccharides (OS)
Oyster mushroom, *see Pleurotus ostreatus*

P

Pale, soft, exudative meat (PSE meat), 443
PBMC, *see* Peripheral blood mononuclear
    cells (PBMC)
PD_{max}, *see* Maximum protein deposition
    capacity (PD_{max})
Pectic oligosaccharides (POS), 318
Pectinase, 462
Pectins, 33, 223, 374–375; *see also*
    Nonstarch polysaccharide
    (NSP); Polysaccharide-based
    structures
  affinity to procyanidins, 35
  inhibitory activity, 224
  pectic substances, 403
  structure of, 223
Peripheral blood mononuclear cells
    (PBMC), 191
Peristalsis, 434
Peroxisome proliferator-activated
    receptor γ2 (PPARγ2), 281
PFS, *see* Prebiotic fiber supplementation
    (PFS)
Phenol; *see also* Polyphenols
  antioxidant capacity of, 37–38
  in plants, 34
  during tissues destruction, 35
  in vacuoles, 35
Phentermine, 369
Phenylpropane units, 404
Phlein, *see* Levan
Phytase, 463
Phytochemicals, 32, 386
Piedade mushroom, *see Agaricus–blazei*
Pili, 331
Plant
  cell wall, 34, 401
  phenols in, 34

polysaccharides of, 33
tissue destructuration, 35
Plantain banana (*Musa* spp.), 334
  characteristics, 336
  plantain fiber effect, 338
  soluble NSP composition of, 336
Plant cell wall polymers, 400; *see also*
    Dietary fiber
  in animal feeding, 401–402
  cellulose, 403–404
  hemicelluloses, 404
  lignins, 404
  pectic substances, 403
  phenolic compounds, 404–405
Plant foods; *see also* Apple; Dietary fiber;
    Nonstarch polysaccharide
    (NSP); Starch
  benefits, 31
  bioactive constituents, 32
  carbohydrates, 208
Plant fructan, 2, 3, 23; *see also* Fructan
  applications, 4
  biosynthesis, 2, 3, 23
  carbohydrate-mediated regulation, 6–7
  in dicot plants, 5
  fructosytransferase gene induction, 4
  inulin accumulation, 5–6
PLE, *see* Pressurized liquid extraction
    (PLE)
Pleuran, 176; *see also* Mushroom
    polysaccharides
Pleurotus ostreatus, 176; *see also*
    Mushroom polysaccharides
PMNs, *see* Polymorphonuclear
    leukocytes (PMNs)
Poliovirus type 1 (PV-1), 162
Polydisperse polysaccharides,
    212; *see also* Nonstarch
    polysaccharide (NSP)
Polymolecular polysaccharides,
    212; *see also* Nonstarch
    polysaccharide (NSP)
Polymorphonuclear leukocytes (PMNs),
    215
Polyphenoloxidases (PPOs), 35
Polyphenols, 34
  antioxidant capacity of, 37–38, 39
  in apple, 36
  bioactive compounds, 36
  in gastrointestinal tract, 35–36
Polysaccharide-based structures, 347,
    362, 363; *see also* Carbohydrate

cell wall remnants and, 356
dietary fiber sources, 362
effects in intestines, 359
on enzyme access to substrates, 350
on fecal parameters, 358–360
fruit and vegetables, 355
and hindgut function, 358
interactions between foods, 355–358
nondigestible structures, 349
and nutritional properties, 350
–OH groups, 348
polysaccharides of dicotyledonous
    plants, 33
retention, 360–362
seeds, 351–355
starch, 350–351
Polysaccharide-K (PSK), 177; see also
    Mushroom polysaccharides
in cancer treatment, 187
Polysaccharide–phenol entity formation,
    34
Polysaccharide–protein complexes
    (PSPC), 177; see also Mushroom
    polysaccharides
POS, see Pectic oligosaccharides (POS)
Potato starches, 122; see also
    Carbohydrate (CHO); Starch
amylose and phosphorus content of,
    109
characteristics of, 108
extraction, 107
gelatinization, 108
granule structural features, 110
production, 107–108
size distribution, 108
swelling power of, 109
yield determination, 107
PPARγ2, see Peroxisome proliferator-
    activated receptor γ 2 (PPARγ2)
PPOs, see Polyphenoloxidases (PPOs)
Prebiotic, 60, 63, 282, 314–315; see also
    Fructan prebiotic activity;
    Health benefits of FOS;
    Probiotic
chicory fructan as, 282–286
effect, 330, 372
high-amylose starch, 122
Prebiotic fiber supplementation
    (PFS), 313
Precision nutrition, 432; see also Animal
    agriculture
Pregelatinization, 111

Pressurized liquid extraction (PLE),
    151, 152
Probiotic, 58; see also Fructan prebiotic
    activity; Prebiotic
bacterial growth in fructan, 58
functional carbohydrates, 59–60
SCFAs by colonic bacteria, 59, 61, 63
Procyanidins, 35
Proteases, 463
Proteinases, see Proteases
Protein deposition, 435
Prowashonupana, 234; see also β-Glucan
on glycemic and insulin responses, 247
PSE meat, see Pale, soft, exudative meat
    (PSE meat)
PSK, see Polysaccharide-K (PSK)
PSPC, see Polysaccharide–protein
    complexes (PSPC)
PV-1, see Poliovirus type 1 (PV-1)
PYY; see also Glucagon-like peptide 1
    (GLP-1); Resistant starch (RS)
chicory fructan on, 287
glucose response, 377
gut motility inhibition, 281

Q

Qsymia, 369

R

Radical-trapping antioxidative potential
    (TRAP), 37
Ragi, see Finger millet
Randomized controlled trials (RCTs), 268
β-glucan effect on glycemic and
    insulin responses, 241–242
on β-glucan from barley, 252
on CRC patients, 390
efficacy of soluble and insoluble
    fiber, 309
RCTs, see Randomized controlled trials
    (RCTs)
Reactive oxygen species (ROS), 190
Reishi mushroom, see
    Ganoderma—lucidum
Renaturing, 160
Resistant starch (RS), 122, 370, 445;
    see also Starch
health benefits of, 372
nutritional classification, 210
and obesity, 371–373

Resting heat production, 459
RGI, *see* Rhamnogalacturonan I regions
    (RGI)
Rhamnogalacturonan I regions (RGI), 33
Rimonabant, 369
ROESY, *see* Rotating frame Overhauser
    enhancement spectroscopy
    (ROESY)
ROS, *see* Reactive oxygen species (ROS)
Rotating frame Overhauser enhancement
    spectroscopy (ROESY), 154
RS, *see* Resistant starch (RS)

S

Satiety hormone homeostasis, 65
Scallion (*Allium fistulosum*), 77
Scanning electron microscopy (SEM), 116
SC-CO2 extraction, *see* Supercritical
    carbon dioxide extraction (SC-
    CO2 extraction)
SCFA, *see* Short-chain fatty acid (SCFA)
sc-FOS, *see* Short-chain fructo-
    oligosaccharides (sc-FOS)
Schizophyllan, 156, 174; *see also*
    Mushroom polysaccharides
  chemical structures of, 175
  immunostimulating properties,
    186–187
SDP, *see* Short degree of polymerization
    (SDP)
SEC, *see* Size-exclusion chromatography
    (SEC)
SEC-LLS, *see* Size-exclusion
    chromatography combined
    with multiangle laser light
    scattering (SEC-LLS)
SEM, *see* Scanning electron microscopy
    (SEM)
SF, *see* Swelling factor (SF)
6-SFT, *see* Sucrose, fructan
    6-fructosyltransferase (6-SFT)
Shallot (*Allium oschaninii*), 77
Shear rate, 159
Shiitake mushroom, *see Lentinus edodes*
Short-chain fatty acid (SCFA), 59, 371,
    392
  production and chicory fructan, 285
Short-chain fructo-oligosaccharides
    (sc-FOS), 272
Short degree of polymerization (SDP), 48
Sibutramine, 369

Size-exclusion chromatography (SEC),
    153
Size-exclusion chromatography
    combined with multiangle laser
    light scattering (SEC-LLS), 157
Sizofiran, *see* Schizophyllan
Smooth region of pectins, *see* α-D-
    Galacturonic acid (GalA)
Solid-gel transformations, 159
Soluble dietary fiber (SDF), 302, 329, 407,
    441; *see also* Dietary fiber
Soluble dietary plant NSP, 328, 339,
    341; *see also* Dietary fiber;
    Nonstarch polysaccharide
    (NSP)
  bacterial adhesins, 331–332
  bacterial toxins, 332
  dietary oligosaccharide use, 332–333
  E. coli inhibition, 333–334
  green plantain composition, 336
  plantain NSP, 334, 336
  S. typhimurium colonization, 337
  translocation blockage, 335–339, 340
Solvent extraction techniques, 151
SOS, *see* Swedish Obese Subjects (SOS)
SP, *see* Swelling power (SP)
Spring onion, *see* Scallion (*Allium
    fistulosum*)
1-SST, *see* Sucrose:sucrose
    1-fructosyltransferase (1-SST)
ST, *see* Heat-stable toxin (ST)
Stabilization of starch, 114
Standard Diet (STD), 65
Starch, 106, 208, 235, 350, 441; *see also*
    Nonstarch polysaccharide
    (NSP); Potato starches;
    Resistant starch (RS)
  acetylated, 114–115
  α-amylase, 118–119
  α-glucanotransferases, 121–122
  amylopectin, 209
  amylose, 209
  annealing of, 112
  arrangement of, 351
  β-amylase, 119–120
  conversion, 116–117
  converting enzymes, 118
  crosslinking, 113–114
  cyclodextrin glycosyltransferase,
    120–121
  digestion of, 122, 351
  ethers, 115–116

gelatinization temperature, 112, 113
glucoamylase, 120
granules, 350
heat-moisture-treatment, 112
heat treatment, 111
history of, 106–107
modifications, 110, 111, 113, 118
phosphates, 115
potential of, 122–123
prebiotic, 122
pregelatinization, 111
product hydrolysis, 118
stabilization, 114
storage, 106
structure, 209
STD, *see* Standard Diet (STD)
Streptozotocin (STZ), 287
STZ, *see* Streptozotocin (STZ)
Sucrose:sucrose 1-fructosyltransferase
(1-SST), 2, 48
activity in roots, 5
into nonfructan-accumulating
plants, 17
regulation, 7
Sucrose, fructan 6-fructosyltransferase
(6-SFT), 9, 48
to synthesize graminans and
phleins, 18
Sucrose into FOS, 139–140
Sugarcane (*Saccharum* spp. L.), 22
Sun mushroom, *see* Agaricus—blazei
Supercritical carbon dioxide extraction
(SC-CO2 extraction), 152
Supercritical fluid extraction,
151–152
SV, *see* Swelling volumes (SV)
Swedish Obese Subjects (SOS), 264
Swelling factor (SF), 112
Swelling power (SP), 109
Swelling volumes (SV), 115

T

T3SS, *see* Type III secretory system
(T3SS)
Tailor-made fructan, 19, 23, 24;
see also Fructan biosynthesis
modification; Heterologous
fructan production
competitive fructan and starch, 20
drought and cold resistance of crop,
21–22

fructan stability in storage organs,
20–21
platform crops for, 22
sucrose on yield of, 19–20
TDF, *see* Total dietary fiber (TDF)
Thin layer chromatography (TLC), 55
TLC, *see* Thin layer chromatography
(TLC)
TLR-4, *see* Toll-like receptors 4 (TLR-4)
TLT, *see* Transplantable liver tumors
(TLT)
TNF-α, *see* Tumor necrosis factor-α
(TNF-α)
Toll-like receptors 4 (TLR-4), 264
Topiramate, 369
Total dietary fiber (TDF), 303, 400, 441
Total nutrition, 436; *see also* Dietary
polysaccharides
concept of, 437
molecules in diets, 436
nutrient conversion efficiency,
436–437
protein deposition, 438
Trametes versicolor, see *Coriolous
versicolor*
Transferase to hydrolase activity, 136–137
Transfructosylating activity, 141–142
Transplantable liver tumors (TLT), 391
TRAP, *see* Radical-trapping antioxidative
potential (TRAP)
Tremmella mushrooms, 178; *see also*
Mushroom polysaccharides
Tumor necrosis factor-α (TNF-α), 184,
265
Tumor therapy, 161–162
Two-step process, 142
Type III secretory system (T3SS), 337

U

UAE, *see* Ultrasonic-assisted extraction
(UAE)
Ultrasonic-assisted extraction (UAE), 152
Ultrasonic-/microwave-assisted
extraction (UMAE), 153
UMAE, *see* Ultrasonic-/microwave-
assisted extraction (UMAE)
Unavailable carbohydrates, 32–33, *see*
Dietary fiber
Uronic acids, 412
U.S. Food and Drug Administration
(FDA), 163, 237, 377

V

Van Soest method, 405, 439, 441
VE, *see* Villus epithelium (VE)
Very-low-density lipoprotein (VLDL),
        162, 250
VFA, *see* Volatile fatty acid (VFA)
VFB, *see* Viscous fiber blend (VFB)
Villus epithelium (VE), 339
Viscous fiber blend (VFB), 305
VLDL, *see* Very-low-density lipoprotein
        (VLDL)
Volatile fatty acid (VFA), 411

W

Water-extractable AX (WE-AX), 219
Water-extractable polysaccharides
        (WEPs), 210
Water fluidity (WF), 117
Water-insoluble cell wall (WICW), 406
Water-soluble
        αβ-glucan, 155, 156
        neutral polysaccharide, 155
Water-soluble carbohydrate (WSC), 47
Water-unextractable polysaccharide
        (WUP), 210
Waxbar flour, 237; *see also* β-Glucan
WAXS, *see* Wide-angle x-ray scattering
        (WAXS)
WB, *see* Wheat bran (WB)
WCRF, *see* World Cancer Research Fund
        (WCRF)
WE-AX, *see* Water-extractable AX
        (WE-AX)
Weende

analysis, 439
    method, 400
Welsh onion, *see* Scallion (*Allium
        fistulosum*)
WEPs, *see* Water-extractable
        polysaccharides (WEPs)
WF, *see* Water fluidity (WF)
Wheat bran (WB), 302
WHO, *see* World Health Organization
        (WHO)
WICW, *see* Water-insoluble cell wall
        (WICW)
Wide-angle x-ray scattering (WAXS),
        109
World Cancer Research Fund (WCRF),
        306
World Health Organization (WHO), 263,
        430
WSC, *see* Water-soluble carbohydrate
        (WSC)
WUP, *see* Water-unextractable
        polysaccharide (WUP)

X

XOS, *see* Xylooligosaccharides (XOS)
Xylanase, 462
    supplementation effect on nutrient
        digestibility, 465
Xyloglucans, 33
Xylooligosaccharides (XOS), 389

Z

ZO-1, *see* Zonula occludens-1 (ZO-1)
Zonula occludens-1 (ZO-1), 280